Sigismund Sutro

Lectures on the German mineral Waters and on their rational Employment

Sigismund Sutro

Lectures on the German mineral Waters and on their rational Employment

ISBN/EAN: 9783337140649

Printed in Europe, USA, Canada, Australia, Japan

Cover: Foto ©ninafisch / pixelio.de

More available books at **www.hansebooks.com**

LECTURES

ON THE

GERMAN MINERAL WATERS

AND ON

THEIR RATIONAL EMPLOYMENT.

WITH AN APPENDIX

EMBRACING A SHORT ACCOUNT OF THE

PRINCIPAL EUROPEAN SPAS AND CLIMATIC HEALTH-RESORTS.

BY

SIGISMUND SUTRO, M.D.

M.R.C.P. LOND.

SENIOR PHYSICIAN TO THE GERMAN HOSPITAL, FELLOW OF THE ROYAL MEDICO-CHIRURGICAL
AND HUNTERIAN SOCIETIES, MEMBER OF THE SOCIETY OF PHYSICIANS OF MUNICH,
CORRESPONDING MEMBER OF THE PHYSICO-MEDICAL SOCIETY OF ERLANGEN, ETC.

SECOND EDITION,

CAREFULLY REVISED, AND ENLARGED.

LONDON:
LONGMANS, GREEN, AND CO.
1865.

TO

CHARLES J. B. WILLIAMS, M.D. F.R.S.

LATE PROFESSOR OF MEDICINE AND FIRST PHYSICIAN TO UNIVERSITY

COLLEGE HOSPITAL, CONSULTING PHYSICIAN TO THE HOSPITAL

FOR CONSUMPTION AND DISEASES OF THE CHEST,

ETC.

IN ADMIRATION OF HIS HIGH ATTAINMENTS

AND DISTINGUISHED AND VALUABLE EXERTIONS IN THE CAUSE OF

MEDICAL SCIENCE,

THIS WORK IS RESPECTFULLY DEDICATED

BY

THE AUTHOR.

PREFACE

TO

THE SECOND EDITION.

IN preparing the second edition of the Lectures I have endeavoured to increase their utility, without greatly adding to the bulk of the work.

Since the publication of the first edition (now out of print for nearly a year), the facilities of travelling have progressed to such a wonderful degree, that distance almost ceases to be taken into consideration in the selection of a health resort. It therefore behoves our profession, not only to be acquainted with Spas that were formerly easy of access, but also with all available natural means of curing or preventing disease.

Wishing to give a concise account of many other Spas visited and explored since, I thought it best to leave the Lectures in their original form, so favourably received by the profession, and to add *an appendix*, which might serve as a short but comprehensive manual of all the important health resorts, not treated of in the previous edition.

I have entirely omitted those portions which might be well suited to an auditory of students, but which would not be missed by the ordinary medical reader, as the lecture on the method of analyzing the waters. Other portions I have re-written.

In treating of the British health resorts, I deemed it useful to give an exact description of the climate of the metropolis. Being one of the most important towns of the world, it is temporarily or permanently inhabited by such an immense number of human beings (probably increasing to five millions in the next generation), that information about the geological and meteorological condition of its various sites might serve to prevent disease, by adapting the choice of a residence to the peculiar diathesis of the inhabitant.

But as the *mode* of reaching the various suburbs ought decidedly to form an element of reflection, I extracted the most essential parts of the report issued by the Lancet Sanitary Commission on the influence of railway travelling. The facts enumerated by the most trustworthy authorities will point out those cases in which *habitual* railway travelling has to be avoided, and also what precautions are required to diminish or prevent any injurious consequences.

This unpretending volume is not intended to supersede larger works on the important subject of climate. On the contrary, I feel thoroughly convinced, that the facts laid here before the reader in a small compass will show him the absolute necessity of a thorough acquaintance with the various sanative and preventive natural agents, and induce him to study the excellent works of Sir James Clark, Dr. Scoresby Jackson, Mr. Luke Howard, Dr. Vetter, Dr. Helfft, Dr. Seegen, Dr. Ewich, and others.

I have availed myself of the most authentic information, and attempted to put the geographical position, the mode of access, and the peculiar *distinctive* indication of each locality, impartially before the reader, whose kind indulgence I wish to claim for the shortcomings he may discover in these pages.

37A FINSBURY SQUARE :
June 1865.

PREFACE

TO

THE FIRST EDITION.

THE following Lectures were delivered last session, at the *Hunterian School of Medicine*. A portion of them have already appeared in a medical periodical, and seemed to meet with so much indulgence, that I am induced to publish the whole in a collected form, after a careful revision. The utility of publishing such a work may perhaps be questioned. It may be asked, have we not already very complete expositions of the virtues of the German Spas by Dr. James Johnson, Dr. Granville, Mr. Edwin Lee, &c.?—and is the subject important enough to require further elucidations?

To these objections I answer—that far from depreciating the works of the above gentlemen, I consider the profession and the public highly indebted to them for the light they have thrown on certain means of cure, formerly little known, and still much neglected. But though they have succeeded in imparting a great amount of information in a very pleasing manner, yet it will happen, that any work on the German Mineral Springs, taken up for the purpose of *choosing* between Spas of analogous properties, will leave the reader embarrassed and undecided by the very variety of the remedial agents submitted to his choice. The task of facilitating such inquiry was that which I principally proposed to myself when personally visiting the various Spas, and comparing their special effects. Hence I thought a faithful description of their claims by an impartial German writer might not prove quite unwelcome to the English profession.

That numerous invalids return cured or relieved from the Spas is not disputed. But those who have not had the opportunity of devoting special attention to the subject, generally ascribe the benefit to the recreation of the journey, to the change of air, of diet, to the absence of the usual toils and cares, &c.

That the enlivening changes of objects, sights, climate, occupation, and diet, greatly assist in disposing the organism to a favourable reception of the waters, I am free to admit, and I do not hesitate to express my conviction, that certain regions must so fill up as it were every pore of the traveller's mind, by their manifold charms and beauties, that many mere functional derangements will give way to the absorbing admiration of God's greatness, as displayed in his creative wonders. We cannot but forget our own littleness for a time, when the vast forests and gigantic mountains surround us with a constantly alternating landscape, and with the gladness of animated beings acknowledging their satisfaction in the air above and in the fields below. The forgotten and unpampered body soon imbibes mental agility and fervour, and responds by increased action of the various contending organs. But whilst I grant the highly important benefit of travelling, no one will expect an indurated liver, a contracted joint, or a paralysed limb, to become restored by the influence of locomotion or the most beautiful scenery. No journey or absence of six or seven weeks will infuse strength and a greater amount of iron into the circulation of a previously chlorotic and debilitated female, without some potent medicinal alteration. No mere change of living or scenery under the most favourable auspices will be expected to cure obstinate gout, rheumatic or neuralgic pains, sterility, or tendency to abortion, &c. Again, how many authentic instances are recorded of incipient phthisis, inveterate pulmonary catarrhs, hoarseness with spitting of blood, and general emaciation, &c., completely cured by a course of four or five weeks at some of the Spas? Can this have been accomplished by mere travelling?—or can it be indifferent which of the Spas are chosen, when we find numerous individuals at each watering-place, who, even while rapidly improving, will inform us how many other Spas of more or less analogous virtues they have previously tried in vain, and who bitterly inveigh against their advisers for not having recommended the present Spa in the first instance? And how can it be rationally conceived that it is of no importance to what region or Spa the sufferer directs his steps, supposing even that no proof existed of their differing results? A glance at the contents of the various springs will satisfy the most sceptical physician that such striking differences of chemical and physical properties must produce strikingly different effects.

A work, therefore, seemed needed, which would not only embody all authentic and available information on the subject, but also furnish a comparison of the curative properties of the various Spas, and thus put the reader in the same position as if he had undertaken the journey and compared the results himself. With this view I have interspersed the volume with cases *illustrating the characteristic* efficacy of each Spa, and sifted the adventitious cures from those properly due to the *prominent* sanative powers of the springs.

Though I have endeavoured to omit no fact or rational theory of importance that has come under the notice of the most competent German Spa authorities, I have sought in vain for precise directions as regards the *choice* between Spas of the same class. I therefore venture to lay down rules and explanatory views for facilitating a precise discrimination of analogous springs, and I submit them with the more confidence to the reader from the fact that they coincide throughout with the recorded cases of success or failure of the various Spas, being deduced from scrupulous and careful observations extending over a number of years.

The best mode of reaching the various Spas is also indicated in the present volume; but for minute descriptions of hotels, price of living, &c., I must refer the reader to other sources, as I thought these matters too transitory to be of permanent value, and somewhat foreign to the principal object of these Lectures.

The necessity in certain cases for avoiding particular mineral waters altogether is here pointed out with the same impartiality as their curative effects. For the Spas are far from being a panacea for all complaints to which the human organism is liable. On the contrary, I would limit their sphere of action to those cases in which the ordinary medical treatment has failed to restore the patient.

They are not only entirely *inapplicable* in acute diseases, where prompter remedial agents are required, but even in chronic disorders I would always advocate the preference of medical treatment amid the comforts of home, and under the care of those who are fully acquainted with the patient's constitution and morbid dispositions. On the other hand, when the sufferer has arrived at that stage in which the usual pharmaceutic remedies cease to forward recovery, so that change of air becomes advisable to increase the prospects of health, then I think it highly useful to consult the respective virtues of the Spas, and to recommend the appropriate one, with due regard to the intrinsic and extraneous properties detailed in the present volume, for which I earnestly request an indulgent consideration.

LONDON:
June 1851.

CONTENTS.

LECTURE I.

Difficulties in the Treatment of Disease—States of Transition—Hints of Nature—Characteristics of Mineral Waters—Carbonic Acid—Its Influence in causing Absorption—Brighton Pumproom—Advantage of genuine Mineral Waters—Duration of the Season—Continuance of Effect afterwards—Batheruption—Contra-indications 1

LECTURE II.

Natural Classification according to Temperature—Advantage of diminished Atmospheric Pressure in higher Situations—Diminution of Warmth in proportion to Height—Changes of the Water by Atmospheric Influences—Difference of local Origin of the Springs, or of their dependence on the general Character of the Mountains—Origin of Acidulous and Thermal Springs—Effects of the Volcanic Processes in the interior of the Earth—Formation of Gaseous Products—Relation between Earthquakes and Thermæ—Origin of the Hot Springs—Cause of inherent Heat—Composition of the Thermæ—Stability of Temperature of Acidulous Springs—Consideration of Climate in the choice of a Spa 9

LECTURE III.

Curative Effects of Sea-air—Bleakness of Climate through neighbouring Mountains—Influence of Narrowness or Width of the Valleys—Effects of Altitude—Proportion of solid Constituents - Difference between loose and intimate Combination of Carbonic Acid—Tension of evaporating Bodies—Solution of Gases—Medical Effects of Temperature—Influence of Warmth on the Digestive Canal—Mechanical Effects of Water—Characteristic Effects of the Chemically indifferent Spas 15

LECTURE IV.

WILDBAD.

Journey to Wildbad—Comparison with Baden-Baden—Climate—Temperature of the Baths—Physical Effects of Bathing—Youth-restoring Power—Assimilative Changes greater than can be effected by more substantial Waters—Reason—Instance of Food—Effects observed during Cholera—Indications—How to distinguish from Pfäfers—Description of the Spa by a Munich Physician 29

LECTURE V.

PFÄFERS.

Road from Wildbad—Canstadt and its Springs—Lake of Constance—Würtemberg Railroads—Rorschach. *Pfäfers.* *Hof-Ragaz*—Attempt to explain the minor efficacy of Ragaz—Chief Indications of Pfäfers—Paracelsus' Opinion—Hufeland's—Explanation of the efficacy of the Spa 40

LECTURE VI.

GASTEIN.

Road from Munich to Salzburg—Effect of the Journey itself—Charms of Nature between Salzburg and Gastein—Deeper Inspirations necessary than in lower Localities—Wandelbahn—Magnetic Power of Oxygen—Renal Crises—Difference between direct and indirect Cures—Walk to Hof-Gastein—Distinctive Indications between Wildbad, Pfäfers, and Gastein 54

LECTURE VII.

ISCHL—TEPLITZ.

Hallein—Salt-works—Road to Ischl—Salzkammer-gut—Soole-baths of Ischl—Swimming-school—Cases sent by d'Outrepont—Journey to Teplitz. *Schönau*—Climate—Prevalence of Nitrogen—Cure of Dr. Wengler from Paralysis—Teplitz as an After-cure—Sudden appearance of Cholera . . . 69

LECTURE VIII.

BITTER WATERS—CARLSBAD.

Origin of Bitter Waters—Carlsbad—Sprudel—Origin of—Relation of Temperature to Height—Reputation in Hepatic Swellings—Difference of Carlsbad purging from ordinary Purgation—Warning to Continental Patients—English Living a Safeguard against certain Epidemic Diseases—Reasons—Franzensbad as an After-cure—Mishaps to be avoided in the selection of Spas 85

LECTURE IX.

MARIENBAD—FRANZENSBAD.

Journey to Marienbad—Abundance of Carbonic Acid - First employment of Gas-baths by Dr. Struve—Use of Mud-baths by Dr. Wetzler—Discrimination between Carlsbad and Marienbad. *Franzensbad*—Goethe's remarks—Comparison with Marienbad—Individualities especially adapted to each of the three Bohemian Spas—Benefit obtained by Frederick the Great—Remarks of Hufeland 102

LECTURE X.

SALINE SPRINGS—KISSINGEN—BOCKLET.

Saline Springs—Iodine Springs—The Ocean Journey to Kissingen—Effects of Ragoczy—Case of Hepatic Induration by Dr. Maas—Maxbrunnen in Renal

CONTENTS. xv

Catarrhs—Direction for distinguishing between Kissingen and analogous Spas —Air of the Graduation Works—Effects of Soolen-sprudel—Its Baths compared with Sea-baths. *Booklet*—Its Reputation in Sterility . . . 119

LECTURE XI.
BRÜCKENAU—HOMBURG.

Brückenau—Environs—Abundance of Carbonic Acid—Dr. Wetzler's Case—Attractions of—Recommended as an After-cure. *Homburg*—Climate—Effects of the Springs—Benefit after Typhus—High Reputation in abnormal Menstruation—In Menstrual Spasms—Contra-indications—Discrimination between Homburg and Kissingen 133

LECTURE XII.
SODEN—WIESBADEN.

Soden—Common Origin of the Springs—Useful in Dyspepsia—Comparison with Homburg. *Wiesbaden*—Mildness of Climate—Scarcity of Fresh Water—The Gaming-Table—Its injurious Influences on Health—Action of the Water—Compared with that of the Bitter Waters—Danger of too high a Temperature—Instance of Hæmoptysis—Wiesbaden as a Winter Residence—Hospital Report of Dr. Haas—Comparison with Wildbad—Comparison with Homburg—Similarity of Constituents—Difference of Results 146

LECTURE XIII.
WEILBACH—BADEN (AUSTRIA).

Weilbach Sulphur Springs—Their Action—Effects on Renal Secretion—On Alvine Evacuations—Results in incipient Phthisis Effects on Pulse and Respiration—Modus Operandi explained—Its Action as a derivative compared with abstraction of Blood—Comparison with Aix-la-Chapelle. *Baden*—Surrounding Mountains—Vöslau—Evolution of Nitrogen—Comparison with Weilbach—Sulphurous Swimming-baths—Advantages in weakly developed Thoracic Organs—Value of Preventives—Contra-indications—Instances in which Baden is to be preferred to Weilbach 160

LECTURE XIV.
KREUZNACH—ADELHEIDSQUELLE.

Kreuznach—Bingen—Elisabethbrunnen—Graduation Works—Difference between Bauer's and Löwig's Analysis—Carburetted Hydrogen—Brine as a Clyster for Hepatic Induration—Effects compared with those of analogous Spas—Individualities to which the Spa is specially adapted—Contra-indications. *Adelheidsquelle*—Comparison of Contents with analogous Springs . . . 175

LECTURE XV.
NENNDORF—EILSEN—MEINBERG—AIX-LA-CHAPELLE.

Journey to Nenndorf—Heating of the Baths—Formation of the sulphurous Water illustrated by Dr. Wöhler—Action of the Water—Decrease of Pulse—Utility in

Rheumatism—Contra-indications—Mud-baths—Simultaneous employment of Sulphur-baths and Inunction—Neundorf compared with Weilbach—Apparent anomaly of Sulphur and Brine-baths being used alternately accounted for. *Eilsen. Meinberg*—Sprudel-baths advantageous as an After-cure. *Aix-la-Chapelle*—Sulphuretted Hydrogen—Mode of its development—Comparison of Aix-la-Chapelle with other Sulphur Springs—Necessity of exhilaration of Spirits—Connection between Anxiety of Mind and Formation of Abscesses—Chalybeate Springs. *Burtscheid* (Borcette)—Mühlenbadquelle the hottest Spring in Germany 190

LECTURE XVI.

PYRMONT—DRIBURG—SCHWALBACH—SPAA.

Journey to Pyrmont—Recommended in impaired sanguification through lengthened sojourn in Tropical Climates—In acute Anæmia—Employment of the Spa by Hufeland—Cures of passive Metrorrhage, Fluor Albus, and Sterility—Mud-baths—Gas-baths—Contra-indications. *Driburg*—Analogy to Pyrmont—Saatzer Sulphur-Spring. *Schwalbach*—The Rheingau—The Valley of the Aar—Bleakness of the Climate—Paulinenbrunnen strikingly effective in the debility resulting from a Tropical residence—Disposition to Diarrhœa favoured by the atmosphere—Liebig's Theory—Results of introduction of Iron on the production of animal Heat—*Spaa*—Pouhon useful in Diseases resulting from intermittent Fever 209

LECTURE XVII.

EMS—SCHLANGENBAD—BADEN-BADEN.

Journey to Ems—Reputation in Laryngeal and Pulmonary Diseases—Hufeland's Recommendation—Congestion of Pulmonary Vessels diminished—Sedative Effects of the Baths. *Schlangenbad*—Cosmetic Influence—Recommended as an After-cure to follow the Course of Ems. *Baden-Baden*—Natural Vapour-baths—Comparison with analogous Spas—Distinction between Cures effected in the Spa and by the Spa 230

LECTURE XVIII.

OEYNHAUSEN—SEA-BATHING—NAUHEIM.

Rehme—Porta Westphalica—Climate—The Water compared with Sea-water—Different Modes of evolving Carbonic Acid—Natural Vapour-baths—Air of the Salt-works—Useful in too rapid Growth of young Persons with Phthisical tendency. *Sea-Bathing*—Solid Ingredients of the various Seas—Causes of the Differences of the Amount—Varying Temperature—Utility of warm Sea-baths, of Sea Voyages—Injury of Sea-air in certain instances—Preference of high Localities—Utility of Sea-bathing in Fluor Albus—In certain Cases of Epilepsy—Instances in which ioduretted Spas are to be preferred—Effects of cold Sea-baths—All the Benefit due to the Reaction. *Nauheim*—Soolensprudel Springs compared with those of analogous Spas—Dr. Benecke's Method of diluting the Drinking Spring, approximating its Composition to that of Ragoczy—His Researches as regards the Effects of the Springs on the healthy Organism—Increased Diuresis and diminished action of the Heart are the main Results of the warm Nauheim Baths, besides decrease of respiratory

CONTENTS. xvii

PAGE

Frequency—The diluted Cure-spring increased general Transformation, and promoted Excretion of Urea, but not of Phosphoric Acid—It ameliorated Biliary Secretion, and produced a more abundant Formation of Gastric Juice at Meals—Artificial Medicated Baths 276

APPENDIX.

ACHSELMANNSTEIN—Edelquelle—Climate—Useful in incipient Tuberculosis—Saline Vapour-baths—Whey 277
AIX-LES-BAINS—Sulphurous and Aluminous Springs—Douches—Recommended against Rheumatism, Eczema—Scotch Douche 277
ALEXANDERSBAD—Chalybeate, very exciting—Baths of Pine-foliage—Roughness of Climate 278
ALEXISBAD—Selkebrunnen, one of the purest Chalybeates . . . 278
ALTWASSER—Alkaline earthy Chalybeate—Restorative after weakening Spas . 278
AMÉLIE-LES-BAINS—Very mild Climate—Reputed in Chronic Catarrh—Sulphurous inhalations 279
APENRADE—Baltic Seaport—Protection through bent of the Coast . . 279
ARNSTADT—Healthy Climate—Baths of Pine-foliage—Powerful *Saline*-baths—Additions of Malt—Poultices of Brine 279
ASKERNE—Spa—Mancr-well—Reputed in Articular Rigidity—More beneficial in Irritable Skin than Harrogate 280
ABERYSTWITH—Welsh Sea-bath—Sheltered Position—Bracing Mountain and Sea-breezes 280
ALGIERS—Excessive Summer-heat modified and violent Atmospheric Changes prevented by the Mediterranean—Higher Annual Temperature than Italian Resorts—Climate not rendered damp by the Rain—Rainfall compared with that of Torquay—Sirocco—Climate not relaxing—Recommended for threatening Tuberculosis 280
ALPINE CLIMATE—Lowering of Temperature in proportion to Altitude—Ascending Currents more capable of absorbing Heat—Air more rarified—A greater amount required for Respiration—The Föhn—Frequency of Thunderstorms—Improved Digestion—Greater soundness of Sleep—Atonic Ulcers cured through Mountain Air—Feverishness produced in some Constitutions—Alpenstich—Utility in atonic diarrhœa, anæmia, and scrophulosis . . 282
BADEN (Switzerland)—Picturesque Situation—Chloride of Sodium chief Ingredient—Inhalations—Recommended in Atonic Catarrhs, Chronic Rheumatism—Duration of Baths from Fifteen Minutes to Three Hours—Administered Cool—Followed by Repose 286
BADENWEILER—Bracing Air of the Black Forest—High Situation . . 287
BAGNÈRES-DE-BIGORRE—Charming Situation—Mild Climate though 1,900' high—The Springs reputed for restoring Bodily and Mental Vigour . . . 287
BAGNÈRES-DE-LUCHON—Altitude, 2,000'—Variety of Springs—Greatest quantity of Sulphuret of Sodium—Recommended in Cutaneous Affections—In Chronic Rheumatism—Development of Sulphuretted Hydrogen different from that prevailing in Germany—Effect more stimulating 288
BARÈGES—Altitude, 4,000'—Most celebrated in inveterate Chronic Rheumatism. 289
BATH—Hot Springs—Commodious Swimming-baths—Recommended for Chronic Rheumatism—Atonic Gout—Dropped Hand—Subaqueous Douche . . 290

a

CONTENTS.

	PAGE
BUXTON—900' high—Bracing Air—Romantic Walks—Public Baths—Highly restorative—Useful in Chronic Gout and Rheumatism	292
BERG—Saline Baths with low Temperature—Useful in Dyspepsia	292
BERKA—Pine-foliage Vapour-baths—Sulphurous and Chalybeate Springs	293
BERTRICH—Eminently useful in Diseases due to suppressed Cutaneous Function	293
BEX (Switzerland)—1,380', high—Charming Situation—Exhalation of Salt-works—Spring with Sulphuretted Hydrogen	293
BOTZEN (Tyrol)—Most pleasant and useful Residence in incipient Tuberculosis—Great contrast of Temperature between sunny and shady Places	294
BIARRITZ (Bay of Biscay)—Fine sandy Beach	294
BOULOGNE—Climate mild—Bathing-ground sandy and sheltered	295
BLANKENBERGHE—Coast gradually sinking	295
BERWICK (North)—Beautiful Scenery—Bracing Air	295
BLACKPOOL—Northern Brighton	296
BOURNEMOUTH (Hampshire)—Valley sheltered—Ground Sandy—Climate mild	296
BRIGHTON—Sheltered by the South Downs—Climate bracing and restorative, especially the Eastern part, the Western more damp and mild—Steyne intermediate—In Winter more suitable to Strumous Persons—Milder and steadier in Autumn than Hastings	296
BORDEAUX—Mild Atmosphere—*Montpellier*—Formerly recommended for Consumptive Patients—Phthisis rather aggravated by the Northerly Winds	297
CHARLOTTENBRUNN—Sheltered by beautiful Fir-forests—Whey-cure—Chalybeate and Acidulous Springs—Resorted to for Chronic Pulmonary Catarrh	298
CLARENS (on Lake of Geneva)—Autumn Residence for delicate Persons—Lausanne and Geneva inappropriate	298
VEVAY—Most charming Scenery—Grape-cure—Whey	298
MONTREUX—Beautiful Views and excellent Protection—Even suitable as a Winter Residence for Consumptive Invalids	299
COLBERG—Baltic Sea-bath and Saline Springs	299
CRANZ—More Northerly	299
CUXHAVEN—North Sea-bath—Different Cars for *Flood*- and for *Ebb*-Sea-baths	299
CASTELLAMARE—One of the healthiest and most pleasant Summer Residences in Italy—Quisisana—Numerous Mineral Springs available besides Sea-baths—Reputed for the cure of Cutaneous Diseases, for Uterine Infiltration—Individualities more suited to this than to a Northern Sea-bath	300
CAUTERETS—3,000' high in a charming Valley—Sheltered and mild—Springs milder than those of Bagnères-de-Luchon—Half-baths—Foot-baths—In Chronic Rheumatism and Cutaneous Diseases	300
CAIRO—Climate mild—Dry—Equable—Exhilarating—Highly favourable Winter Residence for Consumptive Patients—Choice of Habitations—Temperature compared with other Winter Resorts	301
COÏMBRA—Climate peculiarly adapted for Consumptive Patients, but Accommodation extremely deficient	302
CHELTENHAM—Charming Summer Resort—Highly useful Saline and Chalybeate Springs—Especially recommended in Functional Derangements of the Liver	303
CLIFTON—Atmosphere highly elastic, mild, and reviving—Recommended as a Winter Residence for Persons affected with Chronic Pulmonary Irritation	304
DIEPPE—The Brighton of the Parisians	305
DOBERAN—Violence of Waves prevented by the sheltering Dam	305
DÜRKHEIM—Ioduretted Springs—Atmosphere equable and dry—Grape-cure	306
DOVER—Limited Shelter—Exposure to High Winds—Beautiful Views from the Chalk Cliffs	307

CONTENTS.

EAUX-BONNES—Embedded in a Valley 2,100' high—Advantages and Disadvantages of its Climate—Recommended in Chronic Pulmonary Irritation . 308
EAUX-CHAUDES—Great Reputation for Chronic Rheumatism—Sulfuraire. . 309
ÉTRETAT—Sea-bath with very strong movements of Waves . . . 309
FÖHR—Mildness of Climate due to the sheltering Downs of Sylt and Amrum . 310
FÉCAMP—Offers more Accommodation than Étretat 310
GAIS—2,875' high—Pretty equable Summer Temperature—*Whey-cures* in incipient Tuberculosis 310
GREAT BRITAIN—Climate of 312
LONDON—Climate of 313
    Seasons according to *Temperature* 315
    Mortality from Consumption—*Conservative* Character of the British Climate
    —Comparison with the Continent 317
    Choice of a Private Residence preventive or productive of Disease . 318
    Geological Condition of the various Parts of the Metropolis—Its influence
    on different Constitutions 319
    List of Population, Altitude, and Mortality 322
    Influence of habitual Railway Travelling on Public Health . . 324
HEIDEN—2,424' high—Enclosed by Promontories—Charming resort for Whey-cures 330
HEINRICHSBAD—2,410' high—Beautifully situated—Whey-establishment somewhat more sheltered 332
WEISBAD—Altitude 2,524'—Provided with fine shady Walks, and possessing more Protection than the neighbouring Whey-establishments . . . 332
HELGOLAND—Pure maritime Climate without disturbing influences . . 333
HERINGSDORF—Bathing-place protected without impediment to the free breaking of the Waves 334
HAVRE—Advantage of the Flood-tide nearly remaining Three Hours daily . 334
TROUVILLE—More sheltered and rural, with a fine sandy Ground—Danger of Quicksands 334
HYÈRES—Mildness of Climate—Compared with Nice 335
CANNES—Climate milder than Nice—Less humid and relaxing than Pau . 336
HARROGATE—Bracing and charming locality, with Sulphurous and Chalybeate Springs—Particularly efficacious when stimulation of the Emunctories is more called for than thorough alterative action 336
HASTINGS—Lower situations particularly guarded by high Cliffs—During January and December, Climate milder than at the neighbouring Resorts—Air moist and sedative 338
ST. LEONARDS—Less exposed to the Counter-currents from above—More liable to the vicissitudes of Temperature 338
VALE OF GINSENG—Its superior Climatic advantages 339
THE CAPE OF GOOD HOPE—Seasons the reverse of ours—Scarcity of Rain—Death from Consumption rarer than at other Military Stations . . . 339
ILMENAU—IMNAU 340
INTERLAKEN—1,712' high—Climate extremely mild and sheltered—Deficiency of Spring Water—The Föhn—Places to be preferred in oppressive Summer Heat 341
GIESSBACH—2,400' high—One of the most charming and picturesque Whey-cure Establishments—The Lake of Brienz—Illumination of the Waterfalls . 343
MEYRINGEN—1,800' high—Romantic resort for climatic and local Advantages . 344
GRINDELWALD—3,150' high—Summer Atmosphere cooler than in the neighbouring Plains—Particularly recommended in Hypochondriasis . . 344
ISCHIA—Suitable to Persons affected with Nervous Debility—The Hot Springs serviceable for Mercurial Cachexia, after Syphilis—Natural Vapour-baths . 345

CONTENTS.

	PAGE
ITALY—Climate of—Temperature of various Parts compared	346
Florence—Its varied Attractions—Oppressive Summer Heat	349
Genoa—Apparently most protected and suitable for Invalids—In reality perfectly inappropriate through the frequent and trying vicissitudes of Temperature	349
Milan—Altitude, 483'—Beautiful and interesting Town—But the abode of Pellagra—Charming Scenery and Relaxation afforded by the Journey from Milan to the neighbouring Lakes	350
Naples—Unique beauty of the Environs—Climate too treacherous for Pulmonary Diseases	350
Pozzuoli—Milder Atmosphere than Naples	351
Pisa—Mild Temperature due to the Tuscan Hills—Climate relaxing, damp, and soothing	352
Rome—Temperature more steady than that of Naples and Pisa—Less than of Nice—Atmosphere distinguished by a peculiar stillness	352
Palermo—Most delightful Climate—Heat more equably divided between the months than at the other Mediterranean resorts	353
Venice—Climate less Variable than at other Parts of Italy, the Transitions being slow and gradual—Air impregnated with Iodine and Bromine	354
JERSEY—Winter very mild—Characteristics of the Climate: Mildness and Moisture	355
KIRL—Elegant Sea-bathing Establishment, with a mild Climate	356
KÖSEN—Saline Springs in a charming and protected Valley	356
KÖNIGSDORF-IASTRZEMB—Powerful ioduretted Spa	356
KRANKENHEIL—2,467' high—Efficacious ioduretted and sulphuretted Springs	357
KRONTHAL—Saline Springs with a very mild Climate	358
LABASSÈRE—Cold Sulphurous Springs used for Chronic Catarrhs	359
LANDECK—1,398' high—Chemically indifferent Spring with rather a low Temperature—Air bracing and sheltered—Moor-baths against Chronic Uterine Enlargements	359
LANGENBRÜCKEN—Cold Sulphurous Springs—Useful in Chronic Catarrh of the Bladder	359
LEUK—Altitude, 4,351'—Hot Springs, with Sulphate of Lime as chief ingredient —Recommended in Catarrhal Hoarseness, Chronic Rheumatism, Eczema — Climate rough, but bracing—Mixed bathing of the Sexes	360
LIEBENZELL—In a romantic Black Forest Valley—Lukewarm Spring, particularly recommended in Chronic Metritis	361
LIPPIK—*Ioduretted Saline Thermæ*, reputed for the Cure of Uterine Enlargements	361
LIPPSPRINGE—Altitude, 378'—Mild, sheltered Climate, with a deep sandy Soil. *Arminiusquelle*—Specially curative in certain forms of incipient Tuberculosis.	362
Ottilienquelle—Less exciting—Agrees with irritable Conditions of the Mucous Membrane	363
LUHATSCHOWITZ—Altitude, 1,600'—In a charming Valley surrounded by Mountains—A powerful ioduretted Spa	363
LEGHORN—Beautiful Arrangements for Sea-bathing	365
LUCCA—Warm Baths celebrated for the Cure of Chronic Rheumatism	365
LEAMINGTON—Saline, Chalybeate, and Sulphurous Springs	365
LOWESTOFT—Peculiarly bracing and restorative	366
LYMINGTON—Sheltered Sea-bath	366
MADEIRA ISLANDS surpass the Italian Winter-Resorts in steadiness of Temperature—Young persons with a too rapid Development of the Frame and Phthisical Tendency are especially benefited—Incipient Tuberculosis energetically checked—Advanced Phthisis rapidly deteriorated	366

CONTENTS.

MALAGA—Climate warm, equable, with very small Variations—Soothing but not Relaxing—Comparison with Cannes, Madeira, and Nice . . . 368
MENTONE—Climate extremely mild and equable 369
NICE—Having a milder Atmosphere than more southern Localities, but subject to rapid vicissitudes of Temperature 370
MERAN—Altitude, 881'—In a most fertile and protected Valley—Lower Summer Temperature than in all other Towns of South Tyrol—Autumn and Spring best Seasons for Persons affected with Chronic Catarrhs 371
MERGENTHEIM—591' high—Bitter and Saline Springs used against Biliary Obstructions and Lithiasis 372
MISDROY—A sheltered Sea-bath of the Island of Wollin . . . 372
MONDORF—Strong Saline and Bromuretted Spring, lying in an extensive Plateau surrounded by shady Walks 372
MALVERN (Great)—One of the finest and most salubrious spots of Great Britain 373
—Injurious Effects of violent drenching with Cold Water . . . 374
MATLOCK-BATH, in Derbyshire—Resembling the Saxon Switzerland—Singularly Restorative in Convalescence from protracted Fevers 374
MARGATE—Atmosphere cool, dry, and bracing 375
RAMSGATE—Somewhat more sheltered and soothing—Adapted in Summer to Persons affected with Bronchial Irritation 376
NEUENAHR—225' high—Very useful in Chronic Laryngeal Irritation and first stage of incipient Tuberculosis—Its Action compared with that of Ems . 376
NORDERNEY—Climate extremely equable—Bathing Establishment protected by a Mountain-ridge—Bathing-time to be selected according to the desirability of stronger or weaker Wave-strokes 377
OFEN—Warm Alkaline Saline Springs, highly efficacious through their Temperature 378
OSTEND—Equable—Firm and Sandy Bathing Ground—Influence of the situation below the level of the Sea 379
PARTENKIRCHEN—2,434' high—In an extensive sheltered Meadow Valley—Favourable in Tubercular Diathesis 379
PETERSTHAL—1,251' high—Increase of Warmth in Summer through the Rocky Walls—Steel-spring—Gas and Saline Springs 379
GRIESBACH—1,500' high in the narrowest portion of the Rench-valley . 380
PUTBUS—The situation on the southern declivity of the Coast imparts mildness and shelter to the Climate, but the Wave-strokes are weakened through the opposite Island 380
PAU—Wild romantic Scenery—Climate extremely mild and sedative—Recommended to Persons suffering from a dry tickling Cough . . . 380
PLOMBIÈRES—1,310' high—Air bracing and pure, but subject to frequent Vicissitudes—Great range of the Temperature of the Springs—Especially celebrated for the Cure of Chronic Rheumatism, Sciatica—Prolonged Duration of the Baths—Professor Hebra's Ingenious Bed for keeping Patients in Water during a whole Course of Treatment 381
RECOARO—1,465' high—Bracing Summer Residence—Chalybeate Springs . 382
REICHENHALL—1,470' high—Very mild and bracing Climate—Extremely grateful to Persons affected with Bronchial Irritation—Charming Contrasts of Scenery—Concentrated Saline Springs 382
REMAGEN—Climate more congenial and salubrious than the Valleys of the right shore of the Rhine 383
RIGI-SCHEIDECK—5,073' high—Curhaus recommended for Anæmic Persons . 383
RIGI-KALTBAD—4,436' high—Situation more sheltered—Excellent Cow and Goat Whey 384

	PAGE
RIPPOLSDAU—1,886' high—Surrounded by Woody Mountains—Springs *tonic resolvent*—Air pure, fresh and bracing, rendered balsamic through the Exhalations of Fir and Pine Forests	384
ROMERBAD—755' high—Bathing in large Basins (Gebäder)	384
KOMITSCH—In a fertile and lovely Landscape—Climate extremely mild—Principally resorted to in Cases of Abdominal Plethora	385
ROSENHEIM—Chalybeate and Sulphur Springs for Drinking and Bathing, besides Moor-baths and Pine-Foliage Vapour-baths	385
ROYAN—Sea-baths—Protected Position—Mild Climate	385
SAINT MORITZ—5,710' high—Situation extremely romantic and picturesque—Climate of the Canton of Grisons—Chalybeate Spring compared with Schwalbach—Useful in Helminthias, Scrophulosis, Chlorosis—Effect of the magnificent and varied Landscapes—Ride to the Village of Maria	385
SCHINZNACH—1,060' high—In a friendly Valley—Useful in Prurigo, Sycosis, in Scrofula, in Lead and Arsenic Poisoning, in Chronic Rheumatism	388
WILDEGG—Powerful Ioduretted Spring; employed with Iodide of Potassium	389
SCHEVENINGEN—A fashionable Sea-bath in a sheltered Position, with fine Walks and adjoining Forest—Advantages of the proximity of the Hague	390
SODEN—440' high—In the Spessart—Climate moist and equable	390
STACHELBERG—Sulphur Spring—2,044' high—Magnificent Scenery—Position sheltered chiefly by gigantic snow-covered Mountains—Useful in Chronic, Bronchial and Gastric Catarrhs, in Chronic Rheumatism, and Cutaneous Diseases	390
STEBEN—1,786' high—Chalybeate—Climate bleak, but tonic	391
STREITBERG—1,800' high—Sheltered Position in a charming Valley—Climate very mild and equable—Whey-establishment principally used in cases of incipient Tuberculosis	391
SULZA—Powerful Saline Springs—Secluded Locality—Recommended to Scrofulous Patients fond of Quiet	392
SULZBRUNN—2,671' high—Ioduretted Spring—Climate peculiarly favourable	392
SWINEMÜNDE—The 'Plantage' enclosing the Establishment for Warm Baths	392
SYLT—Thorough maritime Climate with strong Wave-strokes	392
SAINT-SAUVEUR—4,620' high—Climate bracing without being bleak—Soothing Effects of the Sulphurous-baths on the Nervous System—Action different from that of Barèges—Recommended in Uterine Infiltrations	393
SALZBRUNN—1,215' high—Extending in a charming wide Valley along the Salzach—Excellent Effects of Whey	393
SALZHAUSEN—461' high—Saline Springs with some Bromine	394
SALZUNGEN—778' high—Climate considerably impregnated with saline exhalations	395
SALCOMBE—Gifted with a mild and equable Winter Climate	395
SCARBOROUGH—The Queen of British Watering Places—North-sands in a better Condition than the South—Sands hard and gradually shelving	395
SIDMOUTH—Sheltered by lofty Hills—Climate mild and relaxing	396
SWANSEA—Frequently resorted to from its beautiful Situation	396
TARASP—4,608' high—Magnificent Landscape—Combination of Saline and Alkaline Springs—Comparison with Carlsbad	396
TEGERNSEE—2,487' high—With an ever-changing Series of beautiful Walks	398
TEINACH—1,223' high—Air permeated with Exhalations of Fir Trees—Springs Tonic, Stimulant, and Antacid	398
TIEFENAU—1,800' high—Hydropathic Establishment resorted to after a Course of Mercury to Strengthen the Reactive Power of the Organism	399
TÖPLITZ—With its Warm Sulphurous Springs in the midst of a Park	399
TRAVEMÜNDE—Bathing Ground firm and gently sloping—Baths of Pine-Foliage	400

	PAGE
TRIEST—Excellent Arrangement for Warm and Cold Sea-baths—Suitable to vigorous Constitutions only—Weather mutable and subject to abrupt Transitions—Social Charms and Advantages	400
VENICE—Excellent Arrangement for Sea-bathing	401
TEIGNMOUTH—Picturesque Position—Highly recommended for Sea-bathing in Summer—Not steady enough for a Winter Residence	401
TORQUAY—The City of Villas—Atmosphere less moist and more equable than the Devonshire Climate in general, through its western Projection into the Atlantic—Highest mean annual Temperature in Great Britain—Comparison with Clifton—Advantage in Convalescence from Pneumonia—Comparison of Temperature with other Health-resorts—Increasing Accommodation—Mutability of the English Climate useful in hardening the Constitution—Distant Climes sought after by advanced Pulmonary Invalids—Consequences	402
TUNBRIDGE-WELLS—289' high—Varying Attraction of picturesque and wild Scenery—Chalybeate Water—When to be Employed—Sound Sleep a Peculiarity of the Effect of the Climate	404
VERNET—With a Climate so mild and equable as to admit Bathing through the whole Year—Vaporarium	405
VICHY—733' high—Enclosed by a mountainous Amphitheatre—King of Alkaline Spas—Comparison with Carlsbad—Indications and Contra-indications	406
WARMBRUNN—1,100' high—Pleasant Appearance produced by the Gardens and Fields surrounding the Houses—Formerly reckoned amongst the Sulphur Spas—Rooms for Inhalations, for Electrial Therapeutics—Greatly reputed for the Cure of Articular Stiffness and of Herpetic Diseases	407
WÄGGIS—1,350' high—Encompassed by the most magnificent Scenery and completely protected against severe Winds—Climate moderately moist and exhilarating	409
WEISSENBURG—2,759' high—Atmosphere distinguished by its Humidity—Temperature changeable—Warm Spring at the Foot of a Rock	409
WEISSENSTEIN—3,949' high—With most magnificent Alpine Views—Cabinets for Whey-drinking and Whey-bathing	410
WILDUNGEN—300' high—Most pleasant and variegated shady Promenades—Particularly recommended in Gravel, Lithiasis, Spasms of the Bladder, and Chronic Inflammation of the Prostatic Gland	410
WIPFELD—Sulphur Spring and Sulphur Mud-baths—Useful in Neuralgia and Chronic Rheumatism	412
WHITBY—Most interesting Sea-view from the West Cliff—Numerous wooded and sheltered Walks—*Bagdale* Spa	412
WIGHT (ISLE OF)—Garden of England—Exhibiting almost every Variety of Landscape in Miniature	413
UNDERCLIFF—Protecting Downs—Air imbued with a certain Dryness and Astringency—Effects of the Altitude of the Undercliff—Peculiar Influence of the perpendicular Rocks—Comparison with Torquay	413
WORTHING—Climate soft and relaxing—Numerous pleasant Walks	415
ZAIZON's Ioduretted Springs—1,700' high—Considerable Amount of Iodide of Sodium—Great Reputation for the Cure of Glandular Swellings combined with Anæmia	415

ON THE

GERMAN MINERAL WATERS.

LECTURE I.

GENTLEMEN,—The subject I have to bring before you claims to be a very important part of Materia Medica; for it treats of remedies, prepared in the womb of the earth by the power of nature alone, and in many instances indispensable to effect a cure.

The mineral springs, though standing on the same ground they occupied years or centuries ago, have come considerably nearer to us through the blessing of the great world-reformers, the railroads. A place, which would formerly have been reached only after a long journey and at a great expense, becomes every year more accessible to sufferers of the middle class; and often in your after-life will you thank the gentlemen at the head of this Institution for having afforded you an opportunity to learn that which many of your fellow-students are unable to acquire.

The spas are not unknown here, for a great many English are found at almost every continental watering-place. The only regret to be felt is, that they do not resort to these fountains of Hygæia by the advice of their medical attendants, but mostly on the recommendation of some lay acquaintance, who has found relief from his ailment at a certain spa, and by merely judging from appearance, of course thinks every analogous morbid affection must be combated by the same means. How often disappointment must follow such advice you may easily imagine, for the spas are at no time indifferent remedies; the patient will either improve or get decidedly worse; nay, his health is sometimes jeopardised if he uses baths or springs on his own account, and without proper discrimination.

In the treatment of disease you will meet with several classes of difficulties. After having carefully investigated the morbid phenomena, and satisfactorily established the nature and cause of the suffering, you proceed to adopt the most appropriate plan of treatment. But at your next visit you find that the remedies which seemed to be clearly indicated, and which confidently promised relief, have failed to answer your expectations. Suppose a case of severe rheumatism claims your care: you have given the patient alkalines, *colchicum* and other approved anti-rheumatics; you have regulated his digestive functions; you have even been induced by the severity of his suffering to employ antiphlogistic remedies; and, according to theory, the patient ought long since to have left his bed and mixed with the healthy. But in sad reality, there he lies, still feeling pain in his joints, still unable to use his limbs, and pursue his avocations, perhaps to the injury of beloved persons depending on his exertions. What is your next step?

You subject all the prominent symptoms to a fresh examination, and you conclude, that, if you could raise the power of the nervous system, by giving *quinine* for instance, the functions of the muscles and muscular organs would be strengthened, and the morbid sensibility diminished. Some relief has been obtained, but only temporarily, and the pain, inconvenience, and disability, still exist or return, to the silent reproach of human skill. You attack the enemy from another point. You give *iron* to improve the strength of the vital fluid, and thus induce a more energetic organic metamorphosis. The contention between diminished irritability and increased nervous sensibility is often removed by raising the former, and thus restoring the equilibrium necessary to health. You may then resort to *iodide of potassium*, which frequently cures similar states of disease, by increasing the power of the absorbent vessels, and causing effete exudations to become absorbed and excreted. You have employed vapour baths, external derivatives and internal revulsives; and though each remedy (when judiciously selected) helped to allay the symptoms, still days, weeks, nay months have passed, the disease has become chronic under your hands, in spite of the most careful and approved treatment. You must not suppose that I fill your mind with imaginary fears. Though fortunately rare, such cases will occur, notwithstanding our daily progress, and the almost hourly discovery of some new remedy. It is at this stage that people throw themselves into the hands of quackery, relating how many bottles of medicine and boxes of pills they have 'swallowed,' as they call it, how they have been given up by the profession, &c., &c. What gratitude will you earn, if, on the point of abandoning treatment, you remember that similar cases have been cured by a certain spa, and you are thus instrumental, by its recommendation, in restoring the patient's health while he is far removed from your sight?

Another class of difficulties ought not to be passed over, for they will occur in practical life. Your advice will occasionally be asked by persons complaining of some deviation in the function of certain organs, and still, after having accurately observed the phenomena, you may find that actual disease does not exist. There are *states of transition* between the normal performance of the harmonising human faculties and disorder. What seems functional derangement is perhaps, in this instance, only morbidly increased sensibility, or momentary predominance of one system or organ over another. A desire arises in your mind to recommend steps, which form the intermediate link between dietetic rules and pharmaceutic preparations. This you can satisfy by ordering a mineral water, the constituents of which act sometimes more energetically than larger doses of the same remedies in the ordinary form. The reason probably is, their greater degree of solution. They enter the digestive organs as more congenial bodies, and their active principles, so finely divided, are fit to be immediately imbibed into the absorbent vessels, and to be assimilated without previously performing the tortuous route of digestion, as is the case with many artificially prepared medicaments. Very frequently, nature gives us distinct *hints* of a tendency to a disturbed equilibrium. Is it not very meritorious to combat these first deviations of natural functions, and thus often prevent the development of actual disease? From the imperfection of everything human, you will not, of course, always succeed. But I can affirm, from the experience I have had in the occasional administration of mineral waters for a number of years, that their effects in this respect are extremely gratifying. Often have I prescribed the one or the other, at first, as an innocent experiment or an expectative remedy, without hoping to find the beneficial results that actually ensued.

A gentleman, about thirty years of age, who began to study medicine, and afterwards turned to mercantile pursuits, underwent much anxiety and mental labour in the year 1846. For twelve years past he has felt daily, a few hours after each meal, a burning sensation in the cardiac region, extending upwards to the shoulder; he was also frequently affected with headache in the occiput, particularly in the evening. He tried many remedies and dietetic changes in vain, and latterly *carbonate of potash*. He resides in a healthy suburb, daily takes much exercise, and lives with the greatest regularity. Finding the subjective phenomena unconnected with any structural or functional disorder, I considered the free carbonic acid, with carbonate of soda, and the other ingredients contained in *Fachingen* water, would improve his condition. I accordingly recommended this water, and was extremely gratified when, after some time, he declared himself entirely free from the inconvenience which had molested him so many years.

The name of *mineral waters* indicates that certain mineral substances are dissolved in the springs. If so, why could we not artificially produce the same combination, and expect similar results?

Because they mostly contain substances insoluble in ordinary water. But what agency keeps them in solution? It is *carbonic acid* gas thoroughly impregnating the water. Were we to employ any fixed acids to dissolve lime, magnesia, or iron, the chemical composition of other combinations would be changed. Carbonic acid not only dissolves the one substance without disuniting combinations of others, but it enters the system charged with these particles, and presents them to the mouths of the absorbent vessels in this highly diluted condition; it further promotes their *direct* absorption by exerting a stimulating power on the vascular and nervous systems. Thus you may understand why six-tenths of a grain of iron imbibed into the lacteals, with the above gas, may be more exciting and strengthening than three or four times the quantity of pharmaceutic carbonate of iron, which has to be dissolved in the gastric juice *previous* to absorption. A great many spas possess similar ingredients, but in different proportions; and their efficacy generally corresponds with the *predominant* constituents. Other ingredients admixed prevent a too powerful action on any organic sphere. Suppose sulphate of soda or magnesia to be the chief ingredient (as in *Püllna, Saidschutz*, &c.) the alvine evacuations might be excited in too high a degree, and the sanguification might become too much weakened to perform the nutritive function of the whole body. But carbonate of lime and of iron present in small proportions, give a certain check to the solvent and liquefying action, and increase the tone and resistance of the blood. Where iron is the chief ingredient, a too vigorous excitement of the vascular system is prevented by the presence of a small quantity of lowering sulphates, and of solvent chlorides. But you will raise the objection, that we have been impressed with the great advantage of simple treatment, and of not employing too great a complication of remedies. It is certainly most desirable, in ordinary treatment, to fix the appropriate remedy in the simplest form, and then both success and non-success will improve your experience and therapeutic knowledge. But though it is necessary to be guided in the choice of the mineral waters by their chemical composition, each spa must be considered as one whole, acting on well-defined abnormal conditions with a more or less certain effect, according to the records of eminent English and foreign writers. Having informed you that a gaseous acid is the chief solvent of the mineral waters, you will at once see the difficulty of artificially imitating them. Nevertheless, the great advantage derived from their use induced several attempts to prepare fictitious mineral waters. Dr. Struve of Dresden succeeded, after years of unceasing labour, in producing fictitious mineral waters, which resemble the natural in taste, colour, specific gravity, and, above all, in the results of chemical analysis. He endeavoured to follow the process apparently employed by nature, and he argued that the effects must be likewise identical. What is called the 'Brighton pump-room' is one of these establishments; and many instances are on record of cures performed by these waters, and of specific effects only belonging to the respective natural waters. Some go even so far as to claim a preference for the artificial waters, from the circumstance of their being more easily obtainable, and of their losing less carbonic acid by distant carriage, &c., &c. But, though our present knowledge of chemistry can discover no perceptible difference, who could assert that some new test might not find substances in the springs, which were unknown at the time of their last analysis? Before the discovery of iodine and bromine, for instance, the efficacy of *Kreuznach* or *Adelheidsquelle* in scrofulous diseases might have been attributed to the presence of chloride of sodium and chloride of calcium. That there are active principles yet undiscovered in some mineral springs, we are justified in surmising, if we take cognisance of the astonishing changes produced by certain spas called 'chemically indifferent,' because their constituents are scarcely distinguished from those of common water. It is a singular fact that these very spas are among the most powerful. Take for instance *Wildbad*, near Stuttgardt, which is particularly renowned for curing inveterate gout, *arthritic* paralysis, and contractions after wounds. What do you suppose its constituents to be? No more than 3½ grains in 16 ounces, and these are about two grains of chloride of sodium, half-a-grain of carbonate of soda, some carbonate of magnesia, of lime, manganese and iron, with some silex. Are these few grains able to cause absorption of substances deposited in the joints, or to restore pliancy and power to limbs, which have for years resisted the manifold means that knowledge and experience have devised? Put the same ingredients into ordinary water of corresponding temperature, and see whether you will obtain results at all approaching those frequently experienced at Wildbad? Is it because the warmth of the water is identical with that of blood, and requires neither heating nor cooling? You have only to think of *Gastein*, in South Tyrol, the temperature of which is about 111° F., and which must be cooled for bathing, and still its reputation for the cure of atonic gout, of paralysis, and of spasms through deficient nervous power, almost surpasses that of Wildbad. What are its constituents? Still less, only 2½ grains in sixteen ounces—viz., 1½ sulph. of soda, then some sulph. of potash, chlor. of sodium, carb. of lime, &c. It is true, an undetermined quantity of animal substance, called *glairine*, has been found in it. But is that to explain the visible transformations happening within a short period before your eyes? Why can the spring of the 'hôpital' in Vichy be freely employed, whilst that of the 'Grande-grille' must be administered with great circumspection, though both possess nearly the same chemical constituents? Probably because the vegeto-animal substance, incapable of imitation, is more abundant in the former.

Another objection to artificial waters may be found in the supposition that many salts obtained by evaporation may possibly have been *formed* through this process, without having previously existed under the same combination; in fact, it may rather be a product than an educt of analysis. Nevertheless, they are excellent substitutes for the genuine waters; although when these latter can be obtained, it is my opinion that they ought decidedly to be preferred. On the other hand, great advantages may be derived from certain imitations; thus, at Gros-Caillou, rue de l'Université, Paris, they produce a solution of magnesia in an excess of carbonic acid, which is so saturated that a pint contains nearly half an ounce of magnesia; about six grains can be given to a child in a table-spoonful of this solution, either as an absorbent, as an antacid, or as an aperient, &c.

The spas themselves are generally resorted to between the months of May and October (inclusive). The course lasts from three to six weeks. Their effects invariably continue for a long period, and the most successful cures frequently take place months after the patients have rejoined their family circles. When immediate improvement ensues, it is often of a less durable character. This lasting efficacy particularly adapts them for the treatment of chronic diseases. In most spas, bathing and drinking of the respective springs take place. Some, however, are merely employed internally, others only externally.

The mineralised mud of some is used separately as a highly curative external remedy; in others, the abundant evolution of carbonic acid serves for general and local gas baths. Where the temperature is too high, ingenuity is taxed for contrivances calculated to lower the heat, without altering the composition of those ingredients partially held in solution by the high temperature. If the temperature is too low for bathing, the *bade-meister* (bath-master) will show you in one place how the *baignoires* are warmed by subterranean steam, so that the spring may not lose its carbonic acid and have important substances precipated by being heated. Another will explain that warm water is mixed in his baths in such a proportion with the spa water as not to impair its properties, &c. At others you have douches of various height and power. In some you will see *ascending* douches, to which many cures are attributed, particularly in several diseases of women. In others again, friction is employed with the douche as a great auxiliary to the medical treatment. (This is particularly well understood and unsurpassed at Aix-la-Chapelle.) In fact, when you visit any spa, you will be astonished at the manner in which every particle of the natural gift is brought to bear upon diseases. If the source be on a higher situation than the baths, you will see this taken advantage of to fill the baths by pressure from below, so that the water flows upwards in a wave-like manner. You see a shaft constructed in which the water rises and is made to splash over and to fill the circumvenient air with its vapour and exhalations for medical purposes. The quantity of the water taken internally varies considerably, and as a rule is gradually to be increased.

Generally, a band begins to play about six in the morning, waking the visitors from their slumbers. In the intervals of drinking, they take walking exercise for about a quarter of an hour. About an hour after a light breakfast, the baths are taken. The diet is regulated according to the nature of the spa. The curative power seems to be evolved by a slow reaction, which the *ensemble* of the healing influences produces in the human system. If this reaction is speedily exhibited by signs of a violent revolution, as headache, giddiness, depression, lassitude, restlessness, want of appetite, obstruction or diarrhœa, distention of the abdomen, feverishness, &c., immediate discontinuance of the course is necessary.

The course might be resumed as soon as a more favourable impression can be reckoned upon. 'Bath eruption,' occasionally appearing after a few weeks, and then disappearing without medicinal aid, is considered a favourable sign.

Both the spas and mineral waters, however useful in chronic, must be entirely avoided in acute diseases, in inflammation of vital organs, inflammatory fevers, &c. They are also contraindicated in hectic fever, in formed tuberculosis, in carcinomatous degenerations, in aneurisms, in congestion of the lungs or brain, &c. In fact, before recommending a spa, the subsequent reaction and unfailing excitement must be taken into almost more serious account than the direct influence itself.

LECTURE II.

The springs furnish a natural point of classification by their varying temperature. The more a spa approaches the temperature of the blood, the less animal heat is withdrawn by the contact, and the greater the perception of warmth. For convenience sake let us designate, with Vetter, those springs having a temperature below 66° Fahrenheit, *krenæ*,* or cold springs, and those of which the temperature exceeds 95° Fahrenheit, *thermæ*, or hot springs. Those that range between 66° and 95° Fahrenheit, may be considered as of intermediate temperature, still depriving the body of some heat, but unable to display the medicinal effect of cold; they are designated as *pegæ*.† Mineral waters, without reference to temperature, are also termed *pegæ*.

Another natural division may be derived from their local variations, which do not fail to exercise a considerable influence on their medicinal efficiency. Their respective altitude modifies the atmospheric pressure, and displays properties of its own.

The diminished pressure and greater purity of the air in higher situations invigorate and stimulate the weakened nervous system, and diminish passive pulmonary blennorrhages, whilst these places would disagree with persons of irritable thoracic organs, and might excite hæmoptysis, congestion, or inflammation, where a tendency to such diseases already exists.

It has been calculated that the warmth of the air diminishes by 1° Reaumur for every 500 feet of height. But however applicable this law may be in the higher regions, it is less so nearer the earth, the temperature being modified by the direction of the mountains, geographic latitude, and many other circumstances.

It has been assumed, that the whole mass of water on the globe remains constantly of the same amount, though undergoing various changes of form by atmospheric influence. The water attracted and imbibed by the surface of the earth, penetrates to

---

* From κρήνη—source. † From πηγή—spring, salient water.

different depths according to the more or less yielding and porous character of the recipient layers. It then collects in the interior and begins its solvent and chemical action on the surrounding strata.

It is of importance to consider whether a spring has a merely *local* origin, or whether it owes its existence to the *general* character of the mountainous formation.

Thus, most acidulous and thermal springs can be traced to certain characteristic mountain chains, whilst sulphureous and chalybeate springs are mostly independent of the general character of a region, and seem to stand as isolated products of local causes.

The volcanic processes in the interior of the earth drive mighty rocks of basalt out of the depth of the sea, inflame strata of coals, inundate whole regions with lava and ignited substances, and shake the highest and firmest mountain ranges, and all this free from the various forces and elements acting in the atmosphere of the surface. Fire alone could not accomplish these processes without the co-operation of water.

The contact of the two powers, however, produces vapours, which, by expanding, burst the opposing layers of the earth and discharge streams of lava and of basalt.

If the vapours are pent up, earthquakes necessarily ensue. Should they, however, find no resistance, they form gaseous products and stream out as *carbonic acid, sulphuretted hydrogen* or *nitrogen*. To these gaseous streams the *thermal* and *acidulous* springs seem to owe their origin.

The volcanic character is probable, from their situation being mostly near active or extinguished volcanoes. Vesuvius is surrounded by thermal springs. The mightiest volcanic mountain chains of Europe are accompanied by powerful thermal and acidulous springs.

A relation, no doubt, exists between earthquakes and Thermæ. It is asserted that those regions are less exposed to earthquakes which possess volcanic springs—for instance, North Bohemia, the Rhine and Taunus regions. Such mountain chains, in which no eruption of lava, basalt, hot vapours, or carbonic acid, has taken place, are said to be more exposed to earthquakes. During the earthquake of Lisbon, that part built on limestone suffered more than the adjoining Belem, partly built on basalt.

Of all the earthquakes that took place in January and February 1824, from the foot of the Saxon mountains to the Elnbogner-kreis, only two German miles from Carlsbad, nothing was felt in Carlsbad itself. On the other hand, whilst an earthquake took place at Lisbon in 1809, the Schlossbrunnen disappeared, but returned in 1823 with a lower temperature.

Through the earthquake of 1692, the water of the Pouhon, one of the springs of Spa, near Liége, became clearer, of a stronger taste, and more abundant. Sometimes, however, earthquakes are only perceived in the environs of hot springs, whilst the flat country is spared.

Most remarkable are the changes that took place on November 1, 1755, when one half of Lisbon was destroyed by an earthquake. Between eleven and twelve in the morning, the chief spring of Teplitz began to get turbid, and to discharge for a few minutes a dark yellow liquid; and after having ceased running a short time, it burst forth with such violence and abundance, that all the basins overflowed. At first it came out turbid and yellowish-red, but regained its former transparency after about half an hour.

A few days later, on the 9th of November, in Canstadt (Würtemberg), near the mineral springs, two such violent concussions took place, that an adjoining house sank several feet with a loud crash.

The hot springs generally arise out of granite, gneiss, and other volcanic kinds of mountain, frequently near basalt or transition rocks of analogous formation and composition, as porphyry, greenstone, and greywacke.

Directly out of gneiss, granite, and greywacke, or in their vicinity, arise the springs of Pfeffers, Leuk, and Bormio, in Switzerland, Warmbrunn, in Silesia, most of the hot springs of Hungary, Styria, Salzburg, &c.

Even when Thermæ seem to spring up out of strata of red sandstone or shell-lime, as happens in several springs of the Vosges, in the ramifications of the Black Forest, and the mountains of Nothern Switzerland, this latter formation only seems to form a sort of covering for the deeper primary mountain-masses.

The warm springs of Baden, near Vienna, arise out of tufaceous* lime.

The primary mountains do not seem, however, to be the proper focus of the thermæ, but rather a means of their connection with the volcanic processes in the interior; for the springs mostly come

---

* Tufa is a clayey fossil, mostly porous, ashy gray, and consisting of loose particles of lime; its origin is volcanic.

to light in such regions, in which volcanic mountains are found near the primary.

In Sweden, with its prevalence of primitive rocks, not one considerable therma is found. At the northern declivity of the Alps, as in Baden, Würtemberg, Bavaria, comparatively few hot springs are found, the greater number being on the southern.

Formed out of melted granite or analogous stones, and violently raised, like lava, from their subterranean volcanic birthplace by vapours, basaltic masses burst the crusts of different kinds of mountains, and frequently attend active or extinguished volcanoes. The warm springs of Bertrich arise out of greywacke slate, interspersed with lava and basalt; the thermæ of Aix-la-Chapelle out of greywacke. This connection of thermal character with basaltic eruptions is clearly shown in the thermæ of North Bohemia, of the Taunus and Eifel mountains (near the Rhine).

As regards the cause of the *inherent heat,* curious notions were formerly entertained. Some explained it from a peculiar process of fermentation in the interior of the earth, others imagined that the springs came in contact with caustic lime, by which heat was produced; according to others, through the action of water on sulphur pyrites. Some ascribed it to subterranean conflagration of strata of coals or peat. It is more rationally assumed, that as the temperature lowers in proportion to the rarefaction of the air in ascending upwards from the surface, the temperature must become higher the deeper the earth is entered and the more the air is condensed.

Others maintained that a peculiar heat constantly exists in the centre of the earth, independent of extraneous influences. That the temperature rises in proportion to depth without reference to geographical latitude, or to season, is an acknowledged fact. The frequent presence of cold springs in the neighbourhood of hot, demonstrating the deep origin of the latter, has been already pointed out.

Let us now consider the *composition of the Thermæ.* Alkalies prevail in combination with carbonic, hydrochloric, or sulphuric acid. The non-volcanic springs possess more earthy salts. Carbonate of soda is very frequently met with in volcanic mountain masses, as in klingstone, basalt, pearlstone, pumice, different kinds of lava, &c. Sometimes sublimated carbonate of soda is found in volcanic regions.

Sulphuric and hydrochloric acids are frequently found near volcanoes. The same holds good of carbonic acid, though it is sometimes difficult to determine whether its evolution is due to the action of heat or of a stronger acid, by which it may be expelled.

Hydrochloric acid gas escapes from Etna. The surface of the lava ejected from Vesuvius in 1794 was covered after a few days with crystals of chloride of sodium and hydrochlorate of ammonia. Chloride of sodium is the prevailing constituent of volcanic productions; the next is sulphate of lime, then sulphate of potash, then hydrochlorate of lime and of potash. Moreover the quantity of nitrogen found in several thermæ seems to refer to their volcanic origin, this gas being often met with in gaseous volcanic evolutions.

Potash is frequently found in volcanic mountains, and also in granite, mica, and other kinds of primary rocks. In a similar manner, the presence of lithia, manganese, and iron, can be explained, as also the phosphates and fluates.

The Riesengebirge and the mountains of the county of Glatz, have only two thermæ; but numerous cold acidulous springs. The same is the case with the mountains of North Bohemia, which form, as it were, one chain extending as far as the Rhine, Taunus and Eifel mountains.

Most acidulous springs originate out of transition lime, variegated sandstone, clay slate, gneiss, greenstone, marl, and very frequently near basalt, and other volcanic products.

Their *temperature* is remarkable, from its stability being very slightly influenced by atmospheric changes, which shows them to possess a much deeper origin than common springs, and a great analogy to the characteristics of the thermæ.

In the Ragoczy spring of Kissingen, for instance, the temperature was 43° F., when the thermometer stood at the freezing point; when in hot summer, the temperature rose to 104° F., the spring had only 52° F. Thus the temperature of the spring only changed 9° to 72° of the atmosphere (from 32 to 104).

As in the thermæ, their ingredients are most intimately combined, carbonic acid and soda being the media of solution. Even the proportionate quantity of solid ingredients is analogous to the thermæ. It is inconsiderable, when they arise in primary mountains. In both, soda is mostly present, with carbonic, sulphuric, or hydrochloric acid. The quantity of *free* carbonic acid deserves particular attention.

Mighty evolutions of gas take place periodically in volcanic eruptions, or appear as results of continued volcanic processes in the interior. In Italy, this not only happens in the celebrated Grotto del Cane, but also in other parts. Permanent evolutions of gas are also met with in the volcanic mountain ranges of the Rhine, especially of the Eifel, near Birresbronn; at Daun, near the shore of the lake of Laach, which furnishes by its environs unmistakable proofs of a former active volcano; at Kissingen and its environs; in the neighbourhood of Pyrmont and Driburg; and near Franzensbad and Marienbad. The gas mostly consists of carbonic acid gas, but sometimes contains sulphuretted hydrogen, and nitrogen mixed, as in Marienbad and Franzensbad : the temperature of the gas naturally corresponding with that of the spring: the quantity somewhat depends on the pressure and temperature of the air, on its movement or quietude, or its electric condition.

The circumstance that carbonic acid gas may become liquid by high pressure, induces the belief that the gas may have originally existed in a liquid state, but become transformed into gas by its issue into the external regions, under diminished pressure.

A very important consideration in the choice of a spa is, further, the variation of the climate. Geographical latitude often fixes the character of a watering-place, though not invariably so. The more easterly or westerly position must also be looked upon as exerting some influence. Thus you find, under nearly the same latitude, *Wiesbaden*, which is renowned for its temperate and mild climate, and *Steben* on the Saale (tributary of the Elbe), and Alexandersbad (on the Main), known for the inclemency of their climate.

The quality of the ground, the nature of the surrounding mountains, the cultivation of the soil, standing or flowing waters, all exercise their influence. In spas surrounded by marshy fields or stagnant waters, intermittent fever is sometimes found endemic. How this injurious influence may be removed by cultivation is shown in Franzensbad, where intermittent fever was formerly endemic. But now, the marshy meadows and ponds having been dried up, this disease is very seldom met with, even in very hot weather.

LECTURE III.

THE mysterious nature of these remarkable outpourings induced many persons to attribute accidental circumstances to their influence. Thus, for instance, the vapours arising out of the springs at Pfäfers were thought a preservative against the plague, because in 1611 and 1629, when the cantons of St. Gallen and Appenzell were devastated by the plague, all those that resided at the time in Pfäfers were spared. This, however, could not furnish a proof of the preserving power of the spa. The non-attack may have been due to the high and isolated situation of the place; being, perhaps, beyond the reach of atmospheric miasma. On the other hand, the salutary effect of sea air was well known and appreciated by the ancients. The cause is, no doubt, the diminished carbonic acid of the atmosphere, and its impregnation with saline exhalations. The same influence is also shown in the character of the surrounding vegetation. A favourable effect, similar to that of sea air, may be expected from the vicinity of salt and graduation works, for a considerable quantity of free hydrochloric acid has been found in the air near the salt-works of Halle. The same acid has also been detected in the rain water of Salzufeln (lat. 52° on the Weser).

If snow-covered mountain peaks are situated in the neighbourhood, the climate will be characterised by a certain bleakness, though the snow may be present only a part of the year.

This is, for instance, perceived in the spas at the foot of the Fichtelgebirge, Thüringer Forest, Erzgebirge and Black Forest.

The climate is further modified, according as the spa is situated on the southern declivity of the mountains, and thus protected against violent north and east winds, or on the northern declivity just exposed to them.

Look at Wiesbaden, being on the southern declivity of the Taunus, below the reach of north and east winds, and enjoying an extremely pleasant and mild climate. Now, behold Schwalbach, only a few leagues to the north, unfavourably known for the bleakness and severity of its climate. What is the reason? It lies on the plateau of the mountain, and the same height that serves as protection to its fortunate neighbour exposes it to the full attack of the north and east winds.

In Barèges, the celebrated French spa of the Pyrenees, the climate is so severe, that it cannot be well inhabited more than six months of the year, whilst in its neighbourhood mineral watering-places enjoy the most lovely climate. A still greater difference exists between the places lying north and south of the St. Bernardino.

Though in the northern situation the climate is very severe, on the southern, luxuriant meadows are seen at a height of 5000'. At Misox (4900'), corn cultivation begins: at Soazzo (3000'), the vine is cultivated; and farther down fig and mulberry-trees flourish.

The circumstance whether the valley of the respective spas be narrow, encircled by steep and high cliffs, or broad and open, becomes of high importance; as, for instance, in diseases of the chest. The partial impediment to the entering rays of the sun causes the narrow valley to be comparatively colder and moister, and patients with weakened thoracic organs will feel oppressed by a long sojourn in it. Invalids of this description occasionally complain of a somewhat impeded respiration, even in the valley of the Tepl, at Carlsbad, or of the Lahn, at Ems. How oppressed and inconvenienced would these persons feel at Pfeffers, which, though it lies 2000' above the level of the sea, is so enclosed by high and steep rocky mountains, that the beneficent influence of the sun is not admitted more than seven hours in the longest days. Thus, supposing the present disease should strongly mark out Pfeffers as the most appropriate spa, you must not send a sufferer there, if his thoracic organs are at all liable to irritation, or disposed to derangement.

The influence of the greater or smaller elevation I have already treated of. I have said that the purity and tenuity of the atmosphere belonging to high situations, possesses tonic and stimulating properties, whilst that of lower situations, being denser and impregnated with more impurities, must produce corresponding depression of the vital functions, or vitiate the circulating fluids, and thus lay the seed of actual disease.

You will have observed some analogy between acidulous and hot springs, as regards their volcanic origin. But you may further notice, that heat and carbonic acid seem respectively to perform the same function of solving and keeping the constituent particles in close union. When you hear, on my treating specially of the waters, that a spa contains so much carbonic acid, it is of the utmost importance to inquire, whether the acid be intimately and firmly connected with the water, or whether it merely seems to stream through it, loosely attached.

Though in general 100 volumes of water absorb only 106 volumes of carbonic acid, we find the drinking spring of Pyrmont to contain, in 100 cubic inches of water, 171 cubic inches of carbonic acid; the Franzensquelle, near Eger, 153 cubic inches; the Ferdinand's spring of Marienbad 145 cubic inches; in fact, a greatly varying amount, irrespective of what might have been imbibed under the ordinary atmospheric pressure.

In some instances, the quantity of volatile ingredients varies according to the electric tension of the atmosphere, or in consequence of unexplored processes in the interior. The cold sulphur spring of Günthersbad, near Stockhausen, in Thüringen, evolved during four months (from November, 1817, to February, 1818) a considerable quantity of sulphuretted hydrogen; suddenly the quantity diminished, and the water exhibited instead a strong taste of iron. When the Ragoczy, of Kissingen, was cleaned out, a source of carbonic acid was found, with a varying quantity of gas. In June, previous to a tempest, at a temperature of $81\frac{1}{2}°$ Fahrenheit, 170 cubic inches of carbonic acid flowed out in a minute. In July, during moist weather, and a temperature of $63\frac{1}{2}°$ Fahrenheit, only 110 cubic inches in the same period, and a day later 140 cubic inches. A similar variation of quantity has been observed in those grottoes in which a continuous evolution of carbonic acid takes place, as in the Grotto del Cane, near Naples, and the vapour cave near Pyrmont. As regards the quantity of ingredients dissolved in the springs, it does not invariably exceed that dissolved in common water; on the contrary, it is often smaller. What constitutes them *mineral waters, is their peculiar composition and distinguishing properties of taste, colour, temperature, and specific gravity, and, above all, their specific efficacy on the human organism.* Several drinking wells of Berlin, Stockholm, Hanau, and other towns, contain from five to ten grains of solid ingredients, dissolved in sixteen ounces, without claiming the character of mineral waters, whilst the powerful spa of Wildbad contains only $3\frac{1}{2}$ gr. in 16 ounces; Teplitz, $4\frac{3}{4}$; Gastein and Pfeffers, $2\frac{1}{2}$ gr.; Brückenau, 2 4-10; Spa, 3 3-10; the sulphur spring of Landeck, 2 6-10. Those which contain chlorides and sulphates have most ingredients. Amongst the German springs, Püllna possesses 182 gr. of solid ingredients in 16 ounces; Saidschutz, 160; Seidlitz, 126; the muriatico-saline spring of Pyrmont, 113; the Soolspring of Nenndorf, 93; Ragoczy, of Kissingen, 85; the sulphur spring near Doberan, 76; the Kreuzbrunnen of Marienbad, 66; the Kochbrunnen of Wiesbaden, 59 gr.

As regards the proportion of solid ingredients of sea water,—

The Mediterranean possesses in 10,000 parts	.	410 grains.
The English Channel	.	380 „
The North Sea near the Isle of Föhr .	.	345 „
„ near Norderney .	.	342 „
„ near Ritzebüttel .	.	312 „
The Baltic Sea near Apenrade .	.	216 „
„ near Kiel . .	.	200 „
„ near Doberan .	.	168 „
„ near Travemünde	.	176 „
„ near Zoppot .	.	76 „
„ near Carlshamm .	.	66 „

When evolutions of carbonic acid or sulphuretted hydrogen overspread whole regions, the common sources are partially impregnated with the gas. But then it escapes very readily, causing iron or other ingredients, previously kept in solution, to precipitate. Thus in the steel-spring of *Brüchenau* the carbonic acid adheres less to the water than is the case in the neighbouring spring of Wernarz: a bottle of the latter was filled and left open the whole night, and still a considerable quantity of carbonic acid was found in it next morning. Again, in the chalybeate of Schwalbach, the wine-well possesses the carbonic acid in a more adherent state than the so-called Stahl-brunnen (steel-well). The mineral water of Steben, in Bavaria, after having been kept three years in a well-corked bottle, was still clear, transparent, and without the least sediment. Some of the chalybeo-sulphurous water of Bocklet was exposed for twenty-four hours in an open vessel to the influence of atmospheric air, and still no oxide of iron was precipitated, and, when shaken, many gas bubbles were developed. Most of the Silesian and Glatzian acidulous springs have their carbonic acid but weakly adherent; and thus they would lose much of their character by being sent to a distance. (Niederlangenau and Obersalzbrunn appear to be excepted.) In the chalybeate of *Driburg* the gas adheres firmly. Pyrmont possesses a similar distinction. This is also the case in Selters-water, though the small quantity of iron it contains becomes easily precipitated. By a very intimate combination are further distinguished—Kissingen, Spa, Franzensbad, &c.

Even sulphuretted hydrogen, which is generally less firmly united with the water, on account of its lower specific gravity, varies as regards its adhesion in several springs. For this reason some powerful sulphurous waters have less sulphur precipitated, and cannot furnish, therefore, materials so appropriate for sulphur mud-baths, as weaker springs with more abundant precipitates.

If the hot mineral waters have lost their heat by exposure to the atmosphere, many of their combinations become disunited or deposited.

The best adapted for distant carriage are waters abounding in soluble fixed salts, and comparatively deficient in volatile ingredients; for instance—bitter waters, saline waters, &c. Though the constituents of most springs are of inorganic character, some, undoubtedly, possess organic substances.

If you find yourselves near the Sprudel of Carlsbad, you perceive the same smell as if you were near a kitchen where soup is being boiled.

The water of Wiesbaden tastes just like weak chicken broth, somewhat over-salted; and if you closed your eyes in drinking it, you might really fancy yourselves taking broth.

In cold springs the adhesion of carbonic acid becomes firmer, through cold, and thus its invigorating property is increased.

By a very high temperature, gaseous constituents are volatilised it is true, but the fixed ingredients are the more firmly united. From this reason, hot springs, though possessing weakening salts, are well assimilated, without irritating the digestive canal, or depressing the organism.

As in the constituents, I pointed out the difference between loose and thorough combination, so in temperature, we have to remark the peculiarity of the *inherent* heat of the springs. Many experiments have been made to compare it with heat artificially produced. It was generally thought, that the natural springs possess a greater capacity for caloric than the artificial ones heated to the same degree.

Some attempted to show, that heated waters, exposed to the atmosphere, lose their heat sooner than naturally hot springs. Others demonstrated the fallacy of these experiments, in which the same ingredients had not been added to the artificial water, as were contained in the natural. No difference was established in the time of cooling between the two, if each contained the same solutions.

Nevertheless we may assume that the caloric produced by

volcanic processes exerts a different influence on the human system than that which has been artificially produced.

It is true, if we observe the effect of a hot spring, we cannot well separate that part produced by temperature from that which the constituent particles may have contributed.

But, finding such strong efficacy in some thermal springs with scarcely any solid ingredients of importance, we are compelled to attribute a portion of their powers to the peculiar inherent caloricity, unattainable by artificial means.

The different physical perception is apparent. Let anyone take a common warm bath at Wildbad, and then bathe in the mineral spring, he will find a certain degree of languor after the former, and even during immersion he will not feel comfortable in staying longer than twenty or twenty-five minutes. How different will be his sensation when he lies on the warm sand in the thermal bath. No shadow of oppression is produced by the heat; on the contrary, he seems to breathe with greater freedom than before, and to become more cheerful the longer the immersion lasts.

We certainly cannot prove by analysis the different character of this caloric: but can we analyse the rays of the sun? and still we see their necessity in the growth of plants. Withdraw these rays, the most blooming and beautiful specimens of the vegetable creation wither and decay. You provide a substitute by the hothouse; but do ever these hothouse plants perfectly resemble the natural ones? They sometimes exhibit a finer appearance; but will they ever be equal in intrinsic value? Will they give out the same odour? will they last the same length of time? Moreover, some thermal waters can be drunk without inconvenience, whilst a common beverage of the same thermometrical heat could not be taken with impunity.

May not we also attribute some importance to the circumstance, that, in a common bath, the different layers of water can scarcely be expected to have all the same degree of heat? The lower strata will always possess a slightly diminished warmth compared with the upper. Besides, how can the water be made to retain the same heat during the stay of the bather? If, on entering, he found the temperature exactly suitable, it must be less so after a few minutes. If, notwithstanding these disadvantages, warm baths are such useful, nay indispensable, auxiliaries of medical treatment, what benefit may you not expect from the influence of this congenial warmth surrounding the body, in company with the involving iquid, gently stimulating the lymphatic and blood vessels to an increased function, promoting the exhaling power of the cutaneous pores, improving the secretions of the dermic follicles, soothing the morbid sensibility of the peripheric nervous ends, and imparting pliancy to rigid muscles?

The tendency of evaporating bodies to assume the gaseous form is called *tension*, and equals in power the pressure of one atmosphere at their boiling heat; viz. each liquid must be assumed to hold part of itself in a gaseous form, which escapes when absorbing greater heat. The expansive power of heat attenuates the circumambient air, and consequently diminishes its resistance and pressure. As soon, then, as the heat has been raised to such a degree that the impeding weight of the atmosphere has been sufficiently diminished, volatilisation takes place. According to the stronger or weaker tension, the boiling point will be at a lower or higher degree of heat under the same atmospheric pressure: for you are aware, in a vacuum where the air is exhausted, water is made to boil considerably below the usual boiling heat. Besides its own gas, water also has the power of binding permanent gases without evolution of latent heat; that is, without increase of temperature, and consequently there is no diminution of heat when the gas escapes.

This binding of permanent gases is called *solution*. It also depends on the quantity of water-vapour contained in the liquid. If you raise the temperature of the whole, the proportion of the absorbed foreign gases diminishes as the watery vapour increases, the expanding homogeneous gas filling out the atomic interstices, and thus-expelling the foreign gas. A strong barometric pressure can cause more gas to be absorbed, but always in the same proportions.

Thus, 100 volumes of pure non-aërated water absorb 253 volumes of sulphuretted hydrogen; 106 of carbonic acid; $6\frac{1}{2}$ of oxygen; 4 6-10ths of hydrogen; 4 2-10ths of nitrogen.

As one volume of nitrogen corresponds with twenty-five volumes of carbonic acid, water saturated with carbonic acid, and coming in contact with air, must expel twenty-five volumes of carbonic acid before it absorbs one volume of nitrogen; the acid escapes, therefore, the slower, the smaller its quantity is in the water; and when, already, other gases are dissolved in the water in their proper proportions. In consequence of this relation, water always absorbs comparatively more of the oxygen than of the nitrogen of the air, and whilst the proportion of the oxygen and nitrogen in the air is as 21 to 79, in water it is as 31 to 69.

The greater the specific gravity of the water, the less it is able to dissolve permanent gases.

For if solid bodies are kept in solution, the whole is smaller than the addition of both volumes. For instance, water in which $26\frac{1}{2}$ parts of salt are dissolved, should have a specific gravity of 1·150, if both volumes were simply added, but in reality it weighs 1·200 at 66° Fahrenheit. What may be the reason of this curious contraction? Ought we not to suppose, on the contrary, that the solid body entering into a liquid state, would occupy a greater space than formerly, rather helping to enlarge than to diminish the volume of the former liquid? The reason is, no doubt, the escape of latent heat out of the water to combine with the liquefied solid, by which means the watery atoms must contract. From the same cause, they offer less surface to permanent gases, which might otherwise be retained in the atomic interstices.

Many masses of lava and basalt contain carbonate of lime, which retains its carbonic acid when melted with other stones under strong pressure, but gives it up when coming to light freed from compression.

Chemical affinity also occasions sometimes its expulsion. Thus sulphuric acid forms gypsum out of carbonate of lime, and bitter salt out of the domite.

Those atmospheric springs which contain carbonic acid must have obtained it by the process of fermentation and vegetation in the external layers of the earth.

Now let us devote a few moments' consideration to the *medical effects of temperature*.

Our organism has not only to create the temperature of the blood, but an excess of warmth, as a regulator of the circumambient temperature, either to heat the surrounding colder media, or to transform the enclosed water into vapour, if the media approach or exceed our own heat. On this account we only feel at ease if we move in a lower temperature than that of our body. For though *perspiration* would relieve the system for some time of the excessive generated heat, if the atmosphere becomes too warm; the irritation of the peripheric nerves would ultimately extend to the central nervous system, and cause over-stimulation, giddiness, headaches, palpitation of the heart, fainting, &c., as results of the impeded escape of the regulating heat of our body. Clothes serve to prevent the too rapid escape of our internal caloric. The nature and form of the capillary vessels dispose them more to transmit animal heat to the exterior, than to spread external cold into the interior. Under the influence of a low temperature they contract their volume, condense their tissue, and close those openings of the secretory surfaces, in which the blood discharges part of its water in the form of liquid or gas. Thus, it requires the very highest degrees of cold to produce immediate paralysis of innervation and gangrenous congelation. In all minor degrees of cold, a reacting process takes place from the central nervous system, and induces increased heat on the surface, as soon as the refrigerating influence ceases. This reaction differs materially in various organisms. An epidermis frequently exposed to cold ablutions, for instance, possesses a stronger degree of nutrition, a denser tissue, and a steadier peripheric circulation, in vessels of larger calibre, than another in which reaction has seldom been evoked.

If the excess of animal heat is rapidly absorbed by evaporation, the blood accelerates its movement to supply the necessary quantity of liquid, and becomes more inclined to obstructions, by being partly deprived of its serum. When in this state the external temperature suddenly lowers, demanding as sudden a withdrawal of internal heat, the superficial nerves become irritated, and necessarily impart this irritation to the central organs, as the tide of circulation will flow more violently towards the interior.

The above will explain the great difference between the action of cold on a body heated by exercise, the cause of such manifold injuries, and the comparatively innocuous application of extreme cold on a person whose *epidermis* merely has been incited to increased heat in a quiescent position, as by vapour baths. The violently irritated exhaling vessels are somewhat soothed by the sudden cold, and the calm function of internal organs the less disposes them to participate in the effects of the sudden change, as the cold is not allowed to act long, if cold douche, for instance, be applied. For reaction from the interior takes place before the deprivation of heat can communicate lesion to the non-excited internal organs. The better a substance conducts heat, the sooner it withdraws our caloric, and the sooner it establishes an equilibrium. This circumstance causes metals to produce a sensation of more than thermometrical cold by contact.

The water having a much stronger conducting power than air, withdraws our heat much quicker. Hence, the temperature of the atmosphere, in which we feel at ease, would cause an intense sensation of cold if it were imparted to water, in which we are immersed.

The effects of baths on the epidermis are in accordance with the horny character of the latter. Heat extends and swells it, and renders it more pliable; cold contracts it, and makes it more rigid. The highest and lowest temperature make it impenetrable for the exhaling substances, and thus raise the cuticle in blisters.

The highest heat borne without injury is 113° Fahrenheit. The normal excess of caloric is not only prevented from further development, but a part of the hot medium is communicated to it; therefore, besides the local sensation of heat, general immoderate reaction ensues, circulation becomes increased, the central nervous system agitated, and arterial function heightened. By the softening of the horny substance, the excretory canals are contracted and closed at the external ends, and thus the subcutaneous watery vapour collects and causes tension of the epidermis, which becomes fragile in consequence, and desquamates sooner or later.

Such elevated temperature may be admissible in very few cases of general torpor, in fact when this external derivation is to be safely employed, to restore diminished cutaneous innervation. But great caution is requisite; for in such general torpor some internal organ is mostly in a state of irritation, forbidding the employment of such a violent remedy.

Hot mineral waters create a somewhat less sensation of heat, because part of the caloric is required to keep the dissolved ingredients in a liquid state. This is particularly the case in mudbaths and in the so-called earthy and sulphurous thermæ; less so in the alkaline or saline thermæ. In the latter, the irritation of heat is supplanted by the chemical stimulus of soda or chlorine.

Baths of a temperature between 77° and 100° Fahrenheit would not produce any influence on the temperature of the organism if the animal heat had not the function of furnishing a regulating excess to the surrounding media. In some individuals this excess is very small, and would be withdrawn by a bath of 95° Fahrenheit. In others, again, of more robust and plethoric habit, this heat would produce effects described as appertaining to baths of 100° to 113° Fahrenheit.

In the lukewarm and cool bath the absorption of internal heat must influence those organs which perform the function of calefaction. The amount of heat which each atom of water requires to put itself into equilibrium with the heat of the body, and the rising of the warmed layers from the surface of the body upwards must materially lower the amount of animal heat, and primarily depress the external innervation; but the consequent reaction induces a powerful impulse from the interior to the circumference, tending to an increased production of heat, and a heightened metamorphosis on the surface.

After a cold bath, the reaction produces such an excess of warmth as to guarantee a certain stability of external innervation and resistance to the changing temperature of the air. The epidermic redness produced by a cold bath certainly resembles the visible effect of a hot one. But whilst the consequence of a hot bath is reaction *to* the interior, commencing with congestive fulness of the eperdermis; in a cold bath, external redness and increased cutaneous circulation are the closing phenomena.

The cold bath will only be beneficial when its effects assume the type of fever—cold, warmth, increased secretions, &c.

Smaller quantities of water rapidly exchange their temperature for that of the blood. Moist bodies under thick covering stimulate the cutaneous system to a greatly increased serous secretion. They act like local vapour-baths, supplied by the body itself with the necessary heat. Such moist applications may be reckoned as powerful sudorifics, and prove beneficial in complaints produced by suppressed perspiration.

Vapours can be used in much higher temperature than water, being worse conductors, and possessing a smaller capacity for caloric. But why should they be better borne than air? Because they require a great amount of heat to be kept in the gaseous form, which is not the case with the permanent gaseous mixture composing our atmosphere. They are very useful where the liquefying process is to be heightened, where perspiration has to be promoted.

Careful experiments have shown beyond a doubt that, during the bath, water is absorbed by the body, while serous and other cutaneous excretions are dissolved and retained by the water. The continued action of the liquid exercises a peculiar stimulus on the sebaceous glands.

Inhaled vapours gently promote the flux of blood to the mucous membranes; but, being charged with moisture, they exert a relaxing and softening influence. Whilst, therefore, they would aggravate deeper affections of the pulmonary tissue, they are useful in passive chronic irritation of the mucous membrane of the lungs.

The greatest utility of the vapour-bath is shown in rheumatic paralysis, due to suppressed cutaneous function, when we require the smallest amount of local irritation with the highest degree of general evaporation.

The characteristic effect of *warmth in the digestive canal* is *pure stimulation* of the nerves of the alimentary tube, without secondary peculiarity.

After the application of this stimulus, circulation becomes slightly accelerated, the pulse fuller, perspiration and urinary secretion increased.

Sometimes a hot beverage causes over-stimulation, and in consequence antiperistaltic motion and obstruction. Generally, bile and gastric juice are caused to flow with greater abundance.

If internal organs are in a state of irritation, hot drinks are liable to produce violent hæmorrhage, plethora of the brain, headache, giddiness, or oppression of the chest, &c.

This congestion to vital organs may be prevented either by keeping off all external influences that might impart cold (for instance, by the patient remaining in bed to induce perspiration) or by gentle exercise. General circulation would be promoted, and act as a derivative from locally irritated tissues.

Cold water taken internally will prove highly useful, if acid gastric juice is secreted to excess, or if venous circulation be retarded by the extended blood-vessels, or if abnormal innervation occasions antiperistaltic motion (that is, vomiting).

As regards the mechanical effects of water, some lay stress on the increased pressure, water being much heavier than air. If a person stands in water up to his neck, the weight is considerably greater on the lower than on the upper part of his body, pressing the circulation upwards. Hence some people feel a sort of oppression when entering a bath. As a general rule, however, less importance is to be attached to this than to the movement of the water, either by suddenly falling on the patient as douches, or by steadily touching and receding from the bather, as occurs in the wavy motion of sea-baths, which are so eminently useful by inducing muscular re-action and counter-movement; vastly superior to any gymnastic contrivances, connected with violent exertion or agitation.

The muscles of the neck and chest being particularly exposed to this increased action, their organic innervation becomes strengthened, and with it the tone of the thoracic organs. Besides, it is the most valuable mode of accustoming ourselves to the evil consequences of atmospheric changes; and thus we may escape the numerous grave maladies produced in the unprepared by vicissitudes of temperature. On that account sea-baths are so eminently useful in preventing, to a great extent, development of tuberculosis and of other pulmonary diseases. Those that cannot go to the coast are recommended to sponge daily the face, throat, and upper part of the chest with hot water first, and then immediately with cold. This would greatly fortify the organism against the injuries arising from unfavourable skiey influences. According to the late Dr. James Johnson, one of the most talented physicians, this process has been successfully applied to young children, to ward off threatening consumption.

The douche acts through its violent shock, according to its height, as a more or less exciting local agent. The shower-bath produces a sort of titillation of the peripheric nerves, and diminishes excessive nervous sensibility.

With reference to the *imbibition of the constituents*, we must bear in mind that organic cells and tissues have sometimes more attraction for one combination than for another, and thus counteract the purely chemical influence.

Some constituents of the mineral waters no doubt possess a restorative power, supplying substances requisite for the proper performance of organic functions; others cause chemical action by displacing particles without undergoing changes themselves. Most spas possess, therefore, the character of *alteratives*.

I shall now bring to your notice the classification adopted by Vetter, who divides all the mineral waters into two large classes, viz. *Akratopegæ* (from a negativum, κρατος power, and πηγη spring), such springs which have as it were powerless constituents, notwithstanding their noted efficacy, and *Synkratopegæ* (from συν with, κρατος power, and πηγη spring), such mineral waters in which the power of the constituents to a certain measure corresponds with the observed effect.

We shall first occupy ourselves with the waters belonging to the former class, also called 'chemically indifferent.' They are clear, tasteless, and generally inodorous (sometimes possessing a slight smell of sulphuretted hydrogen), of nearly the same specific gravity as water, containing in sixteen ounces less than five grains of solid ingredients, and not above the tenth part of the quantity of gas which would correspond to their tension. The constituents are not such as exhibit strong effect in small quantities.

These are subdivided into:—

Akratothermæ, chemically pure thermal springs, as Gastein, Landeck, Pfeffers, Teplitz, Warmbrunn, Wildbad, &c.

Akratokrenæ, chemically pure cold springs.

The *akratopegæ* arise out of primitive mountains or such as are composed of little soluble fossils; they are alkaline or earthy, deficient in gas, with the exception of nitrogen or sulphuretted hydrogen. The more water approaches chemical purity, the greater is its latent heat; therefore they may stimulate more than common baths of the same temperature. Their power of solving animal evaporation and of entering the peripheric vessels is likewise greater. They are particularly useful, where earthy formations are deposited in tissues from a deficient power of excretion, or from diminished circulation. On this account they are especially adapted to old age, by strengthening the innervation, and diminishing the rigidity and weakness of the limbs.

LECTURE IV.

WILDBAD.

To proceed to Wildbad, in Würtemberg, lat. N. 49°, long. E. 8°, we have first to reach Mayence, which we can do from London in twenty-eight hours, thence the railroad takes us through Heidelberg to *Pforzheim* (in 6¼ hours). From here a three-hours' diligence ride through a most beautiful part of the Black Forest brings us to our place of destination.

The road from Baden-Baden, about thirty English miles distant, is highly picturesque. After having enjoyed the views of the surrounding peaks from the acclivities you have to mount, you will descend a winding road to the town of Gernsbach, in the valley of the Murg; you then ascend to the village of Laffenau; the path winds downwards again to Herrenalb, encircled by majestic mountains. Turning to your left, you perceive curious groups of basaltic rocks, with the appearance of a fortress. Ascending, you reach a plateau, which continues for six or seven miles, and offers extensive prospects towards the north-west. After passing a deep wood, you descend to the town of Neuenburg, on the Enz. From here you ascend for eight miles on the right bank of the river, and you will find yourselves in the valley of Wildbad, about 1,300 feet above the level of the sea, whilst the mountains reach on each side the height of 1,500 feet. The fall of the Enz during this short distance is 370 feet. You see the course of the river to be from south to north, consequently the spa is exposed to these two winds, while it enjoys mountainous protection at the east and west.

Cold naturally prevails in its climate, the summits of the mountains being covered by snow from November till May. The heat is correspondingly great in June, July, and August. I need not tell you, as regards Wildbad, that the road from Baden-Baden is nearer still, if you walk through the fields and valleys straight eastward, as is often done by the inhabitants of the environs. The town of Wildbad lies eleven leagues* (thirty-three miles) to the west of Stuttgart, and has about 1,800 inhabitants. Karlsruhe lies at a distance of nine leagues to the north, Calw four leagues to the east, Pforzheim six leagues to the north-east. The wild and picturesque character of the environs is well worthy of admiration. An early walk along the river Enz, which rushes with violence through the spa, led to the following notes in my journal, which I beg leave to quote: 'I cannot imagine anything more romantic and delightful—though shallow and narrow, the river foams and hisses, so that one might suppose oneself near the seashore. On both sides rise the mountains, covered with beautiful fir and pine-trees, of every variety of green. Particularly charming appear the rays of the sun, when they begin to force their way over the peaks of the eastern mountain to gild the yellow waves of the furious little river.' By reason of the almost perpendicular acclivity of the enclosing mountains, the beneficent influence of the sun is obtained an hour later from the east, and departs an hour sooner in the west, than on the surrounding localities. The spa enjoys the reputation of great antiquity; and in the beginning of the sixteenth century its curative powers were already extolled. A remarkable charter was given to the place by Charles V.; viz. 'that all criminals, with the exception of murderers and highway robbers, should enjoy here peace and liberty for a year and a day.' The surrounding mountains consist of ferruginous red sandstone and granite. The springs flow out of cleft granite rocks in four divisions from north to south, forming several independent basins. They vary in temperature from 88° to 99° Fahrenheit. The largest bathing space, also enclosing the warmest springs, is called 'Herrenbad' (gentlemen's bath). On the left we observe a niche, which reaches to a considerable distance into the wall, and is called the 'Hölle,' being the hottest spot, out of which the chief source originates. The basin is separated by boards from another bathing space, called 'Bürgerbad' (citizens' bath). Then there is a space called 'Fürstenbad' (princes' bath); and another called 'Frauenbad' (ladies' bath). The bottom of the baths is covered with sand; and it excites extremely pleasurable sensations to move along on the warm

---

* League, the German 'Stund,' or hour, signifies such a distance as might be walked in an hour; it corresponds to about three English miles. A geographical German mile is rather less than two leagues or 'Stunden,' and equal to about five English miles.

sand, and dig it up with the fingers, causing bubbles of gas to rise to the surface. The temperature of the water being identical with that of blood, neither heating nor cooling is required to adapt it for use. This circumstance must be considered as highly advantageous. Another point of great importance is the constant influx and efflux of the same water, with unvaried temperature and constituents. This would be positively unobtainable by any artificial contrivance. You see the water bubbling up from several holes in the sand, exhibiting a greater heat than the more distant parts. You may thus consider that the natural stimulus of this congenial warmth, instead of acting continuously on the organism, rather divides itself into repeated and constantly renewed stimulating forces. The extent of the basins allowing muscular movement, compensates in some measure for the disadvantages of bathing in common (with separation of sexes) which is generally practised here. The water is let off every night, the sides are cleaned, and the sand is levelled. Before commencing the course, the visitor is enjoined to take a common warm bath. According to the susceptibility and complaint of the patient, the warmer and cooler baths are chosen. A peculiar feeling of comfort and general ease spreads over the bather. Refreshed and invigorated he will certainly feel on leaving the bath, with increased cheerfulness and desire for exercise. After a certain number of baths, however, a sort of reaction sometimes appears, ushered in by lassitude, depression, headache, general languor, loss of appetite, frequent feeling of chilliness, with subsequent heat and other signs of feverish disturbance. Pains of rheumatism, gout, or of wounds, sometimes momentarily reappear, after having been dormant for a long period. These ought not to discourage the sufferer; on the contrary, they are signs of a peculiar power exercised on the affected organs. The apparent systemic counteraction only shows the efficiency of the spa. With properly regulated precautions the course can be continued as soon as the signs of febrile reaction, or bath eruption, have passed away. On the other hand, this must not be looked for as an indispensable condition of cure. Patients sometimes are gradually relieved or cured of obstinate chronic diseases without these rebellious symptoms. This chiefly depends on individual idiosyncrasy. I can conceive the baths benefiting one individual by the titillating contact with the sentient extremities of the nerves, stimulating the cutaneous function, and indirectly promoting the secreting power of vascular and sero-fibrous organs, by which effete and stagnant deposits may be carried off to make room for healthier products, whilst in another this effect is not produced till the vascular system has been put into a more or less violent commotion, whereby a new abnormal state has been created, to serve as a desirable crisis. In case the water should be entirely inappropriate, of course, Nature will give us distinct signs of her ungracious reception of the remedy, and these must not be disregarded on any account.

The constituents of the spring are, in sixteen ounces:—

Chloride of sodium	. . . . . .	1·82
Carbonate of soda	. . . . . .	0·53
,, lime	. . . . . .	0·34
,, magnesia	. . . . .	0·07
,, iron	. . . . . .	0·02
,, manganese	. . . . .	0·02
Sulphate of soda	. . . . . .	0·40
,, potash	. . . . . .	0·02
Silex	. . . .	0·39
	Total . . .	3·61

The gas dissolved in the water contains, in 100 parts:—

12½ carbonic acid.   79¼ nitrogen.   8¼ oxygen.

The gas evolved from the water, however, consists, in 100 parts, of—

2·00 carbonic acid.   91·56 nitrogen.   6·54 oxygen.

Formerly the baths only were employed; but since 1836, a drinking spring has been discovered, which is also made use of, and greatly assists the efficiency of the external treatment. Its constituents, to the amount of 4¼ grains in sixteen ounces, resemble very much the former, with, however, a little more silex, carbonate of lime, and carbonate of soda. The water is perfectly clear, tasteless, and of 1·004 specific gravity. What does then produce these beneficial changes to which I have already alluded? Some have ascribed all efficacy to the inherent caloric, which is supposed to bear greater analogy to our blood than the same temperature artificially produced. It is obvious that the chemical purity imparts to the water a more solvent power on animal exhalations. It may enter the peripheric vessels more easily and cause absorption and excretion of earthy deposits which had previously been stagnant from a deficient plasticity, as so often happens in real and premature old age. To all the 'akratic' spas, the common property of 'Verjüngen' (youth-restoring) is attributed. Some explain the diminished rigidity of the limbs by the kind of soap that may be formed between the alkalies contained in the water, and the oleaginous evaporation of the epidermis. This imaginary soap rinses the ends of the excretory dermic follicles; and freeing the system of effete animal matter, it communicates a stimulus to organic metamorphosis.

Admitting a more unrestrained entrance of the water into the peripheric vessels, we may assume that the small quantity of ingredients being constantly renewed and in motion, the power of penetrating to the assimilative organs must increase with the quantity of water brought in contact with the body. Have we not a right to believe that more chloride of sodium, for instance, is imbibed by a person exposed to the action of this water for a certain time (though less than two grains are contained in sixteen ounces), than by another individual who bathes for the same length of time in water with 400 grains of the same salt in sixteen ounces?

The latter liquid being considerably denser than pure water, of course penetrates with more difficulty. In fact, the beneficial results produced by such water are more sought in the stimulus exercised by the irritating power of the particles, than by their actual combination with the organic fluids. This view will also explain the reason why those springs standing between the akratic and synkratic are the least powerful. They are not diluted enough to enter the absorbent vessels, nor are the constituents sufficiently strong to produce the stimulating effect of the more highly charged waters. I have then a right to attribute part of the utility of Wildbad to the chloride of sodium it contains, whilst I need not be refuted by the minor efficacy of the neighbouring Baden-Baden, which contains a greater amount of the same ingredient.

All along, I have endeavoured to impress the conviction on your minds, that we must not merely look on the quantity of ingredients, but on their more or less intimate combination or intrinsic adherence to the water, and particularly on the manner of their reception by our organism.

Do we not meet this difference daily in common life? We call many an individual ill-fed, though the most substantial diet may regularly be introduced into his stomach; while another, with the healthiest appearance, probably consumes much less nutriment. Even in the very same individual the same food produces a different impression and different digestive results, according to the *period* of ingestion. And it is often less important what a person takes within the twenty-four hours, than at what time.

For instance, I have frequently convinced myself, and particularly during the prevalence of cholera, that substantial food is more easily dissolved and assimilated if ingested four or five hours after a light breakfast—that is, in the middle of the day—than towards the close of the ordinary time of business. The reason is obvious. After you have quite shaken off the fettering weight of slumber, and roused fresh action by a warm stimulating drink, body and mind feel the greatest vigour, which increases towards the end of the morning; in the afternoon, retrogression of animal power takes place; towards the evening you feel incapacitated from performing considerable mental or bodily labour, independent of the work carried on during the day. Then, I ask, is it possible that, whilst all organs open to our perception appear exhausted and debilitated, the stomach, our most hard-working servant, should contract with the same vigour, and excrete gastric juice of the same strength and solvent power, as it would have done at an earlier period? Reason says it is impossible, and daily facts prove the impossibility. I have frequently asked *commercial* gentlemen, who merely take a biscuit in the middle of the day, whether they would feel distressed by waiting for their evening dinner half an hour or an hour later than usual? The answer is invariably in the negative. The craving for the ordinary meal, felt by early diners, if they have to wait beyond their ordinary time, is quite unknown to the former. Is not this the best proof of the want of nature being strongest at that particular period, because she is then most able to perform digestion? Moreover, the want of an evening meal is considerably stronger after a substantial mid-day dinner, than after a mere appetite-deluding biscuit, because in the latter instance, the stomach has become too much weakened for energetic action. I must also mention, that I have found malt liquor to have a much better effect on digestion with the mid-day than with the evening meal. With dyspeptic persons the latter meal is better digested without malt liquor; for the concentrated and stronger gastric juice of the early part of the day bears dilution, and is, perhaps, benefited by it, whilst the weaker juice, a product of exhausted digestive organs, is impeded in its function by a greater dilution. If, from all the above, it is perfectly clear that such a great assimilative difference is produced in the same individual, without reference to the ingested quantity, I have a greater right partly to refer the differing results of the various spas to modified assimilation of their constituents.

Every bathing space has a depth of water of one foot eight inches. Smooth stones are placed in several parts, to enable the bather to sit in a greater or smaller depth of water. Narrow basins adjoin the larger spaces for a small number of persons, or for single baths. The rooms for dressing are conveniently arranged and warm. The action of the water stimulates the vascular, while it calms and strengthens the nervous system. The function of the absorbent vessels increases, secretions are promoted, and the nerves rendered more active. The uterine nervous system is very favourably influenced by the water. The chief indications are *gout, rheumatism, arthritic paralysis, and contractions from wounds.* Unfortunately—or shall I say fortunately?—these very diseases are likewise cured by the other three akratic spas, viz. Pfäfers, Gastein, and Teplitz; some by the halotherma of Wiesbaden; and the difficult question is therefore as yet generally undecided, what forms of the above-named diseases are especially claimed by each spa? I may as well tell you, that till now these four spas have been used almost indiscriminately for the same diseases, and the choice was often more due to accident or local acquaintance than to any difference of properties. You will find arthritic, rheumatic, paralytic, and traumatic patients at each of them; and still there are great differences in their properties and corresponding differences of effects. To arrive at a satisfactory solution of this problem, I made the chief task of my journey last year. It was painful to witness, at every watering-place, individuals who were cured of their complaints by the spas, but who constantly declaimed against their medical advisers for not having chosen this place in the first instance, instead of having previously sent them to several others, where they had found no relief. Geheimerath *Dr. Fricker* recommends Wildbad in rheumatism, after the acute stage has passed, in gout with concretions, in neuralgic pains, in chronic diseases of the uropoietic system, as cramps, vesical hæmorrhoids, in retained and enclosed foreign substances, in contractions and stiffness produced by scars, in paralysis resulting from apoplexy, in hysteria and retarded menstruation. The water, taken internally, is said to promote the action of the liver and kidneys, and gently to increase alvine evacuation. *Dr. Schweickle* found the spa particularly efficacious, also, in atonic ulcers of the legs, in induration of the mammary glands, in hemiplegia after typhoid fevers, &c.

Now, I do not doubt that these diseases may have been cured under the influence of Wildbad; but the question with us must be, 'In what derangements does it afford us the *best chance* of a cure among all the other spas?' Dr. *Fallati*, whom I mention as last, but certainly not least, considers Wildbad very beneficial in such forms of *gout* and *rheumatism*, in which digestion is not impaired (should dyspepsia be present, the disease will, according to him, get worse); also in such paralysis, gout, and contractions after wounds, as are connected with considerable deposits and swelling; in fact, *whenever absorption is to be produced*. The spa is particularly useful when the disease has shown previous tendency to amelioration. In hysteria, and diseases of the bones, he also finds it beneficial. In chlorosis and ulcers he would not recommend it. There is one point almost invariably remarked by the patients, as if by mutual agreement, viz. *that their limbs become more flexible*. Wildbad should therefore be chosen for such cases of *arthritic paralysis* as are based on *articular swellings* or other material cause, when increased absorption forms the chief indication. Dr. Fallati finds the efficacy increase in a direct ratio with the length of stay in the bath; this would strengthen the view of remedial imbibition helping towards the favourable result. I must not forget to mention the beautiful contrivance at Wildbad, by which the patients are let down by machinery from their rooms to the baths without requiring any stairs (it resembles that constructed in the Colosseum). On the ground-floor their chairs are rolled on a sort of wooden railroad to the respective baths. Paralytic and otherwise disabled persons form the greatest number of invalids.

Wildbad is *contra-indicated* in plethora, tendency to congestion, to apoplexy, to active hæmorrhages, in inflammation, internal ulceration, in fever, &c.—in fact, whenever acute disease demands a prompter treatment.

There is an establishment of whey at the place, which is, in many instances, advantageously employed.

Allow me to draw your attention for a moment to the gaseous contents of Wildbad. You perceive no glairine nor baregine amongst the solid constituents, but is not there a certain substitute to be sought in the great quantity of *nitrogen* present? No importance is generally attached to the circumstance, because, forsooth, we live in and constantly inhale azote. How, then, can we expect medicinal results from such an ordinary substance? But how different is the effect of the element when entering the lungs as a mere emollient and companion of oxygen, returning unchanged and unabsorbed to the external world as soon as it has safely delivered the indispensable vivifying agent, oxygen, to the circulating fluid; how different, I say, from its ingestion into the alimentary canal, where it furnishes an indispensable agent for the maintenance of life!

It is true, the gas is only known from its negative properties. But ought we not to seek in it some great and powerful connexion with vitality, if we find its combination with hydrogen to be the most stimulating, reviving, and reanimating substance that can possibly be taken (viz., ammonia NH_3)?

Whilst oxygen is necessary to keep the organic machinery in motion and to circulate vital caloric through all our tissues, forming, as it were, the oil of our living flame, azote is, on the other hand, equally indispensable to restore wasted tissues and fluids. Without the former we should suffocate; without the latter, starve. I should not go so far as to attribute a nourishing property to the azote introduced into the absorbent vessels with the highly diluted water; but when it is admitted that our tissues constantly discharge effete matter from our cutaneous pores in a gaseous form, would it not be reasonable to attribute some restorative function to the contact and combination of the gas with organic particles? We know that, in old age, earthy or inorganic formations prevail in the reproductive sphere. Limbs become more rigid, the joints less pliable, secretions retarded, excretions diminished, vital elasticity and resisting power impaired. Substances ordinarily carried rapidly along the vascular canals in a dissolved state, are now precipitated out of the slowly moving mass, and deposited in spaces where they further impede voluntary movement.

If we see the use of a mineral water, causing distinct retrogression of these anti-vital phenomena; if we perceive gouty concretions to proceed towards absorption; if we observe contracted limbs gradually to try feeble efforts of long-forgotten exercise; if we find cutaneous harshness and rigidity to diminish, and to give way to a former softness; if we behold a resuscitated desire for muscular exertion and for mental work in a prostrate individual, and we know the spa, the originator of these changes, to possess a great quantity of azote, is it not legitimate to attribute to this gas some part of the efficacy?

Whilst the chloride of sodium exercises its well-known beneficial influence on organic metamorphosis, stimulating digestion by forming hydrochloric acid on the one hand, and combining with albumen as soda on the other, counteracting earthy formations, azote may powerfully assist this process, and contribute towards the curative changes.

A highly respected physician of Munich, the late Dr. Öttinger, who visited Wildbad last year, and who, of course, could have no interest in propagating its fame, expressed himself in these enthusiastic terms:—

'*Wildbad*: *July* 1850.—The first month of the season has already passed, and furnished very happy results. Prince T—— could only walk with difficulty on sticks, and was oppressed by physical and mental suffering; now, cheerful and restored, he departs with grateful recollections out of the healing valley of the Enz.

'Many other visitors exchange their crutches for sticks, and walk about without further support. Several persons, bent down by spinal suffering, are daily enabled to approach more the erect posture. Paralytics, who had been unable to leave their beds for years, descend after three or four weeks' course from their garden-chairs, and try the former habitual step with a satisfactory result. But Wildbad must not be thought as affording exclusive aid to the disabled. Deeply-seated internal diseases sometimes are checked here, and become retrogressive, or cured. An emaciated person with impaired digestion, through a gastric ulcer, increases in corpulence and is able to perform digestion after a four weeks' course. Another required the daily application of a catheter for two years, in consequence of an arthritic affection of the bladder, and after the sixth bath he can already dispense with that assistance.

'We have personally witnessed these results, and received confirmation out of the mouths of the respective visitors. The fair sex is very numerously represented here, seeking and finding relief from their Protean nervous complaints. 1,000 guests may be accommodated at a time. The apartments are good; some very elegant; the arrangements for bathing excellent in every respect. The douche is extremely well understood, and managed with highly satisfactory results. Few thermæ offer the complex advantages of a water with the most appropriate temperature, analogous to that of blood, receiving the bather immediately in the bubbling sources, without conducting pipes, without the artificial aid of heat or cold, and thus without volatilisation of its gaseous constituents. Wildbad has been too little appreciated by physicians. The unfortunate term 'indifferent' therma, seems to have served as a privilege to cease exploring either its chemical ingredients or its comprehensive and energetic medicinal efficacy.

'Though no more salts are contained in this therma than in common drinking water, this very circumstance might serve to cause a more intense penetration into the organic tissues. The fact that retrogression of disease and even cure have ensued in incipient spinal softening, in gastric ulcers, in swelling of the uterus and ovaries, in chronic catarrh of the larynx and trachea, &c., justifies the above assertion.

'When larger sums have been devoted to the scientific examination of its imponderable gaseous constituents, and particularly of nitrogen, the most powerful agent of this therma, the spa will be properly appreciated and more frequently recommended. This year's season will be a brilliant one : as a non-resident and unprejudiced observer, I do not think I make too bold a prediction if I prognosticate for Wildbad, that, by the aid of further progress in science and medicine, the period will come when this therma will receive a more determined and well-defined position among therapeutic agents. Then it will not merely be resorted to in such internal diseases as resist pharmaceutical remedies, or where clear indications are wanting. This spring, bubbling out of numerous holes, will then no more be designated as 'indifferent,' but as decidedly and sovereignly efficacious.'

A case of paralysis of the lower extremities, produced by a severe delivery, came under my notice, which was completely cured at Wildbad during the season. Another case was reported to me of a horse-dealer, who was squeezed between two waggons, and lost 'the use of his legs' in consequence. He also found a complete cure in the healing source of Wildbad. I have to add, that the accommodation afforded by the little town of the Black Forest does not reach the luxurious scale maintained at some other more brilliant spas. But real invalids, merely seeking the restoration of their health, will meet here* with every requisite convenience and comfort, at comparatively moderate charges. Physicians:— Dr. Burckhard, Dr. Hausmann, Dr. Fallati, Dr. Schönleber, Dr. Gruel.

* Hotel Bellevue.

LECTURE V.

PFÄFERS.

HAVING left Wildbad at half-past nine A.M., the *diligence* arrived at Stuttgardt in eight hours. The road, as far as Calw, is extremely interesting; it rises constantly, lined on both sides with charming forests. The carriage passes for some time along the brink of a ravine (separated from the high road by stones), down which the timid can scarcely look without a shudder. From Calw to Stuttgardt the prospect becomes more ordinary. The railroad being now open between Pforzheim and Stuttgardt, travellers may return to the former place, and then proceed by rail. From Stuttgardt the rail takes us to *Canstadt* (about four English miles distant), situated on the right bank of the Neckar, which here becomes navigable. The town contains upwards of 4,000 inhabitants, and is connected with Stuttgardt by a handsome park, through which a carriage-road passes. On the 'Wiesenplan,' in the south-eastern part of the town, a rural festival is celebrated every year, on the 28th of September, which is visited by an immense concourse of the surrounding countrypeople. The environs abound in petrifactions. The elevation of Canstadt above the level of the sea is 600 feet. The climate is mild, the environs fertile and well-cultivated, abounding in wine and fruit, and are called by some 'the garden of Suabia.' The mineral springs originate from a ferruginous lime-tufa, superposed by strata of clay and slate. They belong to the class of *saline chalybeates*.

The temperature is 66° to 68° summer and winter. The water is clear, sparkling, and has a saltish piquant taste. That of the *Sulzerainquelle* tastes more agreeably than the others, and exhibits 'Sprudel' properties, its supply increasing and diminishing periodically. It contains about 39 grains of solid constituents in 16 ounces—viz., $17\frac{1}{2}$ of chloride of sodium, $\frac{1}{2}$ grain of chloride of magnesium, 10 grains of sulphate of lime, 2 of sulphate of soda, $\frac{1}{8}$th of sulphate of magnesia, $\frac{1}{3}$rd of sulphate of potash, nearly 6 of carbonate of lime, 1 of carbonate of magnesia, less than $\frac{1}{10}$th of carbonate of iron, carbonic acid gas 21 cubic inches; temperature, 62° F. The other springs are very similarly constituted. The 'Wiesenquelle' contains $\frac{1}{4}$th of a grain of iron. Besides the above, I will merely mention ' *Die obere Sulz*,' a small pond, occupying about a quarter of an acre, and formed by several confluent springs. The surface is constantly covered by gas-bubbles arising out of the depth, and consisting of carbnic acid and nitrogen; temperature, 68° F. The water deposits a great deal of mud, and seems to be in constant motion. Its amount of carbonate of iron is $\frac{1}{4}$th of a grain. There is an ascending douche, very advantageously employed in catarrhal affections of the vagina and rectum; also a whey establishment. The water is considered as tonic and solvent. The celebrated *orthopœdic* institution of Dr. Heine is well worthy a visit. It is built near the 'Frösnerische Bad.' In the 'obere Sulz,' near the gardens of the establishment, the patients are enabled by certain contrivances to bathe in the pond at a temperature of 68° to 70° F.; artificial waves are produced by wheels, to increase the stimulating and tonic effects of the baths. Mud, douche, rain, and shower baths are likewise administered. I would further allude to *Dr. Veiel's* establishment for herpetic diseases, which annually increases in reputation, and in which artificial baths and river baths, with strong afflux, are used with considerable advantage. But I have given these details merely on account of the importance to be attached to Canstadt, from its neighbourhood to the great spa we have just left. If you proceed from Stuttgardt by railroad at eight in the morning, without stopping, south-east as far as Ulm, on the Danube, and then pursue a due southern course, slightly bending westward, you reach Friedrichshafen, on the *Bodensee* (Lake of Constance), in 7½ hours—that is, at half-past three P.M. The steamboat waiting for the trains starts half an hour afterwards, as soon as it has received the passengers and cargo destined to cross the 'Bodensee.' I find in my journal the following remarks:—

'The view on the lake is most delightful, and particularly striking. Whilst hitherto the various modifications of forests, hills, and mountains exhibited their beautiful trees and luxuriant foliage, here nature displays charms of a different kind. The lake presents a green surface, gently moved by slight undulations. On the sides, masses of snow are perceived with the naked eye, covering the peaks of the glaciers in the midst of summer. The gentle movements of the vessel cause a rather agreeable sensation, and do not prevent writing on the open deck in this charming weather. But in storms the boats are said to be tossed about, as if shaken by sea-waves. The Würtemberg railroad appears extremely well managed. It not only forwards the hurrying passengers with considerable speed, but actually encourages traffic by the pleasure it communicates. Every seat affords as much comfort as can possibly be accumulated without identification with the next higher one. The greatest punctuality is observed in starting and arriving. The carriages of the second and third class are so contrived as to give them the appearance of a company assembled on rows of benches in a drawing-room, with an open passage in the centre for the officers and travellers. If, while sitting at one end, you see an acquaintance at the other, nothing prevents you walking up and sitting by him while the carriage is in motion. At every station the name and exact time of stopping is called out. As soon as the train begins to move again, an officer walks through the passage and asks for the tickets of those who have to leave at the next station. Not only is a saving of time thus effected, but the possibility of travellers passing their place of destination is obviated. The great civility of every officer, not only to those of the first class, but to the humblest passenger, is too well known to be dwelt upon.'

I beg forgiveness for this digression; but it is such an important subject for spa visitors, that I could not resist expatiating on its conveniences, with the lurking hope that the simple contrivances of the Continent might perhaps find introduction here.

The steamboat lands the passengers on the opposite shore at *Rorschach* in about an hour and a half. From here the railroad completes the journey in about three hours to Ragaz, which lies at the foot of Pfäfers. You arrive at the post-office, hotel, and bath-house, which are all comprised in one building. The place is comparatively new; the baths are supplied from the chief spring of Pfäfers, and resemble the latter in every respect but temperature, which is here 93° to 95° F. The view on both sides of the house is very pleasant, though not to be compared with that of PFÄFERS itself, to reach which you ascend a winding rugged path along the rapid *Tamina*. On both sides rocky mountains rise almost perpendicularly to a height of 600 feet. The view is most romantic, but becomes truly sublime when, arrived at *Pfäfers*, you pursue the Tamina along the narrow wooden path erected between the rocks, and leading *to the three sources* from which all the baths are supplied. To quote from my journal:—' The rocks here are not only perpendicular, but actually bend towards each other, scarcely admitting the rays of the sun, and presenting cracks, fissures, and promontories, which fill the wanderer with awe. Treading cautiously along, and admiring this wonderful greatness of God's creation, which raises such an insignificant little rivulet into a powerful roaring mass, we entered the enclosure of the chief source after about ten minutes, and found it filled with vapour. By means of a light, after a few minutes we could perceive objects in the disappearing darkness, and we gazed down the cleft whence the steaming fluid issued. Bathed in violent perspiration, we ascended with care and a considerable degree of danger, eight or ten irregular steps, to examine the second and third sources, though these two are not used for the baths, and run down the precipice into the Tamina.'

Pfäfers, lat. N. 47, long. E. 10 (Favières, Fabariæ aquæ), is situated in the canton of St. Gallen, in Switzerland. The Lake of Wallenstedt lies to the north-west, and the town of Chur (Coire) to the south-east. The principal road leads from Ragaz, up a considerable acclivity, and then again by a steep descent into the valley, through the village of Valens. This road is about five miles in length, and is generally chosen for descending, whilst the path described above is more than two miles shorter, and usually serves to bring the visitors to the place. The necessaries of life are partly brought to it by the former road, and partly drawn into the bath by cranes from the high rocky wall of the convent, to which the place formerly belonged.

The walks are obviously limited; they are terraces spirally ascending over each other, and leading to greater and greater heights. At a short distance, however, charming walks may be found by ascending the former convent and wandering through its environs. The Galanda, the Valens Mountains, with the so-called Grauhörner (grey horns), rise to upwards of 7,000 feet, and offer the most variegated tints and contrasts of forests and rocks, of mountain-meadows and snow-fields, of woods and plains, furnishing an *ensemble* of the most sublime and picturesque character.

The rocks from which the springs originate are composed of black limestone, interspersed with veins of white fluor-spar. Formerly the bath-house stood in the grotto of the chief spring. It was erected on beams that were driven into the rocks overhanging the yawning abyss. The patients were let down with cords from the heights of the surrounding cliffs, for a week's course.

Now, human industry has provided a more convenient approach to this remarkable spa, hidden at a height of more than 2,000 feet above the level of the sea, at the foot of the Galanda.

The river Tamina separates Hof-Ragaz from the village of Ragaz, where two high roads meet.

You see the route from the Zurich and Wallenstedt Lake, as well as that from the Lake of Constance, leading through Ragaz and Chur towards Italy.

If you take a survey of the valley at Hof-Ragaz, you perceive on your right the little town of Mayenfeld, the Luciensteig (summit), with the towering Falknis; on the left, the woody declivities extending to the small town of Sargans (north of the spa), over which the Gonzen, the Allvier, and the Kuhfirsten rise, while the youthful Rhine winds through the extensive plain.

Having ascended for about an hour, and reached the convent and village of Pfäfers, you see the mountain-valley extending southward to the Kunkels pass and the Kalfeus valley. To the west rise the Valens Alps, with their ragged summits; to the south-east, the proud Galanda. Near the village of Vättis, the Tamina valley assumes a more westerly direction towards the declivity of the high Ringel, and extends to the *Scheibe*, which rises to a height of 10,000 feet, and forms the centre of the cantons Glarus, St. Gallen, and Graubünden. From the Scheibe the Sardonen glaciers descend into the Kalfeus valley; and from these the Tamina rushes down and flows for about twenty-five miles, fed on both sides by frequent waterfalls. In one of its most awful depths, the thermal healing spring comes to light, and is conducted to a somewhat more open and lighter spot on the other side of the river to the bath buildings, erected on the rocks, and confined by the foaming Tamina on one side, and by the steep overhanging declivity on the other.

The walk to the spring is now less dangerous than formerly, having been provided with balustrades and somewhat enlarged. You start from the drinking saloon, and pass over the Tamina bridge, through a rocky vault, till you reach a little closed gate.

If you take a survey here, you perceive on the right the overhanging rocks; on the left, dark mountain masses covered with the light foliage of marble and beech trees; at your feet, the hissing Tamina; and in the foreground, the bath establishment. In the background is the perspective of the widened gap, sparely illuminated by peeping rays of the sun. On boards, supported by beams, which are wedged into the rocks in a surprising manner, you walk a distance of 1,500 feet. The side rocks are 200 feet high, and at the part where they approach each other, reach 290 feet. The light gradually assumes grayer tints; the moisture and coolness perceived, as you advance, further increase the gloominess of the scene. Under that part where the rocks almost unite, a remarkable marble grotto is pointed out, 35 feet broad and 34 feet high. It lies on the left of the Tamina, and was built some hundred years ago for devotional purposes. After this the rocks open again, and you soon approach the vapour-cave, where the chief spring issues out of clefts in a grotto hewn in the rocks.

Fissures of the Kalfeus Mountains, over the crest of which the Tamina rushes, are probably filled by water from the mountain heights of Galanda. Being closed in winter, they receive no more influx, and therefore cease to supply the spring. The water contained in the subterranean canals then sinks deeper, and the veins of the upper springs begin to vanish, the lowest springs flowing the longest.

The baths are not floored here with sand, but formed in separate basins paved with marble, the water constantly running in and out. Cooling is performed by opening doors and windows and turning the cock off, from which the water runs. The natural temperature of 29° 97′ R. (about $98\frac{1}{2}°$ F.) is lowered according to circumstances to 97°, 95° or 93° F., Persons, particularly of the environs, sometimes remain for hours in the baths, even of the higher temperature, with very favourable results.

The water of Ragaz has lost 1° of Reaumur ($2\frac{1}{4}°$ of F.) by its journey from Pfäfers: all the other arrangements are analogous with the parent spa. The *douche ascendante* is employed with great advantage to assist the course. Though the diminished heat cannot make a difference—for, as I mentioned above, the baths are generally taken at an equally low temperature in both places—I must not conceal from you the fact that Pfäfers, with all its inconveniences and limitations, stands in higher reputation with the profession and the public than the pleasant and commodious Ragaz, which lies about 600 feet lower, but offers the same water to the valetudinarian.

What then is the hidden influence residing in the parent baths, and failing in the filial branch? Ragaz lies about 400 feet higher than Wildbad, and still it is thought of inferior efficacy, while Pfäfers is maintained by many to surpass the spa of the Black

Forest in power. Let us well consider the facts before us, and endeavour to extract a theory from them. It is a remarkable coincidence in the three chief akratic spas—viz. Wildbad, Pfäfers, and Gastein—that the locality of each is confined, and the air consequently impeded in its circulation. But there is another coincidence—viz. in each of the three a violent and foaming mountain torrent rushes through the spa with great fury. A third coincidence consists between the two latter—that of having a new establishment at a more convenient lower locality, receiving the same spring at a diminished temperature. And there is this fourth similarity, that the parent establishments are positively pronounced of considerably greater efficacy.

You will often hear in the common walks of life, even in this stupendous London, that the individuals who have enjoyed for years excellent health, in the circumscribed space of the city, for instance, have found their health impaired after they had exchanged their 'unhealthy' quarter for a more salubrious residence. Such complaints I am occasionally destined to hear myself, after my advice of choosing the open suburbs for habitation has been followed. How is this? Can we not reckon on increased vitality and lengthened life, if we flee from all the injurious exhalations and other deteriorating influences produced by congregated crowds of human beings? Do we not feel more cheerful and more vigorous as soon as we begin to breathe the purer air of the charming fields that a kind Providence spreads out for our use? Physiology promises greater vitality; our sensations confirm the promise; and still, how can we reconcile these contradictory facts? Though, as a general rule, we might continue to advise healthy persons to seek a freer habitation, circumstances must occur in which the latter is actually more injurious. Does nature wish us to inhale as much oxygen as possible? If so, she would not present to our respiratory organs one part of this respirable gas with four parts of the involving irrespirable nitrogen. What do we see in animals that inhale pure oxygen? They live more intensely; all their functions are heightened; but, as an unavoidable consequence, the organs lose sooner the blessing of life. In the same way, with many persons country residence may cause greater vitality, and more intense organic action; but the question is, does not the stronger exertion lead to a quicker exhaustion? I would not receive as an objection the longevity of farmers, who have spent their whole lives in this bracing and pure atmosphere. But we all know how injurious strong contrasts are to health; and the most zealous advocate of temperance will not advise an habitual indulger in spirits to deprive himself suddenly of the usual beverage. If, then, a person has for a long series of years performed the respiratory function under the emollient action of confined space, he will not, without danger, suddenly imbibe the pure but more exciting gaseous mixture. Many a dormant morbid diathesis may and does develope itself into disease; and there is no doubt that many a life would have been prolonged by remaining in a less open situation. A case just occurs to my mind, of a gentleman who has the misfortune of an organic impediment to respiration in a bent spine. For some years he resided at Clapham, and always suffered with a more or less violent catarrhal affection of the lungs. I advised him to remove to the city, near his place of business. For about ten months past he has lived in an airy and commodious house in the same street in which he has to transact business during the day, and he feels himself positively healthier, and his thoracic organs stronger. Some influence is, no doubt, also to be ascribed to his more regular mode of living now. Of course, stagnant waters or other injurious evaporations are hurtful to the immediate neighbourhood. From the above, I wish to conclude that the very limitation of the locality may act healingly in some measure. What patients have we before us? Mostly those in whom nervous power is diminished, perhaps of certain parts only. Vicious metamorphic action has taken place. Substances which should remain dissolved in the circulating liquid, have been separated and deposited in the joints; whilst others that ought to have been secreted, have been retained. Before desiring a stronger vital action to proceed from the circulating organs, by which oxydation and abnormal deposits might increase, we may wish to limit the oxydising function, and to leave freer scope to the penetrating warm liquid from without, for rousing the torpid and weakened peripheric nerves. When this is accomplished, bracing atmospheric influence will be useful in carrying to a successful issue the commenced curative process. The inconvenience that might possibly result from the greater pressure or confinement of the air, may find a certain corrective in the violent fall of the respective rivers, which, through the vigour of their movements, attract atmospheric impurities with more energy, and impart more freshness to the circumambient air, than they would without this rapidity.

The chief indication for Pfäfers is *real nervous paralysis*, through wounds or apoplexy; or *paralytic gout, not based on articular swelling*: the power of the peripheric nervous system is distinctly raised by the spa, and more so than at Wildbad, though, at the latter, absorption and resolution of swellings is better performed.

The temperature of the chief spring is 30° Reaumur (100° Fahrenheit); the deepest spring has $30\frac{1}{2}°$ Reaumur at its issue; the water is clear, tasteless, and inodorous. Sp. grav., 10·003; a small quantity of bath-glue is found, of a yellowish colour, and unctuous to the touch.

Analysis shows $2\frac{1}{2}$ grs. of solid ingredients in sixteen ounces, viz.:—

Carbonate of Magnesia	.	0·87	.	about 4-5ths
„ Lime	.	0·32	.	„ 1-3rd
Sulphate of Soda	.	0·02	.	„ 3-5ths
„ Lime	.	0·37	.	„ 1-3rd
Chloride of Sodium	.	0·21	.	„ 1-5th
„ Magnesium	.	0·16	.	„ 1-5th
Total	.	2·55, with a very minute quantity of iron.		
Gaseous contents:—Oxygen	.	.	.	1·3 cubic inch
Nitrogen	.	.	.	3·7 „
Carbonic acid	.	.	4·15 „	

The bath-glue is composed of silex, carbonate of lime and magnesia, of argilla, and of oxide of iron. Internally and externally the water has a stimulating, solvent, and, at the same time, strengthening and anti-spasmodic effect on the peripheric nervous, and on the vascular system, counteracting venosity of the portal system, and therefore removing obstructions. In spasms, paralysis, and neuralgia, a marked sedative power is exhibited.

Paracelsus, who visited the spa about 300 years ago, expresses himself thus on its caloric:—' You are aware that heat may have a various entity in itself. The heat of the sun is one, that of dung is another; a different heat, again, is that of burning wood, but much is wrought here by the innate warmth, that may be familiarly compared with human nature. What great things are performed by congenial heat is shown by the hens brooding their young ones with it, also as silkworms are bred by such warmth. Thus knowing that such an incorporated heat exists here, Pfäfers would surpass analogous *simplicia*, in which the warmth does not exist.'

Hufeland says of Pfäfers:—' Of all thermal springs, Pfäfers, in Switzerland, contains the smallest quantity of perceptible ingredients. The water tastes and smells like common water, and, nevertheless, it exhibits an efficacy which surpasses the most powerful spas. In this very year a striking instance has occurred to me. A man who has long been affected with hypochondriasis and retarded alvine evacuations, and who had used alternately several spas without effect, even requiring other remedies to strengthen the efficacy, went last year (1825) to Pfäfers; and scarcely had he used the waters two days, when every morning alvine evacuation regularly ensued after drinking a few glasses. His bodily and mental condition visibly improved, and he felt a freedom and mobility in his whole being unknown to him for many years; and, notwithstanding his sojourn in a deep mountain fissure, which only admits light for a few hours a day, he experienced constant alacrity and cheerfulness.'

The spa showed itself efficacious, according to Dr. Kaiser, in dyspepsia, flatulence, acidity and mucosity of the stomach, especially in *gastric cramps*, through repression of piles, of exanthemata or of gout, in habitual diarrhœa, or obstruction in abdominal plethora, &c.

Next, in diseases of the nervous system : hypochondriasis and hysteria, if based on suppressed action of the ganglionic system. If the organs below the diaphragm are impeded in their oxydation and decarbonisation by arterial blood, to the disturbance of the vegetative nervous sphere, the diluted warm liquid penetrates to them, and induces a more vigorous transformation, and subsequently a restoration of the previous equilibrium.

Metastatic gout, particularly in nervous, irritable subjects, and neuralgic pains of the face, are relieved here; also abnormal catamenial flow becomes regulated, &c. &c.

But, as I stated above, the chief reputation of the spa is in *paralysis*, contractions, and local weakness from wounds; but there must be no residue of apoplexia or congestion to the brain, else the spa would be injurious. The paralysed part must not be too emaciated, nor quite insensible, else the so-called 'Ausbade kur' might be required, which consists in persons remaining longer and longer in the baths every day, till several hours' stay, for a consecutive series of days, has produced violent reaction.

Dr. Kaiser, jun., showed me a very interesting case of a young man, twenty-one years of age, who was precipitated about twelve years ago from a hay-waggon, on his head, and the load itself pushed upon him. He became unconscious. A concussion of the cervical vertebræ appeared to have taken place; still he could perform light work for a year with no other morbid phenomena than a stiff neck. After the lapse of this period his right hand began to become paralysed, and some time afterwards the right leg. The left arm and left leg followed in succession; so that, for several years, he was neither able to sit nor stand; urine also was discharged involuntarily, and stool could be promoted only by the strongest purgatives. Artificial sulphur baths and strychnine had been employed without advantage. In this state he arrived, on August 3, 1840, in the establishment for indigent patients at Pfäfers. He had to be carried into the bath, and held there by an assistant. Nevertheless, he received two baths daily, so that he used fifty within a month. At the same time, he drank thermal water *ad libitum*. Improvement was inconsiderable; only the fingers could be moved a little more easily; the digestion showed slight amelioration, the general nutrition being strengthened by wine and substantial diet. Soon after the course a bath eruption showed itself, when he had arrived at his home, and, from this critical phenomenon, marked retrogression of his evil began to show itself. In January 1841 he could move hands and feet, and felt more sensibility in his whole body. In May, he could walk about in the room with two assistants. From June 5th, he repeated a four weeks' course, with frequent douches, on the cervical and dorsal vertebræ. On the 18th day of the course he could walk alone with a stick before the 'Curhaus.' He left the establishment, with the direction to return after a month's repose, and repeat the course. This was done from the 13th of August. In the summer of 1842, he availed himself again of Pfäfers, and continued to do so in successive years, getting gradually, but steadily, better. To-day he can walk perfectly well, without the assistance even of a stick. I examined the patient myself, and the manner in which he described his gradual progress, how he could use one limb and then another, and how he began to sit without assistance, leaves no doubt that his cure from *traumatic paralysis*, in consequence of pressure or lesion of the spine, is solely due to Pfäfers.

The so-called youth-restoring property is attributed to the spa in a high degree. Individuals of eighty years of age, suffering from *marasmus*, are said to have been considerably strengthened and refreshed by the course. Pfäfers is *injurious* in real plethora, in congestion to the head or brain, in active hæmorrhage, in phthisis, in diseases of decomposition (as dropsy), in internal suppuration, in general emaciation, &c.

The constituents being less even than in Wildbad—only $2\frac{1}{2}$ grains in 16 ounces—of course no influence is attributed to their action. But whilst the knowledge of our materia medica would not justify me in choosing these few grains of magnesia, lime, and soda, with carbonic, sulphuric, and hydrochloric acids, for certain diseases presented to me, I feel it, on the other hand, my duty to seek a rational explanation of facts recorded and acknowledged for several hundred years.

If these pure thermal springs *merely* acted through their inherent caloric, then why should there be such a great difference in the species of diseases cured at each? Examine the facts to which I have directed your attention. Whilst in most diseases claiming cure at Wildbad, absorption of effete and stagnant deposits is chiefly carried on, corresponding with the solvent power of chloride of sodium, and assisted by the imbibition of nitrogen (counteracting the prevalent inorganic earthy formation), you see here the chief ingredient to be *carbonate of magnesia and of lime,* with *sulphate of soda.* Taken internally, in great quantities, and brought into a very lengthened contact with the cutaneous pores externally, the magnesia might not be imbibed in a sufficient amount to exert its antacid properties, but it may exert a greatly sedative influence on the nervous system in conjunction with the gently stimulating warm fluid, which rouses the peripheric nervous ends to renewed function.

The lime may partly assist this anti-spasmodic action, and partly enter into combination with the weakened osseous system, allowing a greater degree of exertion, and imparting more stability to the articular movements.

The sulphate of soda may assist in gently promoting the intestinal function, and act as a sort of derivative from the affected nervous system. Join with this the influence of the peculiar atmospheric character incidental to the locality, and we may conceive how this *ensemble* has produced the changes brought to our notice. This view is confirmed by the great utility of the water in the form of clysters in obstinate alvine obstruction, abdominal infarcta, suppressed hæmorrhoids, &c.; also by its great utility, if merely taken internally, in very irritable digestive organs.

An hour is the general length of a bath, and the course usually comprises twenty-one. Persons bathe here separately, in single baignoires, or in larger ones in common with several other persons. After the bath, the invalid generally lies down for a quarter of an hour. The water is conducted by pipes into the bath-vault, and constantly flows into each baignoire. As soon as a certain height is raised, it flows out again. The temperature of the baths in Pfäfers, uncooled, is about $29°$ Reaumur$=97\frac{1}{4}°$

Fahrenheit; in Ragaz, 27° to 28° Reaumur=$92\frac{3}{4}$° to 95° Fahrenheit.

Every evening the water is let off, and the baignoires are cleaned. Some vapour is perceived in the bath-rooms when cold air enters at the opening of the doors, but this is not so perceptible to the bather himself. Where a greater quantity of water flows into the basin, the vapour appears more concentrated, and is employed as a natural vapour-bath with very favourable results.

The tubes out of which the water is discharged serve as weak douches on different parts of the body. But there are besides douches in separate rooms, fitted at a height of twelve feet, and falling down as rain, stream, or drop douches.

What is called *ausbaden* (out-bathing), formerly much in vogue here, consists in enforcing bath-eruption by very prolonged bathing, and is connected with such dangerous processes as to be now nearly abandoned. The bathing was gradually extended to eight or nine hours per day, so that the patient had merely to alternate between his bed and the bath. Between the fifth and ninth day, feverish chill appeared as the precursor of the bath-eruption, which soon followed (between the twelfth and fourteenth day). Bathing was still continued, and prolonged till disappearance of the eruption commenced, when the time of bathing was gradually diminished to the end of the course. Four weeks was its usual duration. The eruption mostly exhibited the miliary character; sometimes mere swelling of hands and feet took place. The paralysed parts were often first affected by the eruption.

Whilst using the bath, the diet should be appropriate to the remedial influence, and the clothing warm. As after-cure, no chalybeate spring nor other tonic treatment ought to be employed, for in the spa the cure is often merely instituted; fresh action may be only awakened, and the salutary crisis may not appear before weeks or months have passed. Beware, then, of disturbing the resumed efforts of nature, unless urged by important morbid phenomena!

Often, however, the so-called ' Trauben-cur ' (grape-cure) is allowed to follow the course with great benefit. The cooling and solvent properties of the grape diminish the irritability of the vascular system, promote retarded secretions of the vegetative sphere, increase bilification and portal circulation, and thus counteract hæmorrhoidal tendency, or otherwise congestive influences.

I ought not to omit mentioning that here, as in nearly all German spas, provision is made to give the foreign and inland poor gratuitous accommodation and treatment, with some necessary regulations and restrictions. In many spas there are even funds to pay the travelling expenses of indigent invalids.

Before concluding, I shall quote a few lines from my journal referring to another subject not devoid of interest for the medical student:—

'Returning from Pfäfers, down to Ragaz, about halfway, a small bridge leads over the Tamina, and then a narrow zigzag footpath winds up to the top of the almost perpendicular mountain on the right of the Tamina. Several times I was obliged to stop for want of breath. When at last arrived at the summit, a wide prospect opened before my eyes. The only footpath appearing to the traveller leads to an ancient convent, transformed into *a county asylum for lunatics*, under the able direction of Dr. Ellinger. His method of treating the patients, though I only observed it for a short period, filled me with admiration. It seemed to consist in two principles—viz. causing the patients to occupy their time by various suitable contrivances, and *speaking with them as if they were perfectly sane*. This latter point is extremely difficult to perform, though apparently easy. For instance, if a patient wishes or utters anything obscure, he neither contradicts it, nor tacitly agrees to it, nor does what is occasionally done by well-disposed physicians—viz. speaks with them as one does vith spoiled children. He enters into conversation with them, and treats the subjects broached as if uttered by sane persons. Of about 150 patients he had under his care for three years, forty were cured, many without any medicine. All his patients seemed deeply attached to him, and readily obeyed him, without murmur or hesitation. Restraint is very rarely resorted to, and only after the failure of all other means. The height of the establishment is 2,700 feet above the level of the sea; and of Ragaz, 1,600 feet. All the arrangements of the establishment I found most appropriate, and the prospects open to the eye on all sides delightful, with a great variety of walks in different directions.'

Physician of Pfäfers, Dr. Dorman; of Ragaz,* Dr. Kaiser.

* Excellent accommodation in the Hôtel Hof Ragaz.

LECTURE VI.

GASTEIN.

To proceed to *Gastein*, the shortest route would be to travel directly east until you approach the Alpine Spa, if it were possible to find a beaten path or road leading through all the inaccessible passes and mountains which separate the two akratic thermæ. You must, therefore, retrace your steps to Rorschach. Thence the steamboat will carry you promptly to the Bavarian town of Lindau. The railroad will continue the journey from here, and take you in a north-easterly direction through Kempten, Kaufbeuern, and Augsburg to Munich, on the Isar. The considerable distance noted on the map shrinks into insignificance as soon as you see these blessed iron links connecting the two spots.

From *Munich*, the eilwagen started formerly every afternoon. Now the railroad performs the journey of thirty-five leagues in four hours and a quarter, the train arriving at *Salzburg*, on the Salzach, the following morning, in time for the Gastein diligence. In passing through *Rosenheim* you might see the celebrated saltworks, with an extensive prospect of the environs. Thence you arrive at the beautiful village of Prien, and might cross the interesting *Chiemsee* (four leagues long) in a steamboat. On the lake a very picturesque view is offered of the romantic ruins of Hohenaschau, of the Kompenberge, and of the high Hochgern (rising to 6,000 feet). You start then for *Traunstein*, on the Traun, also provided with salt-works; thence you might leave the rail and pass through Teisendorf to Reichenhall, on the Saalach, the centre and connecting point of four large salt-mines. The brine is conducted from here by subterranean pipes to Traunstein in the north, and to Rosenheim in the north-west, whilst the place receives the brine from the southern mines of Berchtesgaden. The salt-works are greatly admired by the visitors.

The *Grabenbach* (ditch-river) is particularly worthy of notice. It is a deep subterranean canal, built of brickwork, and destined to receive such sources of the brine as contain too small a quantity of salt. The curious arc carried in boats as far as the river. Though the Ferdinandsberg of Berchtesgaden lies 160 feet higher than Reichenhall, the salt-works had to be artificially raised by water-columns to a height of 179 feet more, in order to fall to Reichenhall; wooden and iron pipes extend to upwards of 100,000 feet between the two 'Salinen.' The brine arises here at a depth of fifty feet, and is pumped up by machinery. One part contains such an abundance of salt, that it is immediately transmitted to the boiling-pans without previous graduation. A most charming road leads from this place through the Ramsau to Berchtesgaden (seven leagues south of Salzburg). You pass between high and interesting mountain-walls to the *Taubensee,* and soon afterwards to the village of Ramsau. The valley now enlarges, and the road passes the 'Illsangmühle,' where Reichenbach's celebrated water-lifting machines are seen, which raise the saturated brine by hydraulic pressure, in pipes 3,500 feet long and 1,200 feet high. A league and a half further you reach the charming and picturesque *Berchtesgaden,* with an antique chateau, annually visited by the King of Bavaria. The salt-works here possess great interest. In the little chateau of Adelheim, you may inspect the 'Klausnerische' collection of ivory and wood-cut wares of Berchtesgaden. The most magnificent views are furnished by the 'König-see,' (King's Lake), south of Berchtesgaden. The encircling high cliffs impart to the whole a solemn grandeur. The water is dark-green, but appears quite black near the shore, through the over-hanging rocks. At the end of the lake a smiling meadow suddenly opens to your view, with a hunting-castle at the foot of the towering Watzmann (9,000 feet high). With a powerful telescope you can perceive the chamois leaping among the glaciers. Good pedestrians may easily wander from here to the 'Eiscapelle,' the lowest glacier in existence. The 'Schreinbach,' falling into the 'König-see' at the southern extremity, with its white foam, forms a curious contrast with the dark water of the lake.

During the presence of the Court, grand stag and chamois hunts take place upon the lake, the animals being driven into the water from the neighbouring mountains. A short walk towards the north brings you to Salzburg. I dwell with greater length and emphasis on this journey than on others, because it forcibly struck me as I proceeded, that such varieties of scenery, such contrasts of atmospheric influences, acting on the senses and faculties of the traveller, must exert a positively healing action in many derangements of physical and mental functions. I defy the hypochondriac to think of his manifold and magnified sorrows when beholding these wonders of creation! The nutrition of the whole frame must become improved, and react tonically on the mind; and thus this cyclus of cause and effect eradicates many an inveterate functional disorder. I do think that travelling certain routes should be advised in many instances, merely for the sake of the journey itself. I transcribe the following from my journal:—' The beautiful town of Salzburg lies in the centre of the so-called " Salzkammer gut" (salt-chamber domain), bounded on three sides by mountains, and divided into two parts by the rapid Salzach, which is crossed by a large bridge. The town contains 15,000 inhabitants, and lies in a valley between the Mönchsberg and Capucinerberg, from which you enjoy magnificent views of the environs. The " Festung" (fortress) of Hohensalzburg lies on a commanding position overlooking the whole town. If you take a survey of the town from that eminence, it appears more charming than it really is. I next visited " Aigen," beautiful and park-like, full of grottoes, waterfalls, rocks, and labyrinths. A spot is pointed out here by the guide as the favourite resort of his Majesty King Louis of Bavaria, who is certainly an excellent judge of picturesque scenery, for it becomes difficult to satiate your sight with the alternating heights and valleys, glaciers and castles, that arrest the eye from different points. Amongst the numerous curiosities of Salzburg, well worthy of inspection, I was particularly struck by the cemetery of St. Petri and its antiquarian monuments; by the interesting gate hewn through the rocks, with the proud inscription, " Te saxa loquentur," &c.* But, however imposing and romantic the views at a distance, the streets are narrow, and many of the houses apparently damp and close, though the place is alleged to be very healthy. Of the great purity and salubrity of the air in the environs there cannot be the slightest doubt. At seven A.M. I took my place in the diligence, and passed through Hallein, Golling, Werfen, St. Johann, Lend, to Hofgastein (where we arrived at half-past eight P.M.) — and Wildbadgastein (at half-past ten P.M.), about thirty-two leagues in fifteen hours and a half. The road, particularly after Golling, is magnificent beyond description. It is more like a fairyland than a reality, particularly the " Lueger-pass," where a small path leads upwards to the " Öfen † der Salzach,"—certainly the most magnificent view

---

* The rocks will speak of thee.
† So called because the Salzach breaks through oven-like rocks.

that the imagination can conceive. It is the perfection of picturesque scenery. The spot which struck me as most admirable is where the Salzach-bridge stands surrounded on all sides by the mountains, as if the world were locked off beyond, and all further passage prevented. And if you now think your admiration has reached the highest point, and that greater natural beauty cannot exist, pass on further, and you will find how mistaken you were in this belief. Rocks, mountains, valleys, verdant fields, and deep ravines perpetually diversify the scene; while the Salzach, coquettishly winding every now and then across your path, and forcing you to cross and recross her silvery current, contributes to render the whole scene so charming and heart-expanding, that none can forbear blessing his Creator, and pouring out his overflowing gratitude!'

Gastein, lat. N. 47°, long. E. 13°.—The valley of Gastein is intersected in its whole length (for eleven leagues) by the rapid *Ache*, which rushes down from the height of 270 feet in the middle of Wildbad, forming a most beautiful waterfall. On the north, a fine prospect opens towards the whole lower valley; whilst on the east and west, mighty columns of primary rocks are perceived, the Tisch, Gamsgarkogl, Thronegg, Graukogl; towards the south, the high plain of Böckstein. The spa lies 3,200 feet above the level of the sea; its filial establishment, *Hofgastein*, nearly 2,700 feet, thus 500 feet lower. The highest peak of the Gastein Mountains reaches an altitude of from 8,000 to 10,000 feet.

The mean annual temperature is 47¾° F.—that of the summer, 56¾° to 59°, being rather lower than in many other spas. Nevertheless, the climate is more bracing than bleak, for the northern storms, as well as the pluvial west and north-west winds, are kept off by the semicircular guard of the surrounding mountains. The easterly winds are partially checked in their violence by passing over the Arleck and the mountains of the Kotschach valley. Even the sirocco from the south, which has such a depressing influence on the nervous system, and mostly appears in spring and autumn, is deprived of its violence by the towering chain, and partly of its heat by the ice and snow-fields of the environs. West-south-west wind is the most frequent. The heat of the summer is rarely oppressive, rapid alpine torrents and neighbouring woods imparting freshness to the atmosphere. The temperature is occasionally subject to sudden changes in the height of summer. If any tempest discharges itself in the mountains above, rain and cold ensue in the valley as a consequence, with a cloudy appearance of the atmosphere. This becomes sometimes more perceptible through the evaporation of the glaciers, after very great heat—as, for instance, when the thermometer has risen to 77° and 86° F. The spring exhibits fewer changes, and is more adapted for courses of the water than is generally supposed. The natural alpine spring-water, colder in summer and warmer in winter than the atmosphere, is considered so advantageous from its excellence and purity, as to be often made use of medicinally in cases of indigestion arising from a weak condition of the intestinal mucous membrane. The barometric pressure is diminished by more than 3 inches (24" 5'''). Thus, if the whole weight of the atmosphere borne by one individual is equal to 28,000 pounds, one inch corresponding to about 1,000 pounds, a diminution of more than 3,000 pounds exists in Gastein. The atmosphere is consequently lighter, and (as it is asserted) more charged with positive electricity. The influence of light is also supposed to be more enlivening and stimulating by passing through a more attenuated aerial medium. It is assumed that alpine heights promote pulmonary circulation and decarbonisation of the blood, and thus diminish the quantity of venous blood.

From the above reasons, you see the animal and vegetable kingdoms develop greater strength and vitality in these heights than in the lower regions. The beneficial atmospheric influence is particularly felt by persons coming from flat countries, from the shores of the North and Baltic Seas, &c. An unusual ease spreads over the whole organism; respiration is more easily performed; the walk is erect, with a certain lightness and elasticity of movement. An instinctive desire for muscular exercise helps to increase the general effect, and induces keener appetite and sounder sleep. The want of a certain amount of oxygen induces deeper inspirations than in low localities, where the compressed air contains a greater quantity in a smaller volume. Patients with weak thoracic organs feel in such heights at first a certain oppression; they have a sensation as if they could not obtain a sufficient quantum of air. This, however, enforces a gradually increased expansion of the chest and deeper inspirations; tubercular diathesis is so greatly counteracted by Kreuth, because the greater dilatation of the pulmonary cells mechanically prevents deposits in the interstitial tissue.

The venous blood being allowed freer reflux by the promoted circulation, obstruction of the portal system is diminished. The intestinal canal exhibits greater tone. Exhalation proceeds with more activity. General nutrition must therefore improve. On the other hand, in confirmed phthisis, or congestion of the brain, or internal inflammation, alpine air must be injurious. The increased pulmonary action increases a speedier exhaustion of the lungs, whilst the stimulated arterialisation heightens the inflammatory symptoms.

The spa has been in repute for centuries. Its annals state that 'more than 400 years ago (A.D. 1436), the Emperor Frederic the Third used it for an open sore in his thigh, and left it completely cured.' The bath hospital, for indigent patients, was founded nearly 400 years ago. Paracelsus said of Gastein, more than 300 years ago—' It opens scars, cures paralysis, dispels contractions and gravel.'

Baths are erected in every house destined for the accommodation of the visitors, with a reservoir of thermal water, possessing the requisite temperature for bathing. The 'Badschloss,' Straubinger, &c., possess large baignoires for persons bathing in greater numbers. The more modern buildings, however, possess merely separate baths, as spaciously and conveniently constructed as possible, so that the patient can move about and be in constant contact with a great amount of thermal water.

Apparatus for douche, shower, and rain baths are attached to all these localities.

Wildbadgastein offers several shady walks to the visitors. Excursions to the Bellevue, or the 'Russian Coffee-house,' furnish fine prospects of the immediate neighbourhood.

Active pedestrians will be well rewarded for walking to the Castle of Hunsdorf, with the charming prospect of the Graukogl, Gamsgarkogl, a glacier lying between the two (the Tischlerkaar), and the Ankogl. Others wander to the neighbouring mines of Böckstein, celebrated for the gold-washing performed there. The 'Schweizerhaus' (Swiss-house), situated between Wildbad and Hofgastein, collects visitors wishing to combine enjoyment of fine scenery with social amusement and rest. In the neighbourhood is also to be found the 'English Coffee-house,' with a fine view of the valley, besides 'Badbrück or Patschge haus,' with its pretty pond of trout. For further excursions, the Anger Kotschach and Anlauf Valley are chosen.

If unfavourable weather prevents outdoor exercise, the guests avail themselves of the beautiful 'Wandelbahn' (walking path), upwards of 400 feet long and 20 feet wide, where you can not only walk about at your leisure, but enjoy charming prospects.

At certain hours of the day music heightens the pleasure of muscular exercise.

The character of the mountain-passes is primitive. The healing springs originate from gneiss, at the foot of the mighty Graukogl, on both sides of the Ache. Towards the elevated southern Böckstein, granite formation appears; whilst towards the northern valley, near Badbrück, mica-slate is found, characterising the Gamsgarkogl and neighbouring mountains. The declivities of the mountain-masses, at the east and west of Wildbadgastein, are superposed by strata of primary rocks, while the deeper valley of Hofgastein is partly covered by the rocks of the surrounding mountains, and partly by alluvial conglomerations. These primitive mountains formerly concealed numerous minerals in their womb, particularly gold, which was obtained to a considerable amount; but now the gold-washing is performed less for profit than to satisfy the curiosity of the visitors.

The order in which the sources arise are—1. The highest, *Fürstenquelle*, 37° Reaumur = $115\frac{1}{4}$° F., furnishing 16,000 cubic feet of water in twenty-four hours, and supplying the baths of the Archduke Johann, those of Straubinger, of the Prälatur, Solitude, &c.

2. The *Doctorsquelle*, lower and more northerly, 36° Reaumur = 113° F. About 3,000 cubic feet of water are furnished daily, and conducted by forcing-pumps into the Badeschloss.

3. The *Schröpfbad*, or Chirurgenquelle,* still more northerly; temperature 36° Reaumur = 113° F. The daily quantity of water is below 4,000 cubic feet, and supplies the baths of the surgeon.

4. *Hauptquelle* (*chief source*), the lowest, but at the same time the most abundant. A new enclosure of brickwork leads to its issue. The temperature of the bubbling spring is $38\frac{1}{2}$° R. = $118\frac{1}{2}$° F.; its daily quantity 100,000 cubic feet. It supplies the baths of Mitterwirth, Krämer, Bath-hospital, and the filial establishment of Hofgastein. The vapours evolved from the water are conducted into a separate locality, and used as vapour-baths.

There is besides, on the right bank of the Ache, the *Ferdinandsquelle*, with 106° F.; then the *Wasserfallquelle*, with 95° F.; and on the left shore of the Ache, the *Grabenbächerquelle*, with 97° F. The water is clear, inodorous, and tasteless. Specific grav. 1.004. It is composed of—

    1·51 sulphate of soda ($1\frac{1}{2}$ gr.),
    0·36 chloride of sodium (about one-third),

* Cupping-bath, or surgeon's spring.

0·36 carbonate of lime (about one-third),
0·05 carbonate of iron (one-twentieth gr.),
0·24 silex (about one-fourth gr.),
with a small quantity of sulphate of potash, carbonate of soda, of magnesia, and *glairine*, amounting together to 2·73 grains in 16 ounces. 100 parts of the gas contained in the water consist of 3·8 carbonic acid, 29·0 oxygen, and 65·1 nitrogen; 100 parts of water contain 0·18 of carbonic acid, 0·90 of oxygen, and 2·02 of nitrogen. Its power of conducting electricity was compared with that of distilled water, and led to the following results:—

1. Distilled water of the temperature of 14·1° Reaumur, caused the needle of the galvanometer to diverge to $3\frac{1}{2}°$.

2. Gastein water, kept nineteen days in an open bottle, with a temperature of 14·4 Reaumur, induced a divergence of 29°.

3. Fresh spa water of 24·4° Reaumur made the needle diverge to 36°, whilst

4. Distilled water warmed to the same heat caused a divergence of 6° only.

The above-mentioned Gastein water, which had been cooled to 14·3°, being heated likewise to 24·4° Reaumur, the divergence of the needle was 36°.

From the above and many other experiments, it is inferred that the water possesses a greater degree of electro-motor power than well or distilled water, as a combined result of its alkaline constituents and heat.

It is thought that owing to the spa water being heated in an enclosed space, beyond atmospheric influence, and without formation of vapour, the warmth penetrates all the particles more uniformly, touching each separately as it were. In water, however, heated by artificial fire, and exposed to atmospheric influence, the warmth is spread by the circulation of the watery particles themselves, so that the calefacient power does not so uniformly act on each atom.

The fact of oxygen possessing magnetic power, lately established by Faraday, may also assist in explaining the great importance of a high position. The same *savant* has proved, that not only heat, but carbonic acid, and other gases, diminish or destroy this magnetic power. Thus we may consider, that in low situations, the protective magnetic force of oxygen is counteracted, both by the warmth of the circumambient animal exhalations, and by the exhaled gaseous bodies. The diminished magnetic tension may then give greater scope and freedom to the development of miasmatic impurities in the atmosphere, which react again in their turn on the living beings from whom they had originally emanated.

Though the temperature of the chief source is only $118\frac{1}{2}°$ F., a sufficiency of vapour is evolved for use. From each layer, as it rises, issues a quantity of steam, whilst in boiling water only the superficial layer develops steam, and must constantly be supplanted by a deeper layer rising from the bottom.

A whitish-grey gelatinous substance, gradually assuming a denser tissue, is observed at the bottom and sides of the effluxes, forming the Gastein bath-mud (*ulva thermalis*).

To the supposition that climatic influences alone produce the observed changes, it is objected that the inhabitants of Gastein are often affected with the fever of reaction when using the baths, whilst this is never observed when bathing in the well-water of St. Wolfgang, warmed to 95° F., in the neighbouring Fusch-valley, which lies 800 feet higher than Gastein. The above analysis shows sulphate of soda to be the chief constituent, with a small quantity of chloride of sodium and carbonate of lime. You have to bear in mind, that the constant renewal of the water, together with the great quantity provided for each bath, may cause a proportionally greater absorption of the ingredients.

The baignoires are four or five feet deep, and hold from 150 to upwards of 300 cubic feet of water (that is, from 8,500 to 17,000 pounds). They consequently contain from three to six pounds of sulphate of soda and other mineral substances. These constituents being presented to the absorbent vessels in such a highly diluted condition, are fit to become absorbed and assimilated.

The bathing basins are constructed of wood, and communicate both with the reservoirs and springs, so as to admit of a constant renewal.

A feeling of general ease pervades the bather; greater elasticity of body and mind is experienced; the circulation becomes more active, the pulse somewhat fuller, and occasionally more frequent. If the stay is prolonged to an hour, relaxation ensues, sometimes a slight chilliness, inclination to sleep, and other signs indicating the necessity of leaving the bath. A short repose on the bed after leaving the bath, brings out a pricking sensation of the skin, particularly in such parts as have been subjected to gentle rubbing. Perspiration is rare.

Healthy persons, after bathing for several days, feel stimulation of the vascular and nervous systems, increased frequency and strength of the pulse; sometimes even giddiness, aridity of the skin, restlessness, and diminished appetite. To plethoric persons in general, Gastein is less adapted than to weakened and anæmic individuals.

Derangements based on vital inactivity, or torpor of the cerebral and spinal nervous system, will find a fitting remedy in Gastein. After the first seven or ten baths the general functions of the muscular and sero-fibrous organs increase. If still continued, reaction sometimes appears with the usual characteristics—as want of appetite, lassitude, headache, mental depression, obstruction, &c. Sometimes these phenomena augment to a state of fever, when the course should be discontinued for a short time, till the undue excitement has passed off with salutary crises. This reaction varies in its time of appearance, between the ninth and twenty-first bath. Old rheumatic arthritic pains often reappear during the course, dormant neuralgiæ are roused, and old scars and paralysed parts become painful.

The solvent power of the spa in inveterate swellings and indurations is *subordinate* to its dynamical and alterative effect on nervous vitality.

The cutaneous system is particularly prone to critical results, having become more susceptible by the alpine climate. Glutinous perspiration sometimes covers the affected parts.

After a certain duration of the course, the back, abdomen, and extremities are occasionally affected with a bath eruption, of either a papular or vesicular character. The bath is to be continued till the eruption disappears, unless the latter be accompanied by fever or erysipelas, when the course must be interrupted.

Renal crises are the most frequent; the urine first becomes watery and more abundant, afterwards sedimentous, and particularly charged with deposits in rheumatic and arthritic diseases, and in lithiasis.

Critical stools after reaction are more rare. The regular flow of hæmorrhoids sometimes follows the course, and removes internal diseases which had been produced by this suppression of the discharge.

Satiety is generally evinced after the twenty-first bath, and requires cessation of the course. In some instances, however, particularly with very torpid persons, the desire for bathing continues longer. Usually, however, after this period, the baths are taken with reluctance and discomfort; the mind becomes peevish and excited, short walks are fatiguing, sleep becomes disturbed, appetite diminished, tongue furred, &c. If, in spite of these symptoms, the course be prolonged, signs of overbathing will be superadded — viz. palpitation of the heart, oppression of the chest, giddiness, restlessness, chills, and at last real fever, which greatly differs in character and intensity from the curative fever of reaction, and requires immediate suspension of the baths, besides careful medical treatment.

Frequently the curative effects of the spa are only exhibited some months after the patient has left the Alps, and returned to his occupation. If no decided indication exists, it would be advisable to leave nature free scope for developing its commenced alteration. The course sometimes merely incites the *vis medicatrix naturæ*, which then gradually progresses till the morbific cause is expelled.

Gastein is recommended, according to Dr. Kiene—

In *chronic rheumatism*, arising through gradual suppression of insensible perspiration, and inducing metastases to internal organs; in rheumatic contractions of the joints; and in rheumatism following the sudden suppression of periodical neuralgia by large doses of bark. In morbidly increased sensibility, the lukewarm baths are used; in great torpor, the warmer ones. The perspirations induced after a certain number of baths display acrid smell and reaction. Urinary secretion shows in its sediment, after some time, increased urate of ammonia. In articular rheumatism, the pains sometimes become extremely violent at first, through using the baths, but only to be followed by soothing effects.

In *gout* and *gravel*, more particularly with anæmic and decrepit persons, or such as have been exposed to harassing mental work, without sufficiently strengthening diet—those persons will be less benefited who possess a plethoric disposition, or who live luxuriously whilst leading a sedentary life, or where there is a natural tendency to expel the morbid matter through the abdominal organs, or where material engorgements are present. Here the cooling and solvent spring of Marienbad, Franzensbad, or Kissingen, will be indicated in some instances; in others, the penetrating thermæ of Karlsbad or Wiesbaden. Gastein is in such cases often resorted to with great advantage as an after-cure, to raise the nervous power, after the exhausting climinations of peccant materials.

Regular local paroxysms of gout are not cured in Gastein, but their frequency and violence are diminished, by preventing new deposits of arthritic concretions. Gout in the articular apparatus of the vertebral column, characterised by dull dorsal pains, and increased by motion, is particularly amenable to the baths and vapour-douche of Gastein. *In arthritic ankylosis*, when the synovial membranes are filled with uric or calcareous sediments, from deficient organic power of transforming and eliminating these substances, the internal and external use of Gastein is very useful. Diarrhœa through arthritic dyscrasia, also gonorrhœa from the same cause, are relieved here.

Gastein is reputed for expelling sand and gravel. When repelled podagra has produced the evil, the former disease becomes localised again. Ischias nervosa, gonorrhœal gout, face-ache of rheumatic or arthritic origin, also if purely nervous without organic change, &c., are all enumerated amongst the category of diseases curable by Gastein.

Writers' cramp * is very often cured here. Habitual spasms of the stomach are only relieved in persons of great nervous weakness. In debility of the abdominal nervous plexus after cholera, in trembling of the limbs produced by general debility of old age, &c., the power of the spa is extolled. *Somnambulismus*, based on predominant nervous irritability of the uterine plexus, with prostration of the central nervous system, is often relieved here. A case is recorded by Dr. Kiene of a young lady of seventeen years of age, who was completely cured by a course of twenty-one baths. The first day the temperature was 84° F., and the stay in the bath five minutes; the next day, temperature 86° F., and stay ten minutes; the following day 88° F., and a quarter of an hour's stay; and all the following 88° F., of half an hour's duration. On the fifth day the paroxysms reappeared, but weaker; again, on the ninth, with still less violence, and subsequently left off altogether.

As regards *diseases of the spinal marrow*, Gastein is not indicated, when inflammation, suppuration, or fever is present; but where exhaustion of nervous power exists, through excessive losses, or weakening diseases, Gastein is eminently curative. Spinal irritation and hyperæsthesis, paralysis of the lower extremities, pure nervous weakness, marasmus senilis, sexual debility, morbid atonic perspirations, *coxarthrocace* (luxatio spontanea), are all asserted to find frequent cures at the spa.

The above array of maladies might easily provoke a smile of

---

* I have myself travelled with a gentleman who was completely freed from this evil at Gastein.

incredulity. 'What!' you will say, 'does Gastein exhaust all these classes of pathology? how can the same remedy cure diseases so diversified in their nature and appearance? If it be decidedly able to heal the one, it must prove inert, or even injurious in the other.'

You have to bear in mind, that a spa of such mysterious properties serves as a last resort in many cases where the ordinary remedial store has been exhausted in vain. Persons suffering with the varied derangements enumerated, have, no doubt, found relief there. The scientific standing of Dr. Kiene, who enjoyed a high repute in Germany, and who practised at the place for nineteen years, sufficiently guarantees the truthfulness of his accounts.

But the question between certain diseases cured there, and what patients you should rather send to Gastein than to other spas, is widely different. Many a sufferer is relieved from disease under a course of certain pharmaceutic remedies, and yet we may sometimes hesitate to ascribe the cure to their agency.

The *ensemble* of Gastein adapts it to those chronic diseases in which the nervous system has been peculiarly weakened or altered in its function. We have to consider the three media from which curative influences may ensue: the inherent caloric, the constituents, and the bracing alpine air with its diminished atmospheric pressure.

I need not tell you what a great number of nervous affections are daily produced by repelled gout, or by retrocession of piles, or of cutaneous eruptions. The general increase of peripheric functions, inducing a derivation from the internal organs, may act healingly in one instance. The roused torpidity of the nervous centres is able, in another instance, to call dormant organs into fresh action, and to elicit imbedded particles from their obnoxious position.

In a third instance, the great quantity of the highly-diluted warm fluid, with its sulphate of soda, chloride of sodium, carbonate of lime, and of iron, may enter into combination with the circulating organic liquids, and partially dissolve stagnant substances, and fit them for elimination. The decided utility of Gastein in gravel would lead to this supposition, for its composition bears some analogy to Karlsbad, where also sulphate of soda forms the chief constituent, and where chloride of sodium and carbonate of lime are in subordinate quantities with carbonate of soda.

In conclusion, I shall quote a few lines from my journal :—

'Aug. 17th.—I was much disturbed the whole of last night by

the roaring waterfall of the Ache. Dr. Kiene, whom I saw in the morning, considers Gastein more particularly efficacious in torpor of the nervous system, *erratic gout, premature age*; in fact, whenever spasms or paralytic affections are produced by deficient nervous power.

' I walked from Wildbad-gastein down to Hof-gastein (about one hour and three-quarters); although it rained, the walk was extremely picturesque and romantic.

' The water of the chief spring is allowed to cool over night, or cooled and thermal water are let from two pipes into the bath, which thereby acquires the desired temperature. From this chief source the water is conducted in wooden pipes down to Hof-gastein, where it arrives with a temperature of about 100° F. Then it runs constantly out of pipes into the baths, which cool down to 95° or 93° F. after a few hours.

' Dr. Sleting (practising at Hof-gastein) considers it an advantage of the filial establishment that the water does not require cooling, that the climate is milder and drier than the parent spa, enjoying the sun three hours longer every day (which must be considered very beneficial in nervous diseases). The walks are more level than in the mountainous regions of Wildbad-gastein. It is more accessible, but less comfortably constructed; in fact, the locality seems rather neglected, and actually looked down upon by its elevated parent. Dr. Sleting related to me several cases of cramps of the stomach, which found a permanent cure at his spa. Also some cases of sterility, and of paralysis through spinal concussions and wounds, that had been cured at Hof-gastein. Sal. H——, of Danzig, who suffered from a kind of chorea (viz. fits of bellowing and imitating various animals), was completely restored here. Schönlein sent to him a remarkable case of an affection of the *vagus nerve*—viz. by seeing others eat the patient got violent pains in the epigastrium, which spread to the throat, and impeded deglutition. This was also relieved. Varicose ulcers are likewise often cured there. The pores become contracted in the bath, the skin paler. Perspiration rarely ensues, whilst diuresis is invariably increased: and Dr. Sleting laid particular stress on the *sound critical sleep* that is enjoyed by nervous patients. He also mentioned a case of *diabetes mellitus*, where perspiration regularly ensued at night, the quantity of urine diminished two-thirds, strength increased, and the patient left greatly relieved, though not cured. As regards lithiasis, particularly in the phosphatic diathesis, it frequently finds relief in Gastein.

'I spoke with a commandant in the free military bathing establishment, who was cured of pain and stiffness in the right femur, where he had been wounded by a ball. I saw many persons who had been cured from traumatic stiffness and spasmodic contractions.

'How, then, is the indication to be fixed, and the choice to be made between the three akratic spas visited?

'*Wildbad* is more indicated in *nodous gout*, and in those cases of paralysis and contractions where absorption is to be promoted, and where resolution of effete concretions and deposits are the chief task of the healing process.

'*Pfäfers* is rather useful in *atonic metastatic gout*, in hemiplegia after apoplexy, and in paralysis connected with the absence of *true* nervous sensibility; also when the disease is more the immediate effect of the concussion or lesion of muscular tendons or nervous centres.

'*Gastein*, however, is more indicated in irregular and depraved nervous action, based on atony. Therefore, it is eminently useful in writers' cramp, spasms of internal organs, affections of the vagus, trigeminus, &c., paralysis with general torpor, and *deficient calefaction*. The water increases the tone of the nervous system, and regulates its power. Persons with seminal weakness, whose irritability has been increased by sea-baths, were cured here, by the increased erectile power, and testicular contraction following the use of the baths, with restoration of the exhausted nervous vitality.'

Physicians of Wildbad-gastein:—Dr. von Koenigsberg, Dr. Pröll, and Dr. von Haerdtl.

Physician of Hof-gastein :—Dr. Pfeiffer.

LECTURE VII.

ISCHL—TEPLITZ.

HAVING remained a sufficient time in Gastein, you will leave at five in the morning by the diligence, to return to Salzburg. On arriving at *Hallein*, the last stage before reaching Salzburg (at about half-past five P.M.), I would advise you to stop and inspect the interesting salt-works. I find the following note in my journal:—'We had to ascend a high mountain, when the guide, for the purpose of shortening our route, led us along a footpath across narrow planks over precipices frightful to contemplate, from the unsafe footing at several spots. The guide walks before with a steady step (for the planks will not admit of two persons abreast), and advises you to hold fast by him, and to look upwards, in order to prevent giddiness, for one false step might hurl you down a fearful abyss. After about ten minutes the depths below me gradually decreased, and I found myself safely arrived at the salt-works. A miner's white dress was put by some official over my clothes, and I was then conducted down the shafts. These are passages hewn out of the salt-rocks, and supported by wood—moist and damp at the entrance, but becoming dry as you descend deeper. Though they are extremely long, not the slightest oppression or inconvenience in breathing is felt, all the main shafts being so constructed as to admit fresh air freely. After having to slide down five times into apparent abysses (without any danger, however), we arrive at last at the principal excavation, with a pool of salt-water in the centre, 40 feet long, 30 feet wide, and 7 feet deep, illuminated by numerous lamps, which beautifully reflected their rays in the still water, and formed certainly a very agreeable contrast with the darkness out of which we had just emerged. The guide stamped on the ground, and a boat approached from the centre of this subterranean vault. We stepped in, and were drawn to the other side very agreeably. It was explained to us that sweet water is conducted into the reservoir, up to the ceiling, where it soon saturates itself with salt (absorbing $26\frac{1}{4}$ per cent.), and precipitates argilla. The ceiling becomes gradually excavated, and the water collects in the pool, which is exhibited to the curious in summer, but boiled in winter for the formation of salt. I was shown very strange kinds of salt-rocks, found in the "saline" at different periods, and some other antiquarian curiosities. We returned to the upper world by a long passage, the walls of which consisted not of salt-rocks but of limestone; they were damp, and of an acrid smell.

'We had to sit across a bench, and were then drawn out at a very rapid pace by a man in front. The passage was so narrow as to leave no spare room. The galloping and clattering made me sometimes fancy, in the half-darkness, that a horse was dragging me along at this furious pace, till I recollected the narrowness of the passage, which did not allow the slightest alteration of position without the greatest danger of being crushed. Although what I saw was very interesting, still I did not feel altogether satisfied, from not having witnessed the preparation of salt in its various stages.'

After about an hour and a half's ride you arrive at Salzburg. Thence the diligence unfortunately leaves at ten P.M. for Ischl, so that you are deprived of the opportunity of admiring the scenery. You pass through Hof and the pleasant village of St. Gilgen, lying on the Aber-or Wolfgang-Lake. Having driven for some time along its banks, you arrive at *Ischl* at half-past five in the morning. The ups-and-downs you have had to experience in the 'eilwagen' sufficiently indicate the mountainous character of the road. Ischl lies in a romantic valley at the foot of the Noric Alps. You see in the immediate neighbourhood the Hallstädter Lake to the south, the Kammer Lake to the north, and the Mond Lake to the west. To the right of Ischl you see the River *Traun* pursuing its northerly direction, to be filtered through the Traun Lake in the north-east. Ischl forms just the centre of the Salzkammergut, and, though upwards of 1,400 feet high, its climate is very mild, from the protection against north winds and violent changes afforded by the surrounding mountains. Comparison with the temperature of Vienna * showed the difference to be only one degree of Reaumur. The romantic valley is intersected by the Rivers Traun and Ischl. From Schmalnauer's garden, situated on an eminence on the other side of the Ischl River, you enjoy a beautiful view of the surrounding mountain-peaks, with the snow-covered towering Dachstein in the background. The Calvarien mountain furnishes another promenade, which will reward you for your ascent by the views from the chapel at its

* Which lies about 900 feet lower.

summit. Ischl is altogether a very charming place with about 2,000 inhabitants, and is almost as much frequented by pleasure-seekers as by invalids. The salt-mountain, from which the brine is obtained, lies at some distance, nearly 3,000 feet above the level of the sea. The drinking-water is obtained from mountain-springs, arising under limestone, and conducted in pipes to Ischl: it is very pure, notwithstanding the superabundance of salt which exists in the locality. The chief virtue of the spa consists in the brine-baths, taken in the new 'badhaus' in single baignoires, where portions of brine, added to warm baths of ordinary water, are frequently prescribed. Here, again, you see all possible contrivances to meet the various contingencies of different maladies. Ischl has only been in repute about thirty years as a mineral watering-place, and I 'might also say was created a spa by the exertions and munificence of the late Dr. Wirer, who spent a large fortune in accomplishing the beautiful arrangements, all tending to one purpose. The brine derived from the salt-works contains, in sixteen ounces—

        223 grains of chloride of sodium
        0·78 ,, of chloride of calcium
        7·10 ,, of chloride of magnesium
        4·85 ,, of sulphate of soda
        1·02 ,, of sulphate of lime
        1·82 ,, of sulphate of magnesia

    Total, 238·591 grains.

A cold sulphur-spring, with a strong smell of sulphuretted hydrogen, but with an undetermined quantity of the gas, is found at the place, but is little used by itself. It possesses sixty grains of solid constituents in sixteen ounces—viz. $44\frac{1}{4}$ chloride of sodium, $12\frac{1}{3}$ sulphate of soda, $1\frac{1}{2}$ sulphate of magnesia, $1\frac{1}{10}$ sulphate of lime, nearly one grain of carbonate of magnesia, and about $\frac{1}{4}$ of carbonate of lime. Into how many remedies did the energy of one mind transform the meagre materials for combating chronic diseases possessed by Ischl thirty years ago! Now you have, beside the salt-baths referred to, douche, rain, and vapour-baths.

The boiling salt-water is used medicinally as a saline vapour-bath. Moreover, you find black moor-baths (containing phosphate of iron, among other ingredients); then, again, there are the saline mud-baths. These two are either used separately or mixed. There is also a swimming-school erected for sanitary purposes. Herbs gathered on the mountain are employed in the preparation of a sort of whey, very agreeable to the taste. On the promenade the visitors will be observed to stop, from time to time, at a certain stall, and quaff their morning beverages; and you will notice the greatest number of drinkers receive the recently prepared whey, brought fresh from the Calvarien mountain. But you will find a goodly number of other bottles standing ready for the numerous patients. These are imported mineral waters. Thus, while one patient uses brine-baths, with whey, for obstruction of the lymphatic glands, another takes mud-baths, and drinks Carlsbad sprudel or Marienbad kreuzbrunnen for some gouty affection of the lower extremities, or engorgement of the liver. Ischl is very much resorted to by the fair sex, and has a great reputation in swelling and incipient induration of the ovaries, if not of a malignant character; also in slighter degrees of hepatic enlargements, sluggishness of the liver, with habitual constipation, and scrofulous diathesis; luxatio spontanea of children is especially expatiated upon as a disease most frequently removed here. Poultices of mountain-mud * are often employed in caries, and, it is alleged, with great advantage. The peat-ground is found at the distance of about half a league from Ischl, and baths are either taken there or the moor is carried to the bath-house, and administered in contractions from wounds or chronic gout, alone or mixed with mud, or with mother-lye of the ' soole,' or with the water of the sulphurspring. There is also an establishment for gymnastic exercises. The mountain strawberries are occasionally ordered to be taken at regular intervals for medicinal purposes. The acknowledged efficacy of saline-baths in certain diseases of the lymphatic and sero-fibrous system, and in obstructed circulation, would indicate that in all such cases these baths might be appropriately resorted to. The late Professor *d' Outrepont* of Würzburg mentions the following case of a lady whom he sent to Ischl. About the period of puberty she was bitten on the left breast. Some hæmorrhage ensued, with inflammation; but as, from a feeling of timidity, she neglected to disclose the accident, induration ensued. She married after some years, and enjoyed perfect health with the above exception. No offspring resulting from the union, the sterility was thought by the husband to be connected with the mammary disease, and therefore many remedies and baths were employed for its cure. Extirpation was recommended amongst others, but was not consented to by the patient, because she had suffered no pain from the enlargement. Sixteen years after her

---

* That portion of humus which precipitates in the salt-mountain during the formation of the salt, chiefly consisting of argilla, sulphate of lime, sulphate of soda, &c.

marriage, Professor d'Outrepont was consulted. He found the left mamma considerably enlarged, the skin very white, and the induration consisting of five different movable tumours. These tumours had given her no pain for many years, nor had they increased in size. There was no trace of scrofula; all the glands were in a perfectly healthy condition, and none of the family had ever suffered with a similar disease; so that the mechanical lesion could alone be the cause of the evil. Iodine having been already administered internally and externally to no purpose, the Professor recommended her to go to Ischl. After three months she returned cured; the tumours had entirely disappeared, whilst the healthy breast had not diminished in size. He would not decide whether the cure was due to the poultices of mountain-mud and peat rubbed into a fine dough with mother-lye, or to the brine-baths employed. Another analogous case is related by the same authority, of a young man who injured one testicle with a hook on putting on his boots. The testicle swelled to the size of a goose egg. After numerous remedies extirpation was advised, but the patient would not consent. The generative functions were not impeded, the patient having become the father of several children. Fifteen years afterwards the Professor saw him, and found the testicle quite hard but not painful; spermatic cord and epidymis perfectly healthy; the scrotum tense, thin, and reddish. The right testicle was healthy. Neither the inguinal nor submaxillary glands were affected. He had never suffered from scrofula, and was quite healthy in every other respect. This patient was also sent to Ischl, and returned cured after ten weeks; but the affected testicle had become atrophied. The physicians of the spa are Dr. Brenner von Felsach, director of the bath establishment, and Dr. Pollack—both of whom have written on the virtues of Ischl works well worthy of being consulted—besides Dr. Kaan and Dr. Fürstenberg. Dr. Pollack considers specially adapted for Ischl affections of the glandular and lymphatic systems induced by an unfavourable mode of living, occupation, or residence; swelling of inguinal glands, or of testicles, as gonorrhœal residues; pulmonary catarrhs after the neglect of the acute stage; hoarseness from over-exertion of the lungs (as in case of clergymen, &c.); adynamic derangements of the heart; hypertrophy of the uterus, or follicular ulcers, with a general anæmic condition; sterility; spinal nervous affections; incipient phthisis, especially of an indolent character, or when hemoptysis seems to act as vicarious of hæmorrhoidal discharge. But let us proceed in our journey. A kind of omnibus leaves at ten in the morning, and takes you in two hours to Ebnsee. Here a steamboat is in readiness to take the passengers over the Gemünder or Traun Lake. In fine weather you will be pleased with the prospects from the water. The passage lasts about an hour. At the mouth of the Traun you perceive the village of Langbath: farther on, and on the right side of the lake, arise the perpendicular walls of the Traunstein (3,000 feet high); while on your left lies the village of Traunkirchen, built on a sort of isthmus in the lake. Lastly, you pass the chateau of Orth, situated on a small island, and ultimately you land at the little town of Gmünden.

Here, after taking refreshment, you avail yourself of the railroad as far as Linz. From this town, which is situated on the right bank of the Danube, you may travel by rail or steamboat to Vienna. If you wish to pursue your northward course, and leave the visit to Baden for a future opportunity, the railroad affords you this facility; for it brings you to Prague, on the Moldau, in sixteen hours, thence to Teplitz in about five and a half hours. The approach to the spa is very striking. After having driven for some time through ordinary fields and plains, your attention is suddenly arrested by the gentle undulations of the scene. The view of distant mountains, covered with a lively green, promises to afford you purer air and a more cheerful locality. You are not deceived. The scenery augments in variety and interest, and every object silently informs you that, from the comparatively barren and unfavoured regions, you are arriving at one of Nature's favoured localities.

Teplitz is situated about 51° north lat., and 14° eastern long., in the Leitmeritzer Kreis (circle) at the north-western extremity of the middle mountains, and at the south of the Erz mountains, in a fertile and charming valley; its elevation over the North Sea is 648 feet. You see on the local map the mountainous semicircle at the north-west and south-east. The village of *Schönau*, to the north of Teplitz, may be considered as a suburb. The valley extends downwards as far as Aussig, and upwards to Kaaden, a distance of thirty miles — the width being sometimes contracted by the Erz mountains to two miles and a half. On all sides you find the town surrounded by hills—the Schlossberg on the east, Wachholderberg on the west. Lower are the Spitalberg on the south (between the two former), Kopfhügel and Kreuselsberg to the west, and Judenberg and Schönauerberg to the north-east. The three former are considerably steeper than the latter, which becomes flattened towards the Erzgebirge. The extensive princely garden begins at the foot of the Wachholderberg, and contains a beautiful chateau. The suburb lies rather lower, at the foot of the Spitalberg. The town counts 3,000 inhabitants. There are some very good private houses between the city and the suburb. Schönau is intersected by the Saubach, with the declivity of the Schlossberg as its eastern boundary, enclosed on the south by the ' Spitzige' (pointed) and Judenberg, and on the north by the Granzer and Dorner heights, and the Hühnerhügel. The climate of Teplitz is very mild, and the vegetation luxurious in the immediate neighbourhood. Besides the numerous houses and mansions for the wealthy invalid, you find no less than eight establishments for the accommodation of military or indigent patients.

One of these (the Saxon foundation of the 26th of July 1811, founded on the anniversary of a princess then in Carlsbad) not only provides Saxon poor requiring the baths with all necessary accommodation during the course, but also pays their travelling expenses to and fro. Patients wishing to avail themselves of this charity must apply to the Commission before March.

The views from the heights around Teplitz are really charming. The eye ranges with pleasure over the cheerful valleys, studded with villages and rural habitations, whilst it enjoys the contrast formed by the sombre forests, antique castles, and citadels of the Erz mountains. In the princely garden you will be particularly struck by two ponds, with canoes for water exercise; by the beautiful umbrageous walks; and by the park-like farm, from the highest point of which you can obtain a view of the distant Mariaschein, Graupen, and Geyersberg. About half a league from the town you may ascend the Schlossberg. Several gentle hills of basalt and porphyry unite into an extensive plain, and then abruptly rise as a steep cone, covered with wood at the northern and eastern side, whilst the southern wall is bald and rugged. The flattened summit bears the ruins of an old chateau with antiquarian relics. The distant Elbe becomes here visible to you, and a great number of mountains as well as works of human industry and skill. Besides, numerous other places invite your visits, such as the shooting-house on the Spitalberg, with its view of the Erz mountains, the woody Lippnay, the charming 'Bergschenke' (mountain inn) with its extensive view, the grotesque Schlakenburg, the Mont Ligne with its view of Schönau, the Judenberg with its distant panorama, the village of Dorn, with its garden, hills of porphyry, and murmuring mountain-river, Probstan, with its garden full of pheasants, or the more distant Mariaschein (about two leagues distant), with its thousands of pilgrims at certain festivals, and the mountainous town of Graupen. When you enter this little town, you will be particularly struck by the strong contrast between the wild mountain scenery of the place itself and the garden-like plain in the distance. Somewhat more to the north (three leagues from Teplitz) you can visit the village of Kulm, with its memorable battlefield, and its memorials of the victory of 1813. In the west you may inspect the monastery of Ossegg (two leagues distant), with its extensive orchards. On a high rock in the neighbourhood are to be seen the ruins of Riesenburg. The little town of Dux, with its castle, and the basin cast out of captured Swedish cannon, is also worthy of a visit. In the village of Seberschen a cold sulphur-spring exists. Two leagues to the west of Dux, on the road to Carlsbad, the little town of Brux is often visited. To the east you may visit Aussig, on the left shore of the Elbe (four leagues distant); to the south the Mileschauer, the highest peak of the middle mountains, 2,700 feet high (four leagues from Teplitz); most extensive prospects are offered on its summit. In the east the eye reaches the Riesengebirge, the towns of Leitmeritz and Theresienstadt; to the south you perceive the Euler mountains behind Prague. From north to west you pursue the Erz mountain from its commencement near the Elbe to its termination near Eger. The springs originate in various places:—

1. *Hauptquelle* [*] issues out of syenite-porphyry in the deepest part of the town, and is enclosed by brickwork. Two pipes conduct the water into the baignoires for men, three feet deep. The temperature of the source is $39\frac{1}{2}°$ Reaumur, about 120° Fahrenheit (thus hotter than the chief spring of Gastein); in the conducting pipe the temperature is $38\frac{1}{4}°$ Reaumur, about 118° Fahr. It furnishes more than 800,000 cubic ft. of water per hour, and supplies the above-mentioned common bath and numerous separate baths.

2. *Frauenbadquelle* [†] arises a few paces from the former, and supplies the baths for females—those for ladies and those for women of a lower class being separated by a wall. Its temperature is 118° Fahrenheit at the issue, and 113° in the basin; its supply more than 400,000 cubic feet per hour.

3. *Frauenzimmerbadquelle*,[‡] near the former, temperature 113° to 118° Fahrenheit.

4. The *Sandbadquelle*,[§] east of the former, temperature 111° Fahrenheit.

[*] Chief spring. [†] Spring of the ladies' bath. [‡] Spring for females. [§] Sand-bath spring.

5. The *Garden springs*, arising in the 'Spitalgarten,' and having a temperature of 76° to 78° Fahrenheit—Trinkquelle, Augenquelle, and Badequelle (drinking, eye, and bath spring). They yield 66,000 cubic feet of water per hour. The village of Schönau possesses—1, *Steinbadquelle*,* lying on meadow-ground at the foot of the Schönauer mountain; its temperature is 100° Fahrenheit, and its supply 500 cubic feet per hour; 2, *Templebadquelle*;† 3, *Wiesenquelle* (meadow-spring); 4, *Militärbadquelle*; 5, *Schlangenbadquelle* (spring of serpent's-bath), temperature of the last three from 95° to 104° Fahrenheit; 6, *Neubadquelle* (spring of the new bath), formerly called sulphurbath spring, with 111° Fahrenheit; and 7, *Sandquelle*, with a temperature of $108\frac{1}{2}$° Fahrenheit. For bathing, part of the water is cooled in reservoirs, and mixed with the thermal water. The water of the chief spring exhibits a greenish appearance in the basin, but becomes clear and transparent when drawn. It is inodorous and tasteless. In cooling, carbonate of iron is found deposited in the conducting-pipes. Exposed to the atmosphere, crenic acid separates as a sort of mucus, and afterwards the so-called Priestley's green-matter developes itself and becomes transformed into oscillatoria. The springs greatly resemble each other as regards their chemical constituents. Carbonate of soda is the prevailing ingredient, and amongst the gaseous contents nitrogen is either evolved in a free state (in the sandstone and serpent's bath), or intimately connected with the water in the others. The chief source contains, in sixteen ounces—

0·43	grains of	sulphate of potash
2·68	,,	carbonate of soda
0·01	,,	carbonate of lithia
0·32	,,	carbonate of lime
0·01	,,	carbonate of strontia
0·08	,,	carbonate of manganese
0·05	,,	carbonate of magnesia
0·03	,,	carbonate of iron
0·43	,,	chloride of sodium
0·10	,,	chloride of potassium
0·05	,,	iodide of potassium
0·02	,,	phosphate of alumina
0·13	,,	silico-fluoride of sodium
0·31	,,	silica
0·09	,,	*crenic acid*

4·84—thus rather less than 5 grains.

Carbonic acid, 0·39 cubic inches; *Nitrogen*, 0·49, *or about half an inch.*

* Temple-bath spring.   † The stone-bath spring.

In 100 parts of gas, the Stadtbadquelle contains about 4·7 of carbonic acid, 0·6 of oxygen, and more than 94·5 of nitrogen. This will remind you of the proportions observed at Wildbad. In former times only the baths were employed, but latterly drinking is frequently added to the external course. Peat-baths are also employed since 1835. The peat is dark-brown, of an unctuous touch, tasteless, and of a bituminous smell. It contains sulphate, muriate, and humate of soda, lime, magnesia, iron, and other bases, with a great quantity of extractive substance and humus. This carbonaceous peat is dried, then mixed with thermal water into a sort of pap, and employed of a different temperature, according to prescription, in movable baignoires; a common thermal bath is immediately taken after emerging from the peat. Teplitz is found very efficacious in chronic rheumatism, in *anomalous gout* with swellings and contractions, in induration of the cellular tisue, in paralysis and stiffness from wounds; also in paralytic diseases, from metastatic eruptions. A very strengthening power is likewise ascribed to the spa in derangement of the sexual system, and a regulating influence in abnormal, catamenial, and hæmorrhoidal flux.

During my visit last year, the cure of a Dresden physician from paralysis as a consequence of typhus fever created so deep an impression, that I am induced to enter into some particulars. Dr. Wengler relates, in his ' Words of Consolation for Paralytics,' that, falling ill in 1848, he was induced to take an emetic. Not finding the expected relief, he resorted to the country, by the advice of Professor von Ammon, of Dresden. The disease soon assumed a typhous character. Six others in the same family were seized with typhus. His sister, nineteen years of age, died. In the beginning of 1849 the doctor's consciousness returned, and then he learned that, during four months, he had mostly lain in delirium, and that his life had been frequently in imminent danger from apoplexy. *He found his legs and one arm paralysed;* he could neither stand nor walk, nor was he able to sit with ease. As soon as summer approached, he was wheeled about in a chair for the benefit of the air. In April he resorted to Teplitz, under the advice of Dr. Schmelkes, a highly respected resident physician. Neither in the pelvic region nor in the vertebral column did he feel any pressure or pain. Nutrition of the thighs was still deficient. But he could now bend and extend his legs; three months before, he had always involuntarily kept the thighs bent, and, brought to consciousness, he had been unable to extend them. Emaciation was greater on the right side; the extensor muscles of the foot were considerably atrophied; the feet were swollen, particularly on the dorsal surface; the toes were bent inwards, so that he could not place the whole sole of the foot on the ground. Professor von Ammon had therefore stated it as his opinion, *that effusion had taken place at the lower part of the spinal marrow*, and was exercising pressure on the nerves of the lower extremities. The Professor particularly thought the ischiatic nerve affected. Dr. Schmelkes recommended the town-baths, and procured a convenient residence for him in the Herrenhaus, where the warmed corridors prevented his taking cold whilst being wheeled to the baths, which he began the second day after his arrival, with a temperature of 28° Reaumur (95° Fahrenheit) for twenty minutes. During immersion the affected parts were rubbed with a long-handled brush. After the bath he was placed in bed again (with the injunction of avoiding sleep), and allowed some Hungarian wine for his second breakfast. He was wheeled about in the air from noon till evening, and then allowed to recline on the sofa. After three weeks the temperature of the baths was fixed at 29° Reaumur=$97\frac{1}{4}$ Fahrenheit, and on the 13th of May the first douche-bath to the spine was administered, under Dr. Schmelkes' personal inspection. Whilst the whole back became rose-red, a small place between the second and third dorsal vertebra assumed *a bluish-red* colour, probably indicating the spot where the effusion had taken place, the absorption of which was now the chief task. The discoloration was greater at the right side.

He took one douche-bath every other day, and afterwards at various intervals; altogether, within two and a half months, nineteen douche and twenty-six general baths. Towards the end of June he returned home, with his mental faculties improved; the previous irritation and tickling of the larynx, with cough, was quite gone, the bowels were regular, and the urine was passed without difficulty. The right upper arm could be moved a little more freely, and the lower extremities were stronger. An eruption had appeared at the back of the foot, of an eczematous character, with small desquamations. Subsequently he resorted to the electro-magnetic rotatory apparatus of Reil for a quarter of an hour every other day, and then every day, altogether twenty-six times. Afterwards he employed *ant vapour-baths*, by causing an anthill to be dug up, and the ants to be covered in a vessel with boiling water. The vapours, passing along his legs, caused a prickling sensation and abundant local perspiration. He now tried crutches, but unsuccessfully; the feet hung down helplessly, and the hands became numbed from the pressure on the axillary nerves.

The following spring he again resorted to Teplitz. Baths of $97\frac{1}{4}°$ Fahr. were at once taken without douches, but the patient used thermal foot-baths of $111°$ Fahr. Double-armed crutches were now tried (distributing the weight to the hands), and this time with success. After every ten to twenty paces, the attendant had to support him with his knees, at first, to prevent his falling. At the expiration of four weeks crutches were the only assistance required. During this stay Dr. Wengler took cognisance of the following cases:—A gentleman thirty-four years of age, *from Zwickau*, whose hands and feet became paralysed in consequence of taking a cold river-bath during a heated state of the skin, was considerably improved after a six-weeks' course, and able to make some use of the injured limbs. But the spa afforded little relief in paralysis of the feet, hands, and neck, occurring in the case of a young lady *of Brunswick*, where nodous gout was considered to be the cause of the evil. In another case of paraplegia of the lower extremities of a *lady from Pilsen*, caused by the death of a married sister and other depressing misfortunes, the baths of Teplitz had not, at the time of the doctor's departure, exhibited any good effects. But in another case great benefit resulted from their use. A government *employé from Berlin* had used the cold-water cure for ischias rheumatica, and had received in exchange for his previous complaint chronic inflammation of both the knees, with considerable effusion, preventing extension of the thighs; walking and standing were thus rendered impossible. When this patient left Teplitz with the doctor, after a course of the baths, the swelling of the knees was considerably diminished, and he could walk with two sticks. In the middle of January 1850 Dr. Wengler could ascend the stairs without holding the balusters, and a week later he could descend them without assistance.

In April 1850 he again sought the spa, from which he had derived so much advantage. On the 5th of May he took the first bath, of $97\frac{1}{4}°$ Fahr. as before, and after twenty minutes he kept his feet for a few minutes in water of $109°$ Fahr. After a few weeks' course, he ascended the Königshöhe, and, to his great surprise, reached the summit without assistance or mishap, and enjoyed the view of the charming valley at his feet. The doctor was rejoiced to meet in this season the lady from Pilsen, greatly improved, and walking without assistance. But the greatest astonishment was created by the healthy appearance of the gentleman from Zwickau, whom the doctor scarcely recognised. He also met the employé from Berlin, very much improved, but less so than the Zwickau gentleman.

During a two months' sojourn, the doctor had used forty-eight baths, and two douche-baths.

Perhaps you may question the utility of the above details, and think the mere statement of the disease might have answered the same purpose.

But in such compound action of remedial, climatic, and dietetic influences, I consider well-authenticated cases of the utmost value for the proper appreciation of the respective spas.

Let us subject the remarks of the doctor to some examination.

It will be admitted that a well-established instance of *paralysis from typhus fever* has been chiefly cured through the power of Teplitz. We have also seen paralysis, through the sudden effect of cold, cured by the same agency; and thirdly, metastatic inflammation of the knees, accompanied with effusion, greatly improved, whilst no perceptible effect was perceived in paralysis of the lower extremities from nodous gout. I may take occasion to observe, that according to the view I offered in the lecture on Wildbad, the latter case was peculiarly fitted for the Wurtemberg spa, where the combined influence of chloride of sodium and nitrogen might have brought about a result unattainable at Teplitz. Taking into account the effect we may expect from thermal water penetrating the absorbent vessels and adding carbonate of soda and of lime with some chloride of sodium to the circulating fluids, we may distinguish cases requiring the spa with predominant carbonate of soda (Teplitz). The nervous system having, in the case of Dr. Wengler, lain so long in comparative prostration with the attendant irritation of the alimentary mucous membrane, the sodaic liquid in the first instance diminished the gastric irritability by neutralising its acidity. In the next place it improved the renal function by diminishing the excessive formation of uric acid. We saw improved vesical action in the first course. By indirectly promoting fluidity of the nutrient liquid, the reflux of venous blood must become facilitated; add to this the local irritation resulting from the douche, forming a revulsive from the internal affection, and you will require no mysterious agency to explain the cure—brought to your notice—giving a sure indication in analagous cases.

The case of paralysis through the cold bath will admit of a similar explanation. In the third case of metastatic inflammation, through the *slow* action of cold, we have already witnessed a less degree of efficacy. The improved action of the nervous system was not sufficient to induce absorption of the exuded particles. It is highly improbable that four spas should be equally curative, while they each possess different ingredients in predominance.

As regards the temperature of the baths, it is necessary to guard against using the hotter ones improperly. Those of Schönau are preferred where cooler baths are required. As a general rule, it is advisable always to begin with the cooler baths, and then only rise in the temperature with great care and circumspection. I need not state that plethoric persons, or those inclined to apoplexy, to congestion, or to obstipation, have to avoid the warmer baths, and often to avoid the spa altogether: as also persons with erethic weakness, or with tendency to thoracic affections. Torpid and phlegmatic individuals will bear the warmer baths better. The country people always prefer the higher temperature, and resort to cupping in order to guard against mischievous consequences. The danger of this habit is too obvious to require further comment. Drs. Höring, Kratzmann, Richter, Seiche, Willigk, Eberle, Hirsch, Karmin, Kraus, practise at the spa, besides Dr. Schmelkes, mentioned in Dr. Wengler's case. Teplitz* is very frequently resorted to as a restorative, after the somewhat weakening course of Carlsbad. Unfortunately, this class of patients consider themselves justified to indulge in the luxuries of the table, which were denied them by the strict dietetic rules necessary at Carlsbad. Carelessness in drinking cold beverages after different sorts of fruit is one of the most frequent occurrences.

At my visit last year, the cholera had suddenly broken out (in August), and carried off several victims very rapidly, and, strange to say, almost exclusively those who had previously used one or other of the pikrothermæ. This caused such a panic that the place was cleared of its numerous fashionable and unfashionable

---

* Hotels: Prince de Ligne, Stadt London, Post.

visitors in a very short time, at the height of the season. Still every death was clearly traceable to the sufferer's own intemperance or want of caution, and especially to the habit just referred to. Not one of the inhabitants was seized by that formidable disease. Both from medical and philanthropic reasons I felt extremely gratified to find confirmation of the notion forced upon me by the observation of the epidemic in London, viz. that no disease can be prevented with more safety and certainty than cholera, and, above all, that unguardedness, especially in *drinking*, is one of the most frequent, if not absolutely the chief provocative of the disease. At least I found those cases the most virulent which could be traced to the imprudence of drinking cold liquids after fatty dishes; whilst, on the other hand, the mere eating of even indigestible or excessive nutriment had not the power of producing that mysterious disease. According to my own belief, it is quite impossible that a specific should ever be found against cholera. From the various cases that have fallen under my observation, I could not help coming to the conclusion, that the disease was not only different in different individuals, but that, in the same patient, you have a series of perfectly distinct, and I might almost say opposite morbid phenomena before you, which so vary in their nature, that a remedy curative of the one series must be rationally considered useless or even injurious to the other. For instance, I have found the stage of collapse (where the extremities exhibit an icy coldness, the face a livid hue, and the wrists absence of or scarcely perceptible pulsation), a disease in which the constant vomiting and purging are not only not to be checked, but this violent intestinal irritation seems actually an effort of nature to prevent life from flagging away under the intense prostration of the whole nervous system. During this period, such remedies only can be of any avail which tend *to restore vitality*, without the slightest regard to the tumultuous alvine action. But the means answering their purpose in this stage will be quite useless in the next, when more power has been recalled and reaction set in. *Now* the morbidity of the abdominal phenomena demands urgent removal. No doubt this circumstance caused so many conflicting reports and such sad disappointments from every possible remedy suggested. Let it be a fixed rule with you, if ever the epidemic should unfortunately revisit this island, that specifics, recommended by whatever authority, are based on delusion too soon to be dissipated. Observe the morbid phenomena, and counteract them out of the ordinary store of healing agents at your command. But to insure success the patient must be seen frequently, and the remedies varied according to the varying stages of the disease. What I state to you here is not mere theory, but the digest of observed facts, and it was God's will that under this method several cases were cured where no hope of recovery existed at the outset.

LECTURE VIII.

PIKROPEGÆ—CARLSBAD.

THE neighbourhood of the spa treated of in our last lecture, leads us to the consideration of another class of mineral waters, viz. to that of the Pikropegæ (bitter springs, from πικρος, bitter, and πηγη, spring), characterised by the predominance of sulphate of magnesia, or of soda, which imparts to them a bitterish and sometimes a nauseous taste. The abundance of free carbonic acid removes the mawkishness or nausea of some, whilst heat modifies the flavour in others. Generally they are transparent and colourless; small quantities of atmospheric air or carbonic acid are found in most of them—rarely traces of sulphuretted hydrogen.

They are called *pikrothermæ*, if warm or hot (from πικρος, bitter, and θερμος, hot), and possess a taste similar to that of chicken-broth, like the weaker halothermæ; and pikrokrenæ, if cold (from πικρος, bitter, and κρήνη, adopted as the appellation for cold springs). The alkaline bitter waters display a less bitter and mawkish taste than the earthy, particularly if impregnated with a sufficient amount of free carbonic acid; for instance, Franzensbad. Contact with organic substances, pieces of straw, &c. whilst the bottles are filling, easily produces decomposition and evolution of sulphuretted hydrogen gas.

The bitter springs originate in volcanic mountains, or in strata of marl, sometimes in secondary layers of gypsum. Their general effect consists in depression of the organic vitality, and they are, therefore, indicated in cases of general irritability, with obstructed abdominal circulation. Of course admixture of iron or other metals modifies this result to a considerable degree.

Coexistence of carbonate of soda in the same spring causes a very powerful combined alterative action on sanguification. From its vicinity to Teplitz, our next visit is claimed by *Bilin*, which we may inspect before reaching the pikropegæ. It is a little town, of nearly 3,000 inhabitants, situated on the river Bila, which meanders through the Middel-mountain, and then enters the Elbe near Aussig. The springs are situated about half a league from the town, at the eastern declivity of the Ganghof. In wandering through the shady walk which leads to the springs, you pass on your left the laboratory, in which magnesia is prepared in large quantities from the chemical interchange between the sulphate of magnesia of Saidschütz and the carbonate of soda of the Bilin spring. The soda of the concentrated Bilin water combining with the sulphuric acid of that of Saidschütz for the formation of sulphate of soda, carbonate of magnesia separates. These works yield a large income to the proprietor (Prince Lobkowitz). Behind the Arhaus, on the right, you descend by stone steps to the chief spring, *Josephs-quelle*; the water is clear and sparkling, with an agreeable pungent taste; temperature, 52° Fahrenheit; specific gravity, 1,006. In the abundance of carbonate of soda, it surpasses all German springs (Vichy, in France, possesses a larger quantity). Analysis, according to Struve, shows it to possess 38 grains of solid constituents in 16 ounces, viz.:—

		Comparison with Teplitz.
22·73 grains of carbonate of soda	. . .	2·68
3·06 „ „ lime	. . .	0·49
1·19 „ „ magnesia	. .	0·28
6·17 sulphate of soda	. . . . .	0·54
2·88 chloride of sodium	. . . . .	0·42
1·73 sulphate of potash	. . . . .	0·43
0·02 basic phosphate of alumina	. . .	0·02
0·35 silex	. .	0·31
Traces of strontia and iron, {	carb. ir.	0·03
	strontia	0·01
Carbonate acid 33½ cubic in.		

A great analogy therefore exists between the two as regards quality.

The water is more drunk at other places than at its source, upwards of 90,000 bottles being annually exported. Compared with *Selters* water it has the advantage of possessing 16 grains more of carbonate of soda, but the latter from its greater quantity of chloride of sodium (17 grains in 16 ounces) has a more agreeable taste, and deserves the preference whenever the properties of the latter salt are more requisite.

Fachingen water bears a great resemblance to Bilin, having only five grains less of carbonate of soda, and about two more of common salt.

Geilnau, which is also frequently used as an alkaline water, contains only 11¼ grains of solid constituents, and of these only six are carbonate of soda, two carbonate of magnesia, and two of lime. *Heppingen* contains the same quantity of carbonate of soda, of magnesia, and of lime, but has, in addition, three grains of common salt and two of sulphate of soda (altogether 15 grains), and thus its efficacy holds an intermediate position between Fachingen and Geilnau.

Without further dwelling on the medical properties of Bilin, which are those of carbonate of soda, referred to in the last lecture, we pursue our course to the south and inspect Saidschütz, situated two leagues to the south-east of Bilin, in the eastern part of the plain of the bitter waters. Deep ditches are dug into the marl, composed of basalt, quartz sand, and carbonate of lime. These gradually fill with atmospheric water, and get impregnated with the soluble parts of their earthy beds. The drier the season, the more concentrated will be their contents.

Before being medicinally employed, these nauseous waters were known in the neighbourhood under the denomination of 'Laxir,' 'Fress,' or 'Fieberwasser' (purging, appetite-making, or fever water).

Saidschütz, enjoying a higher situation, is less exposed to the influx of meteoric water than its westerly neighbour, Seidlitz; and thus its greater abundance of solid ingredients is accounted for. The ridge, gently sinking from Krssina to the Serpina bog, encloses the limited locality of these bitter springs. Saidschütz contains in 16 ounces 178 grains (nearly 3 drachms) of solid constituents—viz.

46¾ grains of sulphate of soda
84 ,, sulphate of magnesia
10 ,, sulphate of lime
2 ,, chloride of magnesium
5 ,, carbonate of magnesia
1 ,, crenate of magnesia
25 ,, nitrate of magnesia
3·100 ,, iodide of magnesium.

You have then sulphate of magnesia as the chief ingredient, with about half the quantity of sulphate of soda, and nearly a third of nitrate of magnesia. Its property as a solvent, aperient, cooling, and antiphlogistic remedy is too obvious from its composition to require any further explanation. Saidschütz salt is prepared by concentration, crystallisation, and separation of the sulphate of magnesia, by means of its greater solubility. It is obtained in the shops under the name of bitter salt, or more commonly under that of 'Englisches Salz' (English salt). *Seidlitz*, about half-an-hour's walk to the north-west of Saidschütz, contains only 126 grains of solid ingredients in 16 ounces (nearly a drachm less than Saidschütz), viz. no sulphate of soda; 104 grains of sulphate of magnesia; 8 grains of sulphate of lime; 3 grains of chloride of magnesium; 3 grains of carbonate of magnesia; 8 grains of carbonate of lime (none contained in Saidschütz); no silex; no nitrate of magnesia.

Analogous to the composition of Saidschütz, it exerts a less aperient power, its sulphates being less in quantity and partially counteracted by the presence of carbonate of lime. The absence of the antiplastic nitrate renders it a still weaker agent in counteracting congestive fulness of internal organs. The real Seidlitz-powder, which I have prepared for this lecture, by evaporation, you will find vastly different from the pleasant and refreshing Seidlitz-powder sold in commerce, with the alkali in white and the acid in blue paper, and consisting of triple tartrate of potash and soda.

Püllna, the furthest to the west, lies on the road to Carlsbad, and possesses several enclosed wells; only one, however, is used, being of such abundance, that 6,000 small bottles might be filled weekly with it. The above three waters are remarkable for their disagreeably bitter taste and their yellowish tint. When drawn, they are clear and transparent. Drunk at the springs, the nausea is partially diminished through the somewhat greater proportion of carbonic acid. When used at a distance, I always find the effect increased, and the assimilation of the water facilitated, by adding an equal quantity of hot water to that medicinally required. Püllna contains in 16 ounces 251 grains (nearly 4 scruples more than Saidschütz); viz. 123 grains of sulphate of soda (about 4 scruples more than Saidschütz); 93 grains of sulphate of magnesia; $4\frac{3}{4}$ grains of sulphate of potash (none contained in Saidschütz or Seidlitz); $2\frac{1}{2}$ grains of sulphate of lime; $19\frac{1}{2}$ grains of chloride of magnesium (only two in Saidschütz); $6\frac{1}{2}$ grains of carbonate of magnesia; $\frac{3}{4}$ grain of carbonate of lime; 17-100ths grain of silex; no nitrate of magnesia; no iodide of magnesium. This analysis at once informs you of its greater power as a derivative, aperient, and solvent, than the two former.

Before leaving the subject of the bitter waters, which are rather to be classed as medical beverages than as mineral springs, allow me to bring to your notice *a fourth*, also frequently employed in analogous cases, though its origin lies some distance from the spot which we are treating of at present. I allude to the *saline bitter water of Friedrichshall*, in the dukedom of Saxen-Meiningen, near the village of Lindenau, four leagues distant from Coburg. The place has been noted for its salt-works for several centuries. Glaubersalt was obtained from the brine, under the appellation of *sal aperitivum Fridericianum*. Dr. Bartenstein, of Hildburghausen, has caused the water to be employed since 1843. To approximate its strength to that of Püllna, it is concentrated by graduating works and filtering processes, and not exported till its specific gravity amounts to 1,022 at $54\frac{1}{2}°$ Fahrenheit. The water is clear and transparent, and contains in 16 ounces $194\frac{1}{4}$ grains of solid constituents (nearly a drachm less than Püllna, and a scruple more than Saidschütz), viz. $46\frac{1}{2}$ grains of sulphate of soda, $39\frac{1}{2}$ grains of sulphate of magnesia, $1\frac{1}{2}$ grains of sulphate of potash, $10\frac{1}{3}$ grains of sulphate of lime, $30\frac{1}{4}$ grains of chloride of magnesium (half a scruple more than Püllna), 3 1-10th grains of carbonate of magnesia, 1-10th grain of carbonate of lime.

Besides the above, bearing analogy to the Bohemian bitter waters, it contains 8-10ths grain of bromide of magnesium, 61 1-10th grains of chloride of sodium, and 5 cubic inches of carbonic acid.

If, then, the bitter waters are generally useful in indigestion, in deficient alvine secretions, in abnormal bilification, in plethora and venous dyscrasia, in thoracic or cerebral congestion, Dr. Bartenstein considers the water of Friedrichshall, from its chlorides, particularly appropriate in various diseases of nutrition, where Püllna would exert a too lowering influence. He found it very useful in dyspepsia, even connected with inflammatory irritation of the stomach, when taken in small doses of two to three wineglasses full, at shorter or longer intervals; in erethic gastrodynia, &c. Even in pyloric induration, he witnessed vomiting diminished by the water taken in doses of a tablespoonful. He also recommends it in flatulence, acidity, and the spasms of childhood, arising from irritation during difficult dentition, in mucosity of the pulmonary mucous membrane, and in hysteria and hypochondriasis, based on abdominal obstructions: in chronic swellings of the spleen he observed rapid cures by a course of the water in small quantities; also in hepatic hypertrophy, after a long-continued intermittent fever. For the habitual venesections of many persons, to counteract apoplectic tendency, the water may be safely substituted. He considers it as holding an intermediate position between the bitter and more tonic saline waters. Its happy combination of chloride of sodium, of magnesium, and bromide, with the sulphates of soda and magnesia, allows us to expect a combined solvent, alterative, and aperient efficacy.

Carlsbad.—But let us proceed on our journey. If you desire to travel uninterruptedly from Teplitz to Carlsbad, you may leave at 6 P.M. by the eilwagen, and in thirteen hours you will reach the so-called king of the German spas. Carlsbad is situated at latitude N. 50°, longitude E. 13°, in the Elnbogner Kreis, of Bohemia, on both sides the Tepl River, in a narrow deep valley, which extends from south to north, at an elevation of 1,100 feet above the level of the North Sea, eighty miles to the west of Prague, ninety to the south-west of Dresden, sixty-five to the south-west of Teplitz.

You see the River Tepl (which means in Bohemian, the 'warm one') originate in the south above Marienbad, about 50° latitude, and entering the Eger River in the north. Carlsbad, a charming little town of 3,000 inhabitants, allows free access to the north winds, as you will perceive from its situation; the temperature is therefore subject to sudden changes, though the climate is generally temperate. You also see the valley devoid of mountainous enclosure in the west. The discovery of the spa is ascribed to a dog of the Emperor Charles IV., who, about four and a half centuries ago, when in pursuit of a stag, leaped into a spring, and attracted the huntsmen by its painful howlings. When they arrived, they found him in the hot spring now called 'Sprudel' (Bubbler), because its steaming liquid constantly rises and falls with a hissing noise. The spot from which that famous leap is said to have taken place, assumed the name of 'Hirschensprung' (stag's leap) to the west of the town.

To the south, you remark the Hammerberg; to the north-east, the Kreuzberg, on the other side of the Tepl. These are the highest mountains. The Laurenz Mountain, or Tappen, to the east, and Galgen Mountain, to the north, are somewhat lower. The rocks consist chiefly of granite. The Schlossberg, leaning on the Hirschenstein, is composed of horn-stone. Immense masses of volcanic origin reach from Schlackenwerth to Engenwall. About a quarter of a league below Carlsbad, the valley widens and allows the Tepl to pour its contents into the Eger River. The road to Carlsbad from the height (if coming from Prague) makes a sombre and yet a grand impression, as you descend into the deep basin. From the western Eger you enter on a plain; both roads join at the Franzensbrücke, and conduct you into Carlsbad on the right shore of the Tepl, where, also, the Sprudel takes its origin. Many bridges join the two parts of the town. The streets are generally narrow, with the exception of those called 'Wiesen' (meadows). Poor patients are provided for, without distinction of country or religion, in the hospital built at the foot of the Bernhard Rock. The environs of Carlsbad are most charming. Picturesque and wild scenery constantly alternates with beautiful park-like clusters of trees; green meadows, with woody hills; dark shady walks, with widely-spread open prospects. By the 'Puppische Allee,' a gravel foot-path leads you to the walks on the ridge and declivity of the Hammerberg on the right, and Laurenzberg on the left. From the 'Neue Wiese,' through an excellent carriage-road, the villages of Hammer and Aich may be reached, with the rapid Tepl between them. The walks to the so-called Himmel auf Erden, to the Posthof, Hirschensprung, Schiessehaus, Antonsgrube, Dichterbank, Belvedere, Augustusplatz, &c. &c. offer many pleasant views. For further excursions you are invited by the town of Elbogen (two leagues to the south-west), situated on a steep rock, and encircled by the Eger River in the form of an elbow (hence its name of Elbogen), to the city of Schlackenwall (a league to the south of Elbogen), with its lead and tin mines, and to Joachimsthal (four leagues from Carlsbad), where silver mines were worked in the sixteenth century. The ruins of Engelhaus (two leagues to the east of Carlsbad), on the summit of a high rock, on the road to Prague, and many other places, furnish a great variety of inducements for pedestrian or carriage exercise.

The springs issue out of limestone, into which wooden pipes are fixed to distribute and equalise the proportion of the rising fluid. This limestone is formed by the water itself, which deposits calcareous sinter in proportion as it loses its carbonic acid. These stony masses extend from one bank of the Tepl to the other, in the middle of the town, and supply foundations for many houses. Wherever you break through these stony coverings, hot water issues. The petrification lies deeper on the right shore, being more particularly fed by the hot source. Out of six apertures the sprudel water issues with a temperature of 59° Reaumur,=

165¾° Fahrenheit, five being near each other, and the sixth, more distant, is the Hygiaeensquelle. About fifteen yards further, in the bed of the Tepl, a larger hole is bored into the sprudel-crust, and provided with a plug, which is only removed on certain occasions. The above openings are walled in, being situated below the level of the Tepl. The wall supports a boarded enclosure, in which you find the chief source, called the Sprudel or Springer (jumper), the water spontaneously jerking upwards in a perpendicular tube, which rises one yard above the boards, and has a diameter of three inches; the height of the water-column from the ground amounts to four yards. About nineteen times a minute the water jumps up and sinks again. This arises from the accumulation of carbonic acid in the upper parts of the sprudel-basin. Its gradually increased expansive power at last breaks a wider passage through the water, which becomes pressed down, in consequence, to admit the issue of the carbonic acid from the water-pipe. As soon as this is partially diffused, and diminished on the surface, the water is allowed free scope to rise again, and thus the process continues, emitting alternately carbonic acid and water. The jerks are not all of equal power; generally after eight or ten weaker and quicker discharges, a stronger and more abundant one ensues, with an accompanying dull subterranean hissing. If the plug be removed from the deeper artificial borehole fixed in the Tepl, only gas escapes from the Sprudel, without any water. The other Sprudel-openings are covered by boards, and cannot therefore be seen. The constantly deposited sinter accumulates to such an extent, that the holes must be bored out four times a-year to prevent their being closed, and inducing sprudel-eruptions in consequence. In former times these eruptions were more frequent than now, less attention having been paid to the safety-holes. One of the most violent happened on the 2nd of September, 1809. On the night of the 1st of September the Sprudel began all at once to jerk its water up with great violence to the height of the wooden ceiling. Removal of the plug in the safety-hole induced a quiet flow again. Some hours, however, after the plug had been refastened, the next day (2nd of September) the Sprudel covering broke in several places, and a new Sprudel (hygiaeensquelle) with the same heat, but more abundant and powerful than the former, issued forth, throwing the water to a height of eight or nine feet. Fissures also appeared in the pavement near the Sprudel, which had ceased to throw its water up, and to emit the usual subterranean hissing. The more distant Schlossbrunnen flowed with less abundance and with diminished temperature, and at last ceased entirely. The new ' Springer ' found about fifteen yards from its predecessor, beyond the 'sprudel wall,' continued to jerk to the above-mentioned height till its opening was con siderably widened, and provided with a large pipe, by which the original spring was restored to its former force, so that the *parvenu* now only flows over alternately, and has scarcely a claim to the title of ' Sprudel.'

The *Schlossbrunnen*, reappearing in 1823 (fourteen years after having vanished) with the decreased temperature of 93° at first, but having now again 113° Fahr., lies farthest away from the Tepl, and issues out of a rocky ground at a more considerable height than the others. This greater distance from the common source out of which all the springs are supposed to arise, accounts for its diminished temperature. The *Mühlbrunnen* lies in a dark corner on the other side of the Tepl, about 400 yards from the Sprudel at the foot of the Schlossberg opposite the Mühlbad-bridge—temperature, 132¼° Fahrenheit. A colonnade extends from this spot along the bank of the river as far as the Bernhard Rock: this spring is much used for drinking. About thirty yards further we perceive the *Neubrunnen*, temperature 141° Fahrenheit. From the stairs that lead to the Wandelbahn (promenading path) you descend on the left to the *Bernhard's brunnen*, the hottest in this region, its temperature amounting to 153° Fahrenheit (12° Fahrenheit warmer than the Neubrunnen). Ascending some stairs from the colonnade we observe the *Theresienbrunnen* (for-merly called the Gartenbrunnen), with a pleasant shady walk, bordered by lime-trees. Temperature, 126½° Fahrenheit (for-merly 133°). Quite at the end of the town, behind the hospital, and on the declivity of the Bernhard Rock, the *Spitalbrunnen* originates, but it is only used for baths. Temperature of the upper spring, 110¾° Fahrenheit, and of the lower, 93°. In 1838, a new spring made its appearance; the *Marktbrunnen*, with a temperature of 130° Fahrenheit; and as late as 1844, a mineral source arose below the Bernhard Rock, and was named *Stephan's brunnen*. Its present temperature is 131° Fahrenheit. The freshly-drawn water of all the springs is perfectly clear, transpa-rent, and inodorous, tasting like weak chicken-broth. Exposed to the air, it assumes a milky appearance, and deposits on the surface a whitish pellicle (bath-foam), and after some time a yellowish precipitate sinks to the bottom, upon which the bath exhibits a more lixivious odour. The water of the Mühl- and

Theresienbrunnen sparkles more than the others. As regards the quantity of the hot liquid poured out by the respective springs, the Sprudel yields annually seventy millions of cubic feet; the Bernhard's brunnen, 800,000; the Neubrunnen, 71,000; the Mühlbrunnen, 41,000; the Theresienbrunnen, 19,000 cubic feet. With reference to the constituents of the various springs, the same proportions are maintained in all of them, thus proving a common origin, whilst the higher or lower temperature is due to their deeper or more elevated issues. The mouth of the Sprudel being nearest to the subterranean caldron, exhibits the highest temperature. The Bernhard's brunnen having a lower situation than all the others, after the two Sprudels, possesses a corresponding higher temperature. The same proportion is shown in the Neubrunnen and Theresienbrunnen, the two last named lying just below each other. The Sprudel contains 41·92 grains of solid constituents in sixteen ounces, viz. 19·86 sulphate of soda (about half of the whole amount), 9·69 carbonate of soda (about one-fourth), 7·97 chloride of sodium (about one-fifth), 2·37 carbonate of lime, 1·36 carbonate of magnesia, 0·02 carbonate of iron, 0·57 silex. Besides some carbonate of strontia 7-1000, of manganese 6-1000, phosphate of lime 1-1000, basic phosphate of alumina 2-1000, and fluoride of calcium 24-1000. Carbonic acid, 11 cubic inches; specific gravity, 1-0049. The Neubrunnen possesses $14\frac{1}{2}$ cubic inches of carbonic acid, the Mühlbrunnen $15\frac{1}{3}$ cubic inches. Theresienbrunnen $36\frac{1}{2}$ grains of solid constituents in the same proportions, and $15\frac{1}{3}$ cubic inches of carbonic acid. Bernhard's brunnen also $36\frac{1}{2}$ grains of solid ingredients, and $13\frac{1}{2}$ cubic inches of carbonic acid. The Schlossbrunnen contains $38\frac{1}{2}$ grains of solid constituents, and amongst them 0·39 of sulphate of potash, and 2-1000 of carbonate of lithia, with $13\frac{1}{2}$ cubic inches of carbonic acid. The Mühl- Theresien- and Neubrunnen, abounding most in carbonic acid, are frequently used for drinking, and exercise a less exciting influence, from the abundance of carbonic acid and from their lower temperature. The Schlossbrunnen, being cooler and not deficient in carbonic acid gas, is generally recommended for commencing the course, and is also used for exportation.

Springs of fresh and sweet water are rare about Carlsbad. As regards the Tepl, I have to add, that its fall from the source amounts to 600 feet in its short course of thirty miles. The granite rocks, from which the springs originate, are partly of large, and partly of small granular structure. Some layers of argillaceous porphyry are found taking the same direction as the thermal springs.

The sprudel-water covers with white, brown, or yellowish incrustations all objects over which it has passed for some time. The colour depends partly on the access or exclusion of atmospheric air. In the former case, oxide of iron will make the crust darker, and in the latter it will be merely calcareous, and display a white colour. Pisoliths (pea-stones) are also products of the thermal water; probably grains of sand formed the nucleus round which calcareous sinter became deposited. It seems somewhat surprising, that this very liquid, with its remarkable petrifying propriety, is the most powerful solvent in hepatic enlargements and abdominal infarcta. Tough, viscid, intestinal mucosity becomes mobilised and excreted; collected and indurated fæces are discharged; the torpid portal circulation is called into greater activity by the removal of acrid obstructing particles. The increased production of animal matter, the source of gout and lithiasis, is powerfully counteracted by the spa. The exciting effect of heat is considerably diminished by the revulsive action, which the sulphate of soda exercises on the intestinal fibres, so that common water of the same temperature as the Sprudel would cause a much higher degree of cerebral excitement and general sanguineous orgasm. The carbonate of soda contributes the chief share in the marked action on incipient lithiasis exercised by the spa. Excessive acidity of the organic juices is neutralised, formation of uric acid diminished, and thus vesical irritation allayed. The addition of chloride of sodium may chiefly perform the function of improving the digestive process by increasing the strength of the gastric juice, through the formation of hydrochloric acid, so that alkalescence cannot reach too high a degree, whilst the soda combines with the albumen of organic pseudo-productions and prepares them for elimination. The carbonate of lime and magnesia assist the antacid and antilithic efficacy, whilst the manganese, iron, and silica, increase the tone of the intestinal fibre, and thus tend to prevent the too weakening effect of the highly-solvent and antiplastic media. Imagine these particles introduced into our organism, with the warm liquid and the accompanying volatile carbonic acid, and you will not be surprised at the remarkable changes wrought in those numerous inveterate diseases which originate from abdominal obstruction and retarded portal circulation. The highest reputation is, however, enjoyed by the spa in *hepatic* or *splenetic enlargement*, the consequence of intermittent fever, in *colic* produced *by gallstones*, &c. ; and from all parts of the globe you may see individuals with puffed-up and icteric appearance, and with unmistakable signs of depraved bilification. Although many are cured, I need not tell you that some are disappointed, and others, particularly if resorting to the spa without due discrimination, even find their complaints aggravated; and this may especially happen if the Sprudel be at once incautiously used. The vascular and cerebral systems often show signs of agitation, as headache, giddiness, lassitude, forgetfulness, disinclination to exertion, restlessness, loss of appetite, sickness, &c. ; these phenomena sometimes appear, in a slight degree, even in phlegmatic individuals, when first using the hot springs—in fact, a sort of mild intoxication is produced. How much more, then, may we expect plethoric persons to be affected, and those disposed to cerebral congestion, apoplexy, inflammation of internal organs, or great general irritability! Such patients must, therefore, never be recommended to resort to Carlsbad, though the state of their hypochondriac organs may appear urgently to demand it. Generally speaking, it is the most renowned mineral water for hypochondriasis, with material basis, or in diseases caused by repression of piles, which are made to flow, and thus relieve the system from the array of metastatic disorders, to which such invalids are liable. On the other hand, a person who suffered from habitual giddiness after an intermittent fever, being sent to Carlsbad, found the fever reproduced, which however disappeared without further medicinal means, and carried its metaschematic remnant with it. That *callus* of previously-united bones often softens again, has been established by several writers. Former wounds, or seats of gouty and rheumatic affections, become painful and appear excited for some time, till crises ensue by the bowels, skin, or kidneys, and restore the former state of health. *Anomalous gout*, connected with deficient hepatic function, is frequently cured here. Besides the state of plethora referred to above, Carlsbad is also *contra-indicated* in actual digestive atony, or in general debility, produced by loss of blood or other weakening causes, in dropsy, scorbutic tendency, in phthisis, and internal suppuration, in lithiasis with great irritation, and such large stones as cannot pass through the urethra, in organic diseases of the heart, in chlorosis, &c. Increased salivary secretion sometimes critically occurs during the course, and lasts for several days, probably caused by reciprocal influence of the stimulated pancreas. Appetite is heightened at first, but as the course proceeds, flatulence, eructation, pressure on the pit of the stomach, tickling, and stitches in the hypochondria, clammy taste in the mouth, &c. now and then take place, and only yield after the critical discharges by the bowels, skin, or kidneys have appeared.

The purging produced by Carlsbad differs from ordinary purgation by very fetid, bilious, mucous, and fatty stools, more charged with actual pseudo-formations or abnormal concretions than with the serum of the blood; it is therefore more an alterative of sanguification than a weakening agent, though, from the above cautions, you may infer that a certain amount of vital stamina is required for undergoing a regular course. But the alvine evacuations are not invariably increased; an opposite effect sometimes takes place, and then the Carlsbad salt is usually added. As regards the choice of the respective springs, you have not only to consider the various effects of heat, but also the difference of the quantity of carbonic acid. Its amount is smaller, and its intrinsic impregnation less adherent in proportion as the temperature is higher; whilst thus, in the hotter, loss of carbonic acid causes the earthy bicarbonates to become sesquicarbonates, and liable to precipitate,—in the cooler the combinations of carbonic acid retain for a longer period the character of bicarbonates, with less liability to deposition. If you wish, then, to produce a deeply penetrating action, and to excite the function of the skin and kidneys more particularly, you will give the hottest, the Sprudel. If you find a heightened alvine function to be the chief requisite, you will recommend the Mühlbrunnen, or Theresienbrunnen; but if you merely desire an alterative action, a check of the abnormal mucosity and pinguefaction, and a remedy against vascular erethism, you will employ the coolest of the thermal springs, the Schlossbrunnen.

A very frequent mode is to drink the cooler springs at first, and after some time to combine them with the hotter in this way: —Supposing the patient receives four to six glasses of Schlossbrunnen first, and increases the number; after some time he substitutes for the last glass of the cool spring one of a hotter spring —then for the last two, for the last three, and so on, till the cool spring is entirely superseded by the hotter one. Of course a great deal depends in this respect on the individual experience of the respective physicians, of whom there are not less than eighteen, viz.:—Drs. Hochberger, Preiss, Fleckles, Professor Dr. Seegen, Drs. Hlawacek, Forster, Osterreicher, Berman, Damm, Anger, Gans, Porges, Sorger, Kronser, Zimmer, Klauber, Stark, and von Juchnowitz.

Though the chief efficacy is expected from the internal use of the springs, baths are also resorted to in the cooled mineral water. The vapour of the Hygiaeensquelle is collected for vapour-baths. Douche-baths, as well as clysters, are likewise employed in appropriate cases.

Not content with all the above media, peat-soil is dug up at a distance of about two miles from Carlsbad, and mixed with Sprudel water for bathing, in cases of chronic rheumatism, anomalous gout, in chronic exanthemata, &c. It is also used as poultices in analogous local affections.

I have still to mention the *Carlsbad salt*, which is obtained by the natural evaporation of the Sprudel water, in vessels fixed to the bore-holes, whence formerly the water ran to waste into the Tepl River. The crystallised salt consists chiefly of sulphate of soda, with an inconsiderable admixture of carbonate of soda, and a minute quantity of lithia. Exposed to a strong heat, it immediately deliquesces. One ounce requires, to effect its solution, about double the quantity of cold and nearly eleven drachms of hot water. The crystals of common Glauber-salt are much firmer, and require longer time for deliquescence. Seventeen hundred pounds of the salt are annually obtained. It acts as a gentle and cooling purgative, without weakening or irritating the intestinal canal. Fr. Hoffman often prescribed it with *dec. tarax. or gramin.* in dyspepsia and flatulence; as a *diuretic* and lithontriptic with nitre; and with bark and cascarilla *in ague*. Before beginning the course of the Carlsbad springs, a preparatory dose of one to two drachms of the salt is often administered for one or two days.

To prepare a salt which should unite all the soluble ingredients of Carlsbad water, Dr. Illawacek proceeded in the following manner:—He evaporated the obtained mother-lye without causing the sulphate of soda to separate in crystals; then he dissolved the dry mass in Schlossbrunnen water, filtered, and evaporated the solution. In the resulting *yellowish-white* powder, chloride of sodium and carbonate of soda maintain the same proportion as in the water itself. He considers it more powerful than the usual Carlsbad salt, and recommends it for exportation and employment with the Schlossbrunnen, especially in lithiasis. He also introduced '*Sprudel*' *soap*. Finding great advantage from the external application of common soda-soap, dissolved into a pappy consistence, in hepatic enlargements, he concluded that the solvent power of the water must be greatly assisted by a soap prepared with Sprudel salt; and his expectations having been realised, he employs it in many instances with very satisfactory results. After the course of Carlsbad is completed, Teplitz is often resorted to by persons of a gouty disposition, to obtain a gentle continuance of the same alkaline action, without the lowering and antiplastic influence of the sulphates. The nervous power is thereby raised, without counteraction of the previous efficacy. More liberal diet is likewise permitted without injury, if used with reasonable care, and with gradually increased allowances. A very important warning to Continental patients is almost superfluous to the English—viz., to avoid drinking water or other cold beverages after taking fruit. This pernicious habit may not always engender the cholera, as it did on the occasion I mentioned in a former lecture, but injurious it must be after such a strict diet and such liquefying beverages have considerably weakened the organic power of resistance, at least for some time. And here I may state, by-the-bye, that the rational manner of English living is one of the greatest safeguards against epidemic diseases.

No wonder that life should be longer here than in many parts of the Continent, with a considerably greater freedom from avoidable diseases during the allotted period, and with comparatively greater physical resisting power, and other unmistakable signs of improved nutrition! As regards food, whilst in this island the most tender flesh from the best-fed domestic animals is simply exposed to the action of heat, just sufficient to increase its solubility in the gastric juice, in many parts of the Continent skilful cooks have to prepare savoury liquids out of the albuminous and gelatinous portions of the meat, and to season them in such various modes as to make a very agreeable impression on the palate. The warm liquid distending the stomach must momentarily diminish the power of its muscular fibres. Nevertheless, the tougher and more fibrinous portion, the parent of the juicy soup, is now introduced, and forces the intestines to unwilling action. Some other dishes make their appearance, with the mere object of recalling the vanishing appetite, and of creating an artificial desire for a greater reception of food. And even now, when the more substantial dishes come before you in their various shapes, art tries to improve on nature and make them more palatable, by sauces and numerous intricate contrivances. However satisfactory all may appear while at table, still on rising, although you may have taken an inconsiderable sum-total of really substantial nourishment, you feel overloaded, your movements are impeded, the physical oppression reacts on the mind; drowsiness, lassitude, and incapacity for exertion naturally ensue. An artificial stimulus, both for abdominal action and nervous power, is called into aid—viz., coffee.

Now, just imagine the consequences. Whilst the one satiated the want of nature, and supplied the organic waste by the simplest substitute, which had merely to be dissolved and reconstituted into its former atoms to produce healthy chyle—the most appropriate for performing the nutrient function of the whole body—the other imposed much greater work on his teeth, on his salivary glands, and his abdominal viscera; and when all is summed up, when the whole mass is sifted for contributing its share towards nutrition, the very purpose of the whole laborious task, why, it is found that very little can be used for sanguification—at all events, less than from the former simple and short repast. Add to this increased work the proportionally advanced inability of performance, and you will not wonder at the thousands and thousands who suffer from piles, at the numerous atonic diseases of a vicious sanguification, at the frequently debilitated constitutions, and at the shortened period of existence affecting so many individuals from avoidable causes. The injurious influence of excessive smoking on the composition and power of the mechanical masticators prevents the proper admixture of saliva, and the necessary comminution of the food, and thus heightens the evil.

But to return to our spa: Franzensbad is used as an after-cure in hepatic derangements, when a combined action of sulphates with tonic remedies is to be continued for the completion of a commenced or progressing cure. A very remarkable instance came to my own notice. When visiting Franzensbad I happened to be introduced to two Hungarian ladies (sisters, and both married), who came from a distance of 150 German miles (about 750 English), with the following complaint:—The younger sister, about thirty years of age, of a small and rather puny but otherwise healthy appearance, had suffered for two years with obstinate intermittent fever and induration of the liver. Large doses of quinine succeeded in relieving the fever, but only for a time, and she could always reckon on a return as soon as her menstruation appeared; then her sufferings in the right hypochondrium were very severe, and refused to yield to antiphlogistic and other remedies. The elder sister related to me that the sufferer's life had become a positive burden to her, all enjoyments being thwarted by these regularly-recurring attacks. At last she was advised to resort to Carlsbad, which she used for five weeks. The induration of the liver diminished, but she felt still frequent pains in the right hypochondrium, and departed, very much debilitated, for Franzensbad. In the latter spa she had used peat-baths for one hour every evening, and drank the *Kalte Sprudel* during three weeks; and at the time I saw her she was completely cured, and about to rejoin her family. I was assured by the patient's sister that I should not know her, so much changed was her appearance. Whether the attacks subsequently returned or not I have no means of knowing, but certain it is that the two sisters left Bohemia with the greatest happiness and gratitude for the restored health. The details of the previous suffering and misery were really so pitiable, that no one could help rejoicing at the patient's recovery and improved mental condition.

But avoid recommending the springs when aggravation of the evil could be foretold by an impartial consideration of all the circumstances. Thus, persons with scirrhus or carcinoma uteri have been sent to Carlsbad, individuals with developed consumption and hectic fever to Ems, rheumatic patients with organic diseases of the heart to Wiesbaden, paralytics with distinct apoplectic tendency to Gastein, &c.

Best accommodation at Carlsbad: in the Goldene Schild, Hotel de Russie, de Hannover, Anger's, &c.

LECTURE IX.

MARIENBAD—FRANZENSBAD.

From Carlsbad, at the right superior corner of the celebrated Bohemian triangle, we journey southward to its inferior corner, Marienbad. The diligence, which leaves the former at 4 P.M., performs the distance of twenty-five miles in six hours; from this tardiness you already perceive that the southern pikropega must be situated in a more elevated position; indeed, its altitude above the North Sea amounts to 1,900 feet (800 feet higher than Carlsbad). Its latitude north is below 50°; its eastern longitude, 12°. It belongs to the Pilsener Kreis (circle), which is chiefly spread over a mountain-plateau, at the foot of which the Tepl arises—a small river, which we have already noticed in its course from the south to the north, through Carlsbad, till it widens and falls into the Eger. Extremely numerous gas and mineral springs are locally connected with layers of peat along its course. Travellers from Eger (twenty-four miles to the west) to Pilsen (in the south-east) have to pass the spa. You see the demesne of Tepl in a due easterly direction (nine miles distant), and Königswarth in the north-west (six miles off). You can enter Marienbad, from the ravine-like opening in the south only—pine and fir-covered mountains forming a towering enclosure from the other sides. In the east the Hamelika rises and mingles with the peak of the Wahrhall, in the north the Mühlberg and Steinhau, and in the west the Schneiderhau. The Hamelika brook, rising at the western declivity of the mountain of the same name, is joined at the extremity of the valley by the Schneiderbach, to form the Auschowitzerbach. The spa is of comparatively recent origin, and the buildings are provided with many modern conveniences. An avenue of poplar-trees leads from the *Kreuzbrunnen* (the chief spring) to the *Carolinenbrunnen*. In the heat of summer many visitors would probably prefer the shade of chestnut or lime trees, but a greater regard to health was displayed by the selection of the present species; as the surrounding mountains deprive this spot of the morning and evening sun, and too much shade might therefore prove undesirable. From the Belvedere, on the Steinhau, the prospect towards the west and south extends as far as the lofty Pfrienberg. Along the banks of the Auschowitzer brook you will find pleasant walks. If you proceed southward, through meadows and green fields, for about two miles, you will observe another spring bubbling up from the fertile ground,—the *Ferdinandesquelle*. The vicarage of Pistan is visited by many, as, from its high position, it affords a magnificent view of the sombre Bohemian forest.

Among the places of resort near Marienbad must be reckoned the Jägerhaus, on the Schneiderrang, near the zoological enclosure of Königswarth, where you can obtain a view of the Eger domains from the Luisenblick. The so-called 'Judenkirchof' (a curious assemblage of stones in an opening of the forest), the monument of Waldstein, and on the Mühlberg, the Friedrichstein and Schweizergang are pointed out. On the Hamelika mountain the Pavilion may be visited, and at its declivity the valley of the Ferdinandsbrunnen, and Böttiger's Ruhe (rest). This frequented spa—so crowded during the height of the season that many must content themselves with very meagre accommodation as regards residence—was a wilderness little more than sixty years ago, only provided with a half-ruined wooden hut, in which two iron caldrons were fixed for the preparation of Glauber's salt (sulphate of soda) out of the Kreuzbrunnen. A rough wooden enclosure of the spring was the only other work of human hands that could be perceived. Not even a footpath led to the spring, which had to be reached by stepping over stones irregularly laid across the numerous bogs and marshy spots. Notwithstanding this difficulty of access, numerous persons visited the spring in summer, and found relief from their ailments by the use of the water; leaving marks of the benefit obtained by writing with chalk, pencil, or charcoal on the wooden boards their names and diseases, with the quantities of water drunk; sometimes even the number of the evacuations was noted down for the edification of the curious. Through the solicitations and partly at the expense of the late Dr. Nehr, the bogs of the environs were drained, and the springs secured.

At the beginning of this century a road was constructed to the little château of Hammerhof (three miles distant). Stagnant waters were led off, hills were dug out, ditches filled up, walks laid on, and, the demand from the frequency of visitors rapidly increasing, new houses and fine buildings arose as promptly as such a limited locality would allow. Thus Dr. Nehr may be considered the creator of Marienbad as a spa.

Its springs present greater variety than those of the therma we have just left. The foremost rank is occupied by the Kreuzbrunnen, bubbling up on the southern declivity of the steep Steinhau from half-efflorescent porphyreous granite. A magnificent colonnade marks its entrance. Only 141 cubic feet of water are furnished in twenty-four hours; but the supply increases in a direct proportion to the quantity of water drawn, more than 300,000 bottles being annually exported. The water is very sparkling, clear, inodorous, and transparent, but exposed to the atmosphere it soon becomes turbid. The taste is acidulous and saline, somewhat bitter; the temperature $53\frac{1}{4}°$ Fahrenheit; specific gravity, 1·0094.

Its solid constituents amount so sixty-six grains in sixteen ounces (a scruple more than Carlsbad), viz. :—

38·11 grains of sulphate of soda (double the quantity in comparison with Carlsbad).
13·56 ,, chloride of sodium (not quite double).
7·13 ,, carbonate of soda.
3·93 ,, carbonate of lime.
2·71 ,, carbonate of magnesia.
0·17 ,, carbonate of iron (only 1·100 of gr. in Carlsbad).
0·03 ,, carbonate of manganese.
0·11 ,, carbonate of lithia.
0·38 ,, silex.
Carbonic acid gas, $8\frac{1}{3}$ cubic inches.

Opposite the Kreuzbrunnen, at the southern end, is situated the *Carolinenbrunnen* (formerly called Neubrunnen), in the centre of an old grove of alder and fir trees. The spring issues out of peat-soil, and is covered by a temple, the cupola resting on eight Corinthian columns. Gas is constantly bubbling up from the opening. The water is sparkling and has an alkaline and ferruginous taste. Some *smell* of sulphuretted hydrogen is perceptible, but not demonstrable by analysis. Its carbonic acid being more firmly adherent, the oxide of iron remains for a longer period unprecipitated than is the case with the Kreuzbrunnen. Its solid ingredients are only $14\frac{1}{4}$ grains in sixteen ounces, being less than one-fourth of the Kreuzbrunnen, viz. :—

2·79 grains of sulphate of soda.
0·82 ,, chloride of sodium.
0·20 ,, carbonate of soda.
3·66 ,, carbonate of lime.
3·94 ,, carbonate of magnesia.
0·44 ,, carbonate of iron (nearly three times as much as the Kreuzbrunnen).
0·46 ,, silica.
0·38 ,, extractive substance.
Carbonic acid, 15·43 cubic inches (nearly twice as much as Kreuzbrunnen).
Specific gravity, 1·0031.

The *Ambrosiusbrunnen* rises about seventy yards to the south of the Carolinenbrunnen, and has a more agreeable piquant taste. It contains only $10\frac{1}{2}$ grains of solid constituents in sixteen ounces (one sixth of Kreuzbrunnen), viz:—

1·86 grains of sulphate of soda.
1·64 ,, chloride of sodium.
1·66 ,, carbonate of soda.
2·89 ,, carbonate of lime.
2·72 ,, carbonate of magnesia.
0·34 ,, carbonate of iron (twice as much as Krenzbrunnen, but less than Carolinenbrunnen).
0·48 ,, silica.
Carbonic acid, 12·9 cubic inches (less than Carolinenbrunnen).
Specific gravity, 1·0023.

About 100 steps from the Ambrosiusbrunnen, the *Marienbrunnen or Badequelle* arises in the peat-soil. The abundant evolution of carbonic-acid gas keeps up a constant hissing sound. The layer of gas spread over the surface of the water is highest before sunrise, lowest at noon, and then increases again towards the evening. It expands in rainy weather, and decreases when the sky is serene. In a very humid state of the atmosphere, the gas reaches as far as the upper boarding ($5\frac{1}{2}$ feet above the level of the water). The carbonic acid is firmly adherent. The water contains only $1\frac{3}{4}$ grains of solid constituents in sixteen ounces, viz.,—about 1-3rd of a grain of sulphate of soda, 1-25th chloride of sodium, nearly $\frac{1}{2}$ carbonate of lime, 3-100ths carbonate of iron, &c., and nine cubic inches of carbonic acid.

After the Kreuzbrunnen, Ferdinandsbrunnen, as already mentioned, claims the highest remedial powers. It arises at about a mile from Marienbad, in a meadow near the left bank of the Auschowitzerbach, and it appears that at some remote period attempts were made to extract salt out of this spring. When dug up, granite nearly efflorescent was found to compose the bed of the water, whilst bubbles of carbonic-acid gas continually issued in great abundance. The supply amounts to 2,900 cubic feet in twenty-four hours. The water sparkles continually when drawn, and holds the carbonic acid so firmly, that even when boiled it will redden litmus-paper. Its taste is piquant, and rather saline; specific gravity, 1·0046. Its solid ingredients amount to 45¾ grains in sixteen ounces (a scruple less than Kreuzbrunnen), viz. :—

22·53 grains of sulphate of soda ⎫
8·99 ,, chloride of sodium ⎬ less than Kreuzbrunnen.
6·13 ,, carbonate of soda ⎭
4·01 ,, carbonate of lime ⎫
3·04 ,, carbonate of magnesia ⎬ more than Kreuzbrunnen.
0·39 ,, carbonate of iron ⎭
0·09 ,, carbonate of manganese.
Carbonate of lithia, 6-100ths.
0·66 silica,
Carbonic acid, 13¾ cubic inches (5 more than Kreuzbrunnen).

Lastly, we have to visit the Waldquelle (forest-spring), at the west of the Kreuzbrunnen, which contains 22 grains of solid ingredients in sixteen ounces (one-third of Kreuzbrunnen),—viz., 5¾ of sulphate of soda; 2 of sulphate of potash (not possessed by another); 2¼ of chloride of sodium; 6 of carbonate of soda; 2¼ of carbonate of lime; $2\frac{9}{10}$ of carbonate of magnesia; no iron; 1-10th carbonate of manganese; more than ½ a grain of silica, and 18¾ cubic inches of carbonic-acid gas. It supplies 37 cubic feet of water in twenty-four hours.

The temperature of all the springs ranges between 47° and 53° Fahrenheit. The Wiesenquelle, near the Ferdinandsbrunnen, is hardly ever employed. Another important healing agent is furnished by the layers of peat found at a great depth behind the bathing-house of the Marienbrunnen. It consists of a brown, bituminous, unctuous mass, intermixed with decomposed vegetable fibre. Sulphates of soda, of lime, and magnesia, with chloride of sodium, oxide of iron, silica, and sand form its chief constituents. The peat is now also brought to the place from the Stänkerhau. After merely removing the grosser admixture of sand and small stones, it is used for mud-baths.

The abundance of the carbonic acid flowing out of the soil in these vast strata of peat lead to the construction of gas-baths, employed either for the whole body, where the patient sits dressed in the gas-basin, with only his head in the ordinary atmosphere— (the penetration of the gas to the epidermis is not obstructed in the slightest degree by the pervious clothes)—or streams of gas are applied locally by elastic tubes, communicating with the gas-reservoir, and held to the mouth, ears, eyes, or otherwise affected parts of the body. Ordinary baths of the heated mineral waters are likewise used. Douche and rain baths are also well contrived and frequently employed.

Marienbad owes its virtues chiefly to the sulphate of soda, and is indicated in plethora, and for persons of luxurious habits. But why should simple purgatives not exercise similarly favourable results? For this reason: they certainly increase the peristaltic motion, and discharge offensive substances; but they also cause a greater quantity of serum to be excreted from the surface of the alimentary tube.

However useful and indispensable a purgative may prove in many instances, a course of purgatives would never be thought of as a remedy for producing beneficial alterative results. The case is quite different if we employ a remedy whose chief agent exerts a peculiarly stimulating influence on the action of the liver, producing greenish, mucous, and fetid evacuations, with distinct evidence of a more than ordinary excretion of bilious matter, while copious serous purgation is avoided through the presence of silica and iron.

The lengthened contact of the dissolved ingredients with the intestinal fibres being thus effected, the subordinate quantity of chloride of sodium finds time to exert its beneficial action on the nutrient organs, whilst the carbonates of soda and of lime assist in preventing the formation of too abundant an acidity in the circulating fluid, and thus *improve* the renal and hepatic action—the latter having been merely increased by the Glauber-salt. Muscular exercise always attending the course of the water, a more active general circulation contributes likewise to counteract too great a stagnation of the portal circulation. Whilst Carlsbad acts, therefore, as a more powerful solvent, and as a more penetrating and lasting stimulant on the liver, skin, and kidneys, Marienbad is the more energetic and exclusive provocator of biliary excretion and of alvine secretions, and is applicable in cases of vascular erethism or local congestion, where the former would be fraught with danger.

From the above you will perceive that I strongly deprecate encouragement of excessive and continuous evacuations, and would advise discontinuance of the course, or decrease of the dose, if such should take place during the use of the water. On the other hand, non-increase of alvine action, or even obstruction (occasionally happening under the influence of Marienbad), should not be allowed to continue. Heating the water will increase its purgative action. Its employment in the form of clysters affords likewise powerful assistance. The separate springs exhibit different properties in relation to the difference of their composition. The Kreuzbrunnen increases the action of all the abdominal organs, and therefore promotes the digestive function and bilious excretion, whilst its carbonic acid increases the nervous tone. Dyspepsia and venous dyscrasia, with all their protean consequences, strongly indicate its employment; acidity, hypochondriasis, hysteria, enlargement of the liver, and morbid bilification all belong to this category. The Ferdinandsbrunnen, with a smaller quantity of sulphate and other salts of soda, and with a greater proportion of lime, magnesia, silica, and iron, naturally acts as a less solvent remedy, and is more indicated when the tone of the secreting organs is to be roused from great torpor, and when the uropoietic system is chiefly to be acted upon. It forms, as it were, the transition from the highly solvent Kreuzbrunnen to the purer tonic, the Carolinenbrunnen, which latter, by possessing nearly half a grain of iron in 16 ounces, with a very small quantity of solvent salts, displays its action more in the vascular system —increasing the tone and resisting power of the circulating fluid, and thus improving the general state of the nervous system; in fact, it is indicated where steel and other tonics are required. Ambrosiusquelle is somewhat inferior to the latter in effect, but quite analogous in its mode of action. The Marienquelle, with its abundance of gas, chiefly used for bathing, induces on entering the bath a sensation of chilliness, which soon gives way to increased heat and circulation over the whole epidermis, with subsequently improved nutrition. These baths are particularly useful in arthritic and rheumatico-paralytic affections, connected with hepatic and intestinal infarcta, or with torpor. The Waldquelle, the only spring which contains sulphate of potash and no iron, with a very considerable amount of carbonic acid, is frequently drunk with warm milk or whey, in chronic pulmonary and vesical catarrh, and in hysteric spasms and vomiting. The importance of potash and magnesia has been proved by the investigations of Liebig, who found that potash and chloride of potassium prevailed in the liquid of the flesh, with magnesia as its predominant earth; whilst soda and chloride of sodium preponderate in the blood, with lime as the predominating earth. The gas and peat baths are powerful supporters of the curative action of the springs, but they also exercise independent properties of their own, belonging to the inherent stimulus of carbonic acid on the peripheric nervous system, and of the peat on the plastic and glandular organs. The gas contains, in 1,000 volumes, 74 of nitrogen, and 26 of oxygen—the rest is carbonic acid; its temperature is rather lower than that of the atmosphere. The incident which led to the separate employment of the gas-baths is too remarkable to be omitted. The same *Dr. Struve*, whom I mentioned in my first lecture as the most successful imitator of the natural springs, and as the originator of the so-called Brighton Pump-room, experienced the result of the first trial in his own person. For many years his left leg was frequently the seat of violent pains, along the course of the ischiatic nerve, from the hip-joint downwards. The chief cause was congelation, of such intensity that the limb was only preserved with difficulty; he also partly ascribed the evil to inhalation of hydrocyanic acid during his chemical operations, which so often induces paralysis of the lower extremities. Torpidity of the lymphatic system was connected with these sufferings. The whole leg, particularly the tibial part, was covered with numerous hardened glands. The lymphatic vessels had the appearance of distended blood-vessels; nutrition was also considerably impaired, the left leg being more than half an inch thinner than the right one. Every little exertion increased the pains, and produced exhaustion. At last he could not walk without a stick, and often required the arm of another person to support him. The portal system was likewise affected. A considerable swelling of the liver had been happily cured the year before (1817), but the left hepatic lobe was still distended. Under these circumstances, he put his trust in the solvent constituents of the Kreuzbrunnen, and in the animating power of the Marienbad, besides using fomentations with warmed peat. For ten days he had employed these three remedial means without perceptible relief. He therefore resolved on making the first trial with the gas-bath. With difficulty and pain, and with the support of his servant, he was conducted over the small hills and declivities to the Marienbrunnen. The suffering leg, denuded only of the boot, was now exposed to the effervescing gas covering the surface of the water. The introduction of a light indicated the exact height of the gas-layer, and its line of demarcation, by its extinction. The first sensation was that of chill. Soon, however, an agreeable warmth took its place, with a peculiar sensation as of ants creeping along the larger nervous ramifications, somewhat analogous to the beginning action of a mustard-poultice. After thirty minutes he withdrew the leg and supported it with a bandage. He began the way back with his habitual precaution, and trust to support. 'But,' he says, 'who could picture the intense joy and gratitude that overpowered me when I discovered, by every new step, that power had returned to the weakened leg, and that the uninterrupted gnawing pain had left it! With agility I walked unassisted over spaces which would have been a work of impossibility an hour ago.' But these blessings of an experimental attempt were not transitory; they still continued for a fortnight after the first trial. The daily repetition of the gas-bath produced invariably the sensations described. Dr. Struve continued these baths for three weeks longer, in conjunction with the internal use of the Kreuzbrunnen and the local application of moor-earth. He then left the spa completely cured. Ever since the gas-baths have been frequently employed. During the use of the mud-baths, Dr. Wetzler observed the skin to become momentarily contracted, and its susceptibility blunted. He had himself suffered from a disagreeable and sometimes painful sensation of the thighs, of rheumatic origin. Neither saline nor steel-baths could relieve the evil, which yielded after the first mud-bath. They are particularly recommended in erethic atony of the epidermis, in tendency to profuse perspiration, great susceptibility towards atmospheric changes, &c. Marienbad is INAPPLICABLE in real digestive weakness, in general atony, whether resulting from loss of blood or from exhausting diseases; in cerebral congestion, internal suppuration, hectic fever, inflammation of internal organs, carcinoma, atonic ulcers, scorbutic dyscrasia, &c. Carlsbad offers such important points of analogy and difference, that it becomes necessary to carefully discriminate between the two, in many given cases which apparently belong to the sphere of action of both. First, we have to take the difference of temperature into consideration. The high temperature of Carlsbad at once excludes all patients of plethoric tendency, with vascular erethism, that may be benefited by the colder springs of Marienbad. Next we have to consider the presence of a larger quantity of iron in the latter as a greater promoter of sanguineous plasticity and reproduction. The larger amount of liquefying sulphate of soda (nearly twice as much) renders Marienbad applicable in cases of abdominal plethora, with a sanguineous constitution, where we should have to avoid Carlsbad. On the other hand, the greater proportion of carbonate of soda and of lime gives the latter more power in renal diseases (as lithiasis, &c.), whilst its heat assists the action on the cutaneous system, counteracts disorders resulting from repelled exanthemata, or from rheumatic and arthritic causes. Carlsbad being invariably useful whenever improved nutrition and circulation of the sero-fibrous or portal system are especially requisite, it stands unequalled in inveterate hepatic induration, gallstones, &c.--in fact, when a more thoroughly penetrating action is desired. But when abdominal secretion and excretion have to be *chiefly* promoted, when hepatic and alvine torpor have to be roused, Marienbad will find its appropriate employment; though we are unable to determine whether its remarkable efficacy be due to a mere mechanical increase of peristaltic motion, or whether the sulphates, particularly of soda, tend to decarbonise the blood by yielding oxygen to its carbon for the formation of carbonic acid on the one hand, whereby the blood becomes partially arterialised, and its circulating force stimulated, whilst sulphuretted hydrogen may be produced on the other, and exert a beneficial action on the ganglionic-nervous plexus. For if, under the influence of vital heat, soda and sulphuric acid allow part of their oxygen to become absorbed by the carbon, we may expect that the newly-produced carbonic acid strives to enter into combination with part of the free sodium. This latter must therefore decompose the water of the gastric juice, and, attracting its oxygen to become carbonate of soda, it encourages the hydrogen to enter into combination with the portion of the deoxidised sulphur, and thus free sulphuretted hydrogen would be accounted for. If we do not generally observe the peculiar effects of sulphuretted hydrogen by the ordinary administration of sulphate of soda as a purgative, this is easily explained by rapid elimination of the remedy with the fæcal impurities. But when a more lengthened contact with the gastric contents affords a greater opportunity for development of chemical attraction, and for interchange of substances according to stronger affinities, with chemico-vital modifications, such a result is highly probable.

Carlsbad containing nearly 2-100ths of a grain of iodine (0·017) may owe part of its solvent power to this ingredient; for scrofulous complications do not contra-indicate its use, but, on the contrary, they are frequently combated by the spa. To sum up, you have to select Carlsbad when the general vitality has to be roused, in persons not devoid of a certain amount of organic vigour, which, however, requires to be coaxed into action; whilst you have to give the preference to Marienbad when general irritability has to be allayed by concentrating a greater focus of action in the abdominal organs. In combating the alvine hyperæmic condition, you will cause the general orgasm to be diminished, and the equilibrium between the sensitive and irritable organic sphere to be restored. *Physicians:* Dr. Frankl, Dr. Opitz, Dr. Herzig, Dr. Schneider, Dr. Lucca, Dr. Kratzmann, Dr. Wolfner, Dr. Kisch, and Dr. Porges.

Franzensbad.—Starting from Marienbad, at 10.25 A.M., the diligence arrives after nearly five hours at Franzensbad (latitude N. above 50°, longitude E. 12°), which you see situated on the north-west, at a distance of twenty miles, 1,500 feet above the level of the sea. The most remarkable place you pass on your road is the town of Eger, on the right bank of the Eger River, one league to the south of the spa. The whole district is called the Egerland, forming the north-western part of Bohemia, near the Bavarian and Saxon boundary. In the town-house of Eger, which is replete with antiquarian curiosities, the halberd is shown with which the celebrated Wallenstein was pierced in 1634, and whose fate forms the subject of the beautiful drama by the immortal Schiller. In speaking of these regions, Goethe says:—' If Bohemia be considered as a large valley, relieved of its waters at Aussig, on the Elbe, the district of Eger may be imagined as a smaller one, which discharges its waters into the river of its own name.' This spot is impacted as it were in an obtuse mountainous angle, the Fichtelgebirg forming the corner, with the Erzgebirg as its superior and the Bohemian forest as its inferior line. *Baireuth* lies forty miles distant to the west, *Hof* thirty to the north-west, and Carlsbad the same distance to the north-east. The encircling mountains consist of primary rocks, with the exception of the easterly Kulmerberg, which is composed of sandstone and slate-clay. The plain exhibits the character of alluvial land. Towards the north you see Teplitz, which enjoys rather more than half the altitude of Carlsbad, being situated near the termination of the Erz mountain-branch that commenced at Franzensbad. Afterwards the Eger falls into the *Elbe*, near Leitmeritz, between Dresden in the north and Prague in the south. As early as the seventeenth century the town of Eger was visited by very high personages, on account of the neighbouring mineral sources. From Eger a very cheerful road, bordered with shady trees, leads to Franzensbad. Passing through a very tastefully laid-out park-like walk, you perceive the Franzensquelle at your left, with its temple-shaped enclosure, and the contiguous colonnade and Curhaus. On the right the Salzquelle (salt-spring) meets your eye, the newly-built packing-house, and the pavilion with the gas-baths. You are now in the so-called Kaiserstrasse, adorned on both sides with chestnut trees, and containing the best habitations of the place. A small park forms the end of the street. The Kammerbühl mountain, a short distance from Eger, with the characteristics of a former volcano, will afford the visitors a beautiful perspective of the environs. Walks to the neighbouring villages of Unter and Oberlohna, Oberndorf, Langenbruck, &c., furnish ample opportunities for pedestrian exercise.

The most renowned of the springs, the *Franzensbrunnen*, yields 275 cubic inches of water per minute. Its temperature is $52\frac{1}{4}°$ Fahrenheit, its specific gravity 1·0058. Small gas-bubbles constantly rise, and cause an undulating motion of the water, which is clear and transparent even for a long time after exposure to the atmosphere.

This spring shows a very intrinsic combination of its constituents. It possesses a refreshing, piquant, and acidulous taste, with some after-taste of iron. The surface of the water is constantly covered with a considerable layer of carbonic-acid gas. The brunnen contains $42\frac{1}{4}$ grains of solid ingredients in 16 ounces (one scruple less than Kreuzbrunnen of Marienbad), viz.—

24·50 grains of sulphate of soda (14 gr. less than Marienbad).
9·23 ,, chloride of sodium (4 gr. less).
5·18 ,, carbonate of soda (2 gr. less).
0·67 ,, carbonate of magnesia (2 gr. less).
1·80 ,, carbonate of lime (2 gr. less).
0·23 ,, carbonate of iron (nearly $\frac{1}{4}$ of a gr. 6-100ths more).
0·47 ,, silex (one-tenth more).

Besides 2-100ths of phosphate of lime, 1-100th phosphate of alumina, 3-100ths carbonate of lithia, 4-100ths carbonate of manganese, 3-1000ths carbonate of strontia, and 40 cubic inches of carbonic acid (five times as much as Kreuzbrunnen), with a distinctly perceptible odour of sulphuretted hydrogen gas. The *Louisenquelle* issues in a north-westerly direction from the latter, in a peat-meadow, and is, properly speaking, a combination of several confluent springs. It has less depth than the Franzensquelle. Constant motion from the turbulent gas-bubbles is likewise observed here. The water appears rather more turbid in the basin : but when drawn, it is clear, transparent, and sparkling. Exposed to the atmosphere, it resists decomposition for even a longer period than the above-mentioned spring. Its chief employment being external, for common baths and mud-baths, I shall content myself with stating, as regards its analysis, that it contains 7 grains less in 16 ounces than the Franzensbrunnen (viz. 35¾ grains), the various ingredients observing analogous proportions, with the sole exception of iron, which it possesses to a greater amount (0·23). Its carbonic acid is likewise less by 8 cubic inches (viz. 32). A few steps to the north of the Louisenquelle will bring you to the '*Kalte Sprudel*' (cold bubbler), so called in contradistinction to the hot Sprudel of Carlsbad, whose heat occupies three-fourths of the thermometric range between the ordinary freezing and boiling points. The constant evolution of gas causes such a violent hissing sound, that it has been invested with the name of Sprudel—rather inappropriately, in my opinion, for a distinct rising and falling of the water-column cannot be observed. When drawn the water is perfectly clear and transparent, and able to resist for a long period the decomposing influence of the atmosphere. It exhibits a pricking acidulous taste, with a saltish after-taste; the odour of sulphuretted hydrogen is strongly marked. The layer of gas covering the surface of the water sometimes reaches to the height of several feet. This spring is used both for drinking and bathing. It contains 44½ grains of solid ingredients in 16 ounces—(two more than the Franzensquelle). It possesses 2 gr. more of sulphate of soda, ½ a gr. less of chloride of sodium, 2 gr. more of carbonate of soda, 3-100ths less of iron, and 1 cubic inch less of carbonic acid; in all other respects the two are similarly constituted.

The *Salzquelle* (salt-spring), to the east of Franzensbrunnen, exhibits a gently alkaline taste, without any astringency. It contains 4 grs. less of solid ingredients than the Franzensquelle (38¼ grs.), 3 less of sulphate of soda, ½ gr. less of chloride of sodium, 2 less of carbonate of soda, rather less carbonate of lime, and only 7-100ths of carbonate of iron; carbonic acid only 26¾ cubic inches (14 cubic inches less). The *Wiesenquelle*, to the southeast of the Salzquelle, contains 46¼ gr. of solid ingredients in 16 ounces (but only 4-100ths of iron). The *Gasquelle* (gas source), formerly known under the denomination of *Polterbrunnen*, evolves pure carbonic acid gas in great abundance, with one per cent. of hydrothionic acid, and is employed for douches, local, and general baths. The strata of peat occupy a great extent near Franzensbad. Within the peat-soil, blackish-brown mud is found impacted in the neighbourhood of the springs, of a fine, soft, and unctuous consistence. If moistened, it spreads a sulphurous odour. The peat is carefully cleaned through a sieve, and then mixed with the water of the Louisenquelle, either for local application or for general baths.

You find in the springs nearly the same constituents as in Kreuzbrunnen of Marienbad; but the inferior amount of Glauber-salt induces a less lowering and antiplastic action, the diminished proportion of chloride of sodium a less solvent power; whilst its greater proportion of iron, silica, and carbonic acid stamps it as a highly valuable, gently-stimulating tonic, displaying its chief sphere of action on the ganglionic nervous system. The happy combination of ingredients promises us increased alvine peristaltic motion, improved biliary and renal excretion, restoration of stagnant or otherwise abnormal portal circulation, without the weakening and exhausting secondary results we might have to fear in some instances, from the fully-developed effects of an energetic course of the sulphates of Marienbad, or of the thermal watery impregnations of Carlsbad. On the other hand, we must consider that the very large amount of carbonic acid which accompanies the curative ingredients here, imparts to them a more dynamic effect, relying for the production of the critical changes more on the roused vital forces than on the chemical changes resulting from the penetration of the more highly-charged Marienbad, or the heated and more violently-acting Carlsbad-water. This must not be considered as depreciating the two latter: on the contrary, the exact knowledge of the primary and secondary effects of each will enable us better to select in various morbid modifications. Franzensbad acts specifically in similar diseases as Marienbad; the whole distinction merely refers to the individuality of the respective patients. If, for instance, you have a torpid, bloated, icteric European, who has been subjected to lengthened attacks of intermittent fever in a tropical climate, and now remains tormented by hepatic or splenetic physconia, with all the signs of abdominal inaction, and without decided inflammatory or congestive symptoms, Carlsbad is alone able to bring about a happy result. But suppose a florid muscular person, of middle age, suffers from indigestion, hepatic engorgement, inaction of the bowels, hæmorrhoidal congestion, or from any of the numerous evils due to luxurious and sedentary living without corresponding muscular exercise, Marienbad will be unsurpassed by any other spa. A third individual presents himself to you, with similar hypochondriacal derangement, but he neither suffers from sequelæ of intermittent fever, nor does he seem to possess a large amount of organic materials of resistance; he probably owes his intestinal derangement to an excessive pursuit of study or business, or to overburdening mental depression; his temper is irritable, his cares and fears constantly surround him, he feels often chilly, particularly at his hands and feet, want of animation being stamped on his whole appearance; for him you have to choose Franzensbad as the most appropriate spring. Of course the many varieties of adjuvants in the three spas must not be left out of our consideration, but the respective chief efficacy of each will be most strikingly unfolded in the described individualities. Franzensbrunnen has the special property of improving digestion and increasing the appetite. Acidity, mucosity, and biliary obstruction are powerfully counteracted, hæmorrhoidal and menstrual flux are promoted if previously suppressed; blennorrhages of the rectum, bladder, and vagina likewise frequently yield to the water. The spa is frequently employed after very solvent and weakening courses, as an after-cure, with great benefit. In fact, it holds a high and undisputed rank in such diseases and conditions in which a pure chalybeate would be indicated, if abdominal venosity and hyperæmia did not require a special remedial complex action. The spa is injurious in plethora, inflammatory diathesis, or inflammation of internal organs, congestion to the brain or other vital viscera, diseases of the heart, induration or suppuration of internal organs; generally speaking, excitable, sanguineous, and erethic constitutions are less benefited here than the chlorotic, lax, phlegmatic, and torpid.

The Salzquelle varies in some respects from the Franzensbrunnen, being less stimulating (through the smaller proportion of iron). Its action on the urinary secretion and excretion is particularly marked; it greatly diminishes increased systemic sensibility and irritability. The Kalte Sprudel, containing more sulphate and carbonate of soda than the above springs, excels in the promotion of all abdominal secretions and excretions, and ought to be employed in preference whenever a more penetrating and solvent action is required; but no vascular orgasm must be present. In many instances, before drinking, a part of the carbonic acid is allowed to diffuse itself, so as not to cause too powerful a stimulation. If the spa be employed as an after-cure, the Salzquelle, as the least exciting, is used first, then succeeded by the Kalte Sprudel, and the course closed with the Franzensquelle. The internal use of the water is powerfully assisted by the baths. The great utility of the gas and peat in many forms of local and general application has already been mentioned.

The constitution of the latter informs you of its highly solvent and tonic properties, wherein it excels that of Marienbad. The sensation caused by a peat-bath is, in my opinion, the most pleasurable that can possibly be excited by any bath. The warm, unctuous, elastic medium gives support, and yields at the same time to our moving limbs. However forbidding the black-broth may look, if you are once seated in the baignoire, the agreeably titillating effect exercised by the semiliquid mass on the peripheric ends of the nerves is extremely agreeable, and you leave it with regret, abridging the luxurious immersion by being warned of the danger connected with a too great prolongation. The stay is gradually increased from a quarter of an hour to an hour. A warm-water bath stands near the other in the same room, and serves to relieve you of the adherent black mass. If you inspect yourselves in the looking-glass after leaving the peat-bath, you may well be frightened by the altered being you behold. After immersion in the water-bath, you observe the skin to have become wrinkled and loosened, as it were, just as if it had become too wide a covering for the body. Increase of appetite may be reckoned upon as an invariable follower of the moor-bath. How useful these baths must prove in excessive perspiration through cutaneous atony, in repelled eruptions, in arthritic and rheumatic disorders, &c., is too obvious to require further allusion. It is desirable, even in cases of completed cure, at Carlsbad, at least after very inveterate and chronic diseases, that the patient should not expose himself to all his former injurious influences by an immediate return home, but that he should rather pass some weeks at Franzensbad, strengthening his health, and guarding it against possible relapse. Though the intrinsic adherence of carbonic acid peculiarly fits the Franzensbad springs for exportation (which annually increases all over the Continent), they are but rarely to be met with in this country, whilst many indications must be furnished for their employment. The imported water acts more as a solvent (by the partial precipitation of iron) than as a tonic, and is therefore very useful in abdominal infarcta and portal obstruction. Where circumstances prevent patients from visiting Franzensbad as an after-cure, they might with great advantage drink the water at their homes, either pure or with wine and sugar, according to the required efficacy. Hufeland speaks of *Frederick the Great* having been freed from a dangerous disease by the use of the Eger water (the former name of Franzensbrunnen), which he then continued annually for the preservation of his health. In 1822—this physician says in his 'Journal of Practical Medicine'—' Men of business or learning, who had been fixed to the writing-table the whole year, and had contracted dyspepsia, abdominal obstruction, hæmorrhoidal or arthritic tendency, were formerly in the habit here in Berlin of using the Franzensbrunnen for four weeks, with a great deal of exercise in the open air, and relaxation from the usual mental exertion. By this annual course they freed themselves from the accumulated morbific matter, and became strengthened for the next year's labours. Thus, notwithstanding injurious influences, many were able to preserve their health to a very great age, and prevent the development of various diseases, by which they might otherwise have been afflicted.' Drs. Cartellieri, Koestler, Palliardi, Boschan, Sommer, Komma, Neidhardt, Meissle, Fürst, &c. are the physicians of Franzensbad.

LECTURE X.

KISSINGEN—BOCKLET.

THE springs now coming under our consideration are called *Halopegæ*, saline springs (from ἅλς salt, and πηγή spring). They generally issue from secondary strata—either from rocksalt, through which they pass, or from the salt strata of the zechstone, of gypsum or variegated sandstone; or, if of alkaline character, out of corresponding volcanic formations, as basalt, lava containing fluor-spar, &c. Their taste varies according to the secondary constituents present, being either saltish or bitterish, astringent, alkaline, or ferruginous. Combinations of chlorine with sodium, magnesium, or calcium form the chief ingredients. In some no perceptible quantity of gas is discovered; in others, carbonic acid, nitrogen, carburetted hydrogen, or common air is admixed—rarely sulphuretted hydrogen. If hot, they are named *Halothermæ* (from ἅλς salt, and θερμὸς hot). Possessing a smaller quantity of saline ingredients (though these are more thoroughly amalgamated), they have a less saline taste and odour, rather resembling weak chicken-broth somewhat oversalted. The cold saline springs, *Halokrenæ* (from ἅλς salt, and κρήνη cold spring), often acquire a piquant and refreshing taste, and a sparkling appearance, from the great quantity of carbonic acid present, which exhibits an action analogous to that of heat in the complete solution and unity of the ingredients. *Salt-springs* and *Salt-lixiviæ* (*Soolen, Salzlaugen*) do not properly belong to the mineral springs, but from their medicinal use we should not omit to mention them in this place. They are more often the products of evaporated saline springs than natural sources. Their specific gravity generally exceeds 1·050; their temperature is low, their taste too nauseous and acrid to be used for drinking or bathing without dilution with another less impregnated water. Their constituents differ from those of the Halopegæ merely in quantity. Minute proportions of *iodine* and *bromine* are contained in nearly all spas of this class. These important ingredients assume a predominant rank in some, and stamp them with the name and character of *Iodepegæ* (iodine springs). We ought perhaps not to pass over the representative of all saline waters—viz., the mighty ocean, with its green colour, its disagreeably bitter and saltish taste, its peculiar aromatic odour, and its specific gravity, ranging between 1·026 and 1·029; with a more constant and moderate temperature than that of the air, and with a quantity of solid ingredients, amounting to 330 grains in some instances, and in others to less than a fourth of that quantity. Inland seas have a diminished amount of solid ingredients, and a correspondingly lower specific gravity. Besides the chlorides of sodium, magnesium, and calcium, invariably present, we meet with sulphates of these bases, some iodine or bromine, and organic matter.

The springs of this class widely differ in their medicinal qualities from the former. They chiefly act on the mucous membranes, which they stimulate to greater activity. The influence of chloride of sodium on the alimentary canal has been too often alluded to already, to require further remark here. Its presence in the saliva shows that it is necessary for the proper performance of the digestive function; its chlorine maintaining the acidity of the gastric juice by the formation of hydrochloric acid with the hydrogen of the liquid, whilst the disengaged sodium appropriates to itself the other element of water (oxygen), and exerts, as soda, a liquefying power on albuminous productions, preparing them for assimilation or elimination. Soda being the chief alkali of serum, the fluidity of the blood circulating in the abdominal vessels becomes promoted by the use of these saline waters, and thus stagnations and obstructions in the portal system are removed. Reflux of venous blood towards the central organ of circulation being facilitated, the arterial movements must become proportionally invigorated, and thus we see organic reproduction considerably improved under their influence. Persons of weakly or irritable constitutions, inclined to disorders of the lymphatic or sero-fibrous systems, are particularly benefited by them. The laxity of fibre and the torpor of nerve, produced by weakening diseases or exhausting excesses, likewise claim the powerful aid of the Halopegæ. The chloride of calcium and magnesium, though only present in a subordinate quantity, exercise a peculiar alterative action on the composition of the organic solids. They will not increase mucous secretion or peristaltic motion, but rather overstimulate and retard alvine excretions after some time. This will furnish a useful indication whenever the abdominal excretions are carried to excess, and of course a counter-indication in the opposite case. The additional presence of carbonates of alkalies will check any excessive formation of acidity, beneficially influencing renal and biliary secretion, and thus helping to remove impediments to normal chylification and nutrition.

Let us now leave Bohemia, with its triangular plains and encircling hills, and seek the kingdom of Bavaria. Leaving Franzensbad at 3·45 P. M. for the north-westerly town of *Hof*, about thirty miles distance, you arrive in six hours. From Hof the train carries you rapidly through *Bamberg* to *Schweinfurt*, and from here the diligence takes you in 2¾ hours to *Kissingen*.

Kissingen, on the Fränkishe Saale, stands 600 feet above the level of the sea (100 above the surface of the Maine at Würzburg, lat. N. 50°, long. E. 10°), in a fertile and charming valley surrounded by orchards and mountains. Würzburg is twelve leagues distant to the south, and Brückenau six to the north. The course of the river indicates the direction of the valley from north to south. The surrounding mountains consist of stratified lime and sandstone, joining in the north the basalt mountains of the Rhön. The extensive salt and graduation works are reached by a pleasant walk of about a mile to the north of the town. Somewhat farther in the north the elevated *Kreuzberg*, with its towering peak, closes the valley.

Towards the south the valley is terminated by the Scheinberg, which is clothed with rich vineyards on its southern declivity. In the north-west rises the *Staffelberg*, the highest of the encircling mountains, covered to its very summit with vines and ancient oaks. From the ruins of the citadel of *Bodenlaube*, on the Steigberg mountain opposite, you have a very interesting view of many castles and picturesque spots of the environs. Towards the east the valley is widened by the flattening of the mountains. A green vale stretches itself hence for about a mile and a half—having a forest of fir-trees rising upon the mountain ridge on the right, and the vine-clad Sinnberg on the left—as far as Winkels, a pretty village studded with fruit-trees, and bordered by hills clothed again with high firs, rising above the vineyards. Thus you look upon a fine landscape, where oak and fir-covered mountains alternate with meadow-plains, vineyards, and abundant orchards, intersected by the serpentine course of the River Saale. The salt-works claim great antiquity. Tacitus is quoted as having made the following allusion to the saline character of the place:—
' In the same summer the Hermunduri and Catti fought a great battle, each wishing to obtain by force a frontier river blessed by the production of salt. Besides the habit of settling all disputes by arms, they were actuated by the religious belief that this region

was particularly near heaven, and that the prayers of mortals were nowhere nearer fulfilment.'

The springs are situated to the south of the town, on the left bank of the Saale. The '*Max*,' or '*Sauerbrunnen*,' lies opposite the 'Curhaus,' in an oval deepening of the 'Curgarten,' to which we have to descend a few steps. This spring issues out of fissures in sandstone rock, with a temperature of 52° F. The water is as clear as crystal, with an agreeably acidulous pungent taste. Numerous air-bubbles constantly rise and burst on the surface, with a hissing noise. It contains $30\frac{1}{2}$ grains of solid ingredients in 16 ounces, and 31 cubic inches of carbonic-acid gas, but no iron. The *Ragoczy*, or Curbrunnen, the most renowned of the springs, rises nearest the Saale, to the south of the Maxbrunnen, in a recess surrounded by stone balustrades, and accessible by steps from four sides. It does not issue from sandstone rock, like the former, but from layers of basalt and sandstone, with a temperature of $52\frac{1}{4}°$ Fahr. The hissing noise occasioned by the rising and bursting gas-bubbles may be heard at a distance. The water is clear and sparkling; the taste saline, bitterish, and slightly astringent. It is only used for drinking. It contains no less than $85\frac{1}{2}$ grains of solid ingredients in 16 ounces; and in this respect surpasses all the springs we have yet had under our consideration (with exception of the bitter waters). Chloride of sodium forms three-fourths of these ingredients, which contain besides more than half a grain of bromide of magnesium (7-10ths) and of carbonate of iron (6-10ths), with twenty-six cubic inches of carbonic-acid gas. The curious name of Ragoczy is said to be derived from that of a Croatian officer who first drank from this healing water, which was discovered in 1738, in the dry bed of the Saale, upon the river being diverted from the 'Curhaus.'

Its neighbour, *Pandur* or Badebrunnen (bathing spring), received its name, according to the same authority, from a more humble origin—viz., from the domestic of M. Ragoczy, who happened to be a Pandurian. It has a subterranean connection with the Rakoczi, and issues out of the same rocky mass, with a temperature of $52\frac{1}{4}°$ Fahr. Its flavour is more saline and less agreeable than that of Rakoczi. It contains 76 grains of solid ingredients in 16 ounces, nearly ten less than its neighbour, but rather more carbonic acid (28 cubic inches). Its constituents maintain the same proportion throughout as those of Rakoczi, though on a slightly diminished scale (bromide of magnesium, 6-10ths; carbonate of iron, 4-10ths; culinary salt, 57 grains).

The *Theresienbrunnen* issues from a deep bore-hole at a somewhat greater distance northwards, about two English miles. The water sparkles very strongly, and assumes a whitish appearance, from the quickly-rising gas-bubbles. Its taste is acidulous, saline, and rather piquant. It exhibits much analogy to the Maxbrunnen, containing $29\frac{1}{2}$ grains of solid constituents, and $28\frac{1}{3}$ cubic inches of carbonic acid. (It possesses no iron, but some bromide of sodium.)

Ascending northwards from Kissingen for about a mile, salt and graduation works suddenly attract your attention, in the midst of charming meadow-ground nearer the Saale. You enter, and are shown the so-called '*Soolen Sprudel*,' or '*runde Brunnen*' (salt bubbler, or round well), of very little importance before the year 1822, on account of its sparing supply. But after extensive boring processes, it discharges now a great abundance of water, with violent subterranean hissing and foaming—viz., every minute forty cubic feet, with $3\frac{1}{2}$ per cent. of salt. The round shaft of this remarkable spring reaches a depth of twenty-five feet, with a width of eight feet. The water possesses a saline bitterish taste, and a temperature of $15\frac{1}{2}°$ Reaum.$=66°$ Fahr. From its name you will be prepared to hear that it does not issue in an uninterrupted stream. But it does not throw its water up in the pulsating manner observed at Carlsbad. The natural phenomena noticed here are quite peculiar. You enter the enclosed space, you perceive a circular glass-covered prominence, with several persons around, and exclaiming, from time to time, 'It does not come yet.' All are perfectly still, and watching. You inquire the meaning of this anxious expectation. Following the throng, and endeavouring to penetrate the subterranean darkness through the protecting glass-covers, you wonder at the absence of all movement or bubbling. After having waited some time, you hear a distant undulatory movement, which becomes gradually stronger and more audible; the foaming and hissing soon become greater, and the eye will now perceive a whitish waving mass of water rolling more and more upwards, till it has reached its greatest height. If there are any boys amongst the visitors, they will never fail to make the experiment of placing a cap on the crown-like top of the enclosure. For a long time the cap rests immovable. You will not, however, have heard the rushing sound long before, suddenly, the cap rises a little, and then is jerked with great force, as if by an invisible hand, into the middle of the room. You examine its former resting-place, and you find a small, scarcely perceptible hole through which the expansive force of the gas performed this feat.

The expectant visitors hurry off now, when you would think it most interesting to watch and listen. But the cause is soon explained. Dr. Pfriem, the superintendent of this establishment, kindly shows the different baths that are waiting for the arrival of the Sprudel water. Here gas-cabinets are gradually receiving their quantum of carbonic acid, conducted by pipes from the covering layer of the well—some for general, others for local gas-baths. There a '*Wellen-bad*' (wave-bath) is filling in a baignoire from a tap below, and we have an opportunity of admiring the constant wave-like motion and formation of white foam in the unheated bath. In another chamber a '*Strahl-bad*' (radiating-bath) is getting ready from the same source for another patient. A third waits for his gas-douche. After having maintained its height for about two hours, the water of the Sprudel sinks back rather rapidly with a distant rolling sound, and then requires a full hour to repeat its rising process. It might perhaps be more appropriately called the *salt-tide*, for the above phenomena are more analogous to a marine ebb-and-flow than to Sprudel jerking.

This spring contains 187 grains of solid ingredients (about three times as much as the Pandurbrunnen) in 16 ounces. Of these 107 grains are culinary salt, 25 chloride of magnesium, 25 sulphate of soda, with about $\frac{1}{3}$ of a grain of carbonate of iron. The following comparative analysis of the five springs will assist in their selection:—

	Rakoczy.	Pandur.	Max-brunnen.	Theresien-brunnen.	Soolen-sprudel.
Temperature	$52\frac{1}{4}°$ Fahr.	52°	52°	$52\frac{1}{4}°$	66°
Carbonic acid	23·25 cu. in.	28·85	31·04	28·35	30·57
Total of solid ingredients in 16 oz.	85·74 gr.	76·39	30·65	29·63	187·68
Viz.:					
Chloride of sodium	62·05	57·00	18·27	18·40	107·51
,, potassium	0·91	0·25	1·00	0·85	0·97
,, calcium	—	—	—	—	3·99
,, magnes.	6·85	5·85	3·10	2·75	24·51
Bromide of sodium	—	—	—	0·07	—
,, magnes.	0·70	0·68	—	—	0·06
Carbonate of soda	0·82	0·03	0·38	0·39	—
,, lime	3·55	5·85	2·59	2·00	1·65
,, magnes.	2·50	1·62	1·82	2·37	6·41
,, iron	0·68	0·45	—	—	0·35
Sulphate of soda	2·00	1·75	1·86	1·35	25·30
,, lime	2·50	0·75	0·65	0.75	
Phosphate of soda	0·17	0·05	0·12		
Silica	2·25	1·55	0·46	0·50	
Oxide of alum	0·18	0·05			
Organic extract	0·15	0·09	—	—	0·86
Loss nearly	0·38	0·37	0·38		

The effect of the Ragoczy water is not generally to increase the alvine actions; sometimes, on the contrary, it is rather obstructing. It agrees, therefore, best with persons suffering from *atonic dyspepsia* and laxity of the intestinal fibre, when excessive mucous secretion impedes the abdominal function.

In fact, a certain amount of weakness produced by age or exhausting disease is necessary for demonstrating the action of the water. It does not depress vital energy like the springs with predominant sulphates, but it rouses the nerves of the reproductive system, counteracts tough mucosity and abdominal scrofula. Vigorous constitutions are less benefited by the water. The abundance of carbonic acid affords no small assistance in strengthening the power of the ganglionic nervous plexus. In hepatic enlargements and passive abdominal congestion, the Rakoczy water shows itself particularly beneficial. Dr. Maass mentions a case of hepatic induration, resulting from hepatitis: constant obstruction, abdominal distention, anorexia, indigestion, and emaciation accompanied the complaint. The complexion of the patient was livid, with yellow colouration of the eyes, the liver considerably enlarged and hardened, the legs and right hand œdematous, besides occasional nocturnal perspirations and febrile orgasm. From three to six glasses of the Rakoczy water, with lukewarm Pandur and Soole baths, induced hæmorrhoidal flux with improved digestive function, but the volume of the diseased liver had not diminished after a week's course. The patient having left Kissingen with little hope of ultimate recovery, surprised the doctor ten years afterwards ('Jahrbücher für Deutschlands Heilquellen,' 1840), by his perfectly healthy and vigorous appearance. The use of the Rakoczy water had been continued by the patient at home until the gradual disappearance of the hepatic enlargement and other morbid phenomena. He was now about fifty years of age, and assured his former physician that he never enjoyed better health, even in his youth, than at that moment. An interesting instance is recorded of a young man, who, after some vexation, had been taken ill with a gastric fever of a slightly nervous character. Two months after his recovery, he was attacked by intermittent fever, which, notwithstanding the use of quinine, did not leave him for six months. Although freed from fever, he found his state of health greatly impaired. His complexion was pale and sallow, his appetite and sleep diminished, eructation and pressure on the pit of the stomach ensued after the mildest food; at the left hypochondrium the spleen was found enlarged and indurated. Action of the bowels was invariably retarded, sometimes from six to eight days. The skin felt dry and harsh, the feet were œdematous as far as the ankles. This patient used for eight weeks the Rakoczy water internally, and the Pandur externally, and was completely cured. As regards gout, for which disease Kissingen is often recommended, no favourable results can be expected in atonic, metastatic, or completely fixed gout, with deposits, contractions, or anchyloses; but when arthritic diathesis proceeds towards development under the influence of vicious and tardy bilification, the spa is often found to possess curative powers. Scrofulous patients are greatly benefited by the spa—not those of a florid erethic character, but rather persons of phlegmatic and torpid constitutions. The Maxbrunnen is recommended in renal and vesical catarrhs, especially if complicated with hæmorrhoidal tendency. *Helminthiasis* is enumerated as one of the principal disorders curable by the Kissingen waters. A lady was freed of a *tapeworm*, eighteen yards long, after a course of four weeks, having been subjected in vain to the ordinary medical treatment for two years; but strict diet was enjoined, and, besides the internal use of the Rakoczy water, clysters of Pandur were simultaneously employed, all fresh from the source, with the smallest possible loss of carbonic acid. Analysis of the Rakoczy water perfectly explains its great utility in systemic atrophy, based on intestinal torpor, and its indication in abdominal derangements with the character of debility occurring in real old age, where a diminished admixture of saliva seems to be rectified by the spa, or in the artificial old age superinduced in young persons by various causes.

You see, then, what different considerations should guide you in selecting either the sovereign of antibilious springs, or one of his neighbouring Bohemian courtiers, or the distant independent chieftain of Bavaria. Hepatic derangement is alleged and proved to be the principal disease curable by the Carlsbad, Marienbad, Franzensbad, and Kissingen waters.

How, then, are we to distinguish between them? If you will bear in mind the individualities which we have pointed out as peculiarly adapted for either of the former three, Kissingen must furnish the greatest chance of recovery, if a person be afflicted with a very tender alimentary tube, with frequent flatulence, eructation, want of appetite, alvine obstruction, general debility, emaciation or scrofulous puffiness; in short, if he require neither the highly-stimulating and penetrating efficacy of Carlsbad, nor the antiplastic and derivatory power of Marienbad, nor the tonico-solvent Franzensbad springs, but improved digestive action and heightened lympathic circulation and nutrition.

Suppose the above patient with splenetic physconia asked your advice previously to visiting a spa : you would consider that there was abdominal inaction, probably more from the absence of certain inorganic materials than from deep, invincible, vital torpidity ; you would find his digestive canal unable to bear even mild nourishment without irritation : to raise his powers, you would not require a remedy producing functional vitality, as the *reaction* of a highly-stimulating and overworking agent, but one calculated directly to improve the elements of nutrition, and to remove the impediments to a proper exercise of the organic functions. But Kissingen offers other curative means besides those enumerated. The mother-lye of the Soole is applied in glandular swellings with great advantage, both locally and by general baths. This contains, in 16 ounces, 1,925 grains of chloride of magnesium, 420 grains of chloride of sodium, 55 of chloride of lithion, the same amount of chloride of ammonium, 246 of sulphate of magnesia, 10 of bromide of magnesium :—total, 2,806 grains. The *salt-mud* is another medicinal preparation, sometimes obtained from the effluvia of the salt-works, and sometimes from a little neighbouring pond, where carbonic acid rises from the ground. The circumambient air of the graduation works is not the least important curative influence reigning in this charming little town. Many patients with weakened thoracic organs, obstinate hoarseness, or pulmonary blennorrhage, find annually relief or cure by drinking Sauerbrunnen with whey, and sojourning a certain portion of the day in the environs of the salt-works. You must have remarked the great analogy between the baths of the so-called Soolen sprudel and those of the sea. The temperature and composition are similar, excepting the additional presence of iron in the Kissingen sprudel. The baths are taken without heating or cooling ; and though chilliness is the first sensation on entering, the great quantity of carbonic acid, with the wavy motion of the sea-warm water, soon causes agreeable peripheric stimulation, redness, and warmth, very similar to the sensations resulting from real sea-baths. We have only to regret that so few persons can avail themselves at the same time of these baths, the difference of extent being so greatly in favour of the genuine sea. Many, perhaps, will smile at this pigmy comparison, and say, What is the use of an imitation sea-bath? Are we deficient in real sea-water or in conveniences for its employment? If baths are required with saline exhalations, and all the healing influences of the sea, let the patient resort to the seaside and bathe in the abundant salt-fluid, instead of waiting here for a puny measure of similar water. This objection seems very plausible, theoretically. But let us examine it in practice, and inquire whether the seaside invariably restores those sunken powers for which it is recommended. Does it not occasionally happen that the powerful shock of the mighty stimulus irritates instead of invigorating? Is not the advantage of sea-bathing often counterbalanced by secondary morbid incidents? However useful and invaluable for combating morbid diathesis, you are well aware how carefully it must be avoided in all erethic conditions, and in many formed diseases. Often, then, when sea-bathing must be forbidden from certain medical considerations, such modification as you find here may prove extremely desirable, particularly with all the other auxiliaries at your command for influencing both the internal and external reproduction in the weakened constitution. You are aware that Kissingen is largely employed abroad, chiefly Rakoczy; but the Maxbrunnen well deserves to be used for exportation, on account of its felicitous combination, and of the close union of its carbonic acid. After having been exposed to the atmosphere for three days in open bottles, and placed in a heated room, a great quantity of carbonic acid is evolved on shaking the bottles. Many consider it preferable to Selters water in its dietetic use. Kissingen gains daily in importance, its efficacy being ranked between that of Carlsbad for abdominal disorders, and of Wiesbaden for derangements of the sero-fibrous and muscular systems.

A case is recorded of a neighbouring physician who was suddenly seized with most violent pains of the stomach and vomiting, so that enteritis was diagnosed, and a corresponding antiphlogistic treatment adopted, but to no purpose. The pains continued, and paralysis of the extremities at last supervened. An eminent Würzburg physician considered the disease as a form of masked gout, and therefore advised Kissingen. Affected with violent palpitation of the heart, he arrived at the spa, after nine months' suffering. After the lapse of a fortnight articular gout made its appearance, with the relief of the paralytic and neuralgic symptoms.

The beneficial influence of Kissingen on the portal circulation will prepare you to hear of its favourable action on abnormal catamenial flux. The majority of the valetudinarians, however, belong to the male sex; and diseases of the hypochondriacal organs annually swell the list of visitors in a preponderating degree. Besides the greatly esteemed German physicians (Dr. Erhard, Dr. Balling, Dr. Welsch, Dr. Bexberger, Dr. Diruff, Dr. Ehrenburg, Dr. Pfriem, and Dr. Gatschenberger), the English visitors enjoy the advantage of the highly valuable services of Dr. Granville and Dr. Travis, who reside at Kissingen during the season.*

Bocklet.—Let us now pursue the northward course of the river Saale, for about five English miles, and we shall arrive at *Bocklet*, situated in a meadow-valley on the left bank of the river, two leagues from Kissingen, six from Brückenau, and seven from Schweinfurth. At the eastern side of the valley, woody hillocks are perceived, less high than those of the opposite side. The meadow-ground presents a very pleasant but rather monotonous appearance. The mountains as far as Kissingen consist of stratified sandstone. Thence layers of stratified limestone commence and extend through the southern part of the Würzburg domain. Towards the Rhöngebirg, on the other side of the Saale, basalt takes the place of sandstone. The springs were discovered, about 130 years ago, by the Vicar of Aschach, Schöppner, who, on passing that way, accidentally remarked a bog filled with yellow water and covered by a variegated pellicle. These peculiar characteristics, besides the unusual taste and smell, and the neighbourhood of Kissingen, excited in the reverend gentleman's mind the idea of its being a mineral water. He had an empty perforated cask dropped into the deepest part, and thus obtained a purer flow of the water, which he tried for his own ailment with success, and then induced many of the neighbouring inhabitants to follow his example and establish the fame of the newly-discovered fountain. A hundred years ago, the spring was enclosed and a bath-house erected near it. Several springs, formerly separate, were found to possess the same origin, and therefore received a common enclosure. The place now contains a chalybeate and a sulphurous spring. The former enjoys a high reputation for its solvent and tonic power. It discharges seventy-nine cubic feet of water per hour, and flows with a considerable hissing noise, sparkling strongly when drawn. Its taste is saline and somewhat astringent; temperature, 50° F.; spec. grav. 1·011^7. The curious tide of the Soolensprudel seems to be

* Excellent accommodation in the Curhaus, Russische Hof and Bairische Hof.

feebly repeated here, for slight ebbing and flowing take place, although without regularity. The source sinks suddenly several inches in the shaft, and rises again with some violence, after a shorter or longer period. On some days no tide is perceived; on others, it occurs several times. It is most marked at the period of full moon, also at the approach of a tempest, and whenever the barometric scale is lowered, carbonic acid gas being evolved at the same time in greater quantities and more energetically.

CONTENTS OF THE CHIEF BOCKLET SPRINGS (COLD).

	Ludwigsquelle. (Ludwig's sprg.)	Schwefelquelle. (Sulphur sprg.)	Stahlquelle. (Steel sprg.)
Carbonic acid	31 cub. in.	21½	39·3
Sulphuretted hydrogen	—	0·2	
Sum total of ingredients	45·9 gr.	5	27·6
Viz. :—			
Sulphate of soda	6·25	0·25	2·54
,, magnesia	—	—	3·23
,, lime	0·50		
Chloride of sodium	27·50	0·25	6·55
,, magnesium	0·75	—	4·43
Carbonate of soda	—	0·50	...
,, magnesia	1·25	0·50	3·36
,, lime	7·25	2·50	6·54
,, iron	0·65	0·40	0·61
Silica	0·50	0·10	0·22

This combination of the sulphate of soda and magnesia with the carbonates of lime and iron, assisted by the presence of the antiscrofulous chlorides, justifies the well-earned reputation of the spa in atonic irritation and mucosity of the alimentary mucous membrane, and especially in diarrhœa based on a scrofulous affection of the mesenteric glands, in anæmia states of the uterus, in blennorrhages, as well as in passive metrorrhage. As a remedy after the use of highly solvent springs, Bocklet is also very valuable, both for internal and external use.

About ten or twelve feet from the chalybeate, the less abundant sulphurous spring comes to light. This is only used for drinking, on account of its sparing supply. In dry, hot summers, the quantity of the water is still more diminished, with a somewhat increased proportion of hydrothionic acid. It displays the characteristic smell of the hepatic gas. On drawing a glass of the water, it loses momentarily its transparency, by reason of the rising gas bubbles. The sulphuretted hydrogen not being closely united to the water, it easily volatilises by lengthened exposure to the atmosphere. The layers of carbonic acid spread over the water are led off, and employed for gas-baths. Ferruginous mud is obtained from the so-called red peat of the high Rhöne, and used for mud-baths. There are two other kinds of moor, of large extent, and forming considerable bogs, which are, however, less appropriate for medicinal use. Motherlye, from the brine of Kissingen, is sometimes added to the baths, or used for local application. From the already explained action of the constituents, the water agrees even with very weak and irritable digestive organs, where other chalybeates would be less easily tolerated, from the want of tempering salts. The chalybeate of Bocklet ranks in its medicinal effects between the more purely tonic Pyrmont, and the more solvent Franzensbrunnen. The atony of the mucous membrane is particularly counteracted by Bocklet.

Whilst assimilation and reproduction are greatly heightened by the use of this water, atonic irritability of the nervous system is allayed. Bocklet enjoys the highest reputation in atonic uterine diseases, in chlorosis, menstrual irregularities, sterility, and blennorrhages; and here, especially, potent efficacy results from the careful employment of the *douche ascendante*. Dr. Kirchgessner detailed to me several cases of sterility and tendency to abortion that had been cured by the internal use of the Stahlquelle and the above-mentioned douche. The liquid is jerked up with different and gradually increasing degrees of force, an experienced female bath attendant directing the machinery. I especially inquired whether erotic sensations resulted from the introduction of this remedy, and was assured by the Doctor, that generally it produced no other physical effects than those of ordinary vaginal injections. Occasionally, however, some sexual erethism is induced, and then the douche is considered as inapplicable, and immediately discontinued. I need not dwell on the importance of this point, for if the excitement of such sensations were continued, it is obvious that the previous atonic irritability and torpor would, after the subsided reaction, increase rather than diminish. When the uterus is chiefly to be acted upon, a stream is led through the douche, whilst for the affected vaginal portion the perforated tube is used to impart an ascending rain-douche. From my own observation, I can state that it is never employed by Dr. Kirchgessner without the greatest care and circumspection; and I can unhesitatingly recommend Bocklet in cases of sterility, where leucorrhœa has formerly existed, and is prone to reappear by any weakening or exciting incident; when nervous susceptibility is connected with abnormal digestive function; frequent obstruction alternating with occasional diarrhœa; when menstruation does not maintain its regular epochs, though the signs of obstinate chlorosis are absent, and there is no positive appearance of anæmia or great debility in the complexion or posture of the patient. Let us imagine her to be every now and then seized with spasms of the stomach, neuralgia of the head, face, or teeth; her mind being extremely excitable for joy or grief, &c. To such a condition the Bocklet water is peculiarly applicable. Patients, however, of great debility, affected with a high degree of chlorosis, and with a greater sexual torpor, but with unimpaired alimentary function, will require a purer chalybeate. When scrofulous dyscrasia is complicated with the sexual disorder, Bocklet claims the preference. In several cases of ovarian tumour, the Doctor used emollient decoctions with hemlock for the *douche ascendante*, besides the sulphurous water internally, and baths of mother-lye, until the complete removal of fluor albus and sterility, which had been connected with the organic disorder. The sulphur spring agrees well even with very weak digestive organs. It exerts a very beneficial influence on the alimentary and urinary mucous membranes, and is used with benefit in vesical hæmorrhoids and catarrh, and in hydrargyrosis. But of course you will not recommend Bocklet when the properties of a pure sulphurous mineral water are required for the cure of disease, having to choose between so many powerful springs of this class: but when you consider Bocklet's muriatico-chalybeate spring useful, complications may exist or arise, which must be counteracted by the sulphur spring. For though weaker than many others, its quantity of carbonic acid, iron, and lime, gives it a preference in many morbid modifications.

Physician: Dr. Rubath.

LECTURE XI.

BRÜCKENAU—HOMBURG.

BY riding westward for a few hours across the Rhön mountain, we arrive at the charming valley enclosing the magnificent spa of *Brückenau*, situated on the little river *Sinn*, which runs from north-east to the south-west, between woody hills covered with oak and fir trees. The height observed on the south is called the *Sinnberg*. The spa lies about half a league from the small town of Brückenau, six leagues from Bocklet, and sixteen from Würzburg. It possesses three springs. The Brückenauer, or *steel spring*, lies nearly in the centre of the valley. Two hundred yards to the south we perceive the *Wernarzer*, and about twenty yards farther, at the foot of the Sinnberg, the *Sinnberger* spring. The two first are separated by the river Sinn, which is here crossed by a stone bridge leading to the Curnplace. Between the town of Brückenau and the spa an umbrageous beech grove borders both sides of the road, which all at once terminates by the unexpected view of the beautiful gardens, walks, and buildings, surrounding the springs. The Curhaus, erected by his Majesty King Ludwig of Bavaria, is one of the most splendid buildings of Europe. The walks and shady resting-places are varied and numerous, and abound in natural charms. The Dreystelz, rising above the Sinnberg, affords a very fine prospect of the environs. The steel spring arises out of the rocks at the depth of fifty feet, and is conducted upwards by a wooden pipe. The water is clear, and strongly sparkling, with an agreeably acidulous, piquant, and slightly astringent taste. When drawn, it quickly covers the sides of the glass with gas-bubbles. If the water be exposed in an open vessel overnight, round, reddish flakes will be perceived at the bottom next morning. Red ferruginous ochre becomes deposited at the sides of the basin into which the water flows from the pipe. Only $2\frac{1}{2}$ grains of solid constituents are contained in a pint of water—viz.,

0·60 sulphate of magnesia.
0·20 sulphate of lime.
0·65 chloride of potassium.
0·35 chloride of sodium.
0·55 carbonate of lime.
0·25 carbonate of iron ($\frac{1}{4}$ of a grain); and
35$\frac{1}{2}$ cubic inches of carbonic acid; temperature between 48° and 50° F. Specific gravity, 1·006.

Brückenau may thus be considered one of the purest chalybeates of Europe, the iron being so finely divided and dissolved, and so little counterbalanced by antiplastics, that it possesses a purely tonic action without any secondary result. The sulphates and chlorides present are just sufficient to cause the chief ingredient to be well tolerated by the digestive organs. The great abundance of carbonic acid assists in directly introducing this invigorating element into the circulating fluids. The spa is therefore applicable in many cases of erethic atony, where other chalybeates would cause too great an excitement in the vascular system. After tedious recovery from exhausting ailments, in chlorosis, profuse perspiration from cutaneous weakness, or tendency to abortion, it is highly recommended. It is often used with great advantage after a course of Kissingen or other solvent waters. The Wernarzer spring is not a chalybeate, but one of the purest so-called acidulous springs in existence, containing 28 cubic inches of carbonic acid, with only 4-5ths of a grain of solid constituents, and among these 1-20th gr. of acetate of potash. The Sinnberger contains less than $\frac{3}{4}$ of a grain of constituents, with 25 cubic inches of carbonic acid. It was found necessary to dig 50 feet through the sandstone to enclose the latter, and the supposition was entertained that it originated out of lava-mass, probably lying here under the sandstone.

This would account for the great abundance of carbonic acid from the lava exhalations, whilst the deficiency of solid ingredients would be due to the small solubility of the superposed rocky masses. The taste of the two latter springs is purely acidulous and slightly pungent. They have been greatly extolled in chronic diseases of the pulmonary mucous membrane, and in lithiac and hæmorrhoidal tendencies. They are also often recommended in such chronic diseases as are based on abdominal obstruction, repressed piles, rheumatism, or gout. In fluor albus and dysmenorrhœa, they are also said to have been employed advantageously. Dr. Wetzler relates the case of a young delicate married woman, who was often affected with spitting of blood, and became so reduced after a severe delivery, that her condition was thought hopeless. She came to Brückenau, and Dr. Schipper, under whose care she placed herself, ordered first the Sinnberger, and afterwards the Wernarzer water, to be drunk, by which means she was completely restored. She had been confined subsequently, and was well at the time Dr. W. mentioned her case. The situation and climate of Brückenau are very favourable for persons with delicate thoracic organs. The variety of natural and artificial attractions here is particularly striking. The fine prospect offered by the Prince's house, standing on an eminence which overlooks the valley with its park-like walks—the gardens between the costly buildings, with their shady groves and well-contrived orchards—the giant oak with its immense horizontal branches, affording shade to more than 100 persons, and often serving as a centre for music and dancing—the manifold walks on the other side in the woods of the Sinnberg, with their green benches or turf seats—all these charms seem little appreciated, for I find that this spa, the favourite seat of his Majesty the late King Ludwig of Bavaria, decreases annually in visitors. When I walked last year through the magnificent Cursaal with its royal galleries and glittering chandeliers, its extensive space and accommodation for great numbers, I was sadly impressed by the absence of the only ornament wanting—viz., a lively throng of human beings. I understood that numerous visitors were attracted by the sojourn of his Majesty, some perhaps from the natural fondness for courtly splendour, others from a desire to petition the king, who was here more accessible than in his capital.

The above shows you that it is necessary to inquire into many circumstances, not immediately connected with the physical or chemical character of a spa, in order to arrive at a just conclusion as to the esteem in which it is held by the public. But what is the cause of the present comparative loneliness of a place offering the purest chalybeate and acidulous spring? This may partly arise from the fact that the supply is rather deficient, for the baths are not given of the pure steel spring, but the Wernarzer and Sinnberger non-chalybeates are heated and mixed with the former. As regards the acidulous springs, with their alterative and stimulating influence on the pulmonary, digestive, and uropoietic mucous membranes, they are probably often neglected in favour of springs which possessing greater combinations, are suited to more complicated morbid conditions. At the time of my visit, an English nobleman (the ambassador at Paris, I believe), had just arrived to drink the waters for a fortnight, after a course of Kissingen; and I do think, whenever circumstances allow the delay, many of the frequenters of Kissingen would be greatly benefited, if, before returning to their usual toils or avocations, they would submit themselves for a few weeks to the tonico-solvent power of Bocklet, or to the purely invigorating Brückenau; they would certainly then carry home a much greater resisting power against morbific causes, by having provided their depurated abdominal organs with the strengthening chalybeate draughts, imbibed amid all the charms that nature and artistic skill can furnish.

Physicians: Dr. Riegel, Dr. Faulhaber.

Homburg.—We have now to direct our way to Frankfort, and for that purpose we go by diligence as far as Gemünden (in $6\frac{1}{2}$ hours). Thence the railroad will convey us to Frankfort in less than three hours ($58\frac{1}{4}$ miles). This beautiful and busy town, full of life, pleasure, and commerce, forms the centre of extremely numerous and varied medicinal springs. They have on the north-west Homburg, on the north Nauheim, on the west Soden, more southerly Weilbach, and due west Wiesbaden, besides the celebrated Nassau Spas at a short distance. Our next visit, however, is intended for Homburg 'vor der Höhe,' which we can reach now by rail in $\frac{3}{4}$ of an hour. This spa was visited by 805 guests only in the year 1837; by 4,600 nine years afterwards, in 1846; and by upwards of 5,000 in 1847. It lies 600 feet above the level of the sea (300 feet higher than Frankfort), on a mountain-ridge, about two miles distant from the south-eastern chain of the Taunus. Woody hills protect the town on the north and west. The highest peak of the Taunus, the *Feldberg*, lies in a due westerly direction. Towards the south-west rises the Altkönig, with the ruins of Falkenstein at its feet. The place is open and unprotected on the south and east. At a greater distance, the Donnersberg is perceived to the south, the 'Bergstrasse' and the Odenwald to the south-east; with these you notice on the map the more easterly parallels formed by the Spessart and Rhön-mountains. The air is considered very bracing and invigorating in the months of June, July, and August. In spring, the temperature is very changeable; and even in summer, it is positively injurious to persons with delicate thoracic organs. The mountain-masses round Homburg consist of quartz-slate, whilst of the Soden mountains chlorit-slate forms the chief foundation. At the foot of the mountains, clay-slate with quartz veins is found. Though tertiary layers of lime are frequent about Soden, no lime can be discovered in the superficial crust of the environs of Homburg. On the other side of the Nied, however, fresh-water shell-lime is found in abundance. Strata of peat exist near Homburg with superposed basalt cones. The mineral sources originate to the north-east of the town, in a meadow-valley within a circuit of a few thousand feet. In boring, a thin layer of gravel was first penetrated; then a considerable stratum of differently coloured clay (150 feet); then a thick vein of quartz was arrived at, out of which the springs issue with their extraordinary abundance of carbonic acid. At a greater depth, efflorescent clay-slate is mixed, here and there, with quartz-sand. The origin of all the springs is shown to be common by their possessing nearly the same constituents. The water merely rises to the surface of the ground, so that deep canals had to be cut, to cause its efflux.

About two hundred years ago, salt was obtained from various bore-holes, but from some cause or other, the graduation-works were discontinued, and the buildings sold to the administration of the Nauheim Saltworks (1740). The place remained unnoticed till some boys, in 1809, discovered an acidulous spring, which was used as a refreshing beverage by the townspeople; but no medicinal employment was thought of before 1834, when Medicinalrath Dr. Trapp tried the now-called Elisabethbrunnen with success, and recommended its further employment. This spring is entirely protected by its enclosure from any atmospheric influence. The others are more liable to slight changes from accidental causes.

The *Elisabeth Spring* comprises several confluent sources, provided with one enclosure. The others are the result of boring trials. It was found necessary to bore to a depth of 140 to 150 feet before a mineral fountain was discovered. The water furnished by the springs is clear and transparent, and issues with a constantly bubbling motion, from the great amount of carbonic acid present, which adds some pungency to the saline, bitterish, and ferruginous taste. Exposed for some time to the atmosphere, turbidity ensues, with a reddish deposit. At the boring-springs, a blackish powder adheres to the sides, chiefly composed of sulphuret of iron. Analysis of the four springs shows:—

	Elisabethqu.	Kaiserqu.	Stahlqu.	Ludwigsqu.
Chloride of Sodium	79·15	117·04	79·86	7·93
,, Magnesium	7·76	7·86	5·32	3·06
,, Calcium	7·75	13·32	10·66	7·28
,, Potassium	—	0·29	0·17	1·71
Sulphate of Soda	0·38			
,, Lime	—	0·19	0·14	0.15
Carbonate of Lime	10·98	11·10	7·53	5·74
,, Magnesia	2·01	—	—	0·09
,, Iron	0·46	0·80	0·03	0·41
Silica	0·31	0·33	0·31	0·10
Total	109·31 gr.	150.93	104·97	86·04
Free Carbonic Acid	48¼ cub. in.	55	46·9	43·35
Specific gravity	1·0115	1·015	1·0108	
Temperature	54½°F.	56¾°F.	54½°F.	55½°F.

The presence of the sulphuretted hydrogen in some of them may be ascertained by the odour, but it is not chemically demonstrable. The effects observed at Homburg quite coincide with the properties of the component parts. The chief ingredient, chloride of sodium (nearly four scruples), not only gently stimulates the mucous membranes to an increased secretion, but also loosens the formed and tough mucus, and thus prepares the alimentary contents for elimination, without actually operating as a purgative. Chloride of calcium (7¾ gr.) has been found to act beneficially in scrofula, being somewhat analogous to chloride of baryum in its solvent and alterative effects. It increases absorption in the lymphatic vessels, and seems to induce resolution in tumefied glands. The isolated remedy is not so favourably received by the alimentary tube as the sodium salt, being apt to over-stimulate and retard alvine functions, if employed to excess. The chloride of magnesium (7¾ gr.) assists the action of the calcium salt. From the circumstance of those springs which contain the greatest quantity of chloride of magnesium particularly increasing bilious alvine evacuations, this salt is supposed to promote the secretion of bile. The rapid removal of mesenteric scrofula by Homburg water, is chiefly ascribed to the presence of these two chlorides. Carbonate of iron to the amount of nearly half a grain (0·46), increases the tone of the blood, and prevents the development of cachectic liquefaction. It enables the organism to carry out the reaction by which the penetrating solvent treatment will be succeeded. The considerable amount of carbonate of lime (10 3-10ths gr.) would rather act as an obstruent in its ordinary form, diminishing serous and mucous secretion by its absorbing tendency; but some modification must be allowed here, from its being accompanied by so great a quantity of carbonic acid. The duration of its contact with the abdominal organs becomes shortened by a prompt imbibition into the circulating fluids, and thus it assists the antacid and sedative effects of magnesia (2 gr). The absence of carbonate of soda in the Elisabethbrunnen is significant. Those combined ingredients might display very different effects, if they were not introduced with an abundance of free carbonic acid (48 cubic inches in 16 ounces), which, according to Professor Liebig, surpasses the quantity found in any other spring in Europe. It is, therefore, not remarkable that a sort of giddiness, and momentary feeling of intoxication, are sometimes perceived by persons of a plethoric habit who drink the water off quickly. The pulse is also often increased during the use of the water, which must be partially attributed to the unusual quantity of free carbonic acid.

The Homburg water causes a sensation of warmth in the stomach, occasionally with some flatulence, which, however, is soon relieved by eructation, or increased alvine evacuations. If renal secretion appears augmented, the action of the bowels becomes less perceptible. Sometimes even obstruction takes place in the beginning of the course. Unless accompanied by unfavourable signs of vascular excitement—as giddiness, headache, abdominal distention, restlessness, &c.—the action of the water alone may be trusted for the production of the necessary eliminations. Should the watchful physician observe any symptoms of cerebral congestion, he will not hesitate to employ an energetic revulsive treatment, by purgatives or otherwise. From two or four tumblers are taken fasting, and ordinarily some fæcal and mucous evacuations follow in a few hours. If they exhibit rather a serous character, they are not considered favourable, and the dose of water should be diminished, or dietetic measures taken to change the diarrhœal disposition. Critical excrementitious stools happen during the course with great relief. Morbid corpulency becomes considerably diminished, and digestion improved. Three weeks is the ordinary duration of the course; prolongation of this period would cause too great an irritation of the alimentary canal. Towards the third week the relief experienced at first generally vanishes, abdominal action slackens, the parietes distend, with general lassitude and languor; appetite, sleep, and temper become disturbed. These signs are merely the beginning of critical reaction, and you must particularly exhort your patient not to be discouraged by them. The alterative process has been commenced, repressed piles or catamenia will be reproduced by the reacting efforts of nature; hardened fæces, and even gall-stones, will be expelled, and the whole reproductive system will often become strengthened after the cessation of these phenomena.

Homburg has been found very beneficial for aged individuals who have undergone typhus or other weakening diseases, and who have an instinctive desire for more nourishment, with inactive intestines and a feeling of discomfort after alvine evacuations. Their blood seems to be deficient in certain materials necessary for a proper innervation, and therefore restoration and cure may ensue by the use of the springs. Experience has shown Homburg to be adapted for *general* scrofulous diathesis without local derangement, and occasionally for swelling of the mesenteric glands, with emaciation; for ulceration of the subcutaneous glands, scrofulous blennorrhages of the eyes or ears, &c. But in the case of infants, no irritation must exist in the infantile digestive canal, if Homburg is to be administered internally; the course is therefore generally commenced with baths. In florid erethic scrofula, the internal use is entirely contra-indicated; whilst in the torpid form, careful employment of Homburg exerts a decidedly curative effect. Whatever analogy may exist between tubercle and scrofula, it has been positively shown that no favourable result can be expected from Homburg in tubercular deposits. Even in cases of hæmoptoë and pulmonary irritation that were relieved during the course, under the appearance of hæmorrhoidal congestion, aggravation of the disease ensued some weeks after the return from the spa. The cause of this important circumstance is not so much to be sought in the climate as in the chemical composition of the water.

The spa is particularly indicated in prevailing venous congestion of the abdominal organs. When scrofulous dyscrasia has existed in youth, mature age is liable to venous predominance in the circulating system. Less arterial blood being required now than during growth, when constant organic additions took place, unchanged sanguification may produce more of this vital liquid than necessary for renewal of the wasted materials. This condition is remedied either by diminishing the quantity of nourishment, or by increasing the function of the emunctories. If, however, luxurious meals are indulged in, and abdominal and cutaneous eliminations are checked through mechanical compression, lengthened sojourn in a confined atmosphere, avoidance of muscular exertion, &c., abdominal plethora must occur, and produce over-filling of the portal system, the impeded venous reflux then impairs the strength of the arterial current. The blood, flowing with diminished force, furnishes a less active stimulus for metamorphic processes. The ganglionic nerves make energetic efforts to counteract this torpidity, and become irritated and weakened in consequence. Dyspepsia, flatulence, irregular stools, colic, headache, mental depression, occasional pains in the back, fulness of the abdomen, and other signs of faulty digestion torment the patient. This state may be relieved by the effort of nature in discharging venous blood through the hæmorrhoidal vessels; but if the causes continue, the abnormal state will be renewed. This morbid state frequently finds a radical cure at Homburg. Although at first the secretion of acid mucus often augments under symptoms of apparent aggravation, this soon yields to relieving evacuations. Gall-stones are frequently removed by the water.

Icteric phenomena are generally aggravated at first, the skin assuming a deeper yellow, till critical evacuations usher in the expected relief. *Melæna* and vomiting of blood are often connected with intumescence and congestion or softening of the spleen. Such cases find a powerful remedy in Homburg.

If enlargements of the liver or spleen be produced by intermittent fevers, these latter sometimes reappear during the course, and require medical treatment; but through the simultaneous use of the spa, the hypochondriacal derangements often disappear with the fever. In diseases of *the uterine system*, especially in abnormal menstruation, Homburg enjoys a very high reputation, probably due to its powerful anti-venous action. A general torpid and phlegmatic state is most in need of this spa. In some cases of *chlorosis*, Homburg will exert a more curative effect than steel springs. Indeed, though the *character* of this disease is generally pretty similar in different individuals, we must allow a great variety of causes. To counteract these must be our aim. There will be, doubtless, deficiency of iron in the composition of blood; but we must inquire how this has been produced. Have hepatic and intestinal functions been previously disturbed? Has not the patient sometimes suffered from bilious vomiting, acidity, or other signs of irritable digestion? So that the attenuation of the blood results more from imperfect assimilation, than from absent elements. The reason why in such cases pure chalybeates are useless, is obvious; and here Homburg acts as a powerful curative agent.

Digestion and bilification improve, mucosity and venous predominance are allayed, and the restored digestive function renders further tonics unnecessary. *The spasms of the stomach*, which often accompany the menstrual epochs, are invariably relieved here. Uterine hypertrophy is diminished, and thus sterility, as well as excessive catamenia, are sometimes cured. Vesical catarrh, and hæmorrhoids, with frequent ischuria and cramps of the bladder, are greatly mitigated.

Homburg is contra-indicated in fever, acute inflammation, congestion to the head or chest, organic diseases of the heart and great vessels, dropsy, internal suppuration, &c. Taking cold is particularly to be avoided during the course, as it materially interferes with the effect of the water. To show the advantageous result of Homburg in digestive weakness, Medicinalrath Dr. Müller records the case of a lady who had been confined to her room for more than a twelvemonth, in consequence of a chronic nervous complaint. Complete anorexia, with a furred tongue and obstinate obstruction, was gradually developing, and resisting various energetic modes of treatment. At last Elisabethbrunnen was resorted to. The water was found to agree with the patient, although it had to be taken without exercise, as she was unable to leave her bed. After a fortnight, the tongue became clean, and alvine action more regular. In the course of five weeks her digestion was perfectly restored. Cases are mentioned of cachectic, emaciated individuals, affected with pertinacious obstruction, occasional cholic, vomiting and diarrhœa, who were restored by using the Elisabethbrunnen during three or four weeks. An individual, with morbid obesity, frequent sleepiness, irregular stools, but unnatural appetite, could not perform the slightest exertion without difficulty. This condition was likewise greatly improved by the spa. In cases where active life has been exchanged for a sedentary occupation, the injurious results developed in the abdominal organs are extremely well combated by Homburg. Several cases are recorded of ladies who had been afflicted with frequent paroxysms of 'cramps of the stomach.' Alvine obstruction was present at the same time, and only yielded after a week's course of the Elisabethbrunnen. An elderly *bon vivant* was suffering from violent and frequent attacks of colic, with obstruction: he used other spas during ten years, with only temporary relief, but was ultimately restored at Homburg. Medicinalrath Dr. Trapp details several cases which may serve as a useful guide for the proper choice of the spa. Mons. de P——, muscular and strongly built, but rather puffy in appearance, had suffered from *febris intermittens* several years ago, when residing on the borders of Holland. Formerly he complained much of obstruction; now diarrhœa is more frequent, with occasional acidity and mucosity, feeling of soreness, and tickling in the throat: after meals, great lassitude and reddened face. His parents also suffered from weak stomachs—the father from gout. Two glasses of Elisabethbrunnen were ordered to be taken in the morning at long intervals, after a bath of $81\frac{1}{2}°$ F., with motherlye. The dose and duration of the bath were gradually increased, and restoration followed. Mr. R., fifty-two years of age, is perfectly healthy, can eat and drink what he likes, sleeps well, but an intolerable pressure on the pit of the stomach never fails to succeed the meals, with eructations and redness in the face; he is inclined to diarrhœa, but has usually one tough, dry evacuation every day, with occasional pain and swelling of the footballs. Three tumblers of Elisabethbrunnen produced from six to eight discharges of green, slimy masses, with great relief, but pulsation appeared in the epigastrium, with a metallic taste in the mouth. The dose was diminished in the morning, but two glasses given at night, with sitting-baths, of $31\frac{1}{2}°$ F., and of five minutes duration. Restoration ensued. Several cases of abdominal plethora, with the characteristic *pulsat. abdom.*, are detailed, which were entirely cured by Homburg water.

In conclusion, Homburg is decidedly useful in abdominal plethora without inflammation or inflammatory tendency, occurring after intermittent fever, engorgement of the liver and spleen, and in *inactive circulation of the portal system*, according to the experience of Medicinalrath Dr. Trapp. Intermittent pulse, with faulty action of the right ventricle, based on abdominal derangements, is frequently cured here; also persons suffering with profuse menstruation (through passive engorgement of the uterus) and periodical cramps of the stomach. Increased diuresis almost invariably takes place, if the result is favourable. Some cases of intermittent fever, which had resisted a persevering employment of quinine, were also cured by the spa. But to act healingly, the Elisabethquelle must be well digested, and therefore requires an *uninjured alimentary tube*. A highly esteemed English physician gives his valuable services at Homburg to those invalids who seek his advice, besides the greatly respected German physicians mentioned above.

To choose between Homburg and Kissingen, we have again to lay almost a greater stress on the constitutional peculiarity of the patient than on the affected organ. You find great analogy in the composition and the altitude of the two spas, but a great difference of climate. The atmosphere of the open Homburg, however bracing and invigorating for the weakened nervous system of the hypochondriac, is injurious to persons with irritable thoracic organs: incipient or latent tuberculosis is more quickly developed. In Kissengen, patients with the same morbid disposition (for the cure of which they were not sent there) find a beneficial influence produced on the organs of the chest; previous irritation is allayed, excessive mucous secretion diminished, and tubercular development retarded.

But let us now review the morbid phenomena which seek direct relief at either of the spas, and for this purpose we must refer in the first instance to the constituents. They both possess chloride of sodium as chief ingredient (Homburg in greater quantity— about a scruple more), some chloride of magnesium (in both the tenth part of the former ingredient); carbonate of magnesia is contained in both (Homburg, 2 grains; Kissingen, 2½ grains); both possess iron (Homburg, 4-10ths; Kissingen, 6-10ths). According to these ingredients, Homburg ought to act as a more energetic abdominal solvent, and as less heating and irritating than Kissingen, yet we find the reverse to be the case. I have shown that digestive atony and hepatic enlargement, find a cure in the use of Rakoczy, whilst I have just stated that Homburg requires an uninjured digestive tube, but with obstructed abdominal circulation. Homburg is contra-indicated in general atonic erethism, where Kissingen is recommended. The explanation of this difference will be easy, if you pursue the chemical comparison further. Homburg possesses chloride of calcium (7¾ gr.), which is absent in Kissingen. It further contains three times as much of carbonate of lime (11 to 3½ grains). This higher proportion of calcium and lime is only to a certain extent compensated by the greater amount of carbonic acid (48 cubic inches to 26). I would not ascribe any therapeutic difference to the sulphate of soda of Kissingen (2 grains), as it is counterbalanced by an equal quantity of gypsum, besides an unusual proportion of silica. A due appreciation of the above analogies and differences will readily explain the beneficial results produced by the use of chlorides, with a great superabundance of the stimulating carbonic acid of

Homburg, on the one hand, and the modified action of the analogous ingredients of Kissingen, on the other, where a smaller proportion of chlorides and carbonic acid is combined with a greater amount of iron.*

Physicians (besides Dr. Müller): Dr. Friedlieb, Dr. Deetz, Dr. Märcklin, Dr. Müller jun., Dr. Bernhard.

---

* Excellent accommodation in Hôtel d'Angleterre and de Hesse.

LECTURE XII.

SODEN—WIESBADEN.

WE now leave the pleasant neighbourhood of Homburg, and return to Frankfort, to direct our steps to *Soden*, in the west. By means of the Taunus railroad (with the *Höchst* branch) the three leagues distance is performed in 25 minutes. Soden lies in a valley (lat. N. 50°, long. E. 8°) at the foot of the southern slope of the middle Taunus, which extends from the west in an easterly direction. Mainz is situated at a distance of five leagues to the south-west (reached in an hour); Wiesbaden, six leagues to the west (reached in an hour and a half); Homburg, three leagues to the north. Orchards and vineyards adorn the hills which enclose the spa on the east and west: to the south, arable land gradually rises. Looking towards the north, the woody promontories of the Feldberg and Altkönig arrest the visitor's eye. The whole appearance is that of a calm, peaceful village. Its altitude above the sea is 437 feet (about 100 feet higher than Wiesbaden). The boundaries described above indicate the extreme mildness of the climate; thoroughly protected as it is, without being, on the other hand, too much narrowed. Violent north and east winds are kept off by the sheltering Taunus, whilst the cheering rays of the sun freely enter from the south. The crust of the valley is partly a peaty soil, and partly covered with rich pasture. It furnishes to the air the necessary humidity without any stagnating bog. In boring, saline springs are invariably met with, so that no sweet water can be obtained without conducting it from the neighbouring mountains. The saline character is likewise communicated to the vegetation, which resembles that of sea-shores. Plantago maritima, Salsola kali, &c., were frequent formerly. Their present rarity is owing to the progressive cultivation of the soil. Insects characteristic of sea exhalations were not wanting, as bledius tricornis, coenia natophila, &c. The evaporation of saline water from the ground is favoured by the warm temperature of several springs. The extreme mildness of the climate is further evidenced by the character of the vegetation. The grass of the juicy meadows admits of being cut three times a year. A great variety of fruits, corn, and vegetables abound in the valley, while vineyards cover the sunny declivities. Endemic diseases are said to be unknown here; but scrófula, though rare, is not completely absent; altogether, the inhabitants appear healthy and vigorous.

The mineral springs arise out of slate-stone. The Taunus itself is composed of two chief groups—the one forming a variety of chlorite-clay, and talc-slate, prevails in the middle and southern declivities, whilst quartz-rock chiefly occupies the northern parts. The numerous Soden springs discovered in this narrow compass show their common origin by a similar quality, though they differ materially in temperature, quantity and supply. It is supposed that water issues warm from the depth, and becomes exposed to different cooling influences, according to the more or less circuitous route it has to perform previous to its superficial outlet. The springs all lie in a plain of 400 feet, by 2,400 feet. Beyond this, neither evolution of gas nor any efflux of mineral water is observed. No less than twenty-three springs come to light in Soden, but only those claim our consideration which are enclosed for use. The water is clear and transparent, constantly agitated by rising gas bubbles. The taste is more or less saline and acidulous according to the greater or smaller amount of salt and carbonic acid. Spring 19 possesses a particularly piquant flavour, and is called the *Champagnerbrunnen.* Some have, to a certain degree, the taste and smell of sulphuretted hydrogen, especially No. 6, called the *Schwefelbrunnen* (sulphur well). The temperature varies considerably; some have only from 52° to 59° F., whilst most of the others are lukewarm, their temperature ranging between 66° and 70° F. Exposure to the air causes the water to become turbid by the disengagement of gas-bubbles, and ultimately a yellow-reddish precipitate of oxide of iron takes place.

Fine flocculent ochre covers the side of the enclosures, forming a yellowish gelatinous mass, hardening into a brownish substance at some distance from the source. It is most abundant in those springs which possess the greatest amount of salt, irrespective of the total quantity of solid ingredients. Ochre, formed by the precipitation of iron, contains, according to the microscrope, infusoria belonging to the class of *gallionella ferruginea*, in different degrees of development, and chiefly composed of iron and silica.

The *Milch*, or *Kurbrunnen* (No. 1), possesses $22\frac{1}{2}$ grains of solid constituent sand $13\frac{1}{2}$ cubic inches of carbonic acid in a pint of water; temperature, 74° F.; specific gravity, 1·003.

The *Winklerbrunnen* (No. 2), 51 grains, $18\frac{1}{2}$ cubic inches of carbonic acid, $64\frac{1}{2}$° F.

Gemeindebrunnen, or Warm (No. 3), $32\frac{1}{4}$ grains, $14\frac{1}{2} \frac{9}{10}$ cubic inches of carbonic acid, 70° F.

Salzquelle unter der Brücke, or *Soolbrunnen* (saline spring under the bridge), (No. 4), $119\frac{3}{4}$ grains, $5\frac{3}{4}$ cubic inches of carbonic acid, 68° F.

Sauerbrunnen neben dem Schulhaus (No. 5), $57\frac{1}{4}$ grains, 15 cubic inches, 57° F. *Wilhelmsbrunnen* (No. 6 A). *Schwefelbrunnen* (No. 6 B). *Wiesenbrunnen* (No. 18). *Champagnerbrunnen* (No. 19). The analysis of the most and least impregnated spring will sufficiently indicate their chemical composition—

	Salzquelle (No. 4)	Milchbrunnen (No. 1)
Chloride of sodium	109·90	17·68
,, potassium	1·07	0·16
Sulphate of lime	0·65	0·19
Carbonate of lime	6·39	2·73
,, magnesia	1·35	1·37
,, iron	0·21	0·16
Silica	0·18	0·16
Alumina	0·62	0·01
Total	120·31	22·51

The diuretic effect of the water is most perceptible after a few days. Feculent evacuations soon follow in moderate quantity. Watery and numerous stools are considered unfavourable, and require diminution of the dose.

According to Medicinalrath Dr. Thilenius, appetite invariably improves under the use of the water. The same spring occasionally appears to the patient to have assumed a more or less saltish taste, when in reality the different perception is only attributable to the improved condition of the drinker's digestive organs. Bilious secretion is considerably increased, and altogether the circulation of the portal system promoted. If carefully selected, the springs are generally well tolerated by the digestive organs, and are recommended for abdominal plethora, dyspepsia, colic, and spasms of the stomach during menstruation; in fact, the same diseases are said to fall under the sway of Soden, as I have enumerated when treating of the neighbouring Homburg. It behoves us, therefore, to weigh the various properties of each before we fix our choice on either. In Soden, cutaneous perspiration is heightened. Should this be impeded by moist or cool weather, the water is less easily tolerated. The increased arterial function produced by the Soden water affords a useful assistance in ganglionic torpidity, whilst it contra-indicates the spring in plethora, congestion to the brain or other vital organ, inflammation, fever, &c.

In the so-called 'molimina hæmorrhoidalia,' or hæmorrhoidal congestion, Soden exercises a very beneficial influence; also in hypochondriasis, hysteria, and in catamenial derangements. Chloride of sodium, the chief ingredient, after being received into the chyle and blood, is supposed to render valuable services by maintaining the liquidity of the albumen and fibrin, and thus preserving the composition and form of the blood globules. The *carbonic acid* is allowed free scope of action as an excitant and stimulant on the intestinal mucous membrane, and as a sedative and anti-spasmodic on the ganglionic nerves.

Tubercular diathesis is powerfully counteracted by Springs 1, 3, and 4, if used with whey, particularly in those cases complicated with anæmic conditions. The extreme mildness of the climate here renders such a recommendation perfectly rational. Chronic pulmonary and laryngeal catarrhs are greatly benefited by this water.

The Springs 6A, 6B, 18, and 19, are chiefly employed in abdominal plethora, whilst 3, 4, and 1, are particularly recommended with whey or milk in thoracic weakness. In the case of weak digestive organs, 6B agrees better than 6A. If obstruction is present, an addition of No. 4 generally removes it.

The Springs 4, 5, 6, and 7, are also used for baths, which are brought to their appropriate temperature partly by the admixture of warm brine, and partly by hot steam. Kreuznach mother-lye is always to be had at Soden, and often employed to increase the strength of the baths. Atonic nervous erethism of the female sex, especially in periods of progression or change, is greatly relieved by the curative influence of the climate, and this spot is often resorted to for that purpose alone. You have then to look upon Soden as upon a modified and milder Homburg, and will recommend it in such forms of digestive irregularities, abdominal plethora, hepatic and menstrual derangements, as require less powerful remedial interference. Again, if Homburg should be indicated by the state of the disease, whilst the general constitution of your patient exhibits tubercular diathesis and great inclination to bronchial catarrhs, or if the cutaneous function be torpidly performed, or apt to be checked by atmospheric changes, or by sympathetic internal disturbances, you will give the preference to Soden, which combines the invigorating, gently bracing action of higher positions with the protection of a sheltered valley, abundantly endowed with saline exhalations.

Physicians: Drs. Thilenius, sen. and junr., Dr. Vogler, Dr. Grossmann, Dr. Pagenstecher.

Wiesbaden.—We shall now resume our westerly course and travel to the neighbouring Wiesbaden. We make a slight detour for this purpose, but the speed of the railroad compensates for the circuitous passage marked on the map, and in an hour and a half we arrive at our place of destination. Wiesbaden lies on the southern declivity of the Taunus mountain, in a deep valley, at a distance of three leagues from Mentz, and eight from Frankfort. It is a flourishing town, and the capital of the dukedom of Nassau, with upwards of 7,000 inhabitants. Forty years ago, there were only 500 residents. Its latitude N. is 50°, and longitude E. 8°. You perceive the Taunus rise on the other side of Homburg vor der Höhe, and extend towards the west as far as the Rhine. Wiesbaden is one of the oldest German watering places. It was well known to the Romans, who left many traces of their sojourn in the shape of coins and bath-ruins, with the inscription of the legion stationed there. The 'Mattiak' sources are mentioned by Pliny, who says: 'Sunt et mattiaci in Germaniâ fontes calidi trans-Rhenum, quorum haustus triduo fervet.' The environs are charming. The 'Platte,' a ducal hunting castle, two leagues from Wiesbaden, at the foot of the 'Trompeter,' affords a most picturesque and extensive prospect of the surrounding landscape. A romantic semicircle of rising forests encloses the spa on the north; in the south and west, fertile plains are intersected by the winding Maine and Rhine, over which the antique Mainz rises with its churches and steeples. Behind this stands the lofty Donnersberg. A view of Mainz and of the picturesque Rhine villages is better obtained from the Geisberg, a promontory of the Taunus, a quarter of a league from Wiesbaden. Gentle fertile eminences on the south and east lead the visitor's eye to the extensive windings of the Rhine. You may judge of the mildness of the climate of this spa from the fact, that with an altitude of 346 feet only, and the mountainous protection against north and east, winds many delicate persons choose it for a winter residence. The exhalations of the hot saline springs contribute in no small degree to deprive the winter of its severity. The vegetation is luxurious, and the abundant products of the soil sufficiently prove the appreciation of the climate by the vegetable kingdom, for almonds, sweet chestnuts, and many other southern fruits ripen here. But fresh drinking water is scarce, so that a stream had to be conducted into the town from the Platte. Historical documents show that the twenty-second Roman Legion, which helped in the destruction of Jerusalem, eighty years after Christ, was sent from Alexandria to Mainz, and fixed its quarters in Wiesbaden. Makrian, a king of the Alemannen, was unexpectedly attacked in the year 371, whilst using the baths of Wiesbaden, by Valentinian, but was fortunately rescued.

It was the chief seat of the Salish Franks, and inhabited for a long time by Charles and Otto the Great, who raised the place in 965 to the rank of a town. As a spa, its reputation has chiefly spread since the sixteenth century. The beautiful walks in the environs offer sufficient inducement for exercise. From the Cursaal a road leads to the old château of Sonnenberg (half a league distant), through a pleasant valley and by the river side. The convent of Clarenthal is situated about half a league from the town, near the road to Schwalbach. About a quarter of a league farther, in a smiling valley, the pheasant-house, with its views of the Rhine, invites the wanderer. The 'Walkmühle' is frequently visited for its alleys and walks.

Biebrich, the ducal summer residence on the Rhine, must not be left unseen. If you ascend the acclivity before Mosbach, you may pursue the Rhine upwards as far as the Melibokus, and downwards as far as Bingen, which would afford you a delightful panorama. The whole beautiful '*Rheingau*' may be embraced in this view.

The Cursaal of Wiesbaden is the place of reunion for the numerous health and pleasure seekers. It lies in a capacious plain, fronting the west. Several walks of plane-trees, limes, and acacias lead to the building, which bears the golden inscription: 'Fontibus Mattiacis, MDCCCX.'

At the principal frontage, a portico of colossal Ionic columns projects, intended for a protection to those who alight from their carriages. A colonnade with ornamented shops joins each side, and two pavilions form the wings. By an extensive hall we reach the principal saloon, which exhibits a length of 127 feet, and a breadth of 67 feet. On both sides a gallery is supported on marble Corinthian columns. In the niches of the sides are placed some magnificent statues in Carrara marble.

This beautiful structure is unfortunately defiled by the gaming-table, which is justly accused of undoing a great amount of the benefit conferred by the bountiful hand of Providence. To display their good effects, all the mineral waters require that the invalid should assist, as much as lies in his power, in a proper assimilation of the imbibed remedy, and in avoidance of any influence calculated to check the healing efforts of nature, bearing in mind the well-known proverb; 'Medicus curat, natura sanat.' Conceive, then, a valetudinarian, with deranged or stagnant abdominal circulation, seated, after a hurried breakfast, in a compressed position round the gaming-table for hours and hours, with depressing emotions, instead of walking in the beautiful green fields and meadows, throwing off all harassing thoughts and impressions, by an undisturbed contemplation of the works of the Almighty. It is astonishing how these pernicious gaming-tables can be tolerated, when so much care is taken to guard against dietetic or climatic injuries. It is with a feeling of deep sorrow and pain that I am compelled to admit the blot on many German spas, at which a pursuit positively immoral, and forbidden among the native inhabitants, is allowed with the poor excuse that it is permitted in other places, or, forsooth, that secret gambling would be resorted to with more injurious consequences. Let the Government do its duty, and not remain blameable for the worldly and physical ruin of many a confiding visitor. No less than 30,000 guests are said to resort, on an average, annually to this unique spa, which would be almost without reproach but for the evil which I have pointed out. Every year some improvement is effected in the town and its baths. The 'Cursaal,' with its magnificent rooms and its adjacent park-like walks, is greatly admired. The mountains consist of gross clay-slate, interspersed with quartz and mica. In the Rhine and Maine-basin it is united with conglomerations of silex, and several layers of clay, enclosing quartz, sand, and horn-stone; in the depth stratified lime is found, and many petrifactions. Basalt and strata of peat are remarked in the immediate neighbourhood of Wiesbaden, continuing as far as the bed of the Maine. The thermal springs owe their origin to volcanic causes. The sulphate of lime or chloride of magnesium present in the basaltic crust may have expelled the carbonic acid, for the formation of that quantity of Glauber or culinary salt which exists in the Wiesbaden water, and thus the production of carbonate of soda may have been prevented. The sources are distinguished by high temperature, great abundance, and a considerable amount of solid ingredients. They supply no less than thirty-two bath-houses (nearly eight hundred bathing cabinets, and fourteen vapour baths). The water is clear, transparent, with a slightly yellowish tint in some (as in the Adlerbrunnen). The smell somewhat resembles that of slaked lime; the taste is saltish, with some resemblance to over-salted veal broth. The pellicle covering the surface of the water is chiefly composed of lime. The red-brownish substance deposited in the pipes consists of carbonate of lime, silicate of alumina, and oxide of iron, with some magnesium, strontium, and bromine. The specific gravity of the water is 1·006 (only No. 3 having 1·005). The temperature of the springs varies from $37\frac{1}{2}°$ to $57°$ Reaumur = $116°$ to $160°$ Fahrenheit.

The *Kochbrunnen* (literally, boiling well) constantly hisses and bubbles, emitting volumes of vapour, which gave rise to its present name; air-bubbles continually rise from the depth and burst on the surface. Its enclosure forms an oblong quadrangle, with a depth of about five feet. It is surrounded by a circle of other bath-houses—on the north side by the 'Römer-bad,' 'weisse Ross,' 'weisse Schwan,' and the 'Engel;' on the opposite side by the 'Blume' and 'Rose;' at some greater distance by the Englische Hof. Another open source is situated behind the bath-house (im Adler). The Schützenhof and gemeing Bürgerbad (common citizens' bath) possess a common source. The latter is mostly used by persons of the lower class. Indigent invalids find accommodation in the hospital founded by the Emperor Adolphus of Nassau. 34,000 cubic feet of water are supplied in twenty-four hours. The analysis of the *Kochbrunnen* shows $59\frac{1}{2}$ grains of solid ingredients; temperature, $57°$ Reaumur=$160°$ Fahrenheit; carbonic acid about $5\frac{1}{2}$ cubic inches, and nitrogen 0·08 cubic inches.

```
45·28 chloride of sodium.
 0·30     ,,      potassium.
 1·30     ,,      magnesium.
 5·78     ,,      calcium.
 0·18 carbonate of magnesia.
 2·82     ,,      lime.
 0·10     ,,      iron.
 1·11 sulphate of soda.
 0·42 sulphate of lime.
 0·07 alumina.
 0·37 silica.
 0·06 bromide of magnesium, with 1,000 of brom. of sodium.
 1·85 organic matter.
```
Total, 59·64 grains.

This great amount of constituents in such thorough combination,

naturally exerts a powerfully curative action in many abnormal conditions. In small doses the water acts as a solvent and digestive remedy. In larger proportions, it is apt to cause diarrhœa, especially in persons whose cutaneous perspiration has been suppressed. When the peripheric function has been roused for some time, or a sediment formed in the urine, the increased alvine motions cease. In general, the hotter the water is for drinking, the less prone it is to cause diarrhœa. In some individuals obstruction is perceived at first; in fact, some alvine disturbance takes place occasionally in the commencement of the course, till the remedy becomes properly absorbed and assimilated. Dyspepsia based on torpor of the muscular fibre is best counteracted by the sulphates; whilst in persons with lymphatic or venous dyscrasy, the same ailment will yield more readily to the class at present under our consideration. As regards Karlsbad, the representative of the spas with predominant sulphates, the principal effect is expected from drinking, a direct action is therefore sought. Here, the most general application is external; thus we seek the chief benefit in a natural reaction following the peripheric stimulation. The baths are taken in separate cabinets, after being carefully cooled to the required temperate. They are constructed of bricks, and covered by 'trass.'*
The thermal water is allowed to fill the baths in the middle of the day, which are then ready for use next morning.

The diseases for the cure of which Wiesbaden enjoys the greatest reputation are, *chronic rheumatism* and *gout*, inveterate contractions, anchyloses, metastatic diseases arising in consequence of repelled cutaneous eruptions, abdominal venous or hæmorrhoidal congestion, &c. The spa is *injurious* in great debility, fever, tendency to hæmorrhage, to abortion, scurvy, during menstruation, &c. At first, old rheumatic pains reappear during the course; this occurrence is considered favourable. In bathing, particular care is to be taken to prevent too high a temperature. Dangerous consequences are to be apprehended from the neglect of this precaution. The atmosphere of the bathing cabinet ought also to be as free as possible from hot vapours, which would partially counteract the beneficial action of the water. Dr. Wetzler mentions the instance of a young lady, in whom hæmoptysis appeared after a few lukewarm baths. When he instituted inquiries at the establishment in which this happened, he found the enclosed hot vapours to have been the cause of the mischief. Among the

---

* A sort of tufa, forming a very hard mortar, if mixed with lime; this combination becomes hardened by the water, and resists its action better than stone.

remedial means must be reckoned the *sinter-soap* introduced by Dr. Peez, and used for poultices and baths with advantage.

The hospital report of Dr. Haas, in ' Gräfe's Jahrbücher,' informs us that 691 patients were admitted in one year. About one-half were treated by the spa-water alone. One hundred and twenty-nine of these suffered from chronic rheumatism, forty-one from arthritic complaints, twenty-five from paralytic affections, &c. Of the first one hundred and twenty-nine, thirty were completely cured (that is, about one in four). Out of the remaining ninety-nine cases, seventy-nine were improved. With reference to the forty-one arthritic cases, thirty-six were relieved. In most of these instances, little or no general reaction was exhibited; eight cases of rheumatic paralysis were relieved, and eight discharged without any improvement. Amongst these was one case of a paralysed tongue; one of paralysed lower extremities of three years' duration, after a miscarriage (patient's age 41); and another of paralysis and atrophy of the lower extremities, &c., induced by neglect of a luxation of the hip joint. In thirteen cases of chronic herpes, only one was discharged unrelieved. In all cases of pains after fractures, relief was experienced.

From the cases treated out of the hospital, he mentions that of a boy, of 14 years of age, formerly healthy, with the exception of a scrofulous habit. By frequent colds, his hearing became affected. Both auditory passages were somewhat narrowed, the tympanum in a more forward direction than usual. On the right side, the ticking of a watch was heard at the distance of two inches, but at the left only on closely applying it to the ear. By the removal of a large quantity of ear-wax, the evil was but slightly diminished. In catheterising the Eustachian tube, air could only be injected with great difficulty. The use of the baths during a fortnight, with local vapour baths, and injections of thermal water, caused the tick of the same watch to be heard on the right side at a distance of twelve inches, and on the left at that of ten inches. Much mucus was discharged from the Eustachian tube by the injections, and the interior of the nose, formerly dry, had become moist.

He further adduces an instance of rheumatic paralysis of the urinary bladder of a female patient. Her physician reported: ' The wife of the burgomaster S——, at H——, ætat. 39, had suffered for several years with violent articular rheumatism, particularly in the left upper thigh. Medical aid was not regularly resorted to. Derivatives were found very efficacious, but as soon as some relief ensued, they were abandoned. I several times urgently recommended Wiesbaden, but from pregnancy and other domestic causes, my advice had not been followed. Since last autumn, the rheumatic complaint entirely disappeared, but in its stead the abdomen became distended, menstruation ceased, strangury occurred, and was rapidly followed by incontinence of urine, and a discharge of dark gravel and mucus. Cantharides, ol. terebinth., &c., were employed in vain. Under these circumstances, I do not expect much from Wiesbaden, but *melius anceps remedium quam nullum.*'

After a fortnight's use of the baths, with douche on the sacral and lumbar regions, and a moderate internal use of the therma, she became so much improved, without febrile reaction or metaschematic processes, that she could hold the water for an hour at a time during the day, and incontinence became restricted to the night. After the second douche, the gravelly appearance diminished, and the urine became gradually clearer. No aperient action was perceived; but menstruation, which had been absent for fifteen months previously, now showed itself, and reappeared afterwards, but irregularly. Her general appearance and strength had likewise greatly improved during a four weeks' course. She now only complained of great thirst. The pains in the vesical region had entirely ceased.

Obermedicinalrath Dr. Franque relates the instance of a man of forty-two years of age, of robust constitution, who had lived to his present age free from dyscrasy and disease, notwithstanding a severe military service of fourteen years. By once sleeping on moist grass, the axillary glands, and afterwards the whole right arm, became swollen and painful. *Stiffness of the elbow-joint* remained, after the swelling had been removed by appropriate treatment. The flexor muscles of the arm were tense. On the upper-arm, above the internal condyles, two moderately deep ulcers discharged a watery purulent matter. The position of the elbow was half-bent. Diaphoretic treatment was first instituted in consequence of a cold, to which the patient was subjected during his journey to Wiesbaden. Subsequently a bath was ordered daily for half an hour, and douches of gradually increased strength on the affected limb. Complete cure of ulcers and anchylosis ensued during the course.

Another instance of rheumatic paralysis is recorded, occurring in a boy of eleven years of age, the child of poor but healthy parents. He fell into a pond; but instead of going home, he undressed, and exposed his clothes to the sun to dry, put them on after some time when still moist, and did not undress again till the evening. Dragging pains in the lower extremities, with rheumatic fever, soon occurred, but medical aid was not sought until the thirteenth day. The lower extremities were found paralysed, and so contracted in the knee-joints, that the soles were only $4\frac{1}{2}$ inches removed from the nates. Anti-rheumatic remedies were resorted to, and succeeded in removing the fever, but paralysis and anchylosis remained. The baths and douches at Wiesbaden produced a complete cure. Other instances of rheumatic paralysis, complicated with repelled itch, are related as having yielded to the beneficial effects of the spa. I attach less value to the cases of icterus, abdominal plethora, &c., because other spas would be more indicated; but let us content ourselves with the principal indication—*chronic rheumatism.* The reputation of the spa for the cure of this disease is European, and the annual influx of valetudinarians is immense.

Those who doubt the efficacy of the mineral waters, or who ascribe the cures to the change of air alone, ought to compare for an instant our present spa with Carlsbad. Wiesbaden possessing one-third more of solid ingredients, and a few degrees less of thermometrical heat, ought to be considered more efficacious when used internally; whilst Carlsbad, with its minor contents and greater heat, seems to be primarily more intended for external application. But what do we find? That just the reverse universally takes place. Moreover, how widely different are the diseases cured or relieved at either, though the baths are cooled to the same temperature in both before being used. I need not give guiding hints for selection between the two, because their indications differ too widely according to experience. But you may have been reminded of another spa while hearing the properties of Wiesbaden detailed. I allude to Wildbad, in Würtemberg. I have shown that its greatest efficacy is exhibited in arthritic and rheumatic paralysis, and in such forms of gouty contractions as require absorption for their cure. You have gouty affections there, somewhat resembling the rheumatic diseases curable here. You remember Wildbad to be one of the akratothermæ, that is, a spa only possessing a few grains of solid ingredients in sixteen ounces, where consequently no power is supposed to exist in the constituents. But if stubborn facts should show analogy in their action, and if on comparing their analyses, you should find both to possess the same constituents in predominance (chloride of sodium), with a proportionate amount of sulphate of soda and carbonate of lime (the chlorides of calcium and magnesium being absent in Wildbad), would it not strike you that some influence *must* be due to the *constituents* of Wildbad, beyond to what is generally ascribed to that water? As I pointed out in my lecture on the Black Forest Spa, water of such high dilution must penetrate into the absorbent vessels, and introduce the dissolved ingredients more easily than denser waters. The amount of culinary salt *absorbed* from the richer Wiesbaden, possibly may not be greater than at Wildbad. The denser liquid finding more difficulty in entering the minutest lymphatic vessels, a great part of its efficacy must be ascribed here to the stimulating action of the warm brine on the peripheric nervous ends. By means of this powerful stimulation of the cutaneous system, the function of the exhaling dermic follicles must be considerably improved, and thus the cause of rheumatism energetically counteracted. The acknowledged advantage of warm baths in rheumatic diseases is here also unattended by the relaxation usually following the employment of these agents; the presence of the chlorides preventing such a result, by means of the reaction they induce. The assistance afforded by the internal use of Wiesbaden cannot be doubted, but its chief reputation having been created by the baths, we are justified in taking their therapeutic results into our more serious consideration. The analogy between the effects of the two named spas is so great in some respects, that careful selection is necessary to decide between them. If you perceive the general nervous power to be in normal condition, but by a regulation of peripheric functions you hope to restore the equilibrium between the nervous and sero-fibrous systems, you will recommend the patient suffering with rheumatic paralysis to resort to Wiesbaden. If, however, the general nervous vitality be diminished—if age or debility does not allow hope of recovery from systemic reaction—if in the contracted or disabled joint, concrete exudations have been deposited, so that to return to a normal condition, not only the cutaneous but the lymphatic and nervous systems must be roused into great activity, you will choose Wildbad. Though, as regards constituents, greater similarity exists betweem Homburg and Wiesbaden, their curative results vary too considerably for any difficulty to arise in discriminating between them; abdominal plethora and menstrual irregularities being the ailments chiefly cured at Homburg. You will observe what importance must be attached to the chemical character of the spas, but at the same time their other inherent qualities must not be lost sight of.*

Several experienced *physicians* reside at this fashionable spa, as Drs. Von Franque, Vogler, Haas, Müller, Gergens, Fritze, Kopp, Reuter, Ebhardt, Mahr, Dörr, Roth, Genth (at Dietenmühle), &c.

* Hotels : The Four Seasons, Rose, de France, Victoria, d'Angleterre.

LECTURE XIII.

WEILBACH — BADEN.

FROM Wiesbaden we turn to the north-east and travel by the railroad as far as *Flörsheim*. From this town an omnibus conveys us in about ten minutes to the Theiokrene (cold sulphur spring) of *Weilbach*. The sulphur springs (*Theiopegae*, from θεῖον, sulphur, and πήγη, spring) are generally produced by the action of water on a sulphuret of sodium or potassium, or on sulphurous acid. Their chief ingredient is a combination of sulphur, which constantly evolves free sulphuretted hydrogen gas. The waters are clear or milky, resembling rotten eggs in their nauseous taste and smell. At Weilbach, the taste and smell are more like those of fresh eggs. By exposure to the atmosphere the waters are easily decomposed. If hot, they are called *Theiothermae* (from θεῖον, sulphur, and θερμὸς, hot), as Aachen (Aix-la-Chapelle) and Baden, near Vienna; if cold, *Theiokrenae* (from θεῖον, sulphur, and κρηνη, cold spring), as Eilsen, Nenndorf, Weilbach, &c. They all exert a beneficial influence on those cutaneous derangements which partially depend on a disordered action of the serofibrous system. Thus they powerfully counteract rheumatic, arthritic and herpetic diseases, by heightening the normal function of the skin, and by causing the excretion of effete substances, which, obstructing the action of secreting organs, act offensively on the sentient nervous terminations. The village of *Weilbach*, lat. N. 50°, long. E. 8°, is situated on a fertile declivity of an alluvial mountain, almost midway between Frankfort and Menz, two leagues to the south of Höchst, one and a half from Hochheim, and half a league distant from the river Maine. The mineral spring rises about 1,000 paces to the south-west of Weilbach, in a sloping field, connected with the village by a footpath. Towards the south the view is open, but to the east a steep hill rises, and affords a charming and extensive prospect from its summit. The luxuriant Maine-valley lies in a southerly direction, with its capacious plain reaching to the Melibokus, the highest peak of the Bergstrasse. Your eye, in glancing to the opposite shore of the Rhine, is arrested by the vine-clad hills on whose acclivities are situated Oppenheim and Nierstein. Towards the north the Taunus peaks of Feldberg and Attking raise their lofty heads. In olden times the Weilbach spring was used by the inhabitants for cutaneous eruptions and ulcers, also as a domestic remedy in thoracic and gastric complaints. It was not until the year 1783 that the Regency of Menz obtained a knowledge of the spring, and caused it to be examined and tested for diseases. The results proving satisfactory, the spring was enclosed. The water is forced into a marble urn and discharged by four pipes. It is transparent, and clear as crystal. The taste is sweetish at first, and afterwards bitter and saline, but not disagreeable. I found it myself very refreshing, and drank it with pleasure. It does not sparkle. Exposed for some time to the atmosphere, it deposits a yellowish-white precipitate of sulphur, carbonate of lime, and organic substance. Its temperature is $56\frac{3}{4}°$ F.; specific gravity 1·007. The supply during twenty-four hours is 2,430 cubic feet. Analysis shows considerable variations at different periods. According to the latest, by Kastner, it contains—

 2·94 cubic inches of sulphuretted hydrogen.
 5·80 ,,   carbonic acid.
 Traces of nitrogen.

4·52 grains of carbonate of soda.
1·80 ,,   ,,   magnesia.
2·17 ,,   ,,   lime.
0·03 ,,   ,,   strontia.
0·35 ,, sulphate of soda.
2·05 ,, chloride of sodium.
1·00 ,,   ,,   magnesium.
0·36 ,, silica.
0·08 ,, organic extractive matter.

Total, 12·40 grains.

The spring was formerly called Faulborn (putrid well), and used in testing wine, vinegar, and brandy, for metallic salts, an evident proof of the abundance of sulphuretted hydrogen contained in it. The chemist Jung found, in his analysis of 1830, $16\frac{3}{4}$ grains of solid constituents in 16 ounces; in 1834, $27\frac{3}{4}$ grains; in 1835, $30\frac{1}{2}$ grains. The ingredients met with in the largest quantities were carbonate of soda and of magnesia, chloride of sodium and magnesium, and silica. The substance deposited in the marble urn adheres to the concave surface, and resembles a sea-green flocculent kind of mud. The surface turned towards the water is covered with a pale-yellowish powder, which is unctuous to the touch, and gives out a hepatic smell at first. When dried, pulverised in a wooden mortar, treated with rectified spirits of wine, filtered, and then evaporated, a peculiar resin is obtained, called *sulphur-resin.*

The water is generally well received by the digestive organs. The diuresis is invariably increased during the course. The matinal urine often appears clearer than usual, strongly acid, and contains neither carbonates nor sulphates. Alvine evacuations are rather retarded at first, but become gradually normal during the course. After some time the fæces assume a greenish colour, chiefly caused by the presence of biliary matter and sulphuret of iron. The alvine retardation noticed above is never found to inconvenience the patients. If required, an aperient effect may generally be induced by repeated draughts of water taken at short intervals. Diarrhœa occasionally happens during cold moist weather, or after sudden atmospheric changes, particularly in the beginning of the course. If inclination to relaxation of the bowels exists, diarrhœa follows, or is augmented, under the use of the water: this also frequently happens in hepatic hyperæmia. Appetite generally improves; pressure and fulness in the pit of the stomach, with teasing flatulence, soon subside. Hæmorrhoidal swellings and blennorrhage of the anus disappear after the first eight or ten days; but Weilbach does not induce hæmorrhage from piles. Many have been entirely cured of this tendency without the least congestion to the brain or other vital organs in consequence.

Most of the invalids at Weilbach suffer from thoracic affections. In certain chronic pulmonary diseases the pulse is invariably found to abate, and the irritation of the bronchial mucous membrane to diminish. The oppression, dyspnœa, and dry cough of incipient phthisis soon give way, unless there be anæmic condition or inflammatory irritation present. The number of respirations diminishes with the abatement of the pulse, enabling the patient to take deeper inhalations. The morbidly-lessened vesicular respiratory murmur characterising this period becomes normal, whilst the cardiac sounds cease to be heard at the parts affected. All these beneficial changes occur more particularly in persons with hæmorrhoidal tendency or dyscrasy—who have generally a slender form, a dark complexion, a dry skin, prominent eyes— and with sclerotica of a bluish tint. Bleeding from the nose spitting of blood, and general orgasm have commonly marked their younger days. Such individuals particularly experience the curative effects of Weilbach if their thoracic organs are affected. Hoarseness through excessive use of mercurials yields to the water. In other tracheal and laryngeal complaints it is necessary to ascertain whether the uvula be reddened and lax, with an abundant venous development in the fauces, accompanied by cough and considerable secretion; for in chlorotic complaints of the same parts, with menstrual derangements, a troublesome sensation of dryness or burning, and a weakened rather than an actually hoarse voice, the evil would rather increase under the use of Weilbach. No benefit will result if scrofulous dyscrasia maintains or causes the affection. With regard to asthma, only such forms are improved as are connected with abdominal infarcta and obstruction. Perspiration is never caused by the water, but rather diminished in cases where an atonic state of the skin had induced profuse nightsweats. Bath-eruption is rare. Chronic muscular or articular rheumatism is relieved, if connected with hæmorrhoidal congestion. Bodily strength and mental cheerfulness visibly increase. The water never causes vascular erethism; generally speaking, the female sex derive less benefit from Weilbach than the male. The *modus operandi* of the water is thought to be the following by Dr. Heinrich Roth, the former highly intelligent physician of the spa:—The water is mostly absorbed in the stomach with its sulphuretted hydrogen. The urinary excretion corresponds to the quantity of water taken. The absence of eructation and flatulence shows that the gas does not pass *through* the alimentary tube, but enters the circulation in unison with the water. On this account no increased evacuations ensue. If, however, in consequence of intestinal irritation, excessive doses, or impeded cutaneous function, diarrhœa should occur, the water ceases to be useful; for the patient becomes too much weakened, whilst the curative particles pass too rapidly through the alimentary tube to produce the metamorphic alterations required. The green excrements mentioned above contain a greater amount of biliary matter than usual, with sulphuret of iron as the colouring principle. If they are dissolved in water and treated with diluted hydrochloric acid, the green colouration disappears under evolution of sulphuretted hydrogen. After filtration the residue exhibits a decidedly bilious colour, and betrays the presence of iron. The same processes, adopted with ordinary fæces of the same individual when removed from the influence of

Weilbach water, elicited no change of colour or evolution of hydrothionic acid, but only a trace of iron and a less bilious colour of the residue. From this circumstance we must deduce an increased bilification. The sulphuret of iron can only have been conducted into the intestines along with the bile, the Weilbach water containing no iron. Being imbibed by the gastric capillary vessels, the water mingles with the blood of the portal vein. Sulphuretted hydrogen, which causes a green colour in ordinary blood by forming sulphuret of iron, combines here with those blood-corpuscles whose vitality has been diminished. Allowing their iron to combine with the sulphur of the gas introduced, they lose still more of their integrant constitution, and are the more fit for separation from their more vital neighbouring corpuscles. Thus by the use of the water a greater amount of material is furnished for the formation of bile. The transformation of the effete corpuscles into biliary matter is further promoted by the presence of carbonate of soda, which constitutes the prevailing solid ingredient. This salt is not discovered in the urine, whilst rainwater containing the same amount of carbonate of soda renders that excretion alkaline. Part of the soda required for the saturation of the choleic and stearic acids is supposed to be derived from the water. Under otherwise favourable circumstances, a more than proportionate quantity of bile must thus be produced. The older blood-corpuscles are naturally most exposed to this chemico-organic metamorphosis.

With anæmic persons the green colouration of the excrements appears late or is not observed at all, the deficient state of the blood-elements admitting of a smaller abstraction of older corpuscles. If hæmorrhoidal swellings exist, the obstructed portal circulation causes vital retrogression of many corpuscles, and renders them more accessible to the chemical action of sulphuretted hydrogen. The characteristic colour of the evacuations appears sooner or later according to the more or less developed hæmorrhoids. After some time this colour ceases, for the generation of new blood-corpuscles does not keep pace with the retrocession and transformation of the older ones. The accumulated material of effete corpuscles being now briskly removed, the normal intestinal function increases. The sallow and yellowish tint of such individuals, due to the incomplete transformation of these overloading materials, gives way to a clear and healthier complexion. The emission of the sulphuretted hydrogen through the lungs and skin proves that it is less apt to attack those blood-corpuscles endowed with a great degree of vitality. Though the circumference of the abdomen decreases, signs of weakness, anæmia, and exhaustion are never observed, notwithstanding the diminished quantity of blood. In chlorosis, however, and during recovery from acute diseases, the previous weakness and anæmia would increase by the use of the water.

The improved appetite perceptible immediately after drinking is likewise ascribed to the more energetic sanguineous metamorphosis; but the liver itself must not be inflamed, enlarged, or otherwise diseased, for then the Weilbach water would not confer its wonted benefit. It would not even be well received, but passing through the intestines it would induce diarrhœa. The characteristic colour of the stools would not appear, and generally the reaction which follows from increased hepatic function would be missed.

The formation of blood-corpuscles is shown to be particularly active in hæmorrhoidal individuals, by their generally bearing hæmorrhages without becoming weakened or anæmic. This may proceed from the insufficient transformation of old blood-corpuscles in the liver. Regeneration of new corpuscles taking place as usual, the blood becomes overcharged with corpuscles, and general circulation is somewhat impeded. The intestinal and other organs perform their functions with less ease; hence dyspepsia, flatulence, distention of the abdomen, languor, headache, &c. inconvenience the patient till the efforts of nature relieve the circulating organs of this surplus of older corpuscles by hæmorrhage. The continuation of the same causes will, after some time, reproduce the same necessity. Weilbach is therefore eminently useful by counteracting the cause of hæmorrhoidal congestion. Excessive catamenia are diminished, and hæmorrhoidal tendency retrogrades; even flow of piles decreases, and ceases entirely by the use of the water, the want of such a reparatory discharge having been obviated.

The course of the blood becoming freer in the hæmorrhoidal vessels, the vascular absorbents are enabled to imbibe more of the liquid intestinal contents, leaving a smaller quantum for fæcal excretion. On this account the evacuations are rather diminished at first, but without any of the ordinary sensations or inconveniences connected with obstruction. The increased absorption of liquid alimentary matter forms some compensation for the heightened elimination of blood-corpuscles. After some time the increased formation of bile will end in a greater intestinal stimulation, and the alvine action will thus become regulated.

The increased elimination of effete blood-globules from the portal system must extend its influence to other organs, because this gradual liberation of obstructing particles enables the portal vein to receive more blood than before. Hence the congested state of the pulmonary tissue diminishes under the use of Weilbach; respiration becomes freer; oppression of the chest, dry cough, &c., decrease perceptibly; hæmoptysis often ceases, the pulse becomes slower, night-perspirations gradually vanish, &c.

Weilbach thus acts as a sort of chemico-vital derivative, but loses its power whenever the laryngeal or bronchial irritation proceeds from other causes than hæmorrhoidal congestion, as in already deposited tubercles, in chronic inflammation of one of these organs, &c. The advantage derivable from Weilbach would be diminished or destroyed by taking too large quantities of the water; for the excessive amount of sulphuretted hydrogen not being absorbed in the portal system, produces irritation in the bloodvessels and ultimately in the lungs, from which it must be exhaled. Chronic bronchial catarrh, incipient phthisis, spitting of blood, congestion to the head, based on hæmorrhoidal dyscrasia, gradually give way here, because the organs of respiration become relieved of a great overcharge of blood without the loss of nutrient corpuscles. Besides the derivation, the composition of the blood becomes more normal, and thus forms a better regenerating agent for the various organs, which in their turn are more fitted for the performance of their regular functions, and thus improvement of health will continue even after the action of the water has ceased. If favourable phenomena do not make their appearance within a few weeks, no cure can be expected. The utility of Weilbach in chronic poisoning by lead or mercury is obvious.

Baths are often employed as an auxiliary to the internal use of the water. Inhalation of the atmosphere surrounding the well has afforded no striking results. The hæmorrhoidal disease is frequently cured here, in contradistinction to many other spas, where the flow of repressed piles is promoted. Chronic rheumatism and cutaneous eruption, accompanied by hæmorrhoids, are likewise often relieved here. The same may be said of urinary or sexual diseases resulting from hæmorrhoidal obstruction. The water must be drunk in small draughts, or the gas would not be so rapidly absorbed, and, consequently, would cause distention of the abdomen and irritation of the lungs.

In filling the glass, certain precautions are necessary—viz., the water should run down the sides of the glass, and the latter should be kept as close to the spout as possible ; for if the glass be held at some distance, and the water allowed to fall with force into the centre, a great quantity of atmospheric air is drawn in with it, whilst the violent agitation causes the inherent sulphuretted hydrogen and carbonic acid gases to escape too soon. From two to six glasses (of six or seven ounces each) are taken in the morning ; sometimes before dinner a smaller dose is repeated.

The diet must be very temperate at first, but more nourishing afterwards. Care must be taken that the liver and intestines be not taxed too much by fatty or indigestible food, or spirituous liquors.

You may perhaps ask whether we can expect such important results from so small an amount of sulphuretted hydrogen—viz., about $2\frac{1}{2}$ cubic inches in a pint of water—and whether we ought to attribute the same action to all sulphurous springs. The answer to this is, that the proportion of the gas is extremely large here, surpassing in this respect all other theiothermæ of Germany : Aix-la-Chapelle, the most celebrated, having only 0·13 cubic inches, Baden, near Vienna, 0·70, Eilsen 2·01, Nenndorf (Quelle unter dem Gewölbe) 1·21, Weilbach 2·64.

Although the same gas stamps their general character, the diseases for which they should be recommended are widely different. Sulphurous springs are generally set down as most useful in chronic rheumatism and cutaneous eruptions, and it might be imagined that we have only to choose between a hot and cold spring. If you visit Aix-la-Chapelle, for instance, you will find most of the valetudinarians there to be suffering from affections of the sero-fibrous or cutaneous system, and in vain will you look for patients who seek relief from pulmonary or laryngeal complaints. But here you will notice the reverse. The spa, however, is very little known, and is not appreciated as it deserves to be. When I visited the chief spas for the first time, it was my intention to pass by Weilbach. I happened to stay at the Post Hotel at Kreuznach. When just on the point of starting, the head-waiter, who heard that I intended to visit Soden, asked me whether I would not pay a visit to Weilbach ; and said I should perhaps feel interested in seeing his principal, who had suffered for several years with spitting of blood, and such an exhausting cough that his friends laughed at him, when, after a fruitless resort to Ems (which enjoys such a European reputation in pulmonary diseases), he rode to Weilbach at the recommendation of some acquaintance; but he persisted, and subsequently found there a complete cure. The landlord confirmed the statement of his waiter, and appeared to me then hale and hearty. The basis of his pulmonary disorder lay in hæmorrhoidal dyscrasy; and as soon as he presented himself to Dr. Roth, that physician informed him that his case was particularly fitted for Weilbach, as it afterwards proved. I at once determined to alter my route, and to examine a remedial agent which had afforded such striking results.

Physician: Dr. Stifft.

Baden, near Vienna.—For the consideration of the next spa, I shall request you to retrace your steps to *Vienna*, the Austrian capital, and thence proceed southward by railroad to Baden, which lies at an hour's distance. Baden was known to the Romans under the name of '*Pannonian Baths.*' The history of this now beautiful town is full of interest. How often were the vineyards and orchards destroyed, the houses burnt, the inhabitants plundered and murdered—now by the Turks, then by the Huns, now by the Turks again, who used to burn those treasures which they could not carry off with them! Then, again, French armies laid contributions on the exhausted treasury of the inoffensive town. Scarcely was one injury repaired when another befel them in the shape of extensive conflagrations.

The discovery of the spa is popularly ascribed to the following circumstance:—At some very remote period, the dogs of a neighbouring nobleman were missed for a few hours every day in the adjoining forest. They were known to be affected with a kind of lepra, and when carefully watched and followed by some huntsmen, they were found to seek some warm springs, in which they bathed for some time, and then returned to their master. Their eruption having afterwards been found to be cured, the nobleman had the surrounding trees cut down, and the source enclosed for the relief of human ailments.

Baden is situated in lat. north 48°, and long. east 15°, on the Schwöchat, four miles to the south-east of Vienna, at the foot of the *Wienerwald*, 638 feet above the level of the sea, and surrounded by very charming landscapes. The Cethic mountains encircle the place from the north and west, whilst to the south-east an extensive open plain stretches as far as the frontier of Hungary. To this position we must ascribe the frequent atmospheric changes to which the place is occasionally subject, amounting sometimes to 34° F. in one day. The environs of Baden are very fertile; wine, fruits, and agricultural products are alike found here in abundance. Baden has about 5,000 inhabitants, and attracts numerous visitors, besides the crowd of valetudinarians that annually resort thither. It belongs to the class of Theiothermæ (warm sulphurous springs), and appropriately follows as a contrast to the last cold sulphur-spring which we have examined.

A great advantage of the Baden water lies in the circumstance that neither heating nor cooling is required to fit it for bathing. The atmosphere of the place is so impregnated with sulphurous exhalations that metallic objects quickly become tarnished and blackened. The surrounding mountains consist of stratified limestone slate and gypsum, and are interspersed with sulphur-pyrites, stalactites, mineral coal, and some curious petrifactions. The climate is generally dry and healthy, with the exception above alluded to.

The whole valley offers a complex of beautiful walks and parks, with rocks and forests beyond. The Alexandrowiczsche Anlage, approached by gardens and vineyards, leads us to the steep rocks behind the Schönfeldish houses. The Carpathian Mountains bound the plain on the south-east. The Langische Anlage, to the south of the Calvarienberg, abounds in rocks ornamented with shrubs, luxuriant foliage winding along the walks, with turf-seats interspersed. The Weilburg stands in its grounds, a memorial of antiquity. The '*Helenen-thal*' extends from Weikersdorf to Heiligenkreuz, and is replete with charming spots and shady walks. The Antonsgrotte, Antonsbrücke (bridge), Krainerhütten, &c. are all objects of great attraction. I will merely add the account of a place situated a league to the south of Baden—viz. *Vöslau*, at the eastern declivity of the Vöslauer *Lindkogel*, remarkable for its swimming-bath and beautiful garden. The water (furnished by a spring) is clear, transparent, inodorous, and insipid—temperature, 75° F.; specific gravity, 1·0005. It contains scarcely $3\frac{1}{2}$ grains of mineral ingredients—consisting of carbonate of lime, sulphate of lime, and of magnesia, chloride of sodium, of calcium, and of silica, besides carbonic acid and nitrogen. This swimming-bath forms an excellent preparation for weakly or irritable persons before the employment of the warmer thermæ of Baden. Not a trace of sulphuretted hydrogen is found in this water, though it seems to derive its heat from the same subterranean process which raises the temperature of the Baden water.

The temperature of the springs in Baden varies from 98° to 81° F.—viz., in Josephsbad the source is 98° F. (the bath, 97° F.);

Frauenbad, 97½° F. (the bath, 96½° F.). No less than thirty-three springs exist in or near the town, of which I have only enumerated the principal ones. They contain 12½ grains of solid and 1½ cubic inches of gaseous constituents in a pint of water, viz.—

  3·20 grains of sulphate of lime.
  1·99   ,,   ,,   soda.
  1·36   ,,   ,,   magnesia.
  1·34   ,,   chloride of sodium.
  0·36   ,,   ,,   magnesium.
  1·75   ,,   carbonate of magnesia.
  1·80   ,,   ,,   lime.
  0·07   ,,   ,,   lithia.
  0·73   ,,   animalo-vegetable substance.
        Traces of phosphate of lime.

Total 12·10 grains.

GASEOUS CONSTITUENTS.

  0·7 cubic inches of sulphuretted hydrogen.
  0·5   ,,   ,,   carbonic acid.
  0·3   ,,   ,,   nitrogen.

Total 1·5

The amount of solid ingredients you perceive to be equal to that of Weilbach, but their quality is different. The chief constituent of Weilbach is carbonate of soda (4½ grains), of which no trace is found in Baden. Sulphate of lime, the principal constituent of Baden (3·2 gr.), does not exist in Weilbach; carbonate of magnesia and of lime, and chloride of sodium, are found in rather smaller proportions at Baden; sulphate of magnesia is absent in Weilbach; sulphate of soda only ⅓ of a grain: thus we have sulphates predominating in Baden and carbonates in Weilbach. As regards the volatile ingredients, Weilbach has three times the amount of sulphuretted hydrogen—viz., 2½ cubic inches to 7-10ths here, and ten times as much carbonic acid, 5 cubic inches to ½; but Weilbach possesses no nitrogen. Besides, you are justified in attributing to the sulphuretted hydrogen somewhat more power than its proportion to Weilbach would seem to warrant, on account of its connection here with thermal water, by which its efficacy and facility of penetration are promoted. The therapeutical results of either spa will be found to coincide with their chemical and physical characteristics. The water of Baden is clear and transparent when drawn, but becomes rather milky when exposed for some time to the air or light. Its taste and smell are strongly sulphurous; the springs all furnish an abundant supply; the specific gravity of the water is 1·004. The yellowish crystals deposited on the sides of the springs are known as Badner salt. The *bath-mud*, the result of precipitation out of water, is to be distinguished from this.

The Josephsbad is a round temple-like building, ornamented with Ionic columns. About sixty persons may bathe in the capacious quadrangular baignoire; it is situated in the Josephsplatz, near the Anger. The *Frauenbad* is situated to the east of the former, at the end of the Frauengasse—its baignoire holds ninety persons. The same source supplies four so-called 'Frauenstundenbäder' (women's hour-baths), containing space for one or two bathers only. The *Carolinenbad*, formerly called 'external women's bath,' forms the southern part of the same building; fifty persons find bathing room in its baignoire. The *Engelburgbäder*, lying on the other side of the Schwöchat, were formerly only used as foot-baths, but are now provided with accommodation for douche, shower, and full baths. The temperature of the baths is 94° F. The *Sauerbad* (so named not from any acid properties, but from its former possessor) is likewise situated on the other side of the Schwöchat, and was newly enclosed in 1821, and provided with an elegant bathing-saloon. The temperature of the baths is 94° F. The *Römerquelle* (Roman's source), commonly called the '*Ursprung*,' arises at the foot of the *Calvarienberg*, with such abundance that it is able to supply the 'Halbbäder, 'Theresienbäder,' &c. By a subterranean passage of about forty-five yards in length, you reach a capacious cavern, in which a cauldron two fathoms deep is constantly filled with the bubbling water from below. It is enclosed by wooden balusters. Formerly the water was drawn here, and carried along the passage to the exterior for use. Now this objectionable mode has been done away with by the erection of a 'Trinkbrunnen' (drinking-well), which receives the spring out of porcelain pipes, and discharges it into a marble basin. A stop-cock is fitted to the spout to regulate the supply. In the above passage artificial bath-mud is prepared, and arrangements adapted for the use of vapour-baths. The temperature of the source is $94\frac{3}{4}°$ F.

At the sides and ceiling the salt-crystals, formed by sublimation, are sometimes redissolved by the exhaling vapours, and fall down as 'acid drops,' destructive of the colour and material of clothes. The salt is dry, yellowish-white, crystallized in fascicular needles, easily friable, and interspersed with minute veins of sulphur, from which they may be separated by solution in water. Taste and reaction of the salt are acid: it loses forty-six per cent. by being heated, and contains, in one hundred parts—

```
37·70 sulphuric acid.
 8·00 alumina.
 7·34 protoxide of iron.
46·00 water of crystallisation.
 0·88 sulphur, and other admixtures.
 0·08 loss.
─────
100
```

This shows a considerable excess of sulphuric acid (for only 18·73 parts are required to saturate the alumina, and only 8·37 for the neutralization of the iron, leaving an excess of about ten parts). Though this phenomenon is not rare in volcanic craters, it is of less frequent occurrence in the thermæ. The sulphuretted hydrogen rapidly issuing in bubbles out of the source, abandons part of its hydrogen to the oxygen of the air for the formation of water; whilst its sulphur, under the influence of heat, partially precipitates and partially attracts the disposable amount of atmospheric oxygen for the formation of sulphuric acid. These acid vapours act then on the ferruginous and argillaceous walls, and dissolve those particles met with in analysis.

The *Herzogsbad* possesses the most capacious baignoire, conveniently holding 150 persons. It receives its water, by leaden pipes, from the Römerquelle;—temperature, 94¾° F.

The *Antonibad*, 93° F., is situated near the latter, and has the same origin.

The Military-bath, Franzensbad, Leopoldsbäder, &c. are sometimes chosen on account of their lower temperature. Vapour, douche, rain and shower baths are also provided in the various establishments. The ascending douche is administered in appropriate cases.

But a distinguishing feature of this spa consists in the newly-erected *sulphurous swimming-baths*, one for ladies and one for the male sex, supplied by springs of 81° F., and cooled down by the extensive surface to 75° F. by the time it is used. The greater number of swimmers I noticed at the time of my visit were youthful patients, and the advantages resulting from this combination of muscular exercise with the free imbibition of this medicinal liquid are said to be very great. Indeed, considering the composition and properties of the water, it would be surprising to find it otherwise. Children affected with rheumatic tendency, with cutaneous acrimony, with weakly-developed thoracic organs, derive great benefit from them; and I doubt not that many a morbid diathesis will be checked and made to retrograde by the early use of these baths.

Besides full baths, half, foot, and hand baths are often exclusively employed at Baden in certain cases. This spa, in general, is recommended in convalescence after weakening diseases (where Weilbach would be injurious), in diminished sensibility or irritability, chronic rheumatism, paralytic affections, swellings of the liver or spleen, in certain chronic eruptions, whenever the function of the skin has been repressed or morbidly altered, in mucosity and cartarrhal irritation of lungs or intestines, hydrargyrosis, and chronic poisoning by lead. The swimming-baths have shown themselves especially *curative* in articular contractions and slight curvatures of the spine. This spa is *contra-indicated* in plethora, active congestion, inflammation, or inflammatory tendency, fever, confirmed phthisis, &c.

The *Badeschlamm* (bath-mud) chiefly consists of argilla, wetted with the water of the Ursprung.

Dr. Rollet related to me the case of a major in the army, who, in consequence of recent injuries, was suffering from painful and stiff joints, which necessitated the use of crutches. This gentleman applied to him with the intention of using the baths. But the doctor considered the symptoms too acute for the spa; he therefore ordered mud-poultices to be applied overnight for a week, at the end of which time the pain was so much diminished that he was enabled to use the baths, and left the place cured after three weeks.

In chronic *emphysema*, resulting from neglected pulmonary catarrh, Baden is asserted to be peculiarly beneficial. Dr. Habel recommends Baden in chronic gout, but neither vascular irritability nor great nervous sensibility must be present. Baden is particularly adapted to that form of gout caused by depressing influences, and exhibiting more the character of arthritic remains: also in scrofula, the deficient chylification and lymphatic absorption are corrected by the spa stimulating the peripheric extremities of the blood-vessels and nerves; secretions are promoted, and morbid products absorbed and removed. Drinking must be combined with the external use for this disease. In cases of children who refuse to drink, clysters of the water must be substituted. For psora and herpes the baths are greatly extolled.

In idiopathic paralysis no advantage is derived. The benefit in syphilis is restricted to the diagnostic value in cases of affections bearing a doubtful psoric, hydrargyrous, or syphilitic character.

The two former are relieved or cured by the spa—the latter would be rather aggravated. In complication of syphilis with hydrargyrosis the latter disease is removed, and the former simplified, so as to be amenable to ordinary treatment. You perceive, then, that Baden should be selected when the functions of the cutaneous and fibrous system have to be regulated, when absorption has to be promoted, when rheumatic, arthritic, or psoric dyscrasy has to be counteracted, whilst heightened function of the bile is only enumerated as a secondary or occasional result. So far from its serving as a derivative or revulsive, it must never be employed where inflammation or even congestion exists. External employment is mostly resorted to. If you compare these peculiarities with its brother theiopege, Weilbach, you will find the character of the Nassau spa almost diametrically opposite. Weilbach is chiefly employed internally. The principal diseases there are hæmorrhoids and pulmonary or laryngeal affections dependent on hæmorrhoidal dyscrasy. The marked activity of the portal and biliary systems exerts a derivative influence upon vital organs somewhat analogous to sanguineous depletion. Menstruation and piles are not promoted, but rather abridged. Exhausted persons become weaker still. Convalescence is prolonged after atonic, nervous diseases or depressing hæmorrhages. Keeping these brief hints in view, you will find no difficulty in choosing between the two.

Physicians: Drs. Habel, Landesmaun, Rollet, Sevegnani, Bratassewitz, Lucas, Mülleitner, and Hirscher. *

* Hotels: Casino, Stadt Wien, Schwan.

LECTURE XIV.

KREUZNACH—ADELHEIDSQUELLE.

AFTER the deviation made for the sake of contrasting Weilbach with Baden, we return westward towards *Biberich*. Here we exchange our confined position in the railroad carriage for the Rhine steamer, which carries us rapidly towards the western curve, on which *Bingen* is situated. At Bingen we leave the Rhine with all its romantic associations, and while most of our fellow-passengers speed onwards to the north, approaching the mouth of Father Rhine, I invite you to accompany me in an opposite direction, and to be carried by rail to the spa (in 38 minutes); or you might travel the whole distance by rail, a line being constructed along the Rhine competing with the river-steamers. *Kreuznach* is situated on the *Nahe*, which rises in the west beyond the Hundsrück mountain, and, after a serpentine eastern course amongst the hills, turns northward, and emerging from rocks, descends into a smiling valley full of picturesque spots, intersects the town of Kreuznach, and passes northwards through fertile fields and green meadows to Bingen, where it pours its stream into the mighty Rhine. The town, containing about 8,000 inhabitants, though situated in the Grand Duchy of Hesse, is under Prussian dominion. Its latitude N. is 50°, its longitude E. 8°: it is three leagues distant from Bingen, eight from Mentz, and ten from Wiesbaden; its height above the level of the sea is only 285 feet. The two parts into which the town is divided by the river are unequal. That on the left bank is enclosed by the Schlossberg and other hills, while the country on the right bank is of a more level character. On both sides of the connecting bridge, green islets emerge out of the Nahe, the upper ones giving birth to the mineral springs at an altitude of 308 feet. Charming gardens, well-cultivated vineyards, rich pasture and cornfields amply testify to the fertile condition of the soil.

The ruins of the so-called 'Heidenmauer' (Pagans' Wall), on the right of the Nahe, prove that the Romans reached the place in their insatiable lust of conquest, and endeavoured to maintain the Rhine boundary by a fortress. Many of the old castles and towers have disappeared; the ancient fortress of the Counts of Sponheim has remained in ruins since its destruction by the French. Vineyards and shady walks cover the side of the mountain, over which a fortified castle domineered at the time of the Thirty Years' War. The excise-buildings now occupy the place in the 'Hohe Strasse' where formerly the mansion of the Pfalzgraves of Simmern stood. A capacious 'casino' was lately built, with tasteful walks, before the Binger Gate. The streets of the town itself are generally narrow. The Nahe Bridge, connecting the two parts of the town, conducts you over the two arms of the river and its islets by seven arches; it is said to date from the fourteenth century; the houses standing upon it give it rather a curious appearance. As a curative agent, this spa has only been known for about forty years.

The *Elisabethbrunnen*, the most celebrated of Kreuznach's springs, rises on the southern extremity of the Nahe islet. About ten feet under the 'dam-earth' the source issues from a borehole, penetrating into porphyry to the depth of thirty-six feet; the enclosing basin guards against the influx of atmospheric water; a strong dam of stone surrounds the spring on three sides, and serves by its colossal proportions to prevent overflow, or ice from disturbing the spring. From the platform you enjoy a pleasant prospect of the river above and below the town. To the west the vineclad sides of the Schlossberg greet your view, and southward are the hills from which the salt-springs arise. The iron balustrade combines elegance with strength. About 1,600 cubic feet of water are supplied in twenty-four hours; a pipe communicates with the basin, and discharges the water in an uninterrupted stream; a pump drives it into the bathing-house, about one hundred yards distant, at times when the spring is not used for drinking.

A second spring, of great abundance, rises in the bed of the river, between the Elisenbrunnen and the left bank of the Nahe. At a depth of ten feet it issues out of numerous fissures of porphyry; a basin and airtight covering of brickwork guard it from admixture with the Nahe water, which passes over it. By subterranean iron pipes the water is conducted into a reservoir near the Elisenbrunn for baths. The daily supply amounts to 3,000 cubic feet.

The islet was connected with the highroad of the 'salimen'

valley by a convenient walk, shaded by a double row of lime-trees. A grand 'Kurhaus' was built, with capacious saloons, refreshment-rooms, bathing-cabinets, and apartments for visitors. Another spring has since been discovered between the Elisenbrunnen and the salt-works near the Oranienhof, and is frequently employed for bathing.

The porphyry rocks of the 'Haart' mountain on the left, and of the 'Gans' on the right bank, form a narrow valley, intersected by the Nahe, south of the town, and give rise to the saline springs of the *Theodorshalle* and *Münster am Stein*, north and south-west, and of the *Carlshalle*, to the east. Their abundance is such that the Carlshalle and Theodorshalle alone afford an annual supply of three million cubic feet of brine. The springs of the Theodorshalle, to the number of eight, arise from various depths. The chief well is situated near the boiling-house, and used for drinking. In its immediate neighbourhood one of the largest 'graduation-works' reaches as far as the Nahe, its covered passage serving as a convenient walk in rainy weather. If you cross the Nahe you perceive, on the right bank near the bridge, the well of the Carlshalle, surrounded by a tower-like building. The water is raised by pumping into a pipe, and is then discharged into a small stone basin for the use of valetudinarians. A more concentrated brine is furnished by a neighbouring borehole. Trees and resting-places adorn the open spot in front of the well.

The saline '*Münster am Stein*,' wedged, as you see it, into the southern corner of the left Nahe shore, supplies also a drinking-well; the spring issues opposite the rocks of the Rheingrafenstein. The adjoining 'graduation-works' also offer a sheltered walk in unfavourable atmospheric conditions.

That in the commencement of the nineteenth century no steps were taken to imitate other ' Salinen' in the erection of contrivances for bathing, is to be attributed to the peculiar political position of the works, which were allotted in the Parisian treaty to Hesse Darmstadt, while the ground is subject to Prussian dominion. It was not until 1820 that foreign visitors began to employ the baths. Between the Elisenquelle and the Carlshaller salt-works you see the grand 'Felnersche Badehaus,' farther on, the capacious buildings of the Oranienhof. The same activity was observed in the erection and embellishment of buildings on the Theodorshalle. In the southern Münster the inhabitants contributed their share in furnishing convenient habitations and bathing arrangements.

The greatest praise, in causing Kreuznach to be so universally appreciated, is due to the personal and literary exertions of the late Dr. Prieger, who first attracted the attention of the medical profession by his phamplet on the 'Iodine and Bromine Springs of Kreuznach,' in 1837. Baths of Kreuznach motherlye began to be tried in distant parts for scrofula and tetter with success, and many were induced to seek the spa itself.

Not only was great benefit obtained from the exported Elisenbrunnen water, but its imitation in Struve's establishments afforded great utility, and swelled the list of patients cured through the agency of Kreuznach. All the springs resemble each other in qualitative properties, although somewhat differing in temperature, according to the respective depths of the boreholes, and according to the greater or smaller exposure of the subterranean reservoirs to atmospheric influences.

The *Elisabeth-*, or *Elisenquelle*, issues at a temperature of $54\frac{1}{2}°$ F. with a specific gravity of 1·004. The taste is saline, bitterish, rather nauseous; the appearance transparent, with a somewhat yellowish tint. Only very few bubbles of carbonic-acid gas rise to the surface in the water drawn. Brownish flakes soon separate themselves, and fall to the bottom of the vessel. According to Professer Löwig of Zurich, the water contains 94 grains (60 grains according to Bauer) in sixteen ounces, viz.—

```
72·88 chloride of sodium.
13·38    „     calcium.
 4·07    „     magnesium.
 0·62    „     potassium.
 0·61    „     lithium.
 0·27 bromide of magnesium.
 0·03 iodide of magnesium.
 1·69 carbonate of lime.
 0·01     „      baryta.
 0·10 magnesia.
 0·15 oxide of iron.
 0·02 phosphate of alumina.
 0·12 silica.
─────
94·02 grains
```

The alumina, silica, and iron become soon deposited. The temperature of the Karlshallerbrunnen is 59° F. at the issue, but higher in the borehole. The taste is less saline, owing to a smaller amount of solid ingredients. It contains 75 grains of solid constituents in sixteen ounces (59 chloride of sodium, $2\frac{1}{4}$ chloride of calcium, 6·6 bromide of calcium, 0·36 carbonate of iron, and nearly 4 cubic inches of carbonic acid).

The chief well of the *Theodorshalle* has a temperature of $70\frac{1}{4}°$ F.; its constituents amount to 87·9 grains.

The chief well of Münster greatly resembles that of the Karlshalle, with a temperature, however, of $81\frac{1}{2}°$ F.; the amount of solid ingredients varies from 64 to 76 grains. It is smallest in winter, when the spring is not in requisition. The green mud covering the bottom of the graduation-works is composed of organic matter.

After the salt has been crystallized and removed from the boiling-pans, the remaining brownish-yellow glutinous liquid is called *motherlye*. The smell bears some analogy to that of *fucus*. The taste is bitter, astringent, and caustic; its specific gravity varies from 1·307 to 1·314. It contains, in sixteen ounces, 2575·72 grains, or about the third of its contents, viz.,—

```
1577·71 chloride of calcium.
 338·72 bromide of calcium.
  92·82    „     potassium.
 154·10    „     sodium.
  60·34 chloride of sodium.
  38·44    „     magnesium.
  17·30    „     potassium.
  35 66 alumina and protoxide of iron.
 216·13 crenic acid, two resinous substances, with traces of iodine.
  44·50 water of crystallisation and loss.
```

The origin of the salt-springs is generally due to strata of rock-salt, into which atmospheric water had previously penetrated; the adjoining layers of lime and gypsum cause the addition of salts of calcium or of sulphates.

The inconsiderable depth of their origin causes the temperature to be comparatively low, and the combination less intimate than in those of a more profound origin. The sources of Kreuznach being confined to the extension of the porphyry between the Elisenquelle and Rheingrafenstein, the comparatively small amount of chloride of sodium, the presence of certain substances not belonging to salt-rocks (as lithion, phosphate of alumina, and chloride of potassium, &c.), and the corresponding analysis of porphyry, led to the belief that this latter rock gives birth to the Kreuznach springs. Professor Löwig obtained from the solution of porphyry an artificial water, containing all the chief ingredients of the sources. Some deposits of salt may, according to Dr. Engelmann, be interspersed amongst fissures of porphyry. The water must have penetrated into greater depths than the mountain-heights would indicate, to dissolve the porphyry; for sweet water issues at the foot of the mountain near the salt-springs—the result of meteoric water merely penetrating a short distance through the superficial layers. The quantitative difference is accounted for by the varying relative contents of the rock itself at different parts. Greater warmth exists in the depth; and if the temperature lowers more in one spring than in another, this depends·on a longer contact with superficial earthy layers before its emission. In the Karlshallerquelle the brine formerly exhibited the temperature of 59° F. when the borehole was 150 feet deep. Boring only 200 feet more produced brine of 68° F.; whilst the present depth of 600 feet furnishes water with a temperature of $74\frac{3}{4}$°F.; the augmentation you will find in greater proportion than you might expect from such an inconsiderable depth.

The general rise is about $2\frac{1}{4}$° of F. to 150 feet, so that it ought to be 9° of F. less, if there were not some counteracting cause. This is sought in the circumstance that porphyry may have retained its volcanic heat longer than the surrounding rocks, of older volcanic origin, amongst which it had to force a passage. The water of the Elisenquelle had formerly the temperature of 50° F. Now, when the depth of the borehole has only been increased to 36 feet, the water drawn in the depth has a temperature of 58° F. and at the issue $54\frac{1}{2}$° F.

The shorter or longer stay of the water in the basin likewise influences its heat. Thus, the temperature of the chief well in Münster only amounts to $79\frac{1}{4}$° F. in the shaft, if pumping has been discontinued for some weeks, whilst the heat rises to $83\frac{1}{2}$° F. during ordinary use. The different degree of cooling in the sides, and the admixture of more or less cooled brine in the side-walls of the boreholes, likewise exercise their influence in this respect. The carburetted hydrogen found in the new borehole of the Karlshalle, and in the chief shaft of the Münster spring, is ascribed to some layers of coal existing in the older coal-sandstone.

If the water appears to have a more saline taste one day than another, this is rather to be attributed to altered state of digestion than to any change in the contents of the water. Though nauseous and bitter, it is borne well by the digestive organs, if the doses are regulated according to the state of the bowels. Appetite improves, but alvine action is not promoted at first; only after gradual increase of the quantity does this result take place. Should the water be taken too quickly, or in too large quantities, the abdomen will be distended, and eructation, pain of the stomach, and diarrhœa will ensue, with a general feeling of chilliness. The same result may follow dietetic irregularities, the partaking of acidifying food, &c., as in Weilbach, where the bowels are more acted upon in unfavourable weather, from the impeded function of the skin. The baths are generally taken lukewarm, with additions of motherlye in larger or smaller quantities, according to the state of the disease. The skin becomes somewhat irritated after a time, and bath-eruption is a frequent consequence. Patients with very tender skin will sometimes bear greater quantities of the motherlye than comparatively inured and healthier persons. The brine is also employed as a clyster, in which form it is particularly effective as a solvent in cases of induration of the prostate gland. The exhalations of the graduation-works are also used for medicinal purposes in similar instances as those of Kissingen. They would of course injure in real plethora or tendency to congestion. After some weeks a sudden sensation of languor occasionally appears, with headache, debility, disinclination to bathe or to drink the water, feverish excitement, &c. These are signs of saturation, and require cessation of the course.

The chief efficacy of Kreuznach must be sought in the chloride of sodium and of calcium, and in the bromine and iodine contained in the springs. The Elisenbrunnen has the strongest effect; the Carlshaller spring acts less powerfully, from the minor quantity of ingredients. If a still weaker spring is required, the Münster well is recommended. In cold and damp weather the warmer water of the latter agrees better with the digestive organs than the colder springs would; the reverse takes place in fine weather. A great advantage of Kreuznach over similar springs lies in the circumstance that we may employ it both internally and externally in appropriate diseases.

The chief indication is *scrofula*. If the lymphatic system be impeded in its function, the secretions become vitiated, reproduction is impaired, and the whole body must suffer in consequence. Dr. Engelmann dissents from the assertion frequently made, that the bromine and iodine springs are more adapted to torpid forms of the disease, whilst to erethic forms alkaline springs are declared as more applicable. Dr. Vogler of Ems supports this objection, and limits the preference of Ems to mesenteric scrofula and tubercular diathesis.

In whatever form the disease may appear—whether the glands of the neck be swollen and indurated, or whether the eyes, ears, nose, mesenteric glands, or bones become affected,—Kreuznach will be found highly beneficial. You meet with patients, mostly in early age, still affected with marked scrofula, or with chronic diseases of the skin, lachrymation of the eyes, nervous tremulousness, or lassitude after inconsiderable exertions: their complexion is florid, their skin tender and very susceptible, their digestion irregular; their appetite often excessive, with a deficient power of assimilation. Scars of former ulcers inform you that scrofulous acrimony still lurks in their blood. By recommending the careful use of Kreuznach water, you will afford such patients a great chance of a radical cure.

The spa is contraindicated in organic diseases of the heart or great vessels,—in inflammation, fever, dropsy, and congestion to the brain or other vital organs. With reference to the quantity required, this depends in a great measure on the nature of the disease and on the constitution. It is advisable to commence in small quantities, and not to drink the next glass before we feel that the last has been properly digested. As is the case in all remedial measures, a slow and gradual imbibition of the healing substances will produce a safer effect than overloading the stomach with quantities of the water poured down in rapid succession. By the latter practice the irritated intestines will rapidly discharge the distending mass, and the lymphatic system will fail to absorb the required ingredients. In some instances the water agrees better if mixed with a little hot milk; or, in cases where an excessive stimulation is feared from the presence of iron, the water should be allowed to stand for some time, till its iron becomes deposited. A further advantage of Kreuznach consists in the possibility of employing it at a distance; and I may bring a case to your notice of a clerk in a foreign counting-house in this city, who laboured for about three years with scrofulous *struma*. He applied to me for advice, after two years of medical treatment. I prescribed the ordinary preparations of iodine and other anti-scrofulous agents for about nine months, with no better result than my predecessors. At last I discontinued all other medicines, and recommended Elisabethbrunnen—a wineglassful only, three times a day, mixed with some warm water. To my own surprise, the first trial proved most successful. One dozen bottles sufficed not only to produce a cure of his present ailment, but his general state of health became greatly improved; his pallid and puffy appearance gave way to a more healthy complexion; the inconvenience in breathing and speaking, so marked in this disease, entirely vanished; and it would now require very close inspection to perceive a slight remaining enlargement of the thyroid gland. I must not omit, however, to mention one fact with reference to this case, which may detract considerably from its therapeutic value—viz., the patient in question was suddenly affected with acute inflammation of the thyroid gland, just after finishing a course of the water, with angina and febrile excitement, necessitating antiphlogistic treatment. After recovery from this attack, rapid absorption and diminution of the enlarged gland to its present almost normal state took place, so that this inflammatory process may have assisted the removal of the struma as powerfully as the mineral water.

Nevertheless, as the Kreuznach water may have increased the function of the gland, and disposed it to take the form of acute disease, probably provoked by atmospheric causes, I feel justified in ascribing the cure in some measure to the Kreuznach water.

Physicians:—Dr. Engelmann, Dr. Trautwein, Drs. Hahn, Jung, Karst, Lossen, Prieger, Wiesbaden, Fouquet, Michels, Stabel, Strahl, Heusner, Kleinhaus, Von Frautzius, Reinhard.*

Now you must again allow me to take you to some distance for the purpose of comparison. Imagine yourselves at *Munich*, the capital of Bavaria, which we passed in our journey to Gastein, the Tyrol spa.

Adelheidsquelle.—About eight German miles to the south of Munich, between the village of *Tölz* and the former convent of *Benedictbeuern*, you enter the small village of *Heilbrunn*. It is nearly two leagues distant from Tölz, and one and a quarter from Benedictbeuern. The height of Heilbrunn is calculated at about 2,400 feet above the level of the Mediterranean Sea, Benedictbeuern being nearly 2,000 feet high. You find it due west of Kreuth, not far from the left bank of the Isar, which descends from the Algauer Alps, and proceeds northward to intersect the artistic city of Munich. Its latitude N. is 48°—its longitude E. 12°. It lies at the foot of an alpine promontory, on an eminence affording very charming and distant prospects. In the north you perceive a beautiful valley, with gently-rising hills, covered with woods, extending to the Würm or Staremberger Lake. Northeast, on the right shore of the Isar, you perceive an immense plain, reaching as far as Munich. Towards the north-west the towering Peissenberg arrests your eye. The southern alpine promontories are easy of ascent, and repay the trouble of climbing

* Hotels:—De Hollande, &c. &c.

them with extremely picturesque and romantic views. Behind these rises the Zwieselberg, and this height is again overtopped by the towering *Benedictenwand*, upwards of 6,000 feet high. The Kochel Lake and Beuedictbeuern lie somewhat lower, to the south and west. The chief mountainous formation of the environs consists in marl-sandstone and peat-sandstone. In the torrents near Heilbrunn several calcareous petrifications are found, besides granite, glimmer, and slate of hornblende. The spring lies between two hills, the vicarage being on the smaller and the church on the higher eminence. It is said to be the oldest of the Bavarian springs. In the year 955 it was destroyed by the Hungarians, together with the convent of Benedictbeuern. One hundred years afterwards the monks caused the place where the well had stood to be dug again. The source was discovered at a depth of four fathoms, but flames arose, and it was thought that the spring originated by a miracle.

The scantiness of supply is a great inconvenience—nevertheless several persons resort there, seeking accommodation in the village-inn or at some of the private cottages; whilst more opulent visitors take up their residence in the convenient Hotel of *Bichel* (one league from Heilbrunn), which enjoys the advantage of being crossed by the high-roads from Munich, Tölz, Tyrol, Weilheim, and Murnau. The water is sent to them in tubs for bathing. An able physician is residing in the immediate neighbourhood (Dr. Vogel of Bichel).

The more distant Tölz, on the Isar, enjoys a charming situation. A large garden adjoins the elegant hotel, and affords a beautiful view of the Isar Valley.

Tölz is celebrated for its beer: the rock-vaults there chiefly contribute to its long preservation.

The Heilbrunn well has a diameter of eight feet above, gradually contracting towards the bottom. The water issues out of three veins of sandstone. The ascending gas-bubbles may be ignited, and burn with a clear flame. The water is clear, colourless, and only sparkling when the well is strongly agitated. The odour is somewhat nauseous (bearing analogy to bromine, carburetted hydrogen, and sometimes to sulphuretted hydrogen); its flavour is similar to that of weak broth, and it leaves a mawkish taste in the mouth. The temperature is about 50° F. It contains 47 grains of solid ingredients in 16 ounces, viz.—

ADELHEIDSQUELLE.

Adelheidsquelle	Kreuznach.	Hall (Austr.)
38·15 chlor. sod. . . .	72·92 . . .	100·72
	(13·27 chlor. calc.) .	2·99
0·20 iod. of sod. . (iod. of mag. 0·03) . . .		5·53
(0·01 according to Fuchs)		
0·40 brom. of sod. . .	0·30	
(0·30 according to Fuchs)		(0·49 brom. magn.)
0·81 carbon. of soda.		
	(0·79 chlor. pot.) .	(0·35 sulph. sod.)
0·23 carb. of potash.		
	(0·25 chlor. magn.)	0·05
0·12 carb. of ammon.		
	(0·29 carb. baryt.)	
0·62 carb. of lime		. 0·31
0·39 carb. of magnesia . . 1·35 . . .		. 0·17
0·05 carb. of strontia . . 0·68		
0·02 carb. of alumina		
0·01 carb. of iron . . . 0·19 . . .		. 0·06
0·25 silica . . . . 0·31 . . .		. 0·16
47·31 grains.	90·68 grains.	114 grains.

And 4 cubic inches of carburetted hydrogen in 100 cubic inches.

The proportions of the constituents (with the exception of the iodine and bromine) bear some analogy to *Selters* water, which possesses likewise chloride of sodium as its chief ingredient (16¼ grains), and carbonate of soda as the next in importance (5¾ grains). The Adelheidsquelle promotes, with reference to its muriatico-alkaline character, the functions of the mucous membranes of the lymphatic, glandular, uropoietic, and uterine systems. The carburetted hydrogen is supposed to diminish the morbidly-increased sensibility of these organs, and to operate as an antispasmodic and anodyne agent. Add to this the very large amount of iodine and bromine (conjointly more than a grain in 16 ounces), only exceeded in this respect by the Haller Kropfwasser (goître-water), and you will be prepared to hear of its powerful effect on scrofulous diseases and complications.

When, besides the highly solvent and antiplastic power of the iodine and bromine, you find an indication for a prominent employment of chlorides, especially of sodium and calcium, your patient will have to resort to Kreuznach.

The quantity of chlorine entering in conjunction with the sodium and calcium must neutralise that acrimonious dyscrasy characterising the circulating fluids of scrofulous individuals; in short, we must consider that Kreuznach penetrates most deeply into the whole metamorphic function going forward in the grandular and lymphatic system. Hall of Austria (near Steyer), which excels the others by its larger amount of iodine (5½ grains of iodide of sodium, according to Von Holger), contains also a considerably greater quantity of chloride of sodium (above 100 grains), and very little chloride of calcium (about 3 grains). Its name of *Kropfwasser* indicates its great reputation in scrofulous struma.

When we desire a simple employment of the two last-mentioned remedies, and have no reason to fear a rebellious reception, by weakened or irritated digestive organs, or on account of general irritability or weakness, we cannot employ a better remedial means than the mineral water of Hall, which unfortunately cannot yet be obtained in this country.

The Adelheidsquelle contains the smallest amount of chloride of sodium (about half of Kreuznach and a third of Hall) no chloride of calcium and magnesium, less iron than Kreuznach ($\frac{1}{100}$ to $\frac{19}{100}$); but it possesses a prominent amount of carbonates instead. Its iodine and bromine being not only more abundant than in Kreuznach, but also more prominent, by reason of the proportionally smaller quantity of other active ingredients, you may expect a series of special phenomena to result from its use, especially if a cure may be reasonably expected by the mere internal use of an iodated water. A few cases, enumerated by Dr. Wetzler, will best illustrate its effects.

Dr. Von Breslau, of Munich, was summoned to consultation on the case of a lady who laboured under such considerable obesity that she could scarcely walk a few steps in the room without dyspnœa. He advised Adelheidsquelle for internal and external use, and it completely cured her. A girl of thirteen years of age had her abdomen so distended and hardened, from affection of the *mesenteric glands*, that she might have been supposed to be pregnant, if her age had permitted such a supposition. At the same time she vomited frequently after taking food, so that Dr. Von Walther considered the pylorus to be hardened and narrowed. Adelheidsquelle being recommended she went to Heilbrunn, and returned cured after six weeks. Dr. Fuchs found highly satisfactory results from the water in gravel and lithiasis, and placed it, in this respect, on an equality with Carlsbad. He recommended the spa to a patient of sixty years of age, who had suffered from a *renal calculus* for about a year, and daily lost upwards of an ounce of blood from the bladder, which greatly reduced and weakened him. Six weeks' bathing and drinking at Heilbrunn restored his health.

Dr. Dietrich says he knows no mineral water which penetrates so deeply into organic plasticity by slowly altering its constituent elements. He cured with it obstinate chlorosis in scrofulous girls, testicular indurations, strictures of the urethra, &c. Dr. Xavier Martin found the Adelheidsquelle extremely curative in mesenteric atrophy of little children. Their emaciated appearance, pale complexion, hollow eyes, pointed noses—their voraciousness, their clay-coloured excretions, and their enlarged mesenteric glands betrayed the evil, and induced the doctor to employ the water in small quantities, with or without warm milk. Success very frequently resulted. In scrofulous ophthalmia he found cold external applications of the Adelheidsquelle highly useful: in amenorrhœa and chronic ovaritis he witnessed decided cures from the spa.

M. Fellerer, from the Hospital of Incurables, states that J. M., thirty-eight years of age, had been affected from his childhood with various glandular swellings. Subsequently, scrofulous ulcers appeared on the right foot, and were complicated with caries; his illness was aggravated by an increasing enlargement of the thyroid gland, so that at his reception his struma was enormous, weighing about four pounds, and impeding respiration and speech more and more. After an ineffectual treatment by pharmaceutic remedies, Adelheidsquelle was ordered (which is furnished gratuitously to the hospital by Mr. Debler). Persevering employment of this remedy for six months effected a complete cure of the goître, and the patient would have been discharged but for the presence of the carious ulcers.

Dr. Horger relates an instance of *incontinence of urine* in a patient of eighty years of age, which was cured by the spa. Dr. Caron du Val cured with the same water several cases of *chronic vesical catarrh*, accompanied by spasms and pain of the bladder; also hepatic hypertrophy, induration of the neck of the womb, and of the mammary glands. Dr. Heigl, of Ratisbon, employed the water with almost specific efficacy in urinary disorders, especially in gravel, dysùria, enuresis, enlargement of the prostate gland, &c.

Dr. Wetzler records an instance of a gentleman who had suffered for eleven years from the most painful dysuria and urethral blennorrhage, resembling gonorrhœa. The patient had to get up several times at night, and walk about for hours in the room, to obtain relief from the violent vesical and urethral pains. Frequent involuntary emissions added to his distress. He was completely cured by Adelheidsquelle, and occasional doses of Püllna whenever his bowels acted too sluggishly. A child of ten weeks, emaciated and wrinkled in appearance, vomited after it had been fed, and had besides twenty to thirty alvine evacuations daily : the tongue was covered with mucus and small ulcers, the pulse almost imperceptible and extremely frequent, the temperature of the abdomen and forehead heightened, and the extremities cold. The first child had died at the age of twelve weeks from consumption, and the mother was desolate at the probable loss of this her second child. Dr. Wetzler recommended her to give it some broth five or six times a day, and almond-milk to drink, and he sent her a bottle of Adelheidsquelle, with the direction to give the child two teaspoonfuls three times a day. After a fortnight half the bottle was used, and the recovery so advanced that further medical treatment was dispensed with.

Increase of urinary secretion and improvement of appetite are considered as the invariable and immediate results of the water. Dr. Schweiger, of Benedictbeuern, communicates a case of scrofulous tuberculosis, with remittent fever, that had been cured at Heilbrunn, besides several scrofulous complaints. The Adelheidsquelle may then be employed with great confidence in scrofula, and in lymphatic struma. Acidity and inveterate mucosity generally prevailing in this habit, the utility of the carbonate and muriate of soda is apparent.

The swelling of hæmorrhoidal vessels round the neck of the bladder, and the mucus formed in consequence, cause the bladder to become very sensitive. Hence, as soon as the irritating liquid arrives from the kidneys, pain is experienced, and contraction of the bladder ensues. But in proportion as this irritation increases the vesical nerves become more susceptible, and thus they react against the irritating particles by spasms of the sphincter, of the bladder, and of the contractile cellular tissue of the urethra. Thus, as soon as the urine collects at night, the patient is awakened by a painful desire of micturition, which he cannot satisfy, in consequence of the spasmodic contraction mentioned. Such cases are extremely distressing, and become more intractable and complicated if treated with cubebs, copaiva, or astringent injections.

The utility of the spa in gravel and lithiasis is due to its carbonate and muriate of soda: for, as most calculous diseases proceed from excess of uric acid or urate of ammonia in the blood, carbonate of soda, which neutralises this acidity, is highly useful—urate of soda being formed and removed out of the circulating mass. The smaller number of calculi formed from oxalate of lime or phosphates are supposed to be favourably influenced by culinary salt, with anodyne and antispasmodic remedies, because, through a chemico-vital process, the oxalic acid may absorb another atom of oxygen, and become transformed into carbonic acid. This acid may yield its place to the chlorine, which forms a soluble chloride of calcium (after the lime has given up its atom of oxygen), whilst carbonic acid becomes attracted by soda. In those calculi formed from insoluble phosphates, the culinary salt is thought to act beneficially by attracting the phosphoric acid, which combines with soda into soluble phosphate of soda, whilst the chlorine may enter into combination with ammonia, and thus break up the hitherto compact insoluble mass before completely hardening. The Adelheidsquelle, containing both these curative salts, is naturally very efficacious in various forms of lithiasis and gravel.

As the blood is thought to owe its stimulating property to the muriate and carbonate of soda, a diminished proportion of these salts, with an abnormal preponderance of phosphates and urates, must engender acrimony and dyscrasy. The wasting of the mammary gland, occasionally observed under the pharmaceutic use of iodine, never occurs in the employment of Adelheidsquelle.

LECTURE XV.

NENNDORF—EILSEN—MEINBERG—AIX-LA-CHAPELLE.

LET us now pursue our journey, and travel as far as Cologne. Hence we cross the bridge and pass by the Northern Railroad from Deutz through Hamm, Minden, &c. to *Haste*-station; near it we find *Nenndorf*, in the Principality of Lippe-Schaumburg. It belongs to Electoral Hesse. Its latitude N. is 52°—its long. E. 9°.

On account of the disagreeable odour proceeding from the well, the inhabitants used to call the locality 'Auf dem Teufelsdreck.' But no particular notice was taken of the circumstance, and even as late as 1784, the learned Erhart complains of the non-appreciation of such a powerful sulphurous water, though some steps had already been taken a few years previously to clean and enclose the well.

The season lasts from the 1st of June to the 1st of September—only three months. Here, again, provision is made for supplying the necessary accommodation gratuitously to indigent invalids. The arrangements of the baths are excellent in every respect. The so-called *Esplanade* serves as a rendezvous for the valetudinarians, who collect in the morning to drink their prescribed draughts, while entertained with music. A pleasant park affords numerous walks for exercise.

In the heat of summer a covered and shady walk leads to a gentle eminence, from which numerous localities in the charming environs may be discerned. Temple-like enclosures and benches for resting are interspersed about the different walks.

You will not find such luxury and pleasure-seeking here as in the Nassau and other spas, the manner of living being on a more moderate scale. Nenndorf possesses four principal springs: three of these arise at the Esplanade, near each other. The seasons exercise a very slight influence on the quantity of the water.

The *obere Brunnen* or *grosse Badequelle*, about 200 feet from the 'Trinkquelle,' supplies 2,500 cubic feet of water in twenty-four hours, chiefly used for the preparation of baths. An extensive reservoir is constructed near the source.

The second spring, the *Quelle unter dem Gewölbe* (source under the vault), lies nearer the drinking-spring, in the neighbourhood of the Arcade and bathing-house: supply, 2,000 cubic feet of water.

The *Trinkquelle* (drinking-spring) has a basin four feet in depth, and supplies about 3,300 cubic feet of water per day.

The fourth spring lies about half a league farther, ' auf dem breiten Felde' (on the broad field); rarely used for baths ; its supply is 2,400 cubic feet per day.

The rocks are chiefly composed of lias-formation, distinguished by petrified remains of antediluvian vegetables and animals, and consisting of alternate layers of sandstone, marl, marl-slate, and limestone, which respectively compose the neighbouring mountains.

The temperature of the three first sources is $52\frac{1}{4}°$ Fahrenheit, summer and winter. The water is perfectly clear and colourless, and no rising of air-bubbles or sparkling can be observed. The smell of sulphuretted hydrogen is very marked in all—the taste bitterish. The water is freely drunk by the inhabitants, even in a heated state of the body, with impunity. If the sulphur-water be left exposed for some time in an open vessel, small air-bubbles arise, composed of sulphuretted hydrogen and carbonic acid. After some time the water becomes turbid, till a deposit of sulphur and carbonate of lime restores the former clearness. To cause as little loss of the efficient gas as possible, the baths are heated with vapour generated by the sulphur-water. As regards the composition of the springs, they vary more in quantity than in quality ; the Gewölbequelle is the most abundant, the Trinkquelle less, and the Badequelle least. For the baths these three are used conjointly.

Sulphate of lime or gypsum is the principal ingredient ($6\frac{3}{4}$ gr.); the next is sulphate of soda (nearly 5 gr.), then carbonate of lime ($4\frac{1}{2}$ gr.) and sulphate of magnesia ($2\frac{1}{2}$ gr.), chloride of magnesium ($1\frac{1}{2}$ gr.), sulphate of potash ($\frac{1}{4}$ gr.). Besides some alumina and bituminous substance, a combination of hydrosulphuric acid with sulphuret of calcium exists in the water. When the sulphuretted hydrogen has been all evolved by boiling, and paper moistened with a solution of acetate of lead ceases to be darkened by it, you have merely to add a few drops of sulphuric acid, and the appearance of (formerly combined) sulphuretted hydrogen will become immediately manifest by a brown or black colouration of the prepared paper. About $4\frac{1}{2}$ cubic inches of free carbonic acid and $1\frac{1}{5}$ cubic inch of sulphuretted hydrogen gas, with traces of nitrogen, are contained in 16 ounces—altogether, in the drinking-spring, $20\frac{3}{4}$ gr. of solid and $5\frac{1}{2}$ gr. of volatile ingredients. The mountains possessing a great quantity of gypsum, it is assumed that part of the sulphate of lime existing in the subterranean water has been gradually reduced by the contact with organic or bituminous substances to sulphuret of calcium. Free carbonic acid, formed in the interior of the earth, permeating the water, causes a portion of the sulphuret of calcium to be decomposed; so that carbonate of lime is formed on the one hand, and kept in solution by the excess of carbonic acid, whilst free sulphuretted hydrogen exists on the other—water having furnished oxygen to the calcium and hydrogen to the sulphur.

Dr. Wöhler illustrated this view by saturating a bottle of common well-water with gypsum, and then impregnating the solution with carbonic-acid gas. A few slips of wood had been introduced as the deoxidizing organic substance, and the bottle was closed and made airtight. After less than three months the water exhibited all the properties of a sulphurous water both as regards smell and taste, and in reference to the precipitation of metallic solutions; when boiled it became turbid, and deposited carbonate of lime.

The Quelle unter dem Gewölbe contains $21\frac{1}{2}$ grains of solid and $6\frac{1}{4}$ cubic inches of volatile ingredients; the Badequelle $12\frac{1}{5}$ of the former and $3\frac{2}{3}$ of the latter. A small quantity of ammonia has also been found in the springs; also some silica—no carbonate of soda, no chloride of sodium, as in Weilbach. The sulphur-water acts as a heating, stimulating, solvent, and alterative agent, gently promoting the functions of the secreting organs. The capillary vessels and their nervous ramifications are particularly exposed to this action. The circulation of the portal system is greatly promoted, and thus abnormal action of the pelvic organs becomes regulated. The observed decrease of pulse so frequently noticed in the baths must be ascribed to the more equable general circulation resulting from the freer movements of the portal system. They act more favourably on phlegmatic individuals, in whom the lymphatic and venous systems preponderate over the arterial. Wherever inflammation exists, or fever, or tendency to cerebral congestion, to active hæmorrhage, to abortion, or to scorbutic dyscrasy, the water is contra-indicated.

The utility of the spa in chronic rheumatism is ascribed to the improvement in the peripheric system counteracting the remote cause of the disease. In chronic exanthemata Nenndorf frequently acts as a curative means, especially in those arising from repressed or neglected itch and other eruptions.

The specific influence of sulphur in the improvement of the cutaneous functions, with its general anti-dyscrasic power and beneficial action on abdominal reproduction, is here called into requisition. In asthma psoricum it is particularly extolled. Pulmonary catarrh appearing during cessation of catamenia is considered as an indication for Nenndorf, particularly if any hæmorrhoidal tendency exists. In varicose ulcers mud-baths have shown themselves highly useful, also in non-febrile hydropic affections, particularly of persons who had been addicted to ardent beverages. Dr. D'Oleire found this spa very useful also in metallic poisoning by lead or mercury: in scrofulous dyscrasy of a torpid character, in tumor albus genu, particularly when the pain is more fixed and the swelling hardened, so that a scrofulous base is to be suspected, local mud-baths and douche of sulphuretted hydrogen have been found useful. Adulteration of wine with preparations of lead is detected by the Nenndorf water assuming a brownish-black colour if three parts of it are mixed with one part of the wine. In atonic anomalous gout, with deposits in the joints, contractions, &c., the external use of Nenndorf is efficacious—also in arthritic diathesis. Catamenial derangements based on disturbed cutaneous function are relieved here.

The *mud-baths* form an important remedial means. The peat-soil is obtained from the neighbouring village of *Algesdorf*, where also several sulphur-springs exist, impregnating the marshy soil. The baths are prepared in a peculiar building with an adjoining reservoir and mud-mill. Sulphur-water is conducted into this reservoir to prepare the mud for use; it is warmed by heated sulphurous vapours. The mud is blackish-grey, and has the consistence of a thick pap with a strong smell of sulphuretted hydrogen. If boiled, the evolution of sulphuretted hydrogen lasts longer than if the sulphur-water be used, and when this separation ceases it will recommence by adding an acid. Milk of sulphur is likewise contained in the mud. The mud-baths highly stimulate the functions of the skin, and generally increase the frequency of pulse. They are said to act as derivatives from the pulmonary and intestinal mucous membranes, and are indicated in chronic rheumatism and gout, in deficient action of the peripheric system, in contractions, exanthemata of a torpid character —as dry tetter, induration of the cellular tissue, varicose ulcers, with hardish livid borders, &c. In obstinate syphilis a cure was several times effected by sulphur-baths alternating with mercurial unction.

A young man of about thirty years of age, with a light florid complexion and exhibiting traces of former scrofula, visited Nenndorf, and placed himself under the care of the late Dr. D'Oleire. He had been infected several times, and subjected to various methods of treatment, with and without mercury, to no purpose. He had ozæna and ulcers of the uvula and fauces, with nightly pains in the bones of the skull, and characteristic humid ulcers on the forehead, arms, and thighs. The internal and external use of the spa made all syphilitic symptoms more prominent. The baths alone were therefore continued, and at the same time grey mercurial ointment rubbed in twelve times daily, according to Rust's method, whilst internally a strong decoction of sarsaparilla was taken. Complete cure ensued. Other cases are recorded where the sulphur-baths were used first, and then inunction for sixteen days, followed by drinking and bathing. The successful simultaneous employment of these two remedies may be explained by the increased power of reaction following the baths and preventing too great an atony of the lymphatic system, which might easily be produced by an energetic course of mercury. Besides, salivation is avoided, and thus a greater amount of mercury may be given with less injury to the system. However specifically mercury may act in syphilis, we occasionally find inveterate cases obstinately resisting the influence of this remedy. It is rational to imagine that the lymphatic system may occasionally become too much weakened to elaborate the metal. In such instances we penetrate the lymphatic system with the stimulating sulphuretted hydrogen, we restore in some measure the natural systemic reacting power, and cure ensues by a subsequent proper reception of the remedy. *Gas-baths* play a very prominent part in Nenndorf. The sulphur-water is made to stream fountain-wise out of a basin, splashing from the height on a copper projection, from which the sulphuretted hydrogen gas spreads about. Scarcely a trace of the gas is found in the water which afterwards collects in the basin, a proof of its efficient separation by the violent contact with the copper. Sofas, tables, and benches are provided for a shorter or longer sojourn of the patient, besides some smaller gas-chambers for separate use. The pulse becomes diminished, and the irritability of the respiratory organs allayed, whilst the secretion of the pulmonary mucous membrane becomes improved. Sometimes giddiness, oppression, headache, trembling, &c. are experienced at first by very sensitive persons, but these symptoms soon subside. Cases of phthisis pituitosa are mentioned where these gas-baths have been useful conjointly with a careful internal employment of the water. Local gas-baths are more especially recommended in deafness and blennorrhage of the meatus auditorius. The gas is here slightly warmed, and applied by means of an elastic tube. These local baths have proved serviceable when rheumatism or gout has formed the remote cause of the evil. Douche of sulphur-water behind the ear is sometimes added. The gas probably acts as a revulsive from internal organs by promoting the function of the skin. Moreover, the admixture of a small quantity of sulphuretted hydrogen with the air may have a certain emollient influence on the bronchial mucous membrane. But the remedial means do not end here. *Brine-baths* are administered; the Soole is led into Nenndorf by subterranean pipes from Rodenberg (half a league to the south), connected with Nenndorf by a beautiful walk. The specific gravity of the Soole is 1·013. It contains ninety grains of solid ingredients in sixteen ounces.

SPRINGS OF NENDORF (COLD).

	Quelle unter dem Gewölbe	Trink-brunnen	Badequelle	Soole of Rodenberg
Carbonic acid	5·2 cub.in.	4·32	2·75	0·14
Sulphuretted hydrogen	1·21	1·20	0·61	—
Sum-total of ingredients	21·4 gr.	20·7	12·19	90·
Sulphate of soda	5·22	4·91	1·11	10·81
„ magnesia	2·83	2·54	1·89	10·01
„ lime	7·15	6·81	5·56	14·82
„ potash	—	—	—	0·10
Chloride of sodium	—	—	—	49·84
„ magnesium	1·63	1·62	0·42	10·01
„ lime	4·30	4·51	3·18	4·61
Silica	0·05	0·06	—	0·20

The brine-baths are sometimes used conjointly with sulphur-baths, sometimes alone, whilst the sulphur-water is taken internally. They especially increase the action of the glandular and lymphatic systems. They must not be employed in congestion of the external skin, great general debility, anæmia, syphilis, painful eruptions, tendency to scurvy, &c. In dry chronic herpes with great sensibility of the skin, they are mixed with sulphur-water and greatly recommended, also in rheumatism and exanthematic metastasis. Some bromine and iodine are contained in the motherlye, which is therefore often added to the baths. Sometimes the saline baths are used as an after-cure, to increase the tone of the skin and diminish the susceptibility to atmospheric changes, or its tendency to profuse perspiration. Whilst the sulphurous water acts as an emollient, the saline liquid engenders reaction, and restores the tone of the skin.

Dr. Grandidier reports several cases of gout, arthritic paralysis, &c., which were cured by mud-baths, vapour-douches, and sulphur-baths—also a case of *aphony* with ulcers in the larynx, occurring in a young person of nineteen years of age who had not yet menstruated. Gargles of the sulphur-water were used, with gas-baths from two to four hours daily, and cure followed.

The baths of Nenndorf being situated below the springs, the water runs in freely and need not be pumped in, whereby loss of sulphuretted hydrogen might take place. Physicians, Dr. Grandidier, Dr. Neussel.

If we compare Nenndorf with Weilbach, a circumstance strikes us very much—viz.: in the former the variations of external applications are extremely numerous and complete, and very frequently employed, whilst in Weilbach the chief mode of employment is internal.

What is the reason? The chief constituents of Weilbach are carbonates of soda, of magnesia, and of lime, with chloride of sodium—a combination which must be well tolerated by the digestive organs, and which, with the abundance of sulphuretted hydrogen absorbed in the intestinal canal, promises the good results which are actually obtained from its use. In the manifold external applications of the Nenndorf water,'I see an attempt at impregnating the organism with the healing sulphuretted hydrogen gas without the concomitant ingredients; for whilst carbonates preponderate in Weilbach, we find sulphates prevail here, and among these nearly a third of the whole is furnished by sulphate of lime, which may be expected to neutralise partially the increased peristaltic motion that might otherwise be induced by the sulphate of soda and magnesia present. Thus the carbonate of lime, instead of assisting the antacid and sedative influence of the soda and magnesia, as in Weilbach, may remain unchecked to a certain extent, and require the digestive organs to be more powerful in order to its being well tolerated. A different class of diseases therefore naturally claims relief at Nenndorf. *Chemico-vital* action is relied upon in Weilbach for the chief curative result in hæmorrhoids, and diseases based on hæmorrhoidal tendency or obstruction of the portal vein; whilst at Nenndorf the *dynamical* and *physical* powers of the sulphur-water, gas, douche, and mud-baths are called into requisition. Hence gout, rheumatism, articular swellings, and contractions are the most numerous class of complaints here. The increased frequency of pulse observed from the use of the mud-baths, and frequently expatiated upon as a peculiarity of Nenndorf in contradistinction to other sulphur mud-baths (as Eilsen, for instance), is probably due to the high temperature at which they are used; for whilst the water-baths are taken at a temperature of $90\frac{1}{2}°$ to $95°$ Fahr., that of the mud-baths is generally ordered between $90\frac{1}{2}°$ to $100°$ Fahr.

Though in obstinate cases of gout or rheumatism, with great torpor of the vascular system, such heat may afford assistance in the cure, as a general rule it is decidedly objectionable. The increase of pulse ought alone to be sufficient to warn us of the danger to which this practice may lead. The body will certainly bear a little more heat in the mud than in the water-bath, because the solid moory mass requires a considerable amount of latent heat to retain its temperature; but if we consider that an increased flow of blood to the chest and brain is primarily encouraged by the compression exercised on the lower part of the body, you must perceive how easily congestion to vital organs may be induced in persons at all inclined to it. It would therefore be greatly advisable to reduce the heat of the mud-baths, and to repress the boasted advantage—which is a great disadvantage in my opinion. To explain the simultaneous use of apparently incongruous remedies, we must assume our organic structures to be engaged in constant struggles with the inanimate substances surrounding us. The oxygen of the air, whilst it maintains the internal process of combustion by its combination with the effete carbon and hydrogen, and thus sustains vitality, will only perform its duty without discomfort as long as the organs of reception have not met with any injury. But let any change of structure or of action take place in these organs, and the life-maintaining virtue of air will hasten the termination of these functions. The digestive canal, destined to elaborate ingredients for the restoration of wasted substances, is too often called upon to receive substances which induce injurious and anti-vital action in the reproductive organs. With regard to the skin, with what admirable wisdom is it spread as a protecting cover over our whole body, designed to prevent any impediment to the necessary movements of the various organic liquids, and to allow egress to such liquid and gaseous particles as have become effete, but have not been removed by the ordinary emunctories of the body! At the same time it is a guardian of the medium in which we breathe. Its numerous nervous ramifications communicate to the superintending brain the slightest deviation from normal contact. To how many attacks is this covering exposed! Whilst Nature permits only a very gradual change of temperature, our civilised habits subject us daily to frequent extremes of heat and cold, rendering the skin more and more susceptible to injurious influences: these dangerous changes are multiplied till repulsion of exhalation and sudden withdrawal of external heat cause congestion of an internal organ.

We return to Bückeburg, and pass cursorily through the village of *Eilsen*, which lies a league distant, 293 feet above the level of the sea, six leagues to the south-west of Nenndorf, two north of Rinteln, and eight north of Pyrmont. Its bath arrangements, as well as the composition of the water, are analogous to Nenndorf (with, however, more sulphate of lime and of magnesia and sulphuretted hydrogen gas). Though less celebrated, it is more frequented than Nenndorf.* Then we direct our course to the charming and fertile plain in which the village of *Meinberg* is situated with its cold sulphur-springs, four leagues to the south-west of Pyrmont, and one to the north of Horn. We have to cross the Weser near Rinteln, to proceed direct to Meinberg, or, coming from the south by the Deutz-Minden Railroad, we stop at *Bielefeld* station, and drive five leagues eastward. This spa is distinguished by possessing steel and saline springs, and a great abundance of carbonic acid, besides the cold sulphur-spring, which stamp it as a highly efficacious theiokrene. The Teutoburger Forest extends in a north-westerly direction past the spa, causing it to possess an altitude of 634 feet. The Battle of Herman, which put a limit to the Roman conquests in Germany, was fought in this neighbourhood. The celebrated rocks of the Externstones are also situated in the neighbourhood. The old

* A detailed description seemed unnecessary, from its great similarity to Nenndorf. The physicians of Eilsen are Drs. Von. Möller and Wegener.

drinking-well is remarkable for the number of ingredients (twenty) which are contained in less than six grains of solid residue. The *Neubrunnen*, with 14¾ grains, contains chiefly Glauber and bitter salt; the *Mineralquelle am Stern*, more abundant, belongs to the chalybeate springs. The saline springs of *Schieder* arise a league and a half from Meinberg, at the foot of the Essenberg, near the high-road between Wöbbel and Schieder: chloride of sodium (50 grains), sulphate of soda (11 grains) and of lime (13 grains), forming the chief ingredients, with chloride of calcium and carbonate of lime (6 grains of each)—altogether 87 grains. There is also an acidulous spring near the Bellenberg, a league to the southwest of Meinberg. Before I mention the composition of its sulphurous springs in comparison with the other theiokrenæ, I must allude to the mighty evolution of carbonic-acid gas taking place with a very considerable tension over the mirror of the Trinkquelle. It is enclosed by an amphitheatre-like building, and provided with benches and seats for patients requiring gas-baths. The strong tension of the carbonic acid, containing a considerable proportion of sulphuretted hydrogen, prevents its mixing so rapidly with the atmospheric air, and affords therefore more potent gas-baths than even Pyrmont. Thus the so-called 'Sprudel' baths are prepared, which become undulated, by a stream of carbonic acid violently rushing through a tap, to the amount of 1½ cubic feet per minute. They are often resorted to with great advantage after a course of the sulphur mud-baths, to obviate excessive susceptibility of the skin.

The local and general carbonic-acid gas-baths are very extensively employed, and are considered as specially sanative in catamenial anomalies, spasms, great weakness of the cutaneous system, &c. In chronic inflammation of the tonsils or uvula, in affections of the meatus auditorius, &c., very happy results from local gas-baths are recorded by Dr. Piderit. In neuralgia of the facial nerves, ozæna, sexual torpor, &c.—in short, where utility may be expected from carbonic-acid gas, Meinberg is especially indicated. The adjoining table will further illustrate the variety of remedial means offered by Meinberg:—

CONTENTS OF THE MEINBERG SPRINGS (COLD).

	Trinkq.	Neubrunn	Quelle im Stern	Schwefel-quelle	Kochsalzq.	Acidulous spring, near the Bellenberg
Carbonic acid . .	34·36cub.in.	—	1·83	2·12	9·74	18·49
Sulphuretted hydrogen	—	—	—	0·55	—	—
Nitrogen . .	0·14	—	—	—	—	—
Total solid residue .	5·96	14·73	23·36	19·48	78·44	7·57
Sulphate of soda .	1·15	4·51	1·34	.5·84	11·01	—·
,, magnesia	1·14	2·52	3·67	1·73	—	0·04
,, lime .	0·28	3·45	15·16	8·33	13·46	0·18
Chloride of sodium	—	—	—	—	40·95	0·07
,, magnesia	0·81 grains	0·98	0·24	1·03	6·31	0·14
Carbonate of lime .	1·45	2·65	1·17	2·14	6·03	5·02
,, magnesia	0·15	0·24	0.17	0·17	0·51	2.04
,, iron .	0·08	0·07	0·01	0·008	0·07	0·005
Silica . . .	0·06	0·25	0·08	0·12	0 05	0·05
Extractive substance	0·57	—	—	—	—	—

Physicians: Drs. Kemper and Kirchner.

Now you must accompany me to some distance again, before we visit the next Westphalian spa. I wish to direct your attention to the hot sulphurous spring of *Aix-la-Chapelle* (*Aachen*) the first German town you passed when travelling from England to visit the distant spas. When you landed at Ostend, the railroad which connects the seashore with the Rhine brings you to Aix-la-Chapelle, so that from London you may reach this celebrated and formerly imperial town in less than eighteen hours. It will be the last sulphur-spring I shall submit to your consideration, but not the least, as you will perceive from its description. It lies in a pleasant valley between the Rhine and the Maas rivers, 450 feet above the level of the sea—fifteen leagues from Cologne, nine from Liége, ten from Spa—at latitude N. $50\frac{3}{4}°$ and longitude E. 6°. The warm springs are said to have been discovered, fifty-three years after Christ, by a Roman of the name of Granus—thence the name of Aquisgranum. The Romans had settled between the Maas and the Rhine when at war with the Germans. Bonn, Cologne, Düren, Jülich, &c. owe their origin to them. Roman coins were often found in cleaning the Kaiserbrunnen. The famous *Charlemagne*, in the year 777, first rediscovered, while hunting, the hot springs and bath-ruins, and was induced by the beautiful environs to build a castle and church there, to reconstruct the baths, and to choose the place for his residence. He declared Aix-la-Chapelle the second town of his immense empire, and the capital of Germany and France, and died there in the year 814, at the age of seventy-two. The German emperors were crowned there for a long time. In the twelfth century the town was so flourishing, and its population so rapidly increasing, that a new town grew up beyond the gates of the old one. Five hundred years ago the town numbered 100,000 inhabitants. It has, however, suffered from extensive conflagrations several times, and on the last occasion (A.D. 1656), nearly the whole town was destroyed, with all the worldly goods of the citizens. From this damage they never recovered. Another great loss had just previously been sustained by the emigration of wealthy and skilful Protestants, in consequence of the persecution to which they had been exposed. When under French government, Aix-la-Chapelle was very prosperous. In the year 1818 the congress of monarchs was held within its walls. It belongs at present to Prussia, is the capital of the Regency of Aachen, and possesses 46,000 inhabitants, and several very fine buildings—as the theatre, the beautiful enclosure of the Elisenbrunnen, the new Regency building, &c. The whole town is pleasantly situated near the Eifel mountain, and is chiefly ancient, with the exception of that part situated between the theatre and the station of the Rhenish Railroad, to the south of the town, which contains modern buildings of very fine exterior. In the centre of the town, on its highest point, is the large marketplace, opposite the antique town-house, with its two lateral towers, one of which (Granusthurm) is ascribed to Roman origin. The palace of Charlemagne is said to have stood here, and to have extended as far as the 'Kaiserbad' and the Münsterchurch. Towards the year 800 he built a cathedral church, and had the marble brought from Rome and Ravenna, and the flagstones from Verdun. This superb church was considerably injured by the Normans in A.D. 882, but was subsequently repaired. The tomb of Charlemagne is shown in the middle of the old dome, with the simple inscription—'Carolo magno.' His skull, ivory hunting-horn, and many other relics are preserved there, and shown to the people every seven years.

The environs of Aix-la-Chapelle are mountainous, with cultivated declivities. The mountains are but of a moderate height, and form only a partial limitation to the openness of the surrounding country. The Luisberg rises to the north of the town, and affords charming views from its eminence. To the south, woody and less fertile regions adjoin, extending westward into the Ardennen, eastward into the Eifel mountain. Towards the north-east the ground becomes flatter, and abounds in corn. The soil of the immediate environs is siliceous, calcareous, or sandy, and in some places as fine as sea-sand. Sulphur-pyrites are frequently found; pit-coal is also dug up in the neighbourhood and used for fuel. Calamine is another production of the environs.

The foundation of the Aachen mountains consists of transition-limestone. This is superposed by grey sandstone intermixed with glimmer, and in some places substituted by strata of coal or clay-slate. The position of Aix-la-Chapelle, and the numerous shady walks, with picturesque country-seats and farms, and alternating hills and valleys, render it a very agreeable resort. Amongst the varied walks, that which leads to the summit of the Luisberg is the most charming. The eye has a wider scope towards the north and east than towards the south and west. It was only with great difficulty that this barren mountain could be ascended formerly, but it is now laid out in the style of a so-called English garden, and easily reached by well-arranged roads. A Belvidere and saloon for company often receives visits from the residents and strangers. A pyramid of hewn stones adorns the top; it was erected in 1807, to the memory of Tronchot and his astronomical labours performed there. The thermal springs are divided into upper (warmer) and lower (less warm). The chief spring *Kaiserquelle* (emperor's spring) has the highest temperature, and contains the greatest proportion of solid ingredients. It supplies the *Elisenbrunnen* (the drinking-fountain), the Kaiserbad, the new bath, and the bath of the Königin von Ungarn: the thermal springs before the Kaiserbad, on the Büchel, have the same temperature as the former—$135\frac{1}{2}°$ Fahr.

The lower sulphur-springs are the Corneliusquelle (with 115° Fahr.), the spring of the old drinking-well (111° Fahr.), and the Rosenbadquelle (115° Fahr). The springs are all surrounded with bath establishments, where the visitors find accommodation for residing and bathing.

The Kaiserquelle issues nearly in the centre of the town, out of several fissures in the rock. It lies as it were at the foot of an eminence, which reaches its highest point on the marketplace. The lower springs lie at about 400 yards distance, in a less elevated position. They come to light between strata of transition-limestone and sandstone with glimmer.

The water is clear and transparent, but has a strong sulphurous smell and taste. The constituents of the various springs are nearly the same, but the amount of sulphuretted hydrogen decreases with the diminution of heat. This is at once a demonstration of the fact, that the sulphuretted hydrogen gas is not evolved from the depth to mingle with the mineral water, as is the case with carbonic acid, for then the colder the spring the greater would be the amount of gas; but, on the contrary, it diminishes with the proportion of glairine, which is smaller in the less warm springs. The amount of this substance is 0·29 gr. in the Kaiserquelle, 0·28 in the Quirinusquelle, 0·27 in the Rosenbadquelle, 0·19 in the Corneliusquelle. The sulphuretted hydrogen is supposed to be due to organic decomposition. Under the influence of heat the glairine enters into chemical action with the sulphate of soda, deoxidising the two component parts and transforming them into sulphuret of sodium. The carbonic acid evolved during the process, tending to combine with sodium, induces this substance to attract oxygen by the decomposition of the water. The disengaged sulphur then combines with the hydrogen of the water, and thus sulphuretted hydrogen results. The sulphuret of sodium discovered in analysis may be the product of the above process. Thus the greater the heat, the more intense the chemical action and the production of sulphuretted hydrogen. The vapours of the springs are employed for vapour-baths; douches are likewise administered with various force, and very judiciously assisted by friction and shampooing.

The analysis of the chief source (Kaiserquelle) shows 31·9 grains of solid and 26½ cubic inches of gaseous constituents; temperature 135½° Fahr., viz. :—

20·71	grains of		chloride of sodium
6·61	,,		carbonate of soda
0·23	,,	,,	lime
0·15	,,	,,	magnesia
0·04	,,	,,	strontia
2·12	,,		sulphate of soda
0·62	,,		sulphuret of sodium
0·14	,,		phosphate of soda
0·47	,,		fluoride of calcium
0·29	,,		animal organic substance
0·54	,,		silica

Total   31·95 grains in 16 ounces

GASEOUS CONTENTS.

8·	cubic inches of	carbonic acid
18·53	,,	nitrogen
0·13	,,	sulphuretted hydrogen

Total   26·66 cubic inches

Quirinusquelle possesses 31·08 grains of solid constituents, with a temperature of 117½° Fahr.; the Corneliusquelle 29¾ grains, and a temperature of 115° Fahr.; and the Rosenbadquelle 29·63 grains, with 115° Fahr.

However inconsiderable the amount of sulphuretted hydrogen may appear (about the sixth of a cubic inch), sulphur deposits itself on the covers of the baignoires, and in all those spots exposed to the rising vapour. At first this covering resembles fine snow, with minute shining crystals. Gradually the first laminæ condense, but remain soft and pappy as long as additional vapours increase their volume, but removed and exposed to the air they become yellowish and hard. The thermal salt obtained by evaporation of the water contains, in 100 parts, 64·84 of chloride of sodium, 20·68 of carbonate of soda, 0·72 of carbonate of lime, 0·47 of magnesia, 0·13 of strontia, 8·57 of sulphate of soda, 0·44 of phosphate of soda, 1·50 of fluoride of calcium, and 1·68 of silica.

The sulphuretted gas was formerly thought to be combined in this spa with nitrogen, instead of with hydrogen. But this turned out a fallacy, and it is now considered as sulphuretted hydrogen mixed with a considerable amount of nitrogen, greatly surpassing in this respect all other sulphur-springs.

If you compare the contents of the Aix-la-Chapelle water with those of other sulphur springs, you will at once perceive the necessity for careful discrimination. In recommending *Nenndorf*, for instance, your patient will imbibe a greater amount of hydrothionic acid, it is true; but whilst sodium and soda form the chief bases here, you have calcium and lime as the prominent bases there. Chloride of sodium forming two-thirds of the solid contents, and carbonate of soda one-fifth, you have, properly speaking, a saline water before you, modified by the presence of neutral salts, and distinguished by sulphuretted hydrogen and a great quantity of nitrogen. That it must be better tolerated by the intestinal tube can admit of no doubt.

I must direct your attention to the circumstance, that (with the exception of the sulphuretted hydrogen) *Wildbad* (in Würtemberg) contains the same ingredients, in the same relative proportions, though in considerably less quantity. You find there chloride of sodium as the chief ingredient, carbonate of soda as the next in amount, and sulphate of soda as the third. If the facts recorded of the peculiar effect of Aix-la-Chapelle water bear a striking analogy to those witnessed in Wildbad (where also nitrogen is the preponderating gas), you may consider it is an additional confirmatory evidence of the views I ventured to express concerning the operation of the Wildbad water. Compare Aix-la-Chapelle with *Weilbach*, and again a very different result is observed. You have only a trace of nitrogen, a greater amount of sulphuretted hydrogen, and as the chief ingredient neither chloride of sodium nor sulphate of lime but carbonate of soda, with carbonate of magnesia as the next, and carbonate of lime as the third important ingredient. It bears therefore more chemical analogy to Teplitz.

Baden, near Vienna, offers more resemblance to Nenndorf, in a chemical point of view, than to Aix-la-Chapelle—with the difference, however, that though sulphate of lime forms its chief constituent, and carbonate of lime the next, every ingredient exists in a smaller quantity; whilst the irritating lime-salts are more than counterbalanced by the presence of gently solvent and aperient salts, as sulphate of soda and magnesia with chloride of sodium. The action of Aix-la-Chapelle water is chiefly displayed in chronic diseases of the skin, in suddenly suppressed itch, tetter, in chronic rheumatism and gout, contractions of the joints with swelling, in acidity, flatulence, menstrual colic, lithiasis, hydrargyrosis, paralysis from metastasis, &c. It is contra-indicated in great weakness, tendency to congestion, to active hæmorrhage, &c. The water is allowed to flow into a reservoir, and not employed for bathing till it has acquired the proper temperature, which ought never to exceed 95° Fahr., but should rather be below this heat. The frictions connected here with the douche-baths and the well-contrived vapour-baths contribute not a little to the success so frequently observed at Aix-la-Chapelle in obstinate cases of rheumatism or gout, in which other spas have failed. In contractions from chronic gout and rheumatism Aix-la-Chapelle has shown itself particularly efficacious, according to Drs. Zitterland, Velten, and Strüter, &c. While rubbing the patient, the frotteur breaks the force of the douche with his hand. In chronic diseases of the liver the action of the water is sometimes assisted by adding Carlsbad salt. According to Dr. Wetzlar, the water acts specifically in all diseases arising from abuse of mercury, or from individual carelessness during its proper employment. Several cases of tertiary and secondary syphilis degenerated by excessive mercurials are so far assisted by the spa that the mercury becomes eliminated and its effects removed, so that the uncomplicated syphilis will then yield to ordinary treatment. Iodide of potassium, or decoctum Zittmanni (in more obstinate

cases), have thus often cured non-Hunterian syphilitic ulcers, when the same remedies have been ineffectually employed before. In chronic poisoning by lead or arsenic the spa is equally useful. As a proof of the utility of Aix-la-Chapelle in herpetic metastases, the case of a lady is mentioned, sent by Professor Andral from Paris. She suffered from symptoms of gastric inflammation, in consequence of a previous 'dartre.' Dr. Wetzlar employed the water with reluctance, as it invariably increases previously existing intestinal irritation. In deference, however, to the high authority of Andral, he administered it, and found the vomiting, pain, &c. disappear as if by enchantment, and after four weeks complete success confirmed the acumen of Andral. Slight prurigo showed itself during the course, but disappeared spontaneously. Erethic scrofula is sometimes relieved by the water. Regular gout is not cured here, but anomalous, wandering, and especially metastatic or metaschematic gout. Count Lubienski presented himself in 1846 with the symptoms of apparent valvular disease of the heart. Dr. Hederus of Dresden, however, ascribing the disease to arthritic diathesis, recommended Aix-la-Chapelle. In this instance also cure ensued, notwithstanding the apparently contra-indicating phenomena. Dr. Wetzlar saw also a case of atrophy of the flexor muscles of the hand, one of rupia, and one of acne sebacea cured here. Dr. Strüter mentioned the following cases among others, which show the efficacy of the springs:—
Mr. B., of Paris, 45 years of age, suffered from paralysis of the upper and lower extremities, without congestion to the head, in consequence of a cold. After six weeks employment of the water, and especially of the douches (from the extremities gradually to the spine), the patient left cured. Mr. H., from Rio Janeiro, through excessive indulgence in fast living, and partly through rheumatic causes, was affected with paralysis of the lower extremities. Steel internally and douches externally produced a cure.

In hæmorrhoidal congestion or otherwise obstructed portal circulation, the Elisabethquelle, with the addition of sulphate of soda, exhibits highly curative results. You see then that hæmorrhoids, which form such a prevailing indication for Weilbach, are here only enumerated as of secondary cosideration. The circumstances mentioned point to the fact, that among all the sulphur springs treated of, Weilbach is the only one where the sanative influence consists chiefly in the internal employment of the water; whilst the agency of heat, the force of the douche, the very skilful and judicious kneading and rubbing of affected parts, form a powerful assistance here. The great advantage of proximity enjoyed by Aachen is in some measure counterbalanced by the less sociable habits of the valetudinarians, who are dispersed in the several hotels and private houses of the town. The association of the Cursaal and bath-houses, with adjoining extensive walks into the open fields of rural spas, is missing here. This must not be taken as depreciating the value of the spa. But it is important to direct your patient's attention to this circumstance, and to request him not to indulge in a secluded mode of living. You must remind him of the necessity of muscular exercise in the free air, connected with social intercourse, not only for a proper elaboration of the water and for inhalation of a purer air, but for greater exhilaration of his spirits.

The very great influence of the mind on the body has been lately demonstrated in a highly interesting clinical lecture by Mr. Solly, of St. Thomas' Hospital, ' On Purulent Absorption.'— (*Lancet*, March 15, 1851.) After premising that there has been a great tendency lately to a low form of gangrenous erysipelas, to carbuncles, and to unhealthy inflammations generally, to which several patients succumbed after trifling operations, he alludes to the observation, that when the vital forces retain their normal power, pus, mixed with blood, coagulates that fluid, and the wound in the vessel is sealed by a firm coagulum of blood while the healing process is going on ; but if the vital power of the blood is diminished by disease, then this conservative coagulating action does not take place in time to plug the vessel and stop the poison at the threshold. The barrier which Nature in a state of health erects to prevent the flow of pus into the veins, is not set up, and the poisonous fluid is carried onward in the current of the circulation. After explaining how this barrier is not only interfered with by disease, but how it is sometimes broken down mechanically, if the limb is not kept at rest, so that the plug is not formed, and phlebitis induced by the generation of pus, he proceeds : ' There is another depressing agent, which I think has not been sufficiently insisted upon : I mean anxiety of mind. I am quite sure that mental anxiety has carried more poor fellows to the grave than any single cause that the surgeon has to contend with. I have repeatedly and for a long series of years observed a connection between anxiety of mind and the formation of abscesses. I have also observed purulent absorption more frequent in patients who, to use their own phrase, have had "something on their minds."

This was certainly the case in the instance of two of the patients to whom I have adverted.'

However remarkable such an observation may be, it ought not to surprise us; for do we not see the best appetite or hunger suddenly checked or destroyed by the occurrence of sorrow or fear? Cheerfulness must be considered as a complete equilibrium of the mental state. The brain possesses then the greatest power, and imparts it by the nerves to the abdominal organs. Reparation of wasted substance proceeds vigorously, the necessary biliary and pancreatic liquids are added in proper time; healthy blood results, and provides the brain with a wholesome stimulus and nutriment. When care or sorrow, however, finds entrance into the mind, and the central power is suddenly depressed, the dependent abdominal nerves are unable to stimulate their subordinate muscles to the required motion. The contractions are therefore more feeble, the gastric juice less solvent, the admixture of digestive liquids less abundant or less timely, the separation of chyle from saburra less complete; hence absorption of bile into the blood, which becomes vitiated and feeble, and reacts again as an unfavourable stimulus on the brain, increasing the former evil. From this the popular but judicious rule not to eat in anger or grief, and to enjoy cheerful conversation during meals.

The cold chalybeate springs found at Aix-la-Chapelle are occasionally used as an after-cure, but they are of too little importance to require a detailed description. The one contains half, the other three-quarters of a grain of iron in sixteen ounces, no sulphuretted hydrogen, but some carbonic acid, besides other ingredients contained in the sulphur-springs.*

Amongst the physicians must be mentioned also Dr. Brandis and Dr. Kilian.

A very short distance to the south of Aix-la-Chapelle, on the declivity of a steep hill, *Burtscheid* (*Borcette*) is situated. The upper (warmer) springs contain no sulphuretted hydrogen, the lower (cooler) do. In other respects their contents are analogous to those of Aachen. One of the upper sources is the hottest in Germany, viz. the *Mühlenbadquelle*, which has a temperature of 62° Reaumur = $171\frac{1}{2}$° Fahrenheit; the others have, respectively, 140°, 138°, and 111° Fahr. The promenade from Aachen to the drinking-well of Burtscheid is very pleasant. The Burtscheid waters are often used, alternately or conjointly, with those of Aix-la-Chapelle.

---

* Excellent accommodation in Hotel Dremel and Hotel Nuellens.

LECTURE XVI.

PYRMONT—DRIBURG—SCHWALBACH—SPAA.

AFTER our deviation from Westphalia, we return to seek the celebrated chalybeate spring of Pyrmont. We alight at the *Herford* station, on the Deutz-Minden Railroad, and then proceed by the diligence through Uffeln, Lemgo, &c. to Pyrmont. The distance of seven German miles (about thirty-five English) is performed in seven hours. Herford station precedes the new saline spring of *Oeynhausen*, near the Rehme station, of which I shall treat on another occasion. Before, however, we enter into a description of the Westphalian steel spring let us consider the properties of chalybeate springs in general.

The steel-springs, chalybokrenæ (from χάλυψ, steel, and κρήνη, cold spring), contain an excess of carbonic acid, which keeps the carbonate of protoxide of iron in solution. Whilst a small amount of iron is contained in most springs, those belonging to our present class possess the carbonate of iron as a predominating ingredient, either in a larger proportion, or in the absence of other powerful constituents. The iron generally prevents too lowering an effect being produced by other weakening ingredients —as, for instance, alkaline, saline, bitter-waters, &c. would produce too great atony of the intestinal mucous membrane; by constant provocation and stimulation of peristaltic action the necessary secretive and assimilative processes would be carried on with deficient tone and vigour, if the corrective presence of iron did not counteract this antiplastic tendency. The advantage of such a combination is frequently experienced by the ordinary administration of aperient extracts with lactate or sulphate of iron in the instance of chlorotic females, or of anæmic patients of our sex, especially if this sanguineous deficiency results from a lengthened sojourn in a tropical climate, as is shown by the admirable writings of Sir J. Ranald Martin. When iron forms the prevailing

P

ingredient, it increases the plastic and stimulating tendency of the blood, and enables it to perform its multifarious functions with vigour. It appears that the less firm the attachment of the iron to its acid or halogen, the more readily it is assimilated. Thus, whilst sulphate of iron, for instance, might be *supposed* to permeate more easily into the circulating channels from its greater solubility, in reality the less soluble carbonate of iron more readily allows decomposition for chemico-vital combinations, when brought into contact with the blood in such a highly-dissolved state (through the excess of carbonic acid). And if we sometimes prefer sulphate of iron in pharmaceutic preparations, it is because we cannot introduce the carbonate with the diluting volatile gas. The non-carbonates seem to require more elaboration before they are allowed to mingle with the blood-globules. For their administration, stronger and less irritable digestive organs are required, as the vital heat seems first necessary to deoxidise the compounds before the iron can attach itself to the organic liquid.

If any tendency to congestion or inflammation exists, iron is of course contra-indicated, as it would increase this morbid disposition. The great importance of iron has been demonstrated by the above authority, who, when treating of *tropical influence* on Europeans, traced the petulance and peevishness of temper, the forgetfulness, inaptitude both for business and recreation, the headache, restlessness, anorexia, alvine obstruction—and even pain and stitches in the right hypochondriac region, with an accelerated but feeble pulse, and symptoms simulating hepatic affection—to an absence of the necessary proportion of iron in the blood, which had lost too much of its serum through the lengthened influence of the tropical sun, so that the overstimulated liver, kidneys, and skin lay in a comparative state of prostration. Apparently inflammatory phenomena (his '*acute anæmia*') were cured in such invalids, not by depletion or weakening measures, but by steel, of course with proper regard to the function of the skin and abdominal organs. The additional light thrown on the nature of these diseases, and the almost certain relief procured by iron and other tonics, ought to induce us to regard with a particularly favourable eye the chalybeate springs which I am about to submit to your notice.

The town of *Pyrmont* is situated at an altitude of 404 feet above the level of the sea (latitude N. 52°, longitude E. 9°), in the Principality of Waldeck, on the left bank of the Weser. It is fourteen leagues distant from Hanover, three from Hameln, and six-and-a-quarter from Bückeburg. The valley in which the springs arise, within and near the town, is very fertile and abundantly provided with cornfields, whilst shady walks intersect the arable land. The environs witnessed the exploits of Arminius, Prince of the Cheruskians, and subsequently the battles fought between Charlemagne and the Saxons. The chief spring was formerly denominated the 'hylige Born' (*fons sacer*), and its immediate circuit the 'heilige Anger.' Though known from great antiquity, their reputation dates from the sixteenth century, especially after the termination of the Thirty Years' War. Upwards of 10,000 visitors are said to have resorted to the spa within four weeks, overcrowding all the adjoining villages and woods. The water was put into tubs, and sent to the expectant valetudinarians around the neighbourhood. In 1681 more than forty royal and princely personages were enumerated amongst the visitors.

Great luxury and convenience distinguish the baths and habitations. Numerous spots in the picturesque environs invite the visitors, as the Mühlenburg, Hünenburg, Gravingsberg, Wilde Schellenberg, with the ruins of Schell-Pyrmont, &c. The earthfalls near Holzhausen, a short distance from Pyrmont, are very remarkable. But the most curious phenomenon remains to be named—viz., the *vapour-cave* to the north-east of Pyrmont, where a constant evolution of carbonic-acid gas takes place, forming a permanent layer of from two to eight feet above the ground, mixed with some atmospheric air and a very small amount of sulphuretted hydrogen gas. According to Humboldt, 100 parts consist of 86·66 of air and of 13·33 of carbonic acid. The cave resembles the Grotto del Cane, near Naples, but the deviation of the magnetic-needle, observed there, was not noticed here. The layer of gas is smallest in winter and highest in summer, just before the appearance of a tempest. The mountains consist of stratified layers and alluvial land. Red sandstone forms the foundation, superposed and surrounded by marl, shell-lime, with the addition of alluvial layers of sand, clay, &c., whilst granite-blocks are sparingly met with here and there. Basalt is found about thirty miles from Pyrmont. The ferruginous drinking-spring (*eisenhaltige Trinkquelle*) arises in variegated sandstone at the beginning of the grand promenade of ancient lime-trees. The water is clear and sparkling—in taste agreeably acidulous, leaving an astringent sensation on the palate. The smell offers nothing peculiar, with the exception of an occasional odour of sulphuretted hydrogen over the surface of the water. Exposed to the air, a brownish deposit of oxide of iron is soon formed, with some manganese and lime. Its temperature amounts to $54\frac{1}{2}°$ F.; its specific gravity to 1·005; and its supply to 22 pounds per minute. It contains $44\frac{1}{2}$ cubic inches of carbonic acid, and above 28 grains of solid ingredients in 16 ounces; sulphate of lime forming the prominent substance (9 grains), carbonate of lime the next (nearly 6 grains), about 10 grains of sulphate of magnesia and of soda, and nearly half a grain of iron (0·49). The *Badequelle*, or Brodelbrunnen (*fons bulliens*), resembles the former, from which it is only a few steps distant. The water is more sparkling, and has a layer of eighteen inches of carbonic gas over its mirror. Carbonic acid and iron are both intimately and firmly united with the water. A bath, tested after having been used three-quarters of an hour, possessed 14 cubic inches of carbonic acid in 13·6 of water, and when filtered the presence of iron was demonstrated by ferrocyanide of potassium and tincture of galls. The *Augenbrunnen* (eye-well), fifty-eight feet to the west of the Trinkquelle, issues out of white clay, analogous in its proportions to the former, but only used externally as a cooling and astringent remedy in certain ophthalmic blennorrhages, &c. The *Neubrunnen* (new spring) issues out of variegated ferruginous sandstone on a meadow near the Emmer, and is very analogous to the drinking-well.

But, besides the above chalybeates, Pyrmont possesses saline springs: the *Soolquelle* originates half a league from Pyrmont, not far from the Emmer, in the deepest part of the valley, in variegated sandstone. Its taste is saline-bitterish. *The muriatico-saline drinking-well* is clear, strongly sparkling, of a marked saline-bitterish taste, inodorous; specific gravity, 1·011; temperature $51\frac{1}{2}°$ F. Besides these, an acidulous spring is found there, clear, transparent, and sparkling, with a piquant taste.

The effect of Pyrmont is chiefly displayed in *real debility*, whether produced by exhaustion of vital power, or by deficient nutrition, debilitating hæmorrhage, severe acute diseases, or too frequent child-bearing; in short, it is a most powerful restorative, whenever a great amount of blood or serum has been lost out of its ordinary receptacle, or when the plastic sphere is originally too weak to engender a sufficient amount of cruor for the performance of the necessary vital functions, as in chlorosis, anæmia, hysteria, &c. You cannot repair the deficiency by the food alone, for the very weakness of the blood causes a corresponding debility of the digestive organs, so that the more repairing par-

CONTENTS OF THE CHIEF PYRMONT SPRINGS.

	Trinkq.	Brodel-brunnen	Augenq.	Neubr.	Soolq.	Mur. sal. q.	Säuer-ling
Sulphate of lime	7·22 gr.	6·07	4·10	—	14·58	5·51	0·31
,, magnesia	2·69	5·53	4·56	3·47	2·33	—	0·60
,, soda	2·14	—	1·71	7·34	5·29	12·24	0·37
Carbonate of lime	5·98	4·52	3·81	7·86	2·71	6·92	1·81
,, magnesia	0·32	0·24	0·25	0 96	0·46	—	0·16
,, soda	—	4·78	0·84	2·62	1·49	6·23	0·30
,, iron	0·49	0·58	0·13	0·75	0·08	0·06	—
Chloride of sodium	—	—	0·44	4·38	61·68	65·49	0·01
,, magnesia	1·12	1·48	0·45	0·97	6·92	12·07	0·12
Silica	0·49	0·25	0·10	0·20	—	—	—
Total	20·02	23·62	16·46	28·98	95·32	108·7	3·72
	cubic in.						
Carbonic acid	44·52	38·51	36·28	39·28	17·46	26·19	21·84
Sulphur. hydrogen	—	—	0·39	—	—	—	—

Temperature, from 51¾° to 54½° F.

ticles the blood claims from the gastric purveyor, the less can be elaborated by that power. Hence we must call medicines to our aid, by which we may strengthen the digestive function, and at the same time supply the want of a certain material in a ready form for immediate assimilation. The great quantity of carbonic acid which introduces the solid particles causes them to be easily distributed and mixed with the existing constituents. But we cannot dictate to our pharmaceutical dose to mix entirely with the chyle, and to abstain from yielding any portion to excrementitious matter. Besides, the carbonic acid has the further influence of rousing the torpor of the languidly-moving mass, and thus it both brings a needed substance, and at the same time stimulates to its *immediate* elaboration and absorption. If the action is once commenced, Nature does not stand still again; otherwise it would be inexplicable how Hufeland could extol the virtues of this spa as the sovereign remedy in all cases of real debility and anæmia. 'Whoever does not believe in the efficacy of mineral water,' he says, 'let him come to Pyrmont and witness the wonderful effects produced by this admirable gift of Providence.' Whenever an individual appears pale, of phlegmatic temperament, of a soft lax fibre, of puffed-up and flabby appearance, the more he is inclined to passive profluvia, to mucosity, the better Pyrmont will agree with him. But if he looks strong, muscular, dark of complexion—if his skin and fibre be dry, tense—if he is more disposed to congestion or active hæmorrhage, Pyrmont and other chalybeates are inapplicable. In most obstinate cases of passive metrorrhage and hæmorrhoidal bleeding, Hufeland witnessed cures by Pyrmont after the useless employment of pharmaceutic tonics and astringents for years, and after the patients had been reduced to a state of deep-seated cachexia and anæmia. But before resorting to Pyrmont in such cases, it is always necessary to examine the phenomena carefully, and to convince ourselves of the presence of *systemic atony*. For should the hæmorrhage be active, or should vascular plethora or general irritability be present, the spa would be highly injurious; the circulating force of the blood would be increased, and with it the hæmorrhage. Besides, alvine obstruction might be induced at the same time, and the general irritability augment in consequence. We must also enquire whether some local irritation be not the cause of the recurring profluvium, as induration of the organ or other degenerations. In this case too Pyrmont would be improper. *Difficult menstruation*, accompanied by colic, vomiting, headache, fainting, spasms, &c., is generally cured or relieved here—as also *fluor albus*, based on an atonic state of the generative organs. *Sterility*, unconnected with organic impediments, forms an important indication for the spa. But the remedial agent must be perseveringly continued for a longer period than usual. The womb sometimes exhibits a great number of abnormal functions by its rebellious reaction after conception, so that a state of ill-health continues during the whole term of pregnancy, and disappears after delivery. Dr. Hufeland mentions the instance of a person who married before her complete bodily development. The uterus having been unable to bear the work of regeneration, feverish erethism, emaciation, colic, headache, stupefaction, constant sleepiness, &c. accompanied her during the whole nine months. At one time the weakness and emaciation reached an alarming extent. But after delivery, to the surprise of all, complete restoration took place spontaneously. Dr. Hufeland then, considering the undeveloped and unstable condition of the womb as the sole cause of the array of morbid phenomena, ordered Pyrmont water to be drunk the first year at home, and the next year (during pregnancy*) at the spring. He had the satisfaction of seeing not

---

* Though he would generally not allow the use in this period, but he could safely recommend it here, from the absence of any tendency to miscarriage.

only this pregnancy run its ordinary course without the former distressing symptoms, but also the next, two years subsequently. But baths and injections should accompany the internal course.

The tendency to abortion likewise belongs to the class of diseases in which Pyrmont shows itself curative. The convulsibility of the womb, which disposes it to contract and expel the fœtus prematurely, is generally due to atonic irritability of the organ. This is powerfully counteracted by the use of Pyrmont whilst the organ is free. *Nervous hypochondriasis* and *hysteria*, resulting from real defect of nervous power, from exhausting diseases, loss of blood, over-exertion, &c., find an excellent remedy in Pyrmont. But should there be a material basis, as abdominal infarcta, &c., Pyrmont would be injurious by increasing the morbific cause. *In nervous spasms of the stomach*, Pyrmont frequently induced cure or relief—also in nervous vertigo; no improvement, however, followed in epilepsy. But in paralytic diseases, connected with general weakness, Pyrmont has been found a powerful remedy. It is also useful in chronic diarrhœa, mucous hæmorrhoids, tendency to helminthiasis, &c. In vesical catarrh and seminal weakness it is likewise highly recommended. Hufeland saw nervous amblyopia, muscæ volantes, &c., frequently cured by the external application of the Augenquelle, with the internal use of the water. The saline springs of Pyrmont find their indication in many complaints where a cooling, solvent, and antidyscrasic remedy is required, and are often used with great advantage as a preparatory course before the employment of the chalybeate. Though numerous diseases are mentioned as indications for Pyrmont, they are all ramifications, diverging from the same central cause. If the nervous power be originally exhausted, the contractions of the heart become enfeebled, the peripheric vessels distribute the blood more slowly, regeneration proceeds more tardily, secretions are performed less promptly; chylification and sanguification therefore suffer. Deficient blood-krasis will then increase the original nervous weakness; or if the cause of debility proceed from unusually excessive secretions, the result will exhibit the same phenomena. Whether the blood be propelled with less force, or whether it be deficient in its required consistency, the consequence must be diminished stimulation and nutrition of the recipient organs. This state then is rationally and practically counteracted by Pyrmont. But when the spa cures diarrhœa, excessive mucosity of the alimentary canal, &c., we must attribute this effect partly to the increased tone of the fibre, and partly to the absorbent power of the lime (nearly two-thirds of the solid ingredients are furnished by sulphate and carbonate of lime). But this utility in heightened serous secretion must warn you against the employment of Pyrmont, whenever the slightest tendency exists to diminished alvine secretion or to obstruction. It is perfectly clear that a very delicate stomach, prone to rebel against any obstruent agent, will not easily tolerate a beverage which contains such a large amount of lime. The alimentary canal would be overstimulated, and either unhealthy diarrhœa or obstinate confinement of the bowels would result, with the natural congestive reaction to the brain. Pyrmont was formerly the most celebrated chalybeate of Europe. If it has lost something of its high repute, the cause must be sought in the great and preponderating importance now so justly attached to the chemical constituents of the mineral waters; and whereas in former times the fashionable Pyrmont was the chalybeate κατ' ἐξοχὴν, its utility in appropriate cases is still willingly admitted; but in diseases unadapted to the combined action of the lime-salts and iron, those spas are selected which promise a more favourable result from the absence of these occasionally objectionable ingredients. That the diet ought to be an object of especial care must be sufficiently obvious, for the good effects of the spa may be easily thwarted by a slight imprudence; and the lime, probably contributing its share towards the restoration of the required strength, if well tolerated and assimilated, must be expected to produce irritation if the digestion be wilfully weakened or overburdened. The chalybeate mud-baths and gas-baths, with all other external appliances, are well contrived and frequently employed to assist the internal use of the water. The physicians of Pyrmont are Drs. Lyncker, Gieseken, Valentiner, Seebohm.

Driburg.—In travelling a short distance towards the south you perceive the town of *Driburg*, at an angle formed by the ' Teutoburger Wald,' pursuing an oblique north-westerly direction, and the Lippe-river, which moves straight from east to west to reach the Rhine near Wesel. It lies 300 feet above the surface of the Weser, about an hour's ride from the *Bucke* station (on the line between Paderborn and Cassel), in an agreeable valley, surrounded by hills of moderate height. The climate is rather bleak in winter. The peat-earth is particularly appropriate for mud-baths, and has the peculiarity of possessing no iron, but a great amount of sulphur. It has a fatty saponaceous touch, is light and free from sand. It gives out a strong smell of sulphuretted hydrogen, and contains chiefly salts of lime, silica, alumina, sulphur, &c. The chalybeate of Driburg bears much analogy to Pyrmont, being distinguished however by a very firm adherence and a great amount of carbonic acid. It offers great inducements for those who prefer a more retired social life to the luxurious and fashionable tone prevailing in Pyrmont.

The *Trinkquelle* contains 41½ cubic inches of carbonic acid, and 26¾ grains of solid ingredients in 16 ounces, viz. :—

```
            8·42 sulphate of lime
            4·25      „      magnesia
            3·88      „      soda
            9·12 carbonate of lime
            0·51      „      iron
            0·53 chloride of magnesium
```

The *Hersterquelle* possesses 32 grains of solid constituents in similar proportions, with the exception of carbonate of iron (only 0·18 gr.) and more gypsum (12 gr.)

The *Saatzer sulphur-spring* possesses 17 grains—no iron, but is in other respects analogous in its proportions to the Driburg water. The close union of carbonic acid causes even the greater amount of iron to be often more easily assimilated and better tolerated than that of Pyrmont. The paramount utility of Driburg (though less frequented) is exemplified by a few cases which occurred in the practice of Dr. Brück. A girl of twenty years of age being forced by her parents to give up an attachment to a dissipated individual, soon changed from a handsome blooming girl into a chlorotic sickly creature. Besides the ordinary symptoms, she was affected with such deep *coma* that she could only refrain from sleeping in the mornings and afternoons by the greatest exertion. The doctor ordered Driburg for drinking and bathing, with cold affusions over the head. After a course of four weeks, complete restoration to her former health had taken place. In a case of peritonitis, affecting a chlorotic girl of nineteen years of age, he was compelled by the urgency of the symptoms to extract blood. Though the peritonitis had disappeared, great prostration and *chlorosis* remained. Twenty-eight baths of Driburg water, with douche and internal employment of the spa, produced recovery. An old Dutch gentleman, formerly robust, was now an emaciated and confirmed hypochondriac. Dyspepsia, languor, flatulence, obstruction, and a feeling of precordial oscillation constantly teased him. With difficulty he was persuaded to persevere for four weeks in the use of Driburg water, and when he departed he stated that he experienced no effect beyond a reddish appearance on the tip of his tongue. The assurance that this slight change promised greater improvement was ridiculed by the incredulous patient, who came however next year greatly altered to his advantage, and happy in reporting complete restoration, with the exception of a slight neuralgia of the plexus solaris, which still remained for a short time. Cases of sterility, sexual weakness, &c. were often cured. In fact, the indications are very analogous to those of Pyrmont. Either the steel-spring is used internally and externally, or the Hersterquelle is taken internally (where less tonic and more solvent treatment is required) with chalybeate-baths; or steel-spring internally, with sulphur mud-baths. A case is mentioned of a corpulent plethoric lady of Ostfriesland, who employed the Driburg mud-baths with great advantage in *arthritic deposits of the hip-joint*, after having been obliged to discontinue the Nenndorf mud-baths in consequence of congestion to the head and metrorrhage, which appeared during their use. The Hersterquelle, with sulphur mud-baths, is recommended in lithiasis, vesical hæmorrhoids, and spasms of the bladder: it contains about 11 grains of sulphate of soda and magnesia, 12 of sulphate of lime, nearly 6 of carbonate of lime, and only 0·18 of iron. This combination quite justifies its reputation in urinary and vesical irritation.

The great abundance of highly important springs in a small compass in the west might remind you of the Bohemian cauldron in the south-east. If you take the 'Teutoburger' Forest as the western starting-point, above 52° north latitude, and pursue the slanting south-eastern line of the Thüringer Forest and Frankenwald, to the Fichtelgebirg, at 50° north latitude, you have the numerous important spas within these two degrees of latitude between the Weser and Elbe rivers. But how different are their characters! Whilst in Bohemia you have thermæ, denoting a great depth of origin, and amongst the constituents salts of soda in preponderance, you perceive here no thermæ (except by boring: Oeynhausen), and salts of lime in predominance. A minor altitude, and the alluvial character of the soil, further indicate a less profound origin. Physicians: Drs. Brück, Hüller, Riefenstahl.

Schwalbach.—In order to examine a highly important Spa, in succession to the foregoing, we must retrace our steps to the Taunus mountain, on the right shore of the Rhine, travel to Wiesbaden by rail, and thence proceed by omnibus to Schwalbach

(10¼ miles in about 2½ hours.) The road passes through the celebrated 'Rheingau,' and is extremely picturesque. The approach to Schwalbach is marked by a rather steep declivity, requiring a steady hand to conduct the horses. The place is properly called *Langenschwalbach*, and lies four leagues distant from Wiesbaden and six from Mentz. The romantic valley of the Aar, with the castles of *Adolphseck* and *Hohenstein*, lies to the north-east. On the west an eminence slants downwards, dividing the valley into two smaller valleys. In the southern arises the *Weinbrunnen*, in the northern the *Stahlbrunen*. Umbrageous walks of beech and lime-trees lead from one valley to the other.

The Weinbrunnen is the oldest spring, and was formerly employed exclusively. It was first brought in repute by the description of Theodor von Bergzabern (commonly called *Tabernæmontanus*), in 1581. Among other properties, he attributed to the spring the virtue of counteracting the effects of excessive indulgence in wine and other spirituous liquors—as headache, chilliness, &c. This circumstance is supposed to have given rise to its name. The bleakness of the climate has already been pointed out in comparison with the mildness of Wiesbaden— Schwalbach lying on the northern declivity of the Taunus mountain, whilst the same height serves as a powerful protection to Wiesbaden in the south. The proper season, therefore, does not commence before the middle of June.

Schwalbach lies 909 feet above the level of the sea. Its average temperature is 6° Fahrenheit lower than that of Wiesbaden (the altitude of which is 586 feet less). If, however, the mean temperature of summer be compared, Schwalbach has only four (Fahrenheit) degrees less of heat. West and south-west winds are most common.

Besides the two springs mentioned above, numerous other springs arise there, as the *Paulinen* and *Rosenbrunnen* (provided with a common enclosure), *Neubrunnen*, *Oberneubrunnen*, &c. The water is clear, sparkling, and has an agreeably acidulous astringent taste. The temperature of the springs ranges between 48° and 50° Fahrenheit. Less solid ingredients are contained in these springs than in the Westphalian chalybeates.

CONTENTS OF THE SCHWALBACH SPRINGS.

	Stahlbr.	Weinbr.	Paulinenbr.	Rosenbr.
Carbonate of lime	1·45 gr.	2·11	2·95	2·95
„ magnesia	0·88	3·12	2·75	0·98
„ soda	0·25	0·17	0·45	0·35
„ iron	0·75	0·83	0.65	0·91
Chloride of sodium	0·34	0·18	0·03	0·32
Sulphate of soda	0·21	0·16	0·02	—
Carbonic acid	28 cub. in.	26	39½	26
Total of solid ingredients	3·83 gr.	6·59	6·86	5·51

The Rosenbrunnen is merely employed externally, and mixed, for bathing, with the Paulinenbrunnen; the others are both employed for drinking and bathing. The baths are heated by steam, which is introduced between the two bottoms of the baignoires—the upper constructed of metal and the lower of wood. Baths may also be obtained in some hotels, but as the water has to be carried there in casks, it would certainly be more advisable to use the bath-house.

It is a matter of great importance which spring is to be used. *Paulinenbrunnen,* the mildest of the three, acts as a solvent and tonic. Its great amount of carbonic acid causes it to be well elaborated. It has been found most strikingly effective in the instance of European invalids, who have been subjected for a long time to a tropical climate. The rigid torpidity of the liver, and the obstinate alvine obstruction, which refuse to yield to mercurials and aperients, give way here. This fact may appear strange, and is even wondered at by the physicians who have observed it. The results of Sir R. Martin's experience perfectly coincide with the effects of the mineral water. As I stated previously, *tenuity of the blood* was found by that distinguished gentleman to be the stubborn cause of the alvine inaction. The furred tongue, the dyspepsia, headache, langour, fretfulness, insomnia, &c. gradually diminish under the employment of pharmaceutic iron with solvents. The blood flows with greater vigour, and is thus a more powerful provocator of central and peripheric nervous and muscular action. Next in frequency of employment is the *Weinbrunnen,* which contains most iron among the drinking-springs; but its carbonic acid is so firmly attached that it agrees better with erethic constitutions than the less substantial Stahlbrunnen, the most exciting of the three. The carbonic acid of the latter being somewhat more loosely adherent, may be evolved in the intestinal canal before absorption, and thus the iron may become separated; hence a greater cerebral excitement may be expected in persons at all disposed to plethora. The paucity of tempering ingredients is another reason why the characteristic stimulant and tonic effect of iron is more distinctly and purely displayed by this spring. With less iron than the Weinbrunnen, this element forms a greater proportion of the whole solid residue—$\frac{3}{4}$ of a grain out of $3\frac{3}{4}$, the fifth part; in the Weinbrunnen, $\frac{4}{5}$ of a grain out of $6\frac{1}{2}$, about one-eighth of the whole. In great general torpidity the Stahlbrunnen is therefore especially indicated.

Medicinalrath Dr. Müller, sen., found the spa curative in diseases produced by anæmia, whether arising from excessive profluvia, or from debilitating disorder, or from exhausting mental labour. That chlorosis, tendency to miscarriage, sterility, catamenial irregularities, seek and find relief here is obvious. But cures of cases are recorded which seem to fall less under this category. An English lady is mentioned, who was cured of *paralysis* of the lower extremities by using Schwalbach water during two seasons. Several painless tumours of the breast—of scrofulous origin—were cured by the baths of the Paulinenbrunnen. Paralysis of the upper extremities, after a violent attack of influenza, has also been removed here. In short, when the articular disability seems to result more from atony than from any arthritic or rheumatic cause, Schwalbach is often resorted to in preference to those spas which professedly act against paralysis, as I detailed when treating of the akratopegæ. Persons whose abdominal organs have been weakened by excessive use of purgatives, and who are inclined to constipation, acidity, mucosity, or to diarrhœa, seek relief here. In hot weather the atmosphere somewhat inclines predisposed individuals to *diarrhœa*. Whenever this occurs the course must be stopped, and appropriate remedial means are to be employed. But precautions should be taken to prevent this ailment. Careful clothing, especially of the feet and abdomen, should not be neglected. The climatic peculiarity of the spa admits of frequent changes of temperature; hot days are sometimes followed by cool nights. How easily profuse cutaneous action may then be checked by carelessness, and a vicarious profluvium be brought about in the intestinal canal!

Moreover, the valetudinarian should beware of *drinking* cold water *intemperately* and indiscriminately between and immediately after meals. During meals, both in consequence of the chemical and mechanical action going forward, the animal heat of the stomach is naturally heightened. Cold water, poured in ad *libitum*, from its theoretical innocence, suddenly diminishes this necessary heat, and interferes therefore with the chemico-vital action. Besides, the strength of the gastric juice is impaired, its solvent acid becoming too diluted to perform its function properly. If water is introduced after fatty or oleaginous substances, these immiscible bodies may be separated by the water from the other digestible morsels, and thus be removed for some time from the solvent influence of the gastric juice. To avoid drinking water after fruit is a popular rule too well known to require repetition. I wish I could persuade my continental friends to abstain from this prevailing habit of apparently innocent water-drinking, in which case the records of the spa would not mention so many instances of diarrhœa interrupting or annulling the course; nor would the advice be necessary to select an earlier period of the summer than the hot July and August, in order more securely to avoid this baneful complaint.

Dr. Genth very judiciously recals to mind the observation of Liebig, concerning the part played by iron in the human economy. That great chemist found iron in no other part than the hæmatine of the blood. The protoxide of iron having a strong tendency to absorb an additional atom of oxygen, gives up the carbonic acid with which it may be combined to gratify this propensity. On the other hand, peroxide of iron coming in contact with substances strongly attractive of oxygen, as carbon, hydrogen, &c., easily yields this additional atom, and then absorbs the carbonic acid, for the formation of which it has just furnished one constituent. This simple process forms, according to Liebig, the whole basis of life. The red globules of arterial blood contain the highly oxidised iron, and are propelled rapidly through the larger vessels with little chemical change; but when the globules are detained by the minute peripheric tortuous capillaries, the organic parenchyma tends to combine with the plastic fluid, and the most exhausted particles allow their elements to be decomposed in order to enter into chemical action with the newly-introduced warm and stimulating liquid. The carbon deprives the peroxide of iron of its less firmly attached portion of oxygen for the formation of carbonic acid, and then combines with the reduced protoxide to form carbonate of iron; the hydrogen absorbs a portion of the oxygen for the formation of water. Not to speak of the other compounds formed, it suffices to bear in mind that a double purpose is served—combustion and generation of vital heat on the one hand, elimination of effete particles and reproduction of new ones on the other. The carbonate of protoxide of iron flowing in the venous blood, gives up its carbonic acid when acted upon by the atmospheric oxygen entering the lungs, and exchanges it for a greater amount of oxygen, so as to become arterialised, that is peroxidised. The quantity of the oxygen of the blood depends, therefore, on the amount of iron present. If we introduce more iron into the chyle and venous system, a greater quantity of oxygen will be attracted from the air, retained in the arterial course, and given up again in the capillary metamorphosis. The calorification must be more intense, and the elimination of effete particles more profuse. Hence a greater appetite during the employment of the chalybeate, because a more extensive waste takes place. Anæmic persons feel chilly (especially in the extremities), inanimate, and easily excited to increased cardiac action, because nature endeavours to correct the deficient sanguineous consistency by more numerous propulsions. Obstruction is another natural consequence of anæmia. The sparing amount of oxygen causes a less active chemical combination, and thus the ordinary emunctories are less often called upon to rid the body of effete substances. The skin feels clammy, flabby, and inelastic; the urine is pale, deficient in nitrogenous compounds; the alvine action rare. This state must continue as long as the sanguineous deficiency remains unrepaired—otherwise a hectic condition would necessarily ensue. Positive experiments prove the increase of red blood-globules through the employment of iron. In one case they amounted to 95·7 parts in 1,000 after the exhibition of iron, whilst beforehand the proportion was only 46·6 parts. The fibrine of the blood diminishes, by its adaptation to new organic productions in consequence of a more active combustion. Whenever the internal use of the water is not well borne the baths alone are used, and the specific effects of the absorbed ingredients are well marked. To prove the absorbing power of the epidermis, several experiments are adduced which clearly demonstrate this point. The hand immersed for a quarter of an hour in water of 112° F. had imbibed 98 grains. After a full bath of half an hour, of the temperature of 82° F., the weight of the body increased 570 grains; in a bath of 95° F., at several occasions, 552, 503, and 465 grains. Another experimenter found the weight of his body increased by 2,550 grains in an hour, when the temperature was 79¾° F. ; the increase was only 638 grains at a temperature of 90° F. ; pulse and animal heat were unchanged. In a bath of 99½° F. there was neither increase nor diminution of weight, whilst the pulse became accelerated and the animal heat augmented. In another experiment at 98¼° F., for half an hour, the perspiration broke out in torrents, the pulse was 98 per minute, and *the loss of weight* 1159 grains.

The great importance of temperature is thus shown. As long as the secretive tendency of the skin is not called into violent requisition, not only absorption of water and its ingredients takes place, but the circulation is not accelerated. As soon as that limit is exceeded (which varies in different individuals) the heat causes a great turgidity of all the cutaneous sudatory glands, the retained animal heat receives an additional impulse, and the heart's action must naturally participate in the excited state of the organism. The more vigorous, plethoric, and inclined to congestion patients are, the sooner will this limit appear, where excretion takes the place of absorption, and where the former sedative influence of the bath is exchanged for the dangerous orgasm alluded to. The more anæmic, weak, and exhausted persons are, the better will they bear a somewhat greater heat, for calefaction proceeds less energetically in their organism, and we may establish it as a rule that imbibition will continue as long as the circulation remains undisturbed.

In general, at Schwalbach, the temperature of the baths is gradually lowered in proportion as the strength of the patient and plasticity of the blood increase. The period of immersion is likewise regulated according to the susceptibility of the patient, and, as a rule, gradually prolonged. The great amount of carbonic-acid gas in the water must never be lost sight of. However curative and useful its stimulating and reviving action, it naturally induces too great an irritation and subsequent relaxation of the nervous system, if its employment be carried to excess. The baths are justly recommended to be taken during calmness of the vascular and nervous system. The best period is about one or two hours after a light breakfast. Gentle exercise is usually taken afterwards, except with very weak individuals, to whom rest in bed is permitted for a short time. The symptoms of saturation are to be looked for during the course, as an indication for its termination. They consist in languor, giddiness, headache, restlessness, bleeding from the nose, præcordial oppression, want of appetite, &c. To prevent a too early occurrence of this satiety, pauses are enjoined in the use of the baths (as an intermission every third or fourth day), and a careful regulation of the dose, so that the normal condition of the blood may be brought about gradually and imperceptibly. For it is apparent that the weaker and more attenuated our circulating fluid happens to be, the less it is able to elaborate and assimilate considerable proportions of stimulating liquids. A stormy inroad of foreign substances may sometimes produce striking sanative effects, but more often the well-intentioned friend will be repelled by the organism as an enemy, if a too rapid amelioration is sought to be enforced.

This warning refers to all the spas, and should be conveyed to your patients, who often attempt to make up for a shortened sojourn by excessive doses of the waters, with results easily imagined. As in the scales we shall not obtain an equilibrium by *throwing* substances on the deficient side, but by gradually adding the necessary weight, so it is in Nature. When we see the various systems acting as safety-valves for each other, we cannot do better than follow the same tract. In jaundice, for instance, we see the kidneys excrete biliary matter, and thus act vicariously for the liver. In fever, when assimilation and nutrition are impaired, a greater amount of urea is excreted by the kidneys, to prevent a dangerous accumulation of nitrogenous substances in the circulating fluids. A certain check of the cutaneous function through cold is sometimes relieved by increased action of the bowels. Many other illustrations might be adduced of this beautiful and wise provision of Nature, but those mentioned suffice to show that you cannot induce violent action of one system without materially interfering with the functions of others which ought to remain unaltered.*

Before concluding this lecture I should wish to bring to your notice a chalybeate which formerly enjoyed a very great reputation, and which is still frequently visited with great advantage in appropriate cases: I allude to *Spaa*, in Belgium, scarcely belonging to the German mineral waters, but still so near Aix-la-Chapelle that it may well be included in our course. When you travel from Ostend towards Cologne you leave the railroad at *Pepinster* station, between Liége and Aix-la-Chapelle, and then proceed by an omnibus to the neighbouring *Spaa*—lat. N. 51°, long. E. 6°. It is situated at an altitude of 1,000 feet above the level of the sea, in a pleasant valley of the Ardennes. There

* Superior accommodation in the Hotel—Duc de Nassau.

are in all no less than sixteen springs. The chief spring, *Pouhon*, arises in the centre of the town out of ferruginous clay-slate, and is frequently used for exportation. About a league to the south, in a somewhat more elevated position in the midst of umbrageous walks, the *Geronstère* is situated. On the road to Malmedy rise the springs called *Sauvenière* and *Groesbeck*, half a league to the south-east of Spaa, and about three-quarters of a league from the Geronstère. The two *Tonnelets* lie half a league from the town, to the north-east of the Sauvenière. In a marshy meadow between the Tonnelets and Sauvenière the *Watroz* and other springs were formerly in use, but they are now nearly abandoned. The temperature of the springs is 50° Fahr.; their taste is acidulous and rather piquant, with a marked ferruginous after-taste ; their odour is somewhat peculiar, analogous to a hydrogen compound of iron. The *Pouhon* contains 3·37 grains of solid constituents, and eight cubic inches of carbonic-acid gas, in sixteen ounces—amongst these four-fifths of a grain of iron ; the other springs contain rather less iron and solid substances. Spaa agrees with some weak and irritable digestive organs, which would not tolerate a more substantial chalybeate. The occasional sudden changes of temperature incidental to its geographical position must not be left out of consideration. On the other hand, the hilly walks in the immediate environs invite to pedestrian exercise, indispensable

CONTENTS OF THE CHIEF SPRINGS OF SPAA.

	Pouhon	Geronstère	Sauvenière	I. Tonnelet	II. Tonnelet	Groesbeck
Carbonic acid	21 cu. in.	14	20	22	19·7	21
(According to Struve,	8)					
Gaseous hydrogen compound of iron }	—	0·04 c.in.	0·02	0·01	0·004	—
Total of solid ingredients	3·37 gr.	1·65	1·28	0·96	0·58	0·83
Sulphate of soda	—	0·04	0·07	0·02	—	0·02
Carbonate of soda	0·90	0·45	0·30	0·21	0·08	0·22
,, magnesia	0·31	0·16	0·10	0·08	0·06	0·08
,, lime	0·75	0·33	0.22	0·15	0·12	0·16
,, iron	0·87	0·45	0·43	0·39	0·25	0·24
(According to Struve	0·37)					
Carbonate of alumina	0·03	0·01	—	—	—	—
Chloride of sodium	0·20	0·09	0·06	0·04	0·01	0·04
Silica	0·28	0·10	0·07	0·04	0·02	0·04

for the relief of hepatic sluggishness. The springs act as solvents and tonics. From the Geronstère some sulphuretted hydrogen is disengaged. The Sauvenière contains more steel than the Geronstère, and less than the Tonnelets. The air is very salubrious and bracing. The springs are particularly recommended in atony of the uropoietic organs—in acidity, dyspepsia, and tendency to gravel. In anæmic conditions generally they possess great efficacy, and deserve to be more employed than they are.

Considering that nearly every severe and prolonged ailment produces a certain state of debility and anæmia, and thus leaves a greater susceptibility for the germination of morbific tendencies, it is obvious that chalybeates will very frequently be required, and that their adaptation to the respective individuals must be of the utmost importance. Though no blood may have been actually abstracted during an acute disease, an indirect loss of blood has taken place, the metamorphosis of vital structures into effete particles having proceeded as usual, whilst the required assimilation of ingested food for the reparation of the loss was impeded. Overexertion of any organ or system, without derangement, is another source of weakness, for we may assume that a limit is placed to the action of each organic sphere.

If the circulating force be merely weakened by depression of the nervous system, the same injuries will result as if the quantity of blood were deficient; for unless propelled with a certain vigour it will afford a less powerful stimulus for reproduction and for generation of heat. This circumstance is probably one of the reasons why we may give pharmaceutic preparations of iron for months to exsanguine and weakened nervous females without obtaining results so often following the use of chalybeate springs during three or four weeks. Though less iron was ingested in the latter instance, the remedy was accompanied by the highly-stimulating carbonic acid, so that the moving force of the blood must have been augmented, and its power of provoking metamorphosis. But the important question remains, what chalybeate shall we choose, if we find its tonic action indicated?

The analysis will serve as a guide in a great measure, but you must by no means wholly depend upon it. Thus in Spaa, the last chalybeate mentioned, without an explanatory difference being afforded by the chemical constituents, the Sauvenière is particularly renowned for cases of sterility, more than the Pouhon; whilst to the Groesbeck a very powerful diuretic action is ascribed, and its utility is extolled in gravel and lithiasis: the two latter are especially recommended in such cases of debility and anæmia as result from moist and damp habitations, from previous intermittent fever, and from scarlatina, especially in leuco-phlegmatic flabby individuals. The Pouhon is, on the contrary, recommended in obstructed portal circulation, in deficient bilification, in congested liver and spleen following intermittent fever; also in flatulence, digestive weakness, acidity, tendency to diarrhœa, passive hæmorrhage, &c. To relieve the consequences of intermittent fever, you find Pyrmont, Schwalbach, and Spaa recommended. In tropical climates, where the function of the skin is excessively stimulated, and in low marshy regions, where the same function is inordinately impeded, the same morbid states often result—viz., intermittent fever and subsequent engorgement of liver and spleen. How is this? Probably because impaired sanguification is the consequence of both abnormal influences.

In the tropical regions the skin assumes, as it were, the work destined to other organs. Without the due proportion of muscular exercise, circulation and vital combustion are promoted. This undue exaggeration of certain organic functions *must* ultimately produce great relaxation and atony of the overworked organs. The serum of the blood being greatly diminished by the constant drain of perspiration, the blood can no more circulate with its wonted rapidity. Though the propelling force of the heart suffices to send it to the peripheric capillaries, its return through the portal vessel will be retarded, the more so as the liver has been likewise overexerted and weakened, by partially performing the function of the lungs—rarity of the air permitting a minor entrance of oxygen for ordinary inspirations. An impaired chylification cannot but result. Thus a constant loss takes place on the one hand, without a sufficient reparatory sanguification on the other. The anæmic state of such invalids is better counteracted by chalybeates which powerfully promote the action of the liver, and remove the atony and susceptibility of the skin—as Franzensbrunn, Pyrmont, &c. The amount of carbonic acid, *inter alia*, must have a decisive weight in the choice. In *marshy and damp* places the ordinary function of the skin is somewhat checked by the watery exhalations of the circumambient atmosphere; the effete nitrogenous and carbonaceous particles repelled to the central organs claim a greater amount of work from the abdominal viscera. The caloric generated in our organism is quickly abstracted by the surrounding atmosphere for the evaporation of the suspended watery particles. The diminished heat of the surface causes a revulsion of the blood towards internal organs, and especially a retarded reflux from the centres of venous circulation. In the latter instance those spas are useful which counteract the debility and anæmia, without materially increasing the circulation of abdominal organs, as Spaa in Belgium, where, more especially, the energy of the uropoietic and cutaneous systems is called into requisition, and where the bracing air of the Ardennes Forest greatly contributes toward a successful result. The services of a very scientific English physician (Dr. Cutler) are available for English visitors at the latter place, besides several Belgian physicians of repute, as Dr. Lezaak and others.

LECTURE XVII.

EMS—SCHLANGENBAD—BADEN-BADEN.

To-day I must request you to follow me as far as Coblentz. You perceive the River Moselle entering the Rhine on its left shore. The River Lahn terminates its westerly course a short distance below, on the right.

Our present destination is a very celebrated spa, situated on the right bank of the River Lahn, three leagues to the east of Coblentz, viz. *Ems*, on the railway between Coblentz and Giessen. It lies about eight leagues to the north of Schwalbach, and is enclosed in a narrow valley between high mountains, about a quarter of a league from the village of Ems. The opposite bank is considerably wider, and covered with gardens and meadows. The river, though large, flows so slowly that scarcely any movement is perceptible in it. The surrounding mountains consist of clay-slate, interspersed with quartz; greywacke and layers of shining coal are met with at greater depths. To the east of the spa a curiously-shaped group of rocks rises almost perpendicularly to a great height; to the west the *Bäderberg* is perceived, contrasting with the opposite mountain by being cultivated to the very summit. Vineyards and orchards clothe its slopes. On the other side of the river the mountain-heights are intersected by valleys, and rise like colossal pyramids, covered with wood and verdure. The highest peaks are formed by the *Winterberg* and the *Molbuskopf*.

In contradistinction to the village, the spa is called 'Bad Ems.' The houses destined for the reception of the valetudinarians are built along the river. The Curhaus is most conveniently arranged, both for residence and sanitary purposes, with water and douche-baths, &c. About half a league from the village of Ems the so-called 'Silberhütte' invites the attention of visitors. On the opposite bank the mines of 'Lindenbach' are perceived. About an hour's walk along the dam of the Lahn brings you to Nassau, with its antiquated castle. On the other side of the river a mountain rises, covered with trees and shrubs, and bearing the ruins of the old châteaux of Nassau and Stein.

Walks and roads are laid out to supply the invalid with means of exercise. Donkeys are generally used for ascending the distant hills and mountains. Though the valley offers many romantic spots and natural charms along the serpentine course of the Lahn, its confined position, the frequent blasts and winds, especially in the morning and evening, and the consequent vicissitudes of temperature make it an undesirable locality for those who do not positively require the sanitary use of the waters. No temptations are offered to the pleasure-seeker for a prolonged sojourn.

The Bäderley is considered as the focus of the thermal springs which originate at its foot. The spa is one of the oldest in Germany, and was known to the Romans, according to undoubted testimony: it belongs now to the domains of the Duke of Nassau. The various springs differ greatly in their temperature, the constituents being nearly the same in each. Though the number of visitors has considerably increased of late (to 4,000 and upwards in one season), the former quiet tone is preserved, and no opportunity given for noisy amusements. This is chiefly due to the serious nature of the complaints of those seeking relief here—partly also to the peculiar local disposition. A covered colonnade now adjoins the Curhaus, for walking in unfavourable weather.

The 'Steinerne Haus' and 'die vier Thürme' are private property, but also serve for the accommodation of invalids. The former adjoins the Curhaus. In the 'Armenbad' indigent patients receive gratuitous accommodation. The water has a weak, alkaline, saltish taste. Its colour is transparent. In the canals through which it flows a reddish bath-stone is deposited, consisting of ferruginous lime-earth. Of the numerous springs I will merely mention the principal ones:—

I. The thermal springs of the Curhaus:
  The *Kesselbrunnen*, $117\frac{1}{2}°$ F.
  The *Kränchen*, 91° F.
  The *Fürstenquelle*, 95° F.

II. Springs of the Steinerne Haus:
  The *warm* one of 100° F.
  The *lukewarm* one of 77° F.

III. The thermal springs of the Armenbad have a temperature of 109° F.

The highest temperature is possessed by those of the Pferdebad—viz., $133\frac{1}{4}°$ F.

Several warm springs originate in the bed of the River Lahn, near the Pferdebad, communicating to the water a heat of $104°$ F., with a constant development of bubbles of carbonic acid and nitrogen gas, so that warm river-baths might be constructed with great advantage to the patients.

The *Bubenquelle* (boys' spring) deserves also a special notice. It bubbles up a few steps from the chief spring, with a temperature of $117\frac{1}{2}°$ F. This spring is merely used in cases of sterility; an *ascending douche* drives the water with some force into the vagina of barren women sitting over it. The great reputation of this spa in cases of sterility must be accounted for partly by the stimulating mechanical agency, and partly by the alkaline effect of the water. The carbonic acid and nitrogen are present in an inverse proportion to the heat of the water. The chief constituents are carbonate of soda and chloride of sodium.

According to Kastner, the Kesselbrunnen contains thirty-one grains of solid ingredients in sixteen ounces, viz. :—

20·01 carbonate of soda.
1·97 „ lime.
1·19 „ magnesia.
0·03 „ iron.
7·02 chloride of sodium.
0·03 „ potassium.
0·54 sulphate of potash.
0·40 silica.
0·07 extractive substance.
13 cubic inches of carbonic acid, and half a cubic inch of nitrogen.

The *Kränchen* contains twenty-nine grains of solid constituents, —viz., seventeen of carbonate of soda, two of carbonate of lime, and $7\frac{3}{4}$ of chloride of sodium; in other respects analogous to the former, but it contains $18\frac{1}{2}$ cubic inches of carbonic acid, and two of nitrogen. The altitude of Ems is 188 feet above the level of the sea. You are aware that Ems enjoys its greatest reputation for the cure of *laryngeal* and *pulmonary* diseases. Since the urgent recommendation of Hufeland, patients without number resort to the spa, expecting confirmed tubercular consumption to be cured there. Many are certainly disappointed, especially after considerable progress has been made by the disease—the whole system showing its participation by emaciation, nocturnal perspirations, hectic fever, &c. The waters are unable to arrest the destructive process rapidly going forward. Though, on the authority of Hufeland, no deterioration ensues in this spa, still, when no rational judgment can promise relief, the exciting journey and the stimulating baths should be avoided in such advanced stages. It is however quite otherwise in the incipient stage of phthisis, or in mere diathesis, of persons of florid complexion and characteristic frame, greatly inclined to pulmonary or tracheal catarrh, or to hoarseness. If these phenomena appear as a reflex of abdominal mucosity, hepatic sluggishness, or tendency to acidity, lithiasis, irritative dyspepsia, &c., Ems offers itself as a unique and unrivalled remedy. Whilst the chloride of sodium tends to improve the digestive process, the chief ingredient, carbonate of soda, exerts its antacid and solvent power. It softens the tough viscid mucus of the intestinal and uropoietic passages, causing therein a more normal secretion and a less embarrassed capillary circulation. The congestion of the pulmonary vessels is thus diminished by an improved abdominal metamorphosis; the expectoration becomes looser, and mucus more abundant and normal. The confined state of the atmosphere might cause an inconvenient oppression, without the use of the waters, but during their therapeutic action the pulmonary weakness is not aggravated; on the contrary, the denser state of the air renders deep inspirations less necessary—consequently less exercise of the lungs is needed to obtain the required amount of oxygen. When the beneficial changes have been effected by the springs, then a more invigorating and bracing atmosphere is wanted. The above remarks are necessary to explain an apparent contradiction concerning the great advantage of high positions in tubercular diathesis. The cure is there to be produced by the mechanical dilatation of the lungs, but here through the chemically alterative process instituted in another part of the system, when it is desirable that the secondarily affected lungs or trachea should remain as inactive as is compatible with health.

Less cutaneous irritation is produced by the Ems baths than by those of many other thermæ; indeed, an allaying sedative effect is exercised on the nervous system, and an inclination to repose and sleepiness is frequently felt, but it must not be indulged in on any account. Moving about, friction, or a moist cold cloth on the head, are frequently recommended to the bather. This shows how dangerous the baths are in any tendency to congestion, plethora, active hæmorrhage, &c. When the skin is less irritated through the small amount of culinary salt, a greater scope is left to the action of heat, and considerable caution is therefore demanded, especially in *warm* bathing, and *more particularly* by that class of patients usually resorting to Ems. The energetic flow of blood towards the circumference soon reacts, and returns with greater vivacity to the internal organs—especially to the lungs, heart, brain, or any other organ in a state of irritation or congestion. The Kesselbrunnen is most frequently drunk; the Kränchen, from the very scanty supply, is used less frequently. The former is preferred where a greater peripheric action is desired. Vascular erethism is diminished, especially in the mucous membranes of the air-passages. Alvine action is, however, not promoted, but rather retarded.

The *Kränchen*, from its greater quantity of carbonic acid, has a more stimulating, solvent, and tonic power on the intestinal canal, energetically ameliorating the uterine and uropoietic functions. It is therefore more enployed in abdominal sluggishness. The thermal springs of the Steinerne Haus are used as a transition between the two. The water is frequently employed with great advantage in the form of douche in neuralgic, rheumatic, and arthritic complaints; also as clysters and injections in hæmorrhoidal spasms, menstrual anomalies, fluor albus, &c. In cases of great pulmonary irritation the Kesselbrunnen is administered with asses' or goats' milk. Persons subject to nervous erethism often find great benefit from undergoing a short course of eight or fifteen baths at Schlangenbad after having finished the cure at Ems. A few cases will best illustrate the action of Ems. Miss P., twenty-six years of age, of a slender and delicate build, had lost her mother, a brother, and one sister by tubercular consumption. She was well up to her twenty-first year; from that time the catamenial flux began to diminish in quantity, and to be accompanied by most violent abdominal spasms. These phenomena gradually deteriorated, so that she was ultimately confined to her bed during that epoch. Dyspnœa and oppression of the right side of the chest became now always associated with this period. These symptoms regularly reappeared every four weeks, till at last *pulmonary hæmorrhage* ensued each time, with violent spasms. Her bodily strength now began to decrease, respiration became less free, and cough with spitting of blood formed the climax at each monthly epoch. This state had lasted from the autumn of 1837 to the spring of 1838, when the patient was first seen by Dr. Franque. Physical examination exhibited weaker respiratory murmur at the upper part of the right lung; there was no dulness on percussion, no suspicious expectoration, nor nightly perspirations, during the intermission; the bowels were rather confined, though the appetite was unimpaired. The conclusion was arrived at that no actual tuberculosis had developed itself, but that a merely congested state of the lungs existed, and would probably be developed to the fatal malady, unless checked in time. Ems was therefore advised. She arrived on the 6th of June, after having undergone one of the above-mentioned attacks. The Kesselbrunnen was ordered, with goats' milk, and lukewarm half-baths every other day. A few days before her expected menstruation, leeches were applied to the inner side of the upper thigh, and for the first time this dreaded epoch passed without spasms or spitting of blood. The course was continued for eight weeks, and the patient left without experiencing any more attacks up to January of the next year, the time when this report was communicated, being altogether greatly improved in health and spirits.

Mr. T., thirty-five years of age, showed a distinct phthisical disposition by his whole build, and also by the husky tone of voice, easily getting hoarse by any exertion. Two of his sisters had died from pulmonary consumption, as also his mother. Travelling and the use of saline baths had succeeded in strengthening his health in some degree, and enabling him to perform his professional duties with cheerfulness and energy; but catarrhs appeared now and then, and became more and more frequent, alternating with toothache or other rheumatic affections. An issue and appropriate internal treatment alleviated these evils, but only for a short time, so that their return in winter and spring could always be anticipated with certainty. At last a violent catarrh was developed with a hollow cough, tickling and burning sensation in the larynx, hoarsenesss, restlessness, strong matinal perspirations, and great nervous excitability. The expectoration was mucous, liquid, free from blood, but sometimes containing small conglomerated greyish lumps. Appropriate treatment induced amelioration, but great exhaustion was left behind, with mental depression and tendency to profuse nocturnal perspirations. Traces of piles, which had showed themselves at the commencement of the next year, left no permanent effect on his state of health.

When he arrived in Ems, in the month of July, his pulse was of moderate frequency, his skin inclined to profuse perspiration, his voice husky; cough and expectoration inconsiderable; digestion normal. The Kesselbrunnen was commenced, and after some time baths were added. Gentle douche to the neck was subsequently employed, as the morbid irritation seemed specially fixed in the larynx. The result was highly satisfactory, and when he left he had merely to complain of a certain general languor, which frequently follows the prolonged use of Ems. The next autumn, winter, and spring passed with undisturbed health. He returned to Ems the following summer, to complete his cure. In this he succeeded, though the course was interrupted by intercurring diarrhœa, with inflammatory symptoms. From the numerous cases recorded, I purposely select those of minor severity for in these Ems may almost be considered as a specific, whilst in instances of more advanced pulmonary disease the chances of relief diminish. Drs. von Franque, Döring, Spengler, Vogler, von Ibell, von Söst, Busch, &c., are amongst the most reputed physicians of the place.*

Let us now proceed to *Schlangenbad*, after having passed through Schwalbach, from which latter place it is only two leagues distant. Wiesbaden lies to the east, at a distance of three leagues—Mainz at four leagues to the south-east. If you take the curvature of the Rhine at Bingen as the corner, and draw an oblique line from Coblentz to Bibrich, you see first Ems, then Schwalbach, and at last Schlangenbad. This will at once indicate to you the route to be taken when coming from London. If your destination be Ems, you disembark at the upper termination of the line, viz. Coblentz. If you wish to visit Wiesbaden, Schlangenbad, or Schwalbach, it is more convenient to retain your places till you have reached the inferior angle, viz. Biberich. From this spot the railroad takes you to Wiesbaden or Frankfort, whilst horse-conveyances bring you through the pleasant Rheingau to Schlangenbad or Schwalbach. Those fond of picturesque scenery, and possessed of sufficient leisure, would certainly do well to travel by land from Coblentz through Ems to the southern spas of Nassau. Schlangenbad lies in a pleasant valley surrounded by woody hills, with many romantic spots. The neighbouring shores of the Rhine are frequently visited: the Niederwald, the height between Wiesbaden and Schwalbach, and other very picturesque mountain and vale-scenery invite the valetudinarian.

There are several springs, of a temperature ranging between 77° and 88° Fahrenheit. Their water is clear and perfectly tasteless. The chief use is external. The baths are very capacious and covered by ' Traas,' a substance bearing some resemblance to

* Hôtels—d'Angleterre, des Quatre Saisons, and de Russie, afford excellent accommodation.

asphaltes. Heated water is let in to cover the bottom of the baths before the natural thermal water is introduced, because the cold bottom would otherwise reduce the heat too rapidly. The chief bath, however, is filled by the thermal water alone without admixture, the bottom being heated by steam. The *Schachtbrunnen* is the principal spring, having a temperature of 88° Fahrenheit. The water sparkles little when drawn, but feels very soft, and is often exported as a cosmetic. According to the latest analysis, it contains $8\frac{2}{5}$ grains of solid constituents, viz. :—

       3·36 grains of carbonate of soda.
       1·70   ,,   ,, lime.
       1·19   ,,   ,, magnesia.
       2·15   ,, chloride of sodium.

Only a few cubic inches of carbonic acid or other gaseous contents are present—viz., carbonic acid $1\frac{3}{4}$ cubic inches, and nitrogen $\frac{1}{5}$.

The baths have a peculiarly sedative influence on the nervous and vascular systems, and they are especially reputed for the beautifying power they exercise on the skin, to which they impart a satiny softness. In pure hysteric or hypochondriacal irritability, or spasmodic tendency without structural change, the spa shows itself highly efficacious. Its cosmetic influence is to a great measure to be attributed to the combination of its carbonate of soda with the fatty cutaneous secretion, by which means a sort of very fine soap-water is generated, which rinses out the pores of the skin, whilst the lukewarm water enters the cutaneous absorbent vessels to dissolve and mobilise effete particles, and prepare them for elimination. The small amount of carbonic acid induces a very slight general stimulation, and may be the cause of the thermal ingredients chiefly confining their contact and efficacy to the skin and subcutaneous tissues, without penetrating to the central organs and provoking their reaction. Very irritable individuals have to begin with a somewhat higher temperature. For this purpose there are two taps attached to each bathing-space, the one admitting the unheated and the other the heated thermal water, so as to communicate the required temperature to the whole. The position of the spa is peculiarly favourable for giving tone to the weakened nervous system. Whilst its neighbour, Schwalbach, lies on the north-eastern declivity of the Taunus, Schlangenbad is situated on the south-western declivity (at an altitude of 897 feet), and protected by three considerable mountain-groups from the blasts incidental to valleys. The mild atmosphere of the southern declivity is therefore partially enjoyed with the bracing mountain-air, and acts tonically and soothingly on the depressed or irritated nervous system. The soil is chiefly gravelly, abounding in quartz, and partially clayey; so that after rain-showers the ground soon dries again, and invites the invalid to wanderings in the charming environs and verdant fields and meadows. Dr. Bertrand, the present physician, found the spa extremely beneficial in neuralgiæ of the skin and joints; for it both strengthens the functions and diminishes the morbid irritability of the affected organs. The female sex form the greatest number of patients. Its beneficial influence on the uterus and uterine nerves is especially remarked.

Hufeland says that he knows of no spa so adapted to retard or repress the articular stiffness and exsiccation incidental even to healthy old age, or prematurely induced by 'fast living.' 'I know by experience,' he continues, ' that a regular annual use of the spa imparts to old age cheerfulness, agility of the joints, and prolonged strength. If we consider all its qualities, it is peculiarly fit for a lady's bath; for it beautifies the skin and renders it more juvenile and elastic, whilst it gives greater mobility to the limbs. Besides, the extremely romantic situation and the beautiful climate of those regions must be considered as auxiliaries.'

To illustrate the special indication of the spa, I would direct your attention to the following case mentioned by Dr. Reuter, of Eltville:—Mrs. S. v. B., thirty-seven years of age, married fifteen years, and mother of six children, had previously suffered with hysteria, at one time with profuse catamenia, subsequently with rheumatism, then with nervous headache, and when she arrived at the spa, with *neuralgic pains in the loins*. She was greatly debilitated, especially in the lower extremities; convulsions of the abdominal muscles appeared, and inability of turning from side to side, besides great difficulty of sitting or of walking erect. The complexion was pale, the appetite and sleep diminished; occasionally chilliness seized her, with a creeping sensation of the skin, frequent desire of micturition, and a peculiar feeling of fulness and weight in her vesical region. Before her arrival she had been cupped near the sacrum, and rubbed with aromatico-balsamic liniments. At the spa she took nothing else but thirty baths of $90\frac{1}{2}°$ F.; an aromatic plaster was applied to the abdomen after each bath, to counteract the enteralgiæ, from which she suffered after the disappearance of the lumbar pains. She was discharged completely cured. The utility of Schlangenbad, after a course of Ems, will be the more obvious from the above remarks.

I have to request your company to a spa crowded by the greatest number of visitors, and well worthy of being considered as the world's exhibition of all the varieties of the human race: for scarcely a country of the old continent is there unrepresented, nor a language or dialect. The modern philologist will sometimes be puzzled by the different sounds and words that strike his ear within a short walk. The name of the spa is perhaps already guessed. We were led by the course to defer its consideration, notwithstanding its title of *Queen of the German Spas.*

You know, therefore, that I invite you to return to Frankfort, and to avail yourselves of the expeditious railroad to reach the beautiful and universally-admired spa of *Baden-Baden.* The particulars of the journey I have already described in the fourth lecture, when treating of Wildbad, its easterly neighbour.

The town of *Baden* lies on the River Oos, in one of the most charming valleys of the Black Forest. To distinguish it from spas of the same name it is designated abroad Baden-Baden. The Rhine is two leagues distant to the west, Karlsruhe eight leagues to the north, Strassburg twelve to the west. ' When coming from the village of Os, flourishing vineyards border the road to the left, and dark fir-trees, with mighty rocks, and the picturesque ruins of the old castle; to the right verdant fields and luxuriant meadows charm the eye, hills are covered with oak and beech-trees, and alternate with private mansions, farms, and the tower of the Yberg. In the midst Baden is perceived, with its château and pinnacles, and in the background the blue summits of the distant mountain-heights. Part of the town is built at the foot of the hill, the other portion being situate on the hill itself, overlooked by the château at its summit. High mountains surround the town (the highest is the Mercuriusberg), and protect the charming valley against tempestuous winds. The distant prospects offered from the summit of the castle are really delightful. If the sky be serene, the eye may reach as far as the Vogesen mountains beyond the Rhine valley; to the south the high mountains may be seen which separate the dukedom of Baden from the kingdom of Würtemberg. In the environs the efforts of Art rival the beauties of Nature. The walks and rides that may be undertaken by the valetudinarian for his amusement and recreation are varied and beautiful. With an altitude of 616 feet above the level of the sea, and the mountainous protection, the climate is equally favourable to an abundant vegetation and to the human inhabitant.

The air is pure and mild, and heightens the pleasure to be derived from the variegated and enchanting spots which are so profusely spread over Baden and its environs. It was known to the Romans under the name of 'civitas aquensis.' It is one of the most brilliant and fashionable spas, rivalling the celebrated Wiesbaden in elegance and luxury. Upwards of 20,000 visitors resort there during the season (between the 1st of May and the 1st of October).

The springs are numerous, and supply a great abundance of thermal water.

The chief spring (*Ursprung*) possesses a temperature of 161° F., and issues from a rock consisting of horn-stone and quartz. The *Brühbrunnen* lies a few paces off, near the two *Iudenquellen*.

The *Höllenquelle* enjoys the highest position, and lies behind the Ursprung. The temperature ranges between 161° and 117$\frac{1}{2}$° F. The baths are chiefly supplied from the principal source, whence the water runs down into reservoirs. After being cooled, it is admitted by a tap into the baignoires, which receive from another reservoir uncooled thermal water, till the mixture reaches the appropriate temperature. The water is clear, transparent, of a somewhat saltish taste, inodorous, and little sparkling.

After some time a calcareous deposit, with some iron, becomes precipitated. A soft, unctuous, dark-greenish bath-mud is used for discutient applications. The vapour of the chief source is led into an adjoining building through a vapour-pipe, and employed for natural vapour-baths.

The chemical constituents are nearly the same in the different springs. About 22$\frac{1}{3}$ grains are contained in 16 ounces viz. :—

        17$\frac{1}{2}$ grains of chloride of sodium.
        1$\frac{1}{2}$,,   ,,   potassium.
        $\frac{3}{4}$,,   ,,   magnesium.
        2$\frac{1}{2}$,,   sulphate of lime.
        $\frac{1}{10}$,,   carbonate of iron.
        and less than half a cubic inch of carbonic acid.

The spa belongs thus to the warm saline springs, but analysis and experience class it amongst the weakest. The scantiness of chloride of sodium (nearly 30 grains less than Wiesbaden), and of carbonic acid (four cubic inches less), must prepare you to find it a considerably less efficacious remedy in cases of severe rheumatism or rheumatic paralysis, in which Wiesbaden affords such powerful assistance.

On the other hand, frequent instances will occur of slight rheumatic or arthritic affections—of chronic torpid mucosity of the intestinal canal, general irritability and atony of the nervous system, morbid susceptibility of the vesical mucous membrane, &c., in which you might find the peculiar alterative, digestive, and solvent power of saline springs indicated, but without requiring the more intense action of the powerful spas: in that case Baden will be very appropriately recommended. On account of the great advantages offered by the locality, its climate, and environs are of high importance to those who are not seriously disabled. As Wetzler says, 'The air is so pure, the climate so mild, the landscape so rich in variegated beauties: high mountains with distant charming prospects here, smiling valleys there, ruins of antique châteaux, blooming villages, and luxuriant fields alternating with superb vineyards, sunny plains and hills, and dark shady walks. The region is indeed paradisiacal, and blessed days may be passed here! Hastening away from confined chambers, resting from the troubles and toils of life, you may gather there renewed forces in the enjoyment of purer air and purer nature. Let him resort to Baden who has entered the retrogressive period of life; an annual sojourn of a few weeks in this terrestrial paradise may help to prolong his days. Let the citizens wander here who wish to enjoy the charms of rural life, and to contemplate Nature in its finest attire. But let them participate in the pleasures of the luxurious table with moderation. They may also bathe with profit—for strengthening, refreshing, and purifying the skin. But whoever suffers from *very serious* ailment, and expects to be chiefly cured by the agency of the mineral water, must not be sent to Baden.' To sum up, if the patient is too unwell to profit by the numerous resources of climate and locality, his case is not adapted to Baden. There are now very well-contrived *Russian vapour-baths* at the Goldene Hirsch, which assist materially in the cure of rheumatic diseases, but of course the relief has then to be effected *in* but not *by* the spa. Hofrath Dr. Gugert records an instance of scrofulous ulcers of the ankle occurring in a child of five years of age, which were cured by the thermal vapours of the chief spring, after the ineffectual employment of anti-scrofulous remedies and spas. He enumerates some other cases of scrofulous eruptions, of gout, and of pulmonary and laryngeal catarrhal irritation, as cured or relieved by the thermal vapours. In and near the town (Lichtenthal) chalybeate springs originate, and are effectually employed after a course of Baden. They contain 2 grains of solid ingredients in 16 ounces— viz., $1\frac{1}{2}$ of carbonate of iron, $\frac{1}{10}$ of carbonate of soda, $\frac{1}{10}$ of carbonate of lime, $\frac{1}{4}$ of chloride of magnesium, but *no carbonic acid*; hence you may beware of confounding them with chalybeates containing less iron, but accompanied by the indispensable volatile gas. Though the chief employment of Baden be external, the water is also frequently ordered internally—pure or with whey. To render it more efficacious in torpid venous obstruction of the abdominal vessels, an imitation of Karlsbad water is artificially prepared, by adding, according to *Kölreuter's* prescription, sulphate and carbonate of soda, so that about 50 grains of solid constituents impregnate a pint of the water. The physicians seem all greatly occupied during the season (Drs. Rüff, Müller, Gaus, Schrauder, Wilhelmi, Berton, Füsslin, Brumm, Schmidt, Brandis, Jörger, Berg, Heiligenthal), though a very numerous portion of the visitors seek only recreation amid the charms of the surrounding scenery.

LECTURE XVIII.

OEYNHAUSEN—NAUHEIM.

To-day I shall bring to your notice the two most recently discovered German spas, viz. *Oeynhausen* and *Nauheim*.

Oeynhausen (long. east 9°—lat. north 52°), the youngest member of the family of spas, may be reached from Cologne in eight, and from London in about twenty-four hours. It is within sight of the Rehme Station,* near the junction of the Werre and the Weser. It owes its origin to the salt-works, to which it is contiguous (*Neusalzwerk*); and though the last discovered (since 1845), it already enjoys a high reputation in the cure of diseases in which the saline springs are indicated.

It is situated between Minden and Herford, at an equal distance of ten miles. To obtain a fresh supply of salt, a hole was bored (now 2,220 feet deep), when, unexpectedly, a warm salt-spring flowed out in great abundance, giving rise to the spa under consideration.

The borehole and its adjoining baths are situated to the southwest of the salt-works, in a fertile valley, extending beyond the Werre and joining the valley of the Weser. It is bounded on the north by the Weser Mountains (900 feet high) which can be seen for several miles, and which the River Weser intersects in the *Porta Westphalica*, near Hausberg (five miles from Neusalzwerk).

The steep Margaret and Jacob Mountains (constituting the Porta Westphalica) are invested with a pleasant appearance by groves of beech, and the tower built upon the former mountain affords a charming panorama of the environs. The Demberg and Kappenberg constitute, respectively, the southern and eastern frontiers. Behind these rise the Steinegge, Ebenöde, &c., enclosing Vlotho in a deep valley. From the highest point (the Bonstapel), the town of Minden can be discerned in a due northerly direction through the Porta Westphalica. The spa is thus protected by the surrounding mountains from violent extremes of temperature, without being exposed to the foggy exhalations of

* The last station before Minden.

the Werre and Weser, these rivers lying below its level. A mild and healthy climate prevails, though sometimes subject to sudden changes. The mean temperature of the soil is 50° Fahrenheit. The mountain-masses of the environs belong to that class formed of horizontal layers. The lowest stratum is composed of shell-lime. Above this appear the white and red sandstones, then variegated layers of marl (mostly red); a peculiar layer of white calcareous marl then follows, frequently employed for manuring the fields, and containing numerous crystals of sulphur-pyrites. Towards Neusalzwerk it is covered by black slate and pebble-stones, which former may be considered as the transition into the lyas-formation that occupies the south. We moreover find tertiary marl in the Demberg, with remains of testaceous animals, and a considerable stratum of tufaceous lime between Valdorf and Vlotho. The borehole lies 217 feet higher than Amsterdam, and thus extends to 1,994 feet below the level of the sea—probably the greatest depth ever reached. The salt-water was first perceived at a depth of 574 feet, containing $1\frac{5}{8}$ per cent. of salt, and supplying $\frac{2}{3}$ of a cubic foot of water per minute; thence the quantity of water, the temperature (about one degree Reaumur for 120 feet of depth), and proportion of salt gradually increased. At 600 feet the temperature was $12\frac{1}{2}$° R.; at 1,004 feet, 15° R.; at 1,100 feet, 18° R.; at 1,586 feet, $19\frac{1}{2}$° R.; at 1,595 feet, 20° R.; at 1,951 feet, 25° R.; and at 2,219 feet, $26\frac{1}{2}$° R. = 92° Fahrenheit. From $1\frac{5}{8}$ per cent. the proportion of salt increased to $4\frac{1}{2}$, and the flow of water from two-thirds of a cubic foot gradually augmented to fifty-four cubic feet per minute.

The upper part of the hole is now enlarged to a width of nine inches (as far as 1,600 feet). Analysis of the water compared with that of the Mediterranean (by Professor Bischoff of Bonn), shows in 10,000 parts:—

	Oeynhausen salt-water.	Water of Mediterranean.
Chloride of sodium	333·850	251
„ magnesium	10·783	52·5
Sulphate of potash	0·47	—
„ lime	29·947	1·5
„ magnesia	26·038	62·5
Carbonate of lime	8·686 ⎱	1·5
„ magnesia	5·021 ⎰	
„ iron	0·668	—
„ manganese	0·014	—
Silicic acid	0·466	—
Bromine	quantity undetermined	
Total	415·944	369

In 16 ounces, the thermal brine of Oeynhausen contains 319 grains of solid ingredients, viz:—

$256\frac{1}{2}$ gr.	chloride of sodium.	$3\frac{3}{4}$ gr.	carbonate of magnesia.
$8\frac{1}{4}$,,	magnesium.	$\frac{1}{2}$,,	iron.
$\frac{1}{3}$,,	sulphate of potash.	$\frac{1}{100}$,,	magnesia.
$22\frac{8}{10}$,,	lime.	$\frac{1}{3}$ Silicic acid.	
$19\frac{9}{10}$,,	magnesia.	Specific gravity, 1·017.	
$6\frac{1}{2}$	carbonate of lime.		

No trace of iodine has been found, but a considerable amount of bromine, though its precise quantity has not yet been determined. In the chemical manufactory near Neusalzwerk, the bromine is procured from the mother-lye of the salt-water. According to the above analysis the ' Soole ' (salt-spring) may be considered as sea-water modified by the addition of bicarbonates and carbonic acid, besides a higher natural temperature. The water remains clear and transparent, as long as it is conducted in pipes; but exposed for some time to the atmosphere, it gradually loses its carbonic acid and becomes turbid, depositing oxide of iron and carbonate of lime. Three cubic feet of free carbonic acid and other gases (the latter at the rate of six per cent.) escape per minute from the borehole. The absorbed carbonic acid amounts to $\frac{1}{10}$ of the volume of brine, so that forty-three cubic feet of the acid are obtained per minute with the water. Only at the depth of two feet the carbonic acid begins to be evolved—at a greater depth it is completely absorbed. The proportion of the free to the combined acid is as one to fifteen. A weak bitter spring near the ' Soole' is frequently used for drinking. It contains in 1,000 parts $19\frac{1}{2}$ of solid ingredients—($7\frac{1}{2}$ sulphate of soda, $2\frac{1}{2}$ sulphate of magnesia, $3\frac{1}{2}$ chloride of sodium, 2 chloride of magnesium, 1 chloride of calcium, 3 bicarbonate of lime, $\frac{1}{2}$ bicarbonate of magnesia).

At present there are sixty-seven baths of different classes, the baignoires of which are fifteen feet below the level of the borehole. The water rises in the bathing-house in a perpendicular shaft to the height of twelve feet, and fills the basins under the pressure of its column from below. At the sides of the baignoires the filling pipes are so contrived that a wave-like motion can be communicated to the bath, so that the stream can be made to enter in one spout, or in numerous fascicular spouts. The carbonic acid can be evolved near the bottom or at the surface of the bath, with quite a different effect on the bather. The mouthpiece of the filling-tap is provided with screw-windings, to which a copper tube may be attached, reaching nearly to the bottom of the basin, or a bent tube with a leather pipe, or a sieve-like head-piece, according to the intended use. A great importance is attached by the physicians to the kind of bath employed, for one baignoire may exhibit four or five baths of perfectly different physical effects, and these modifications are made use of in the treatment of the respective diseases. For a *quiet bath*, the side-tap must be closed; the water flows in imperceptibly from the bottom, with a comparatively diminished evolution of carbonic-acid gas, and flows out again as soon as it reaches a certain height, at the other end of the bath. The effect is again different, if the filling-tube be merely held and not screwed to the tap. Atmospheric air entering the water with carbonic acid, the latter rises, continually hissing and foaming; by an ascending tube, wave-like motions are formed on the surface. If the leather pipe or short bent tube be fixed to the side-tap, the stream and evolution of carbonic acid can be directed to any layer of the water or to any part of the body (as douche). If the water is allowed to fall from the tap into the basin, a lively wave-like motion is communicated to the whole mass, with constant development of foam and hissing, and the most complete disengagement of carbonic acid.

Though the energy of the sentient nerves is greatly heightened, and the general metamorphosis and muscular tone stimulated, still no injurious effects are perceived from the carbonic acid, unless some contra-indicating circumstances forbid the use of this form of bath. An extremely pleasurable sensation is created by the water constantly moving to and fro with white foam and hissing. But the titillation produced by the sieve-like douche is certainly the most agreeable sensation that can be imagined, and must inevitably be of great therapeutic value in many diseases of the nervous and sero-fibrous system. A different result is also expected from applying the douche under the water, when the force is diminished, or beyond the level of the bath. The douches are generally followed by the use of rubbing-brushes.

The 'Soole' is further made use of for a natural 'vapour-bath.' In consequence of the fall of thirteen feet, to which it is subjected at this distance (thirty-six roods from the borehole), it rises in a shaft to the height of twelve feet, and constantly splashes over, filling the chamber with exhalations of saline ingredients and carbonic acid: the latter tending to move towards the bottom from its gravity, whilst the former remain suspended in the upper strata of the room, exercising their grateful influence on the respiratory organs. The chest seems inclined to expand more freely, with a certain feeling of ease, and to inhale a greater quantum of air. Though the temperature of the room be from 81° to 86° F. (or lowered to 70¼° F. by opening the window-valves, at the ceiling, if required), no oppression or inconvenience is felt: in fact, I could only *perceive* the increased temperature by the contrast when coming into the air. For drinking, imported or factitious mineral waters are used to assist the external treatment—also the ' bitter-brunnen ' mentioned above is occasionally employed.

The *weaker* 'Bulow-brunnen' (containing in 16 ounces 180 grains of chloride of sodium, 16 grains of sulphate of soda, 7 grains of carbonate of soda, 4¾ grains of carbonate of magnesia, 6¼ grains of carbonate of lime) is separated from the stronger ' Soole' for occasional use. The air of the neighbouring salt-works is also made use of for sanitary purposes. The strong ' Soole' of the 'Bulow-brunnen' is dispersed over the thorny walls of the graduation-works. The different layers are composed of various precipitates from the dripping saline mass. This ' Soole' contains, in 16 ounces, 825 grains of solid constituents— viz., 754 grains of chloride of sodium, 22 grains of chloride of magnesium, 25 grains of sulphuret of calcium, 19 grains of sulphate of soda, $\frac{9}{10}$ of a grain of carbonate of iron, 1 grain of carbonate of lime, and $\frac{9}{10}$ of a grain of resin and extractive substance. In *catarrhal affections* of the air-passages, in *emphysema* of the lungs, &c., deeper and more calming inspirations are produced, to the great relief of the patient. The tone of the respiratory muscles seems to be increased, and the irritation diminished. The salt obtained at the chemical manufactory, from the mother-lye of the salt-works, contains, in 16 ounces, 261 grains of chloride of sodium, 4,874 of chloride of magnesium, 630 grains of sulphate of soda, 172 grains of sulphate of magnesia, 19 grains of bromide of potassium and magnesium, and 1,531 grains of hygroscopic water. This motherlye is applied externally with great advantage in glandular enlargements.

As regards the effects of the baths: the pressure of the water exercises a mechanical stimulus on the tissues and vascular net of the skin, and promotes the power of imbibition, whilst its motion peculiarly stimulates the nervous system. The greater mobility of the water, the more carbonic acid is evolved. Neither heating nor cooling being required, any loss of constituents is obviated. Chemically considered, the ' Soole ' is distinguished by its abundance of carbonic acid and of carbonates. In 13½ cubic feet of water (the quantum of one bath), 37 pounds of solid ingredients and 10 cubic feet of carbonic acid exercise their influence on the bather. The constant renewal of course considerably increases this quantity. The ingredients may either produce direct changes in the various tissues of the body, by affording restorative stimuli, or enter into immediate combination with the diseased substances, or may promote absorption and resolution of exudated matters, or excite certain secretory and excretory organs to an increased function. The layer of carbonic acid on the surface of the bath, mixed with atmospheric air, and the exhalation of the saline ingredients, seem to exercise a calming influence on the air-passages. The tone and mobility of the muscles and muscular organs is invariably heightened. The muscular tissues become denser, morbid perspirations diminish, the *skin loses the great sensitiveness towards changes of temperature*, and the nervous centres regain in many instances their lost energy. It is maintained that the mental and physical functions, depending on the integrity of the central nervous system, are restored to their normal condition, if no organic derangement forbids the use of the spa. There is one peculiar evil for which Dr. Von Möller considers this spring as an unfailing specific---viz., the *too rapid growth* and incomplete development of young persons *with hereditary phthisical disposition*, and already beginning signs of the impending calamity. Oeynhausen restores the equilibrium by causing the muscular system to be more invigorated and developed, and the thoracic organs to be strengthened by the influence of the saline exhalations. If employed to excess, or under contra-indicating circumstances, lassitude, depression, headache, giddiness, want of appetite, restlessness, &c. will be the consequence of bathing. On the other hand, the cures on record did not invariably ensue after using some baths, nor even after completing the course, but in many instances some weeks or months after the patients had quitted the place, and perhaps under feeling of disappointment. It is even considered as a more favourable sign if the disease remains apparently stationary during part of the course, or if momentary aggravation of certain symptoms mark the influence of the spring on the affected parts. Bath-eruptions are rare. I omit the directions for the various modifications in which the soole-baths and vapour-chambers are to be used, for these must be determined by the difference of the diseases and other circumstances. The duration of the bath is from five minutes to half an hour. After a few weeks an interruption of some days is recommended. Baths of long duration are more easily borne by children than by adults.

Signs of saturation, lassitude, anorexia, depression, pains in different parts of the body, chilliness alternating with heat, oppression of the chest, &c. require an immediate discontinuance of the bath.

The following cases, furnished by Dr. Von Möller, will illustrate the peculiar efficacy of Oeynhausen :—

A gentleman 52 years of age, exposed to many bodily exertions and changes of temperature, probably also indulging in spirituous liquors, suffered for some time with intestinal catarrh, vomiting of water in the morning, obstruction, *paralysis of both arms and legs*, and general trembling (particularly in the neck, hands, and knees), violent throbbing pains in the forehead and occiput, and absolute insomnia. Twenty short baths, with interruptions, and internally Selters-water with Carlsbad-salt, freed him from the above-mentioned severe complication of morbid symptoms.

A girl of fifteen years is mentioned, resembling in physical appearance a child of twelve, emaciated and pale, of feeble muscles, with a flat narrow thorax, and disposition to febrile symptoms, hæmoptysis, palpitation of the heart, and other signs indicating *incipient tuberculosis*. She took short 'quiet baths,' with intermissions; was exposed to the exhalations of the vapour-chamber, and to the air of the graduation-works; internally, simple whey at first, and afterwards with an addition of Franzensbrunnen water. After six weeks, the respiratory organs and general nutrition of the muscles assumed a very improved character, and a year after the course, the body was normally developed, with a tendency to corpulence.

A merchant, thirty-six years of age (married), through early excesses affected with impotency and frequent seminal discharges at the slightest sexual excitement, dull pains in the occiput, emaciation, general debility, coldness of the hands and feet, violent pains in the lumbar regions at night, with chilliness and subsequent profuse perspiration, deep depression, loss of memory, restlessness, inability to follow a connected train of thought, or to write letters requiring mental exertion, &c. He used quiet baths for four weeks, and drank Franzensbrunnen water. The muscular system gained gradually in strength, the pains of the head and loins with the accompanying symptoms diminished, the genital system lost its abnormal erethism, and the mental faculties became restored.

Swellings of the spongious ends of bones, with distention of the synovial sac, and muscular atrophy, have been removed by long baths with flowing water, whilst internally Marienbad Kreutzbrunnen, and afterwards Homburg Elisenquelle were taken. Chronic inflammation of the knee-joint, with contraction and stiffness, and even carious exfoliation, are said to have been cured or relieved by this spa. Cases of rachitis scrofulosa, osteomalcia, &c. are also reported, in which the baths afforded great relief, particularly with children.

Mr. Papst, of Petershagen, reports several cases of hypertrophy of the womb, hydrops ovarii, &c., which he brought to a successful termination by the spa of Oeynhausen, in connection with other remedies—viz., in robust persons, with swellings and pain of the womb, he applies eight leeches twice a-week; afterwards a bath is ordered; then a ball composed of equal parts of grey mercurial ointment, lard, and yellow wax, is introduced into the vagina, so as to touch the cervix and os uteri. This is renewed after twenty-four hours. Afterwards he substituted iodine ointment for the mercurial. Internally he employed, according to circumstances, either tonics, solvents, or iodine. In Oeynhausen he ordered baths from a quarter of an hour, to be gradually prolonged to an hour. Then an injection of the soole, four times a-day, besides some tumblers of it morning and evening internally, with proper diet and exercise. He details several instances of severe *subacute inflammation* and *swellings* of the *uterus* and *ovaries*, which were cured or relieved in the above manner. The *vapour-chamber*, which may be considered a remedy of itself, requires a few words of further notice. The constant precipitation and renewal of warm saline exhalations with carbonic acid, exercises such a soothing influence on the pulmonary mucous membrane, that whenever increased respiratory movement, or entrance of fresh air, produces cough, pain, or oppression, these distressing symptoms will be unperceived or diminished in this chamber. Whether the good effect be due to the increased tone of the capillary vessels, or to the sedative power of the vapour, or to the absorption of the dissolved particles into the circulating fluids, must remain undecided for the present.

Patients with hoarseness, tickling in the throat, impeded deglutition, with irritation and cough, chronic inflammation of the follicles of the mucous membrane of the larynx, and tendency to ulceration and incipient laryngeal phthisis, are said to have been cured by the sole use of this natural vapour. The voice and thoracic muscles are exercised in the chamber. Whey-cures are often combined with the vapour-course, and equestrian exercise recommended. The catarrhal affections resulting from *whooping-cough* are particularly asserted to be often cured by this remedy. A case of *tubercular phthisis* is reported of a girl of thirteen years of age—parents of arthritic diathesis. The child was brought up in the country, and appeared well fed, but had suffered with bronchial catarrh since her childhood—also *enuresis nocturna* to the end of her twelfth year. In the autumn of 1848, after an attack of scarlatina, circumscribed pneumonia and pleuritic affection were superadded to the bronchial catarrh, besides emaciation and diarrhœa; the thorax ceased to expand to its normal extent, consonant and cavernous rhonchi were discovered by auscultation, and corresponding dulness and tympanitic sound by percussion. Considerable dyspnœa and debility were exhibited on any attempt at exercise; voice hoarse, cough violent and continuous; expectoration tough, purulent, granular, and often mixed with blood; fever, with evening exacerbations and profuse perspirations. This was her state after eight months of suffering. She used the vapour-bath twice a day from one to two hours, with interruptions; and as soon as her muscular strength was sufficiently improved, she spent the greater part of the day near the graduation-works. Complete recovery ensued. The right subclavicular region, depressed to a considerable extent, only raises itself towards the end of a very deep inspiration. Physical examination showed, after a year, partial condensation of the pulmonary substance, containing vesicular tissue, but no subjective signs of disease.

The chemical analogy which the ' Soole ' bears to sea-water (with, however, more common salt and sulphate of potash, and less magnesia) must prepare us to find *improved nutrition* amongst its chief effects. From the circumference the stimulus to increased energy must be transmitted to the nervous ganglia, inducing resolution and absorption of abnormal productions, and a freer action of the lymphatic system.

Different forms of *scrofula* claim, therefore, the first place in the category of diseases to be subjected to its influence. In our experience of *sea-baths*, we find that they restore the tone of the muscular system, increase the contractile power of the blood-vessels, and ameliorate the functions of the glandular organs, indirectly raising the strength of the cerebral and spinal nervous system.

But in many instances, when their useful application is impracticable, from the violent reaction they produce in the nervous system, this spa might form an excellent substitute, particularly with very sensitive, anæmic, and debilitated individuals, who require for their cure both stimulating and integrant curative agents. Hence the great utility of Oeynhausen in many forms of gout, rheumatism, and arthritic paralysis, *with muscular atrophy.*

The advantages of the vapour-chamber in irritation of the thoracic mucous membrane and of the subcutaneous follicular tissue, are obvious; and though some enthusiastic appreciation of the spa may be imagined on the part of some of the resident physicians, still its physical and chemical properties fully justify us in believing that it possesses a considerable curative power in combating many chronic diseases, otherwise intractable.

Physicians (besides Dr. von Möller), Drs. Alfter, Lehmann, Clostermeyer, Rinteln, and Braun.

AMOUNT OF SOLID INGREDIENTS IN SIXTEEN OUNCES OF SEA-WATER.

	Chloride of Sodium	Chloride of Magnesium	Sulphate of Magnesia	Sulphate of Lime	Sulphate of Potash	Bromide of Magnesium
The *Atlantic* in four places:						
Minimum	203·6	1·3	4·5	12	11·5	2·25
Maximum	215	29	8·2	15·7	13·9	3·6
Near Havre	198	21·9	—	9·3	0 72	0·95
The *North Sea*: 51° 9′ N. Lat. 3° 8′ E. Long. (from Farro)	195·8	34·2	5·4	12·4	11·7	2·56
At Ostend	179	41·5	35	6	Traces	11·05(?)
Scheveningen	196	30·7	9·5	4	2·7	—
Heligoland	165	26·3	21·5	8·5	9	—
Föhr	193	21	16·5	3·8	3·6	—
Norderney	174	66·17	—	1·27	—	—
The Baltic:						
At Travemünde	70·51	22·8	—	5·4	—	—
Doberan	87·67	37	0·7	4	—	—
Kiel	92	30	6	3·5	—	—
Puttbus	72·72	23·5	0·56	3·22	—	—
The *Mediterranean and Adriatic*	209	47	50	—	—	—
At Venice	171	24	19	4·6	7·5	—
Livorno	262	37·4	22	8·9	13	—
Nizza	240	24	34	30	—	—
Marseilles	288·4	80	63	6·2	6*	4†

Traces of Iodine are often found in sea-water; the quantity of Bromine is variable.
* Carbonate of Lime.   † Carbonate of Magnesia.

The great analogy of the Oeynhausen brine to sea-water induces me to make a few remarks on sea-bathing. The saline contents of *sea-water* are due to many external influences, modified by light, temperature, winds, influx of sweet water, &c. You perceive that the inland seas (as the Baltic) with a temperature sometimes approaching the freezing-point, and with the influx of so many streams of sweet water, must have a less powerful effect than the large oceans. The Mediterranean, being most exposed to evaporation through its high temperature, contains the greatest amount of salts. But in selecting a sea-bath we have also to pay attention to the climate. The Baltic and North Sea ought only to be resorted to for bathing late in summer or autumn. The Baltic especially extends so far to the north as to be partly covered with ice in winter, to melt which a great amount of summer-warmth is expended. The colder water sinking downwards is impeded in its flow towards warmer regions, and thus keeps the south coasts cool till every vestige of ice has disappeared; then the heat of the sun is enabled to warm the water fully. Consequently the air must assume and maintain a high temperature for a considerable time before the sea becomes thoroughly warm. In the Mediterranean, on the contrary, bathing may be resorted to in the hottest season, the cooling influence being especially marked in summer—probably because, the sky being serene and the sun powerful, evaporation is most energetically carried on. The Italians bathe, therefore, from the middle of June to the end of August.

The following Table shows the respective temperatures of the various European seas:—

	Annual Temperature	Summer Temperature	Winter Temperature
Mediterranean	59° to 68° F.	72½° to 80° F.	59° to 66° F.
Bay of Biscay	59 ,, ,,	73¼ ,, ,,	44 ,, ,,
Adriatic	54½ ,, 59 ,,	72¾ ,, 80 ,,	44 ,, ,,
Atlantic (from Bay of Biscay to the Channel)	50 ,, 59 ,,	68 ,, 73½ ,,	35 ,, 44 ,,
North Sea (from the Channel to Bergen)	41 ,, 50 ,,	61 ,, 68 ,,	25 ,, 35 ,,
Baltic	41 ,, 47 ,,	60 ,, 64 ,,	26 ,, 33 ,,

Warm sea-baths are very useful in obstinate gastric catarrhs, especially in the case of scrofulous children or weakened old persons. Metamorphosis and bodily warmth standing in direct relation, where the former is impaired, through the deranged digestion and deficient assimilation, the latter must suffer likewise. Hence such patients frequently feel too chilly to bear cold sea-baths; they ought to seek the coast of the Mediterranean or Adriatic for sea-bathing (as Nizza, Spezzia, Venice, &c.) A transition might be made after some time from warm sea-baths to bathing in the sea itself.

Sea-voyages are very beneficial to persons of impaired digestive organs; sometimes *sea-air* alone, inhaled on the coast, is of more importance than the bathing. Though the metamorphosis is greatly heightened, excretions of uric and phosphoric acids are diminished according to Prof. Beneke's researches (showing a diminished waste of the body), whilst new organic formations increase. Valetudinarians ought to avoid *fatiguing* bodily exercise : a certain quiet, alternating with gentle muscular exertions, assist most in ensuring a happy result. If sea-air alone can produce a cure, your patients will not require foreign ingredients to be incorporated into their economy. Some of these might not be well borne by the weakened digestive organs, others might directly counteract reparative assimilation (as the alkalies). The temperature of the heated sea-baths ought to be gradually lowered from 88° Fahr. to 72° Fahr. The duration from five to ten minutes, gradually increased up to twenty or thirty, but with careful watching of the patient's condition.

If catarrhal affections of the intestinal mucous membrane be present, the want of food (through frequent exercise) often exceeds the power of digestion. Hence the intestinal canal must neither be overloaded nor supplied with indigestible food— as fat pastry, sea-fish, salted meat, &c. Delicate patients should only bathe every other day, and rely on the bracing air for effecting a cure, with more bodily rest than exercise.

Sea-air is, however, altogether injurious in cases characterised by *irritation* and hyperæmia of the gastric mucous membrane. A pure bracing highly-situated locality is preferable in such instances—as *Kreuth, Achselmannstein, Interlaken, Gais*. Milk or whey-cure to be employed at the same time. Those who are great admirers of the beauties of nature might resort to the *Kalte Bad* on the *Rigi*, or to *Weissenstein* in the Canton of Solothurn, 3,950 feet high, where a very frequented whey establishment exists, with a large elegant hotel and ' Curhaus' (the pension only costing four francs daily), easily reached from Berne or

Basle. The neighbourhood abounds with forests and gardens for promenading.

Females whose nutrition has been impaired by a long-continued fluor albus may employ sea-baths with advantage, but they must not commence as soon as they arrive. They ought first to acquire a certain amount of strength by the invigorating sea-air. Then they should commence with warm sea-baths, and gradually, as they feel their health improved, resort to cold sea-bathing: but only stay a few minutes at first, and omit the bath every fifth or sixth day.

Local vaginal douches are often employed with advantage besides the baths. In Ostend *Marjolin's* douche-apparatus is used. In many uterine diseases, patients would be injured by constant repose, the blood being made to accumulate still more in the pelvic organs and especially in the womb, whilst gentle walks on the seacoast improve nutrition and general innervation. But the strand ought to be as much as possible separated from the land—in fact, an island-climate is the most useful for a course. The diet ought to be substantial but light. For breakfast tea or coffee ought to be preferred to cocoa or milk, as the latter impart too little stimulus to the nervous system, however excellent they may prove in other cases. The skin must be guarded both against excessive and diminished action. Hence warmer dresses must be worn mornings and evenings than in the middle of the day.

Sea-baths have in some instances been useful in *epilepsy*, when the disease had only been of one or two years duration. The evil is said to have been mitigated and even cured by their agency. They are especially recommended if the fits arose from a fright or after a cold, or before puberty. But great care is requisite as regards diet and the mode of bathing. The patient has to bathe at once in the open sea, without preparatory lukewarm baths. He is to remain only one or two minutes at first in the water, gradually extending the time to five or six minutes. He should dip his head under several times. Advantage is derived not only from the shock of the cold liquid on entering, but also *from the breaking of the waves*, as a powerful stimulant of the cutaneous nervous system. A sensation of a pleasant glow over the surface after bathing, shows a healthy reaction of the whole economy. But a feeling of chilliness proves the excitement to have been carried too far. In this case the patient should drink directly some warm broth or tea, and make short but not too fatiguing walks. Spirituous and stimulating liquors ought to be avoided. Meals ought to be very regular—dinner midday, and supper early in the evening. A second bath in the same day ought never to be taken when the digestion is slow, and obstruction frequent. From forty to eighty baths are necessary to obtain a satisfactory result.

In general scrofulous cachexia, a residence on the seacoast is recommended, with warm baths at first, and open sea-bathing subsequently. Nothing improves general metamorphosis more energetically than *sea-air*. The more powerful reflex of light on the sea-shore, the freedom of bodily movements, the absence of the depressing vitiated air of crowded towns, the vast expanse of the heaving and foaming mass open to our view, all contribute to stimulate the assimilative functions of our system.

Children from two to three years old are to use warm sea-baths, (81° to 83° Fahr.), or ablutions with cold sea-water. Cold sea-bathing mostly disagrees in this tender age. Children from three to eight years of age should use cool tub-baths, with subsequent exercise in open air.

After eight years of age bathing in the sea itself may be resorted to, unless the patient have a strong aversion to the sea, which must not be combated by threats or force.

Digestion ought invariably to be finished when the bath is taken. The children ought to go to bed at sunset, and rise early after eight or ten hours' rest. In daytime sleep ought to be avoided. Excursions *on the sea* are generally to be abstained from, as the undulatory movements of the waves sometimes causes anxiety, vomiting, and even convulsions.

Notwithstanding all precautions, sea-bathing sometimes occasions general uneasiness, oppression, or persistent chilliness. Bitter or ætherial remedies, wine and other stimulants, are then indicated. Congestion to the head or chest also occasionally ensues when the ordinary treatment for such affections has to be resorted to.

Sea-bathing ought to be avoided, and saline or iodurated spas to be employed, when swellings of the cervical glands exist; inflammation or abscess of the meibomian glands, exudations in the subcutaneous cellular tissue, or chronic inflammations of mucous membranes, ophthalmia with formation of phylyctænae, otorrhœa, or chronic cutaneous eruptions.

Delicate patients would sometimes be benefited by rubbing the chest and epigastrium with a piece of flannel dipped in Eau de Cologne before entering the sea The sense of oppression felt at first would thereby be diminished, and also the subsequent necessary reaction promoted.

The hair ought not to be enclosed in water-tight caps, which prevent transpiration, and often induce neuralgia or ophthalmia. Nets with wide meshes are to be used in preference. The drying of the hair after the bath is particularly important, as many neuralgic affections are apt to result from neglect in this respect. The hair should be dried with an unwarmed towel, then thinly covered and exposed to the air, and not dressed nor touched with pomatum or hair-oil before complete dryness; otherwise it might glue together, and exhale unpleasant odours.

In general, cold baths always occasion a determination of blood from the capillary vessels of the skin to the internal vessels of the body; but a slight reaction, or glow, soon appears, in proportion to the preceding retrocession from the surface.

When we plunge into the ocean, the sensations on the surface are so overpowering, from the rapid abstraction of heat, that we become almost breathless for a few moments. The heart beats rapidly; the pulse becomes small; the muscles tremulous; the surface shrinking, cold, and pale. With a tolerably vigorous constitution, we soon get reconciled to the frigid element; reaction commences after a few moments; the heart and large vessels drive the blood back to the capillaries of the skin, distending them inordinately, and producing a general glow of the surface, flushing of the face, and increased insensible perspiration. The internal organs become more relieved of the circulating liquids than before, and hence impart a feeling of elasticity, animation, strength, and cheerfulness. The secreting organs participate in the more vigorous central activity. The intestinal mucous membrane, with its innumerable glands—the liver, spleen, portal vein, and absorbents—all are enabled to act with greater energy. Effete materials are more readily eliminated from the system, and replaced by newly-formed healthy particles. The tissues become less clogged with tarrying blood, and with particles of low vitality. The whole resisting power of the economy is heightened. Thus we have in sea-bathing one of the most potent preventives of disease.

But you see all the benefit due, *not* to the act of immersion, but to the succeeding *reaction*. This at once explains why numerous individuals injure themselves by sea baths. They look upon sea-bathing *itself* as the most salubrious proceeding, and think the benefit will be greatest in proportion to the longest contact with the bracing sea waves. I have seen young ladies affected with inflammation and abscesses of the auditory passage several weeks after having left the coast. On enquiry, I learnt they had found it extremely pleasant to float fifteen to twenty minutes on their backs, without any momentary inconvenience or injury. Many others date their failing health from sea-bathing, 'which had disagreed with them.' On closer examination, it was never difficult to ascertain that the injury did not arise from the innocent ocean, but from the *mode* of enjoying its advantages. Of course, if any internal organ be previously over-distended with the plastic fluid, the sudden afflux of blood might aggravate the morbid condition, and the recoil towards the surface might not be sufficiently strong to produce the former equilibrium. In such cases, sea-bathing must be avoided altogether, as injury might arise *before* the beneficent reaction can set in. Also, persons with a leuco-phlegmatic temperament, languid circulation, and a chilly, clammy state of surface, sometimes get chilled by merely walking from the cabinet into the sea, and fail to obtain the subsequent salutary reaction. Fever is then a not unusual result. How, then, should you advise your patients to avail themselves of this most pleasant and universal pastime, without any subsequent injury? Simply by enjoining them to dip in, *and emerge again immediately* at first, and only prolong the stay *by degrees*, always keeping in mind that the *measure of reaction* experienced after the first immersions must be kept up. If the glow of the surface be diminished after the bath, the stay was too long, and the benefit derivable will be less; if chill appears in or after the bath, no advantage, but decided injury, will accrue.

If we plunge into a hot bath, say of 100° F., the sensations are generally very pleasant; the whole cutaneous surface expands, wrinkles vanish, all the capillaries become distended, the face flushes, the temples and the heart throb, the secretions are augmented. After leaving the bath, the blood gradually and slowly recoils to the interior, if the constitution be healthy; but if there is any change of structure, or congestion, or inflammation, the inward current will appear too quickly after the bath, and produce injurious consequences. Hence, bathing in general should only be resorted to if no active morbid process prevails. But in those numerous uninflammatory deviations of health due to wear and tear of body and mind, to prolonged diseases, to exhausting effluvia, &c., careful sea-bathing is extremely restorative. In every bath, impressions are produced on the cutaneous nervous system, which must influence the functions of the internal organs by the sympathy existing between the interior and exterior. This sympathy rouses the languor and allays the agitation of the great viscera (when there is no internal disease), and thus gives a healthy impetus to the whole human machine, and establishes harmonious co-operation between the various organic spheres.

Nauheim, another spa of recent discovery, is distinguished by a remarkable phenomenon, called the ' Soolen Sprudel,' a pyramid of white foam, bubbling up to the height of two or three feet above the surface of the spring from which it rises.

The place has been favourably known for many years through its excellent salt-works; it is situated on the Main-Weser railroad, at the south-eastern declivity of the Johannisberg, 670 feet above the level of the sea, and may be reached from Frankfort-on-the-Maine in an hour and a quarter. When arrived, we see a pleasant village, with 1,500 inhabitants, and the little river Usa meandering through the surrounding fields.

A large and deep pool, with two isles, forms the northern boundary; to the east, a small mountain ridge is perceptible; to the south, the plain extends as far as Friedberg. Giessen lies about six leagues to the north, and Frankfort the same distance to the south. Behind the Johannisberg rises the Winterstein, with luxuriant foliage. The graduation works extend to the other side of the high road. The white, grey, and reddish quartz of the Johannisberg is interspersed with single strata of talc, which forms a transition into clayey talc slate, by receiving clay and quartz. In the Usa valley these are superposed by clay, argillaceous sand, and ferruginous nodules.

The thermal saline springs of Nauheim flow out of the rugged transition strata on both sides of the Usa, and partly in the Usa itself, from the north to the south. Several of these have been allowed to fall into decay, on account of the power and abundance of the Artesian wells about to be mentioned.

Five saline thermal springs are now available for therapeutic use; three exclusively for bathing, viz. :—

1. *Frederik-William Sprudel* (foaming bubbler), bored in 1855, which possesses the greatest amount of water and of carbonic acid, and exceeds all others in its height of bubbling (44 feet); temperature, 96·4° Fahr.

2. *Great Sprudel* (bored in 1846); temperature, 90·3° Fahr.

3. *Small*, or *Gas Sprudel*; temperature, 82° Fahr. Internally, the *cure-spring* and *salt-spring* are employed.

The analyses of the bathing-springs, by Professor Bromeis and Mr. Avenarius, compared with those of analogous spas, furnishes the following result in 16 ounces :—

GERMAN MINERAL WATERS.

16 OUNCES (7,680 GRAINS) CONTAIN:—

Constituent Parts	Nauheim Frederik-William Sprudel (Avenarius)	Nauheim Great Sprudel (Bromeis)	Nauheim Little Sprudel (Bromeis)	Oeynhausen (Rehme) Saline thermal Spring (Bishop)	Kissingen Foaming Sprudel (Kastner)	Oranien Spring (Liebig)	Kreuznach Karlshall Spring (Prüsdnarf and Osann)	Kreuznach Theodorshall Spring (Düring)
	Grains	Grains	Grains	Grains	Grains	Grains	Grains	Grains
Chloride of sodium	265·42	181·24	152·45	256·39	107·616	108·705	59·675	57·191
Chloride of potassium	1·46	4·02	2·07	—	0·98	0·46	0·41	0·297
Chloride of calcium	21·96	14·86	13·17	—	3·99	22·74	9·16	14·70
Chloride of magnesium	3·91	2·60	2·67	8·28	24·51	—	3·31	4·41
Bromide of magnesium	0·072	0·077	0·014	0·0049(?)	0·062	1·780	1·367	?
Iodide of magnesium	—	—	—	—	—	0·0124	—	—
Iodide of sodium	—	—	—	0·361	—	—	0·043	0·031
Sulphate of potash	0·437	0·390	0·838	22·99	—	—	—	—
Sulphate of lime	—	—	—	19·99	—	—	—	—
Sulphate of magnesia	—	—	—	—	—	—	—	—
Sulphate of soda	—	—	—	—	25·307	—	—	—
Bicarbonate of lime	18·201	16·38	14·138	6·67	1·65	0·255	0·611	2·142
Bicarbonate of magnesia	—	—	—	3·85	6·412	0·130	9·490	0·199
Bicarbonate of iron (protoxyde)	0·384	0·507	0·290	0·513	0·355	0·356	0·364	0·218
Bicarbonate of manganese	traces	0·164	0·070	0·010	0·0008	—	—	traces
Silicium	0·192	0·161	0·103	0·357	—	0·999	0·033	0·099
Organic substances	traces	traces	traces	—	0·864	—	1·471	—
Total	312·045	220·416	185·908	313·440	171·851	135·541	75·572	79·350
Temperature	94·44° F.	90·32° F.	82·04° F.	87·08° F.	67° F.	54·5° F.	77° F.	70·25° F.
Carbonic acid escaping in the form of gas, in 24 hours	48000 c.f.	45000 c.f.	17000 c.f.	4737 c.f.	30·737 c.f.	?	?	?
Carbonic acid fixed under atmospheric pressure in 25 cub. feet of brine	7·47 c.f.	13·32 c.f.	23·5 c.f.	21·27 c.f.	21·28 c.f.	?	?	?

At the baths the water is somewhat cooler than at the respective sources—viz., Frederik-William Sprudel is lowered to a temperature of 94·10° Fahr., the Great Sprudel to 88·55° Fahr., the Little Sprudel to 79·88° Fahr. This *variety* of heat within the short space of 400 feet gives a great advantage to Nauheim over analogous spas, especially over Oeynhausen, which possesses otherwise similar constituents.

The baths are employed in the following modifications:—

1. As *full baths*, with temperatures of 80° to 94° Fahr., filled before they are used.

2. As *stream baths*, fresh brine running in at one end and out at the other during the whole time of bathing; they exert a peculiarly exciting effect on the cutaneous nerves by the repeated contact with the saline and gaseous constituents.

3. As *hip baths*.

4. As *external* and *internal douches*.

5. As *local fomentations*.

The great quantity of carbonic acid gas is likewise made use of for therapeutic purposes, as in the employment of full gas baths or of douches.

In some instances, when it is thought that the patient might be too powerfully affected by the natural baths, especially at the commencement of the course, common warm water is added.

When the amount of carbonic acid appears contra-indicated, the bath is ordered to be filled early and stirred, whilst windows and doors are opened to diminish the gaseous contents.

In some cases motherlye is added to the bath, to increase its exciting effects; but this should never be resorted to without great caution. *Dr. Beneke* * witnessed injurious consequences on several occasions from this indiscriminate addition.

Cold *shower* or *rain douches*, and *hip* and *rain baths* are likewise frequently employed.

Drinking Springs. — Dr. Beneke having found occasionally gastric catarrh and dyspepsia resulting from the use of the drinking springs, conceived the idea of *diluting* them with pure water in exact proportions. This modified beverage not only resembles Ragoczy in its composition, as will be seen by the subjoined analysis, but likewise in its well-ascertained effects. The diluted spring possesses on an average a temperature of 59° to 60° Fahr.

* The Warm Saline Springs of Nauheim; their Action on the Healthy and Morbid Organism; and their Employment in Scrofulous, Rheumatic, and Uterine Diseases. By F. W. Beneke, M.D., Privy Medical Councillor, Physician of Nauheim, and Lecturer at the University of Marburg, &c. Williams & Norgate.

GERMAN MINERAL WATERS.

SIXTEEN OUNCES (7680 GRAINS) CONTAIN:

Constituent Parts	Nauheim Curewell (Bromela)	Nauheim Curewell artificially diluted	Nauheim Saltwell (Bromela)	Nauheim Saltwell artificially diluted	Kissingen Ragoczy (Lieblg)	Kissingen Pandur (Lieblg)	Homburg Elizabeth-spring (Liebig)	Homburg Ludwgswell (Will & Fresenius)	Kreuznach Elisenspring (Ludwig & Bauer)
Chloride of sodium	109·923	58·413	141·822	74·363	44·713	42·399	79·154	84·161	72·883
Chloride of potassium	4·047	2·024	5·479	2·739	2·203	1·835	—	2·198	0·624
Chloride of calcium	8·215	4·243	10·714	5·192	—	—	7·756	9·506	13·389
Chloride of magnesium	2·155	1·173	2·102	1·146	2·333	1·625	7·767	6·001	4·071
Bromide of sodium	—	—	0·400	0·200	0·064	0·064	—	—	Jodmag. 0·035
Bromide of magnesium	0·295	0·148	—	—	—	—	—	—	0·278
Sulphate of soda	—	—	—	—	4·508	4·590	0·380	—	—
Sulphate of magnesia	0·740	0·548	0·775	0·565	2·990	2·307	—	0·225	—
Sulphate of lime	—	—	—	—	0·071	0·027	—	—	—
Nitrate of soda	—	—	—	—	0·043	0·040	—	—	—
Phosphate of lime	—	—	—	—	—	—	—	—	1·693
Bicarbonate of lime	11·558	7·540	11·904	7·713	8·148	7·793	10·982	9·726	0·199
Bicarbonate of iron (protoxide)	0·199	0·269	0·199	0·269	0·242	0·202	0·460	0·390	0·009
Bicarbonate of manganese (protoxyde)	0·027	0·014	0·061	0·030	—	—	—	—	1·361
Carbonate of magnesia	—	0·194	—	0·194	—	—	2·011	0·046	0·613
Chloride of lithium	—	—	—	—	0·153	0·120	—	—	0·129
Silicium	0·115	0·119	0·153	0·137	0·099	0·031	0·315	0·125	—
Sum total	137·274	74·702	173·609	92·848	65·702	61·299	108·829	112·752	94·023
Temperature	72·05° F.	59·00° F.	72·3° F.	60·11° F.	51·12° F.	51·12° F.	50·00° F.	50·86° R.	54·6° F.
Carbonic acid escaping in the form of gas	?	?	?	?	?	?	?	?	?
Carbonic acid fixed under the pressure of one atmosphere by atmospheric pressure	14·267 Gr.	12·319 Gr.	17·267 Gr.	13·818 Gr.	17·5 Gr.	20·2 Gr.	21·48 Gr.	18·42 Gr.	?

A third drinking spring, called *alkaline acidulous spring*, contains very few solid ingredients (about 7½ grains in 16 ounces), principally carbonate of soda, of lime, and carbonic acid.

Dr. Beneke's Researches with reference to the Effects of the Springs on the HEALTHY Organism.—Though a remedy will produce a different *reaction* from a morbid than from a healthy organism, still the vital principles invariably obey the same laws. As a remedy introduces a new condition of life into our economy, we can only fully appreciate its influence on the morbid frame by carefully ascertaining its action on the normal state of our body. Hence Dr. Beneke instituted experiments on three different persons (including himself), at two seasons (April and September 1858). Each series lasted three weeks. In each series, the first period of *six days* was devoted to ascertain the respective normal conditions; in the first series, the *second* period to examine the effects of the *simple warm saline bath*; the *third period* to the study of the *saline bath mixed with motherlye*. In the second series, the *second period* was devoted to study the effects of the 'Cur-brunnen;' and the *third period* served to investigate the *combined effects of the Cur-brunnen and the simple saline bath*.

Effects of the Simple Nauheim Bath.—1. In general, little increase of organic metamorphosis is produced; for whilst considerable acceleration takes place in the morning (bathing time), an analogous retardation ensues in the afternoon.

2. The increased metamorphosis induced an increased desire for food. A greater organic waste having taken place during the morning through the bath, there was a greater want of introducing nourishment to supply the loss of the effete and excreted materials. The organic acids, which are particularly calculated to impede normal assimilation, will be the first to undergo decay and excretion, as they most readily admit of oxydation. To supplant their loss by a *carefully-selected* diet must greatly assist the general reproductive process, and frequently determine the success or failure of the course.

3. Heightened metamorphosis is principally shown by the increase of renal excretion, the amount of urea being invariably increased but to a very small extent, while that of phosphoric acid is constantly diminished. The difference in the other ingredients of urine are inconsiderable. The *diminished excretion of phosphoric acid* shows a proportionate gain to the organism; for this diminution is *not* due to a diminished excretion of phosphates of alkalies, or of magnesia (according to the experiments of Dr.

Wimmer), but exclusively to a *lessened excretion of phosphate of lime*. We thus see transformation and excretion of effete particles promoted, whilst the greater quantity of *retained* phosphate of lime demonstrates an increased formation of new tissues.

Hence the nutrition of the organism and the *relative weight of the body* became favourably influenced by the saline baths.

If the increased excretions be supplanted by a corresponding increase of ingested food, the weight of the body remains unaltered; but if the food exceeds the waste, *the weight may decrease as well as increase*. Dr. Beneke has shown by previous experiments that luxurious living *impedes* metamorphosis; for oxalic acid (consisting of two atoms of carbon to three of oxygen) being an imperfectly oxydised agent, it allows the phosphates of the earths to be *excreted* in a morbidly *increased* proportion—which means, impaired and diminished formation of new tissue.

If the supply exceeds the waste in a small degree, increase of weight takes place under the influence of the simple saline bath.

The saline baths seem to have a corresponding effect with the air and baths of the North Sea, in increasing the retention of phosphates by the organism.

The present experiments do not show an increased weight; for whilst B. gained 10 grammes during each bathing day, M. and Ma. suffered a daily diminution. But other circumstances may have influenced the weight, as increased alvine secretions of Ma., increase of the water retained by B., and decrease as regards Ma.

No light being consequently thrown on this subject by the experiments, Dr. Beneke obtained the desired information by carefully weighing the patients who came under his observation at Nauheim.

These investigations, made with the greatest care, showed increase in many, decrease in some, and no alteration in other instances.

But even if no present gain of weight takes place, the increased retention of phosphates must benefit the organism in future. The body having exchanged a great quantity of effete particles for a corresponding amount of healthy tissue, the further nutrition and assimilation will continue to be improved long after the course of the bath has ceased. The cure of scrofulous ulcers, caries of bones, &c., resulting from the employment of these baths, is due in a great measure to the increased gain of phosphate of lime.

4. The quantity and solid ingredients of the urine experienced

a uniform *increase* during and after the bathing hours (during the morning). This is a certain proof of increased metamorphosis. Decrease took place during the afternoon. This might partly be due to heightened cutaneous action, in consequence of the great atmospheric heat. At any rate, the loss experienced by the organism in the morning was repaired in the afternoon or night, when metamorphosis was again slightly increased.

The effect of the baths must not be sought entirely in the general increase of metamorphosis, for a more considerable increase may be brought about by drinking saline springs, the water-cure, and many other modes. But the peculiarly curative influence of the saline bath is shown in *the greater fluctuations of the organic nutritive process*. The solid ingredients of urine invariably increase after the introduction of food, and diminish during a state of inanition.

During the normal experimental days (that is, without baths), a slight degree of inanition was shown in the forenoon; but if a saline bath was taken for half an hour, the body decreased still more, with a proportionate increase of the solid ingredients of urine. Thus *a greater amount of organic substance was transformed into effete materials, and eliminated in the bathing days, than in the non-bathing-days.*

5. The frequency of the pulse is diminished in the bath; but it is higher in the afternoon than in the normal days. Irritation of the vagus causing retarded action of the heart, the cutaneous contact with the exciting saline particles may transplant the irritation to the ramification of that nerve, and thus retard the pulsations; the increased pulsations afterwards may be due to a weakened action of the vagus, as a necessary reaction.

Ingestion of food likewise causes an increased frequency of pulse. As an increased state of inanition in the bathing days required increased ingestion of new materials, the heart's action was proportionally heightened.

6. Frequency of respiration is diminished by the bath, and continues so during the whole day.

In general, the respiratory frequency depends on the accumulated oxydable substances experiencing a want of oxygen, or on the tension of carbonic acid in the blood. Hence pulse and respirations are augmented two or three hours after meals; accelerated metamorphosis having taken place after the bath, less oxygen may be required by the economy afterwards.

Possibly the increased excretion of carbonic acid through the skin may also have some influence in retarding respiration; unfortunately, the amount of carbonic acid excreted by lungs and skin could not be determined.

7. *The effect of the simple saline bath is neither caused by the absorption of the saline particles, nor of the water.* The experiments have demonstrated that no chlorides are imbibed into the system; at the utmost, some carbonic acid. Moreover, very little or no water is absorbed by the body. The result of the baths must thus mainly be ascribed to the irritation of the cutaneous nervous ends, transplanted to the central nervous system.*

On the Effects of the Saline Baths combined with Motherlye.— The following deductions were the results of the experiments :—

1. If the nervous system is powerful enough to tolerate the increased irritation, all effects of the simple bath are heightened; but if the nerves are not endowed with sufficient resisting power, symptoms of general over-excitement arise injurious to the constitution.

2. Metamorphosis in general becomes accelerated, if the baths are well borne.

3. This is especially shown by a greater want of food and a decidedly augmented renal excretion. *Urea and sulphuric acid* are especially increased, whilst uric acid and chloride of sodium appear rather diminished.

Cutaneous excretion is not increased through the bath, which must therefore be simply regarded as a powerful diuretic.

4. The proportion of phosphoric acid excreted ceases to be *constantly* diminished (as in the simple saline bath); it is even sometimes increased. This latter circumstance generally took place when the motherlye bath disagreed by producing too great an irritation on the skin.

Dr. Neubauer's experiments having shown that many organic nutriments exhibit *oxalic* acid, if treated with permanganate of potash (which somewhat imitates the natural process of oxydation), it becomes probable that oxalic acid is as regularly formed in the organism itself. If, then, this acid meets with phosphate of lime, its strong affinity with lime will cause it to displace the phosphoric acid by forming oxalate of lime. The longer, therefore, oxalic acid remains in the system, without being more oxydised (that is, transformed into carbonic acid), the more phosphoric acid will be liberated from lime. Small quantities of oxalate of lime are kept

---

* This does not militate against the partial *absorption* of *highly attenuated* waters WITH their contents, as explained in p. 23.

in solution by phosphoric acid; but as soon as the amount becomes considerable, it has to be eliminated by the kidneys, and indicates a proportionate loss of tissue. If in a later period of metamorphosis part of oxalic acid becomes oxidised into carbonic acid, the affinity to lime becomes thereby weakened, and the connexion is dissolved by the now stronger attraction of phosphoric acid expelling the carbonic acid and forming phosphate of lime. Whatever weakens the nervous system retards organic oxidation, and thus favours the excretion of oxalate and phosphate of lime.

5. The changes in the urinal secretions are similar to those following the use of the simple saline bath.

6. The direct effect of the motherlye-baths on the frequency of the pulse is similar to that of the simple saline baths; but indirectly, different influences are observed individually.

7. The decrease of the frequency of respiration is invariably more considerable under the influence of the motherlye-bath than under that of the simple saline bath.

8. The feeling of case experienced under the use of the motherlye-baths is enduring with some individuals, whilst with others it is succeeded by a sensation of fatigue.

9. Neither water nor any of its ingredients are absorbed by the organism through the use of the motherlye-baths.

On the effects of the CUR-BRUNNEN *(cure-spring), mixed with an equal quantity of water.*— The drinking of 600 cubic centimetres of diluted cure-spring in the morning, does not diminish the weight of the body, but mostly increases it. The excretions increase in the morning and diminish at night (principally by the retention of water). No distinct diuretic properties can be ascribed to the cure-spring; intestinal excretions are, however, increased. But, in endeavouring to influence the intestines, we should always first consider whether the secretory function or the muscular action of the alimentary canal impede the regular evacuations. No increase of biliary secretion could be observed. Whilst taking the *cure-spring*, the body remains the whole day more saturated with water than on normal days. Urea is excreted in an increased proportion (showing accelerated metamorphosis of nitrogenous substances),—also sulphuric acid. But as regards uric and phosphoric acids, the effects of the cure-spring vary: nevertheless, a *relative* increase of *the* phosphoric acid retained in the system is established. The chlorides introduced by the cure-spring were not only completely excreted, but apart from this a greater proportion of chloride of sodium was excreted than in the non-drinking days; the metamorphosis of organic particles was more considerable in the drinking than in the bathing days.

But in the former, the excretion of phosphoric acid was not diminished as in the latter; thus the organism did not experience an absolute gain. However, its proportion to albuminates was increased, inasmuch as a greater amount of nitrogenous particles were excreted, whilst the excretion of phosphoric acid remained unchanged. We may therefore expect that after the termination of the course, when these eliminated materials have to be replaced by new tissue, an increased weight will take place.

Dr. Genth's experiments showed that an increased imbibition of 2,000 cubic centimetres of ordinary water raised the excretion of urea from 40 to 46 grammes in 24 hours, whilst in the present observations the small quantity of 600 cubic centimetres already produced an increase of 4 to $5\frac{1}{2}$ grammes of urea: thus analogous effects are produced by a considerably smaller quantity of water.

A further period of experiments was instituted to study the effects of the combined use of the cure-spring and *simple saline bath*: the result showed that their effects partially neutralise each other. The bath causing a strongly diuretic effect, most of the water taken in the morning leaves the organism after the bath. On the other hand, a greater desire for food at midday is produced by the bath (in consequence of its accelerating influence on the metamorphosis) than under the exclusive influence of the spring. In the afternoon, instead of accelerated metamorphosis (consequence of the cure-spring) retardation takes place (effect of the bath). The excretions are not invariably augmented under the combined use, as under that of the Brunnen alone.

The increase of weight observed in the combination-days is chiefly due to the retention of water.

Excretion of chlorides is less in the combination-days than in those in which the cure-spring alone was used. The excretion of *uric acid* is somewhat diminished. As regards the *phosphoric acid*, the relations are similar in the combination-days to those of the cure-spring days: it was also found that the more distant the bath was after the last meal, the more considerable was the retardation of respiratory frequency.

To sum up—the main result of the warm Nauheim bath consisted in increased diuresis and diminished action of the heart. Persons endowed with a strong nervous system will find the chill from entering the bath followed by a pleasant sensation of warmth; but nervous and weak individuals will retain the feeling of chill-ness for some time, and consequently will not be benefited by the spa, as it does not belong to the class of tonics.

The constant *decrease of respiratory frequency*, from the saline bath, is probably due to diminished tension of carbonic acid in the organism, to accelerated transformation of non-nitrogenous organic acids into carbonic acid, and to the increased excretion of the latter acid through the skin. The preponderance of the above organic acids may stand in connection with the production of various cutaneous diseases (as ecthyma, impetigo, acne, &c.)—hence the diminution of those acids cannot remain without important therapeutic effects. The best time for bathing is two hours after breakfast.

In such cases in which *retrogressive* metamorphosis is required (as of fibroid tumours, ovarian enlargements, rheumatism, &c.), it is often advisable to bathe fasting, and breakfast an hour afterwards. But only strong individuals are permitted to bathe thus, for the shock to the nervous system would be too powerful with weak persons.

As the principal reparative process takes place in the afternoon, every great exertion ought to be avoided at that period.

With regard to the effects of the diluted cure-spring, its natural temperature may be advantageous in some cases. It is known that the introduction of chloride of sodium into our stomach increases the secretion of gastric juice: increased general transformation follows, as shown by the increased excretion of urea. But the excretion of phosphoric acid is not increased, and that of chlorine is even diminished after some part of the course.

It was hitherto considered as a normal consequence of the saline purgative waters to produce emaciation; the present experiments have refuted this opinion. On the contrary, if the general wellbeing was not disturbed, no decrease of weight took place, but often an increase—either due to the retention of water, or occasionally to an increased reparative assimilation of new tissues.

Till now the principal curative action of the saline springs has been sought in their purgative effects; but whether purgation takes place or not, we have to expect improved biliary secretion, as a known consequence of an increased imbibition of water, besides a more abundant formation of gastric juice at meals. With reference to the numerous chronic constipations cured by the saline springs, many of these derangements are more due to faulty muscular function and innervation than to disturbed secretion of the intestinal mucous membrane.

The great advantage of the spring lies in retarding the waste of albuminates and diminishing their excess. Hence persons emaciated, notwithstanding the most generous diet, experience a particular improvement by drinking small doses of the cure-spring.

Though in general the morning hour has to be selected for drinking, conjoined with exercise in the open air, weakly persons may take their draughts about two hours before dinner, or an hour and a half before supper; or they may drink a cup of tea or coffee before going out.

If it is desired to diminish rather the non-nitrogenous compounds than the albuminates of the organism, whilst we wish to increase its phosphoric acid (as in the case of scrofulous or chlorotic individuals), the bath alone ought to be used.

If, however, the albuminates and non-nitrogenous compounds have to be diminished with a *relative* gain of phosphoric acid and of chlorides, the spring alone is sufficient—as in catarrhs of the respiratory organs, hyperæmia of the liver, &c.

If an addition of phosphoric acid is not called for, but rather an increase of chloride of sodium and of water, the so-called indication of diluting the blood (as in rheumatism, gout, &c.), bath and spring have to be used; if decided decrease of new formation is required, motherlye may be added to the bath.

Pathological and Therapeutical Remarks.—The material character of *scrophulosis* consists in retarded metamorphosis, with a morbid increase of the organic compounds, and decrease of phosphates. This is shown by the weakly and slowly-developed osseous system, by the considerably increased urinary excretions of phosphates and urates in certain forms of the disease, by the great tendency to swellings (as of lymphatic glands), which shows arrested development.

If to this basis other faulty conditions are added, a variety of disorders will arise. If the scrofulous phenomena are combined with general debility, Nauheim is *contra-indicated*, and sea-air to be substituted.

If a high degree of chlorosis co-exists, Nauheim is again inapplicable; but milder degrees of chlorosis, which often accompany scrophulosis, are benefitted by the baths under the simultaneous use of mineral acids or of bitter tinctures and iron.

If the nervous system be moderately powerful, and the complexion not very chlorotic, Nauheim becomes very useful.

With regard to the so-called 'resolvent or absorbing effects' of the saline springs, apparently exhibited by the disappearance of glandular or other swellings, the explanation must be sought in the changing temporary fluctuations of metamorphosis; the proportions of individual diffusion seem to have a *self-preserving* tendency. Thus we find fibrin increase in the blood after venesection and during inanition. If, then, the blood be deprived of a portion of its albuminates by increased excretions, an equivalent amount leaves the tissues to supply the loss, while afterwards chloride of sodium is received as another equivalent of diffusion.

The transitory *hyperæmiæ* produced in the intestines, skin, and kidneys serve as *derivatives*, and do not fail to add to the general result.

But the curative action of the spa on scrofulous eczema and on articular swellings, Dr. Beneke considers principally to be due to locally accelerated metamorphosis.

Eczema may be looked upon as an atonic dilatation of the vessels, resulting from a locally retarded nutrition, favouring epidermic pseudo-formations. By the improvement of the general nutrition through the spa this ailment frequently gives way.

In *general debility* Nauheim is absolutely inapplicable, and patients who employed it of their own accord, especially of the female sex, were sometimes affected with lumbar-pains, uterine colic, and different indications of reflex suffering.

The varicose distension of the veins permeating the rectum and neck of the bladder (*hæmorrhoidal complaints*), with their attendant changes of the lining membranes, are either due to a disturbed general circulation or to deficient innervation. For removal of the local derangement, often so distressing, Nauheim offers great chances.

In chronic *gout* and *rheumatism* the increase of organic acids shows the process of metamorphosis to be arrested; hence the great utility of Nauheim, with its various resources. Organic cardiac disease produced by previous rheumatism does not contra-indicate the use of the spa; on the contrary, the saline bath has often been able to prevent deterioration and relapse. Hyperæmia and neuralgia of the womb, based on general rheumatic disposition, are frequently removed by the spa. In diseases *of the central nervous system* so many cures have been observed by the analogous spa of Oeynhausen, that many patients affected with paralysis of the extremities flocked to Nauheim.

If the affections are based on inflammatory derangements of the *coverings* of the nervous centres, Nauheim will be useful, especially if a general constitutional ailment as rheumatism forms the prevailing characteristic. Paralysis following scrofulous inflammations of the vertebræ are often relieved here; but if the disease proceeds from derangements of the nervous substance itself, either exhibiting new formations or atrophy or degeneration, no benefit can be expected. Their diagnosis frequently offers great difficulty ; but the striking derangements of nutrition associated with them clearly point to their origin. Many cutaneous diseases seem to depend on affections of the nervous centres.

As regards *uterine diseases*, it has to be stated that Nauheim almost invariably induces the premature appearance of menses, probably in consequence of a temporary hyperæmia of the uterine mucous membrane and of the uterus itself.

Nauheim is useful in all cases of retarded development of the genital system—in deficient menses, sterility, uterine infarcta, impeded involution after pregnancy; also in leucorrhœa, based on periodical hyperæmia. But no advantage will arise in such morbid conditions as are based on atony of the womb—as chronic leucorrhœa, persisting uterine hæmorrhage, erosions, &c. Here the greatest benefit was derived from the cold uterine douche, cold rain sitting-baths, &c. Also uterine douches of *carbonic acid* have proved serviceable—probably through the primary excitement of the sentient nerves, and the consequent momentary paralytic dilatation of the vessels. But they require great caution, as, according to Bernard, absorption of carbonic acid by the vaginal mucous membrane may produce giddiness, headache, nausea, disturbed vision, &c. Experiments made by Dr. Beneke showed a slight expansion of the capillaries and accumulation of blood-corpuscles, resulting from the local application of carbonic acid.

As regards *chronic eczema*, the most undoubted curative results have shown themselves as *after-effects of the course*. This must not be considered at all surprising, for it has been shown that the *proportions* of the single integrating constituents have been altered in the blood by the bath and brunnen; hence nutrition of the whole organism must improve subsequently, and the diseases based on malassimilation will gradually enter a retrogressive route. Sometimes the local ailment improved so rapidly during the course, especially with scrofulous children, that the effect had to be considered as almost exclusively due to the baths. The stimulation of the cutaneous nerves counteracting the slight local obstructions and inflammatory processes, induces a more healthy nutrition of the epidermic layer. Probably some water may be absorbed by the epidermis itself, though the constituents need not enter the circulation of the blood.

In *difficulty of hearing*, the local treatment, by douches of carbonic acid gas, enjoys a special reputation. But though salutary in some instances, disappointment follows their employment in many others. Out of ten cases of difficulty of hearing, Dr. Beneke only recollects one which was cured through the employment of brunnen and bath. Of course a great deal depends on the cause of deafness. If the derangement is produced by a general rheumatic catarrh, deficient intestinal function, scrofulous swellings of tonsils and mucous membrane of the fauces, Nauheim may be useful. But if pathological changes have taken place in the mucous membrane of the internal as well as of the external auditory meatus, or if chronic catarrh of the tuba eustachii and of the middle ear exists, no improvement can be expected here.

As regards *chronic inflammation of the joints*, if a carious process had commenced, very little change was observed. But if articular inflammations were recent, the simple saline bath and external application of brine or motherlye at night have proved highly salutary, especially when the local complaint was connected with a general scrofulous or rheumatic cachexia.

In *pulmonary tuberculosis*, Nauheim is in general inapplicable, as a state of debility mostly prevails in this disease. But in incipient stages of consumption, patients have sometimes been benefited who sought the aid of the spa against chronic rheumatism or scrofulous glandular swellings.

Kreuznach possesses the advantage of containing iodine, and therefore exercises peculiarly curative powers in the diseases of the glandular and lymphatic system, and in many pseudo formations; but Nauheim has to be selected in many instances from its warm temperature, the great abundance of carbonic acid, the greater quantity of chloride of sodium, of calcium, &c., and especially from its carbonate of iron and of lime.

Amongst the diseases for which Nauheim is especially recommended, *scrofula* takes the chief place. In this peculiar dyscrasia the blood becomes abnormally altered, and unfit to supply those particles consumed or lost by organic metamorphosis.

Nauheim shows itself particularly useful, according to Dr. Bode, in scrofula of the mesenteric glands, with a distended and hardened abdomen, emaciation, pallid and puffed up complexion, obstruction alternating with diarrhœa of acrid fœtid evacuations, tendency to mucosity, to helminthiasis, and in *retarded development* connected with precocious appearance, &c. In very young children, equal parts of Kurbrunnen and milk are administered; sometimes decoction of *malt* is added, with great advantage, to the baths. If the disease has lasted beyond puberty, it becomes more obstinate, though less dangerous.

Tubercular disease is very rare amongst the inhabitants. Nauheim is also very efficacious in scrofulous ophthalmia; the photophobia and characteristic ulcers of the cornea are said to disappear in a very short time, without leaving spots. The spa is less useful in palpebral inflammation.

But though the temperature and ingredients of the spa may fully justify a belief in its superior efficacy as regards some of the diseases mentioned above, still you must be aware that several morbid states of analogous character will have a better chance of recovery in other spas. Even in scrofula itself, the question must frequently arise whether you have to recommend to the patient Kreuznach or Nauheim. Whenever, in parenchymatous swellings or indurations of glandular organs, you require the powerful intense action of iodine and chlorine both internally and externally, you have to select *Kreuznach* as the most vigorous anti-scrofulous alterative. If an internal imbibition of iodine and bromine be chiefly required, with a smaller amount of solvent chlorides, but with some carbonate of soda to act against such forms of scrofula as are connected with profuse acidification, vesical or uropoietic irritation, abnormal prostatic enlargement, &c., you will select the *Adelheidsquelle* of Heilbrunn. But if the chief requisite be a powerful action of the cutaneous system, and an increased function of the peripheric absorbent vessels by warm baths, which do not create cutaneous relaxation, but have the described favourably modifying effect on depraved metamorphosis, you have to choose Nauheim. This applies in scrofulous diseases of the joints; in catamenial deficiency; in females with retarded development of maturity, of a tense and harsh epidermis; in rheumatism and gout produced by repressed perspiration (especially of scrofulous individuals); in scrofulous diseases of the organs of the senses, &c. You have here a greater quantity of carbonic acid and of iron than in any other of the anti-scrofulous spas. But how are we to choose between Oeynhausen and Nauheim, both children of the modern epoch, both results of boring trials, both attached to salt works, both offering nearly the same temperature and very similar ingredients?

The answer will again confirm the statement, that the chemical constituents must not be solely relied upon for determining the therapeutic value of a spa; for however similar the two modern competitors for fame may be, the few contrivances mentioned, when speaking of Oeynhausen, impart to the latter spa such peculiar efficacy in certain pulmonary diseases, that its antiscrofulous ingredients almost recede into the background. I allude to the vapour-chamber. Further, the manner of filling the baths from below, by pressure, all contribute to deviate from its original application, and to render it useful in thoracic and neuralgic complaints, for which it would not have been recommended if left to its ordinary resources. On the other hand, we must not disregard the chemical difference between the two spas—viz. the greater amount of carbonic acid, the presence of chloride of calcium, and the absence of sulphates (with a slight exception) in Nauheim; whilst Oeynhausen possesses more chloride of sodium and of magnesium, and, besides, it contains sulphate of lime and magnesia. It thus bears greater analogy to sea baths; its iron is also more abundant than in the Sprudel of Nauheim. All this combines in rendering Oeynhausen a powerful and, I might almost say, unique remedy in diseases caused by *imperfect development* of the frame through a too rapid growth. However, to return to Nauheim; I will just allude to a neighbouring acidulous spring, which is often used in connection with it.

Schwalheim lies about half a league to the east of Nauheim, in the valley of the Wetter, near Dorheim. The chief well was reconstructed in 1831, and analysed by Würzer; latterly by Liebig, who found it to contain in 16 ounces, 18·61 grains of solid constituents—viz., chloride of sodium, 11·94 grains; chloride of magnesium, 1·08 grains; sulphate of soda, 0·62 grain; carbonate of magnesia, 0·41 grain; carbonate of lime, 4·31 grains; carbonate of iron, 0·08 grain; silex, 0·14 grain. Traces of bromine and crenic acid. It contains, besides, 22·72 grains = 49·44 cubic inches of free carbonic acid.

Its specific gravity is 1·002; its temperature, $51\frac{1}{4}°$ F., summer and winter. If left exposed to the air for some time, a brown flocculent mass is precipitated, but in well-corked vessels the composition remains unchanged for years. Though 150,000 bottles are annually exported, a great part of the spring flows unused into the Wetter. The taste is piquant, agreeably acid, and cooling; it is often drunk with wine and sugar as a dietetic beverage, especially as an after-cure, when the course at Nauheim is completed. By itself, it is recommended in catarrh and hæmorrhoids of the bladder, in renal pains, and tendency to lithiasis. Taken in time, it may prevent the formation or progress of these diseases, calculi being unknown in this neighbourhood. In chronic bronchial catarrh it acts beneficially, if drunk with warm milk. In several forms of scrofula it is taken internally, whilst the soole baths of Nauheim are employed, thus increasing, to a certain extent, the sphere of utility of the Nauheim water.

Physicians—Drs. Beneke, Bode, and Erhardt.

Artificial Medicated Baths.

Of Acids.—½ ounce of nitro-muriatic acid for foot baths.
Of Alkalies.—3 to 6 ounces of carbonate of potash or of soda for a bath.
Of 'Boules baregiennes.'—Consisting of 8 parts of sulphuret of calcium, 2 of chloride of sodium, 1 to 1½ of Extract. Saponariæ and coll. animalis. 1½ ounces of this mass are used for one bath.
Of Bran.—1 to 3lbs. of wheat bran in a bag boiled with water; for children ¼ to 1lb.
Of Glue.—1 to 2lbs. of colla animalis dissolved in boiling water.
Of Iodine.—2 to 4 ounces of iodide of potassium.
Of Malt.—4 to 6lbs. of barley malt boiled for half an hour in water.
Of Motherlye.—2 pints of motherlye of Kreuznach, Kösen, Rehme, or Wittekind, for a bath in which 1 to 2lbs. of sea salt are dissolved.
Of Pine-needle-foliage.—½ to 1lb. of the extractum pini sylvestris.
Of Salines.—2 to 6lbs of sea salt dissolved in a bath.
Of Soap.—Sapo domesticus, sapo viridis, sapo aromaticus, from ¼ to 1lb. of each. From 2 to 4 ounces of spiritus saponis are added to the bath.
Of Steel.—1 to 2 ounces of sulphate of iron for adults; 2 to 4 drachms for children.
Of Sublimate.—1 drachm of bichloride of mercury for a general, 10 to 20 grains for a local (hand or foot) bath.
Of Sulphur.—2 to 4 ounces of sulphuret of potassium, to which ½ ounce of crude sulphuric acid is often added. In the latter case it is advisable to add also ¼ to ½lb. of colla animalis.

APPENDIX

EMBRACING A CONCISE ACCOUNT OF THE

PRINCIPAL EUROPEAN SPAS AND CLIMATIC HEALTH-RESORTS.

ACHSELMANNSTEIN (BAVARIA), near Reichenhall, a league and a half from Salzburg, 1,407 feet over the level of the sea, possesses very abundant brine springs (the Edelquelle contains 1,723 grains of chloride of sodium in 16 ounces, besides 13 grains of chloride of magnesium, and about $\frac{1}{4}$ grain of bromide of magnesium, &c.). The climate is mild and equable, especially useful in *incipient tuberculosis* and in convalescence from exhausting diseases. The saline particles from the graduation works impregnate the surrounding atmosphere, and exert a soothing influence on the air passages, whilst they stimulate the functions of the cutaneous nerves. Besides the saline baths, *saline vapour-baths* are employed here with great advantage, particularly in derangements of the uterine system. Moreover, excellent whey is prepared here, and greatly assists the benefit derivable from the climate.

Physicians—Drs. von Liebig, Geeböck, Schneider, Ris.

AIX-LES-BAINS (SAVOY), eight miles north of Chambery, station on the railway from Lyons to Mont Cenis, near the lake Bourget. Population, above 4,000. There are sulphurous and aluminous thermal springs; temperature, 108° to 116° Fahr.; also excellent douches. Aix is particularly useful in chronic rheumatism, sciatica, and obstinate eczema. Altitude, 768′. The situation is charming, the climate mild. The 'Royal House,' built in 1783, is a most appropriate and well-contrived building. It contains two common warm baths, sufficiently capacious for swimming (for the two sexes separately), a number of douche-cabinets and vapour-chambers (called bouillons), a vaporarium which exhibits a peculiar combination of vapour and warm foot-baths, and two drinking springs. Dr. D'Espine's so-called *Scotch Douche* has to be mentioned here. It consists in directing an ascending douche towards the neck of the womb, either *gradually* lowering or heightening the temperature. When the warmest or coldest degree has been reached, a rain douche of opposite temperature is

278   APPENDIX.

directed externally to the body. Through this opposite action a congestion or derivation is produced in the uterus according to the requirements of the case, with very salutary results. Solid ingredients scarcely more than 3 grains in 16 ounces, with a small quantity of nitrogen, sulphuretted hydrogen (0·04 cub. inch), and carbonic acid (0·02 cub. inch) in the sulphur spring. Aix has to be avoided by plethoric, apoplectic, and phthisical patients.

Physicians—Dr. Despine, Dr. Vidal, Dr. Forestier, Dr. Blanc.

ALEXANDERSBAD.—A chalybeate of south-west Germany (in Bavaria), near Wunsiedel in the Fichtelgebirge, 21 miles ENE. of Bayreuth. It possesses an altitude of 1,754′, and abounds in beauties of scenery. As it contains only $2\frac{1}{2}$ grains of solid constituents in 16 ounces, above $\frac{1}{4}$th of a grain of carbonate of iron with 28 cub. inches of carbonic acid, it has a very exciting tonic effect, and is especially recommended to chlorotic, weakly, and nervous individuals. There is also a hydropathic establishment, and, in addition, baths of *pine-foliage* (Fichtehnadelbäder) and vapour-baths, which attract numerous rheumatic and gouty patients. The roughness of the climate, however, contra-indicates the place to all those whose thoracic organs are delicate or inclined to disease.

Physician—Dr. Fickentscher, of the Hydropathic Establishment: Dr. Pfeiffer.

ALEXISBAD, in the romantic Selke valley (Duchy of Anhalt-Bernburg), in the Harz mountains, about 10 miles from Ballenstädt. The *Selkebrunnen* contains a considerable quantity of hydrochlorate of iron (0·97), sulphate of iron (0·31), and sulphate of manganese (0·37) in 16 ounces. As the whole of the solid ingredients only amounts to $3\frac{3}{4}$ grains, this spa must be considered as one of the purest and most powerful chalybeates, and has to be resorted to in extremely profuse leucorrhœal discharges, and in cases of great atony of the mucous membranes. That strong digestive powers will be required for its elaboration must be evident from the almost total absence of free carbonic acid. *Alexisbrunnen* contains some sulphates, nearly $\frac{1}{2}$ grain of carbonate of iron, some carbonate of manganese, and about 8 cub. inches of carbonic acid gas. There is also a hydropathic establishment, and in the immediate neighbourhood the Beringer saline spring.

Physician—Dr. Richter.

ALTWASSER, a village of Prussian Silesia, district of Breslau, 2 miles north of Waldenburg, between Salzbrunn and Charlottenbrunn, 10 miles from the Schweidnitz station. Altitude, 1,255′. Population, 1,600. It lies in a charming valley, surrounded by mountains, and possesses a mild and bracing climate. The springs belong to the class of alkaline earthy chalybeates. *Georgenbrunnen*: temperature 70° Fahr. Solid constituents, $6\frac{1}{2}$ grains in 16 ounces—viz., carbonate of iron about $\frac{1}{3}$ of a grain, with carbonate of lime $2\frac{3}{4}$ grains, and carbonic acid 106 vol. in 100 vol. of water. For baths, the *Oberbrunnen, Mittelbrunnen*, and *Friedrichs-*

brunnen are used. The place is frequently resorted to as a restorative after the use of weakening and resolvent spas, especially as an aftercourse by valetudinarians who have taken the baths of the neighbouring Salzbrunn.
Physicians—Dr. Rau and Dr. Scholz.

AMÉLIE-LES-BAINS, in the south of France, $2\frac{1}{2}$ miles from the *Arles* station on the Lyons-Marseilles railway, département des Pyrenées orientales, south of Perpignan. It lies at the foot of a considerable mountain ridge, in one of the most romantic landscapes, and enjoys a very mild climate. *Manjolet spring* (108° Fahr.) contains about 3 grains of solid constituents in one litre (two pounds) of water. The spa is especially reputed in chronic catarrh of the respiratory mucous membrane. *Hygiea* spring (temperature 88° Fahr.), and the cooler *Galerie* spring (78° Fahr.), are preferred for very delicate persons with irritable digestive organs. *Inhalations* are employed in the so-called *sulphur-room* into which the gas is conducted as it issues from the source, whilst through ventilators at the top of the room care is taken to ensure a proper renewal of the air. Season lasts from May to October.
Physician—Dr. Pujade.

APENRADE, Baltic seaport, town, and bay, in the Duchy of (and 35 miles north of) Schleswig. Lat. N. 55°, long. E. $9\frac{1}{4}°$. Population, 4,100. Climate mild, resorted to for sea-bathing from June to September. Through the southward bent of the coast and in consequence of a chain of woody hills surrounding the town from the northern to the southern shore, the place is protected against north and north-east winds. The neighbouring island of *Alsen* assists in this shelter. More warm than cold sea-baths are used here. There are also appropriate contrivances for rain and douche baths.
Physician—Dr. Hundewald.

ARNSTADT, in the forest of Thuringia (valley of the Gera), between Gotha and Erfurt, 926' over the level of the sea, enclosed by mountains, offers a very healthy climate with inconsiderable changes of temperature. It possesses baths of pine-foliage and very powerful saline baths. Its brine contains 1,825 grains of solid constituents in 16 ounces, and amongst them 1,723 grains of chloride of sodium, $49\frac{1}{2}$ of chloride of calcium, 39 of chloride of magnesium, 13 of sulphate of lime, and 0·39 of bromide of magnesium. The valetudinarian has to take plain warm baths before commencing the cure. Of course the baths are taken in a diluted form, with varying strength and temperature, according to the greater or less sensibility of the individual patients. With persons of a very irritable skin, or with emaciated scrofulous children, decoctions of malt or bran are added to the baths. In glandular swellings, struma and affections of the osseous system, poultices of brine or mother-lye are applied. The brine is too strong for internal use. Season from middle of May to middle of September.

Physicians—Drs. Niebergall, Hartmann, Nicolai, Franke, and the director of the saline works.

AUSSEE, 3 leagues to the SE. of *Ischl*, has excellent saline baths and good accommodation for visitors.
Physician—Dr. Pohl.

ASKERNE SPA, county York, West Riding, 7 miles NNW. of Doncaster (162 miles from King's Cross station; 4½ hours' journey). The village is built on the edge of a rocky declivity bordering on a plain. The smell of the springs is sulphurous, the water bright and clear when first drawn, but becoming covered with a slight film after standing some time. The water discolours all substances containing lead or silver, which shows the existence of sulphuretted hydrogen gas. The solid contents of the *Manor-Well* amount to 179 grains in the gallon—viz. sulphate of lime 110; carbonate of lime 6; chloride of calcium 3; sulphate of magnesia 34; carbonate of soda 26. The composition of the spring shows that its aperient properties must be considerably inferior to those of Harrowgate. The spa is principally reputed for the cure of chronic rheumatism, especially where articular rigidity is the prevailing symptom, and of cutaneous diseases such as impetigo, eczema, lichen, &c. Where the skin is very irritable it is considered more beneficial by Dr. Lankester than Harrowgate, on account of its smaller amount of saline ingredients. The water is used internally and externally.

ABERYSTWITH, seaport of Wales, 33 miles NE. of Cardigan, on the Ystwith, at its mouth in Cardigan Bay. Lat. N. 52¼°; long. W. 4½°. Altitude, 146 feet. Population, above 5,000. It enjoys a pleasant situation at the most receding depth of the bay, and is sheltered by surrounding hills of considerable height. After a winter sojourn in a mild climate, the mountain and sea breezes are found particularly refreshing and bracing in summer. There is excellent accommodation for sea-bathing, with a gently sloping beach. A mineral spring exists in the neighbourhood, somewhat analogous to that of Tunbridge Wells. The place may be reached by rail, viâ Oswestry or Shrewsbury, from Paddington or Euston Square.

ALGIERS (capital of Algeria), seaport and city, built on the slope of a hill in the form of an amphitheatre on the western side of the bay of Algiers, south of the Mediterranean, in Africa. Lat. N. 36° 47'; long. E. 3° 4'. Mean temperature of the year, 66½° Fahr. Rainfall, 36 inches. Rainy days, 95. Population, 58,000 (37,000 Europeans, 21,000 natives). It has two rocky islands in front (whence its name *Al-jezair*, the islands) connected by a mole with the mainland. It lies between Oran on the left, and Bona on the right, and almost opposite to Marseilles (on the north coast), with which a regular communication by steamers is kept up three times a week. Whilst the excessive summer heat is modified by the Mediterranean, the same cause prevents violent vicissitudes of temperature in winter. Hence the mean annual temperature exceeds that of the Italian and French winter resorts; there is also less difference between winter and spring than at most other places. The annual barometric range is likewise very inconsiderable. Notwithstanding the high number of inches, indicating the rainfall, the climate is not made damp or relaxing thereby, because the rain generally falls in heavy showers of half an hour or an hour's duration, and scarcely is it over, when the ground becomes dry again from the rapid evaporation and the sloping position. The temperature of the air, however, becomes invariably reduced after the rain. The greatest fall of rain prevails in November, December, and January. The number of rainy days is smaller than at other places of a less considerable rainfall. In Torquay, for instance, where the rainfall only amounts to 28½ inches, the annual number of rainy days amounts to 132. Winter fogs are seldom in Algiers. North-west winds are the most frequent and disagreeable, but though generally dry and cold, they are tempered by passing across the Mediterranean. The sirocco coming from the great desert in the south is very oppressive, but occurs rarely. However, when it did arrive, Dr. Jackson found it less overpowering than in Naples or Rome. Approach of rain is generally indicated by the south-west winds. Though the Atlas mountains are covered with snow during the colder months, they do not impart such piercing blasts to the surrounding atmosphere as is witnessed in several Italian towns, the geographical distribution of sea and land being different. Algiers has seen snow only once in seven years. It must be remarked that the above observations only refer to an average of several years; but, however favourable the climate, vicissitudes sometimes arise. Thus in the winter of 1856–1857 the rainfall very nearly reached the whole amount of an average year, between November and 7th of February, to the great disappointment of the visitors, who expected nothing more unpleasant than an occasional heavy shower. In 1857, Dr. Jackson found the valetudinarians to be very few, in consequence; but from November till April there was not one day in which the doctor could not get some outdoor exercise, though in many days the rain fell like sheets of water. For threatening tuberculosis of northern Europeans, Algiers is highly recommended. Far from being relaxing, the climate is considered to combine decidedly bracing and strengthening properties with its usual equability and mildness. Patients who are afflicted with a deposit of crude tubercle will be greatly benefited by spending one or more winters at Algiers; but when the morbid mass has entered the active process of softening and ulceration, the fatal issue will only be hastened by a resort to this or any other distant locality. Dr. Mitchel's tables show, as regards mortality from phthisis compared with that from other diseases, that, of all classes of the population, 1 death is caused by consumption to 27·6 from other causes in Algeria; whilst the proportion in Gibraltar, Malta, and Ionian Islands, is 1 to 3·8; in Marseilles, 1 to 4; in Paris and the French army, 1 to 5; in England and Wales, 1 to 5·3; in London, 1 to 8·1; in Genoa, 1 to 5·4; in Boston, 1 to 6·6; in Charleston, 1 to 6·9; in New York, 1 to 7·2; in Nice, 1 to 7; in Naples, 1 to 8. The town has a magnificent appearance from the sea: the lower part is laid out in the French style, with arcades for foot-passengers, the native quarters being on the upper part of the hill. The environs are very picturesque. Cabs and omnibuses ply all day. There is an excellent theatre; season, from October till May.

Alpine climate.—It is well known that elevation diminishes the temperature, but the degree of diminution varies considerably. Thus in the northern temperate zone an altitude of 250 feet lowers the temperature by 1 degree Fahr., whilst in the torrid zone 330 feet are required to effect the same decrease. Moreover, a proportionally greater diminution of heat takes place in the higher regions of mountains than is experienced during the first part of the ascent. The ascending currents of air, being less condensed the higher they rise, have more capacity for absorbing heat, and thus greater cold is produced. The diminished barometric pressure at the greater heights causes us to inhale a more rarified air—that is to say, air containing in the same volume a smaller amount of oxygen than in the lower regions. As the principal object of breathing is the desire of our organism to get rid of the accumulated carbon, by its combination with the oxygen of the air and its elimination in a gaseous form, it follows that we require a greater amount of air for each respiration than in lower localities. Hence we feel an instinctive propensity of raising our heads and expanding our chests in order to supply this want. Herein lies the great benefit of mountain air in phthisical tendency. The necessity of deeper inspirations strengthens the muscular apparatus, increases the elasticity of the pulmonary cells, improves the nutrition of the thorax, and checks the formation of new tubercular deposits.

On the other hand, the quantity of rain or snow falling on the average, at certain localities, must be taken in account for the choice of a situation. In Southern and Central Europe, the mountains between 4,000 and 6,000 feet of altitude receive more rain and snow than the plains. At higher situations the moisture becomes probably diminished, St. Bernard forming an exception to this rule. Moreover, greater power of evaporation exists in elevated situations. This is shown by the rapidity with which articles of dress become dry. Probably the increased thirst on high mountains and the tendency to dryness of the lips is due to the same cause.

The motion of the air is also greater in elevated localities than in plains (with the exception of the sea-coasts). This becomes modified, however, to a considerable degree, by the part of the mountain on which the place lies; if in a valley, by the direction in which it opens, or is sheltered by surrounding heights. In the same day, and at the same time, neighbouring valleys sometimes exhibit different winds and different temperature. The impeded movement in the air renders some Alpine valleys warmer in summer than the adjacent plateaux and mountain sides. The reflection of the heat from the rocks and deep declivities may also contribute to their higher summer temperature.

In general, there are two regular currents of wind in mountainous countries—viz., one *ascending* from the valley in the warmth of the day, and another *descending* from the mountains in the coolness of the evening and at night.

The 'Föhn' is a very hot and violent wind, melting the ice rapidly. Though it carries a great quantity of moisture, rain is kept off during its appearance, but generally falls in abundance when it is supplanted by a cooler wind. The Föhn has a depressing effect on the nervous system, and disturbs sleep and digestion. North and east winds generally prognosticate favourable weather; south-west and west winds rain.

Thunderstorms are supposed to prevail to a greater extent in mountainous régions than in plains. They occur more frequently in moderately-elevated places (from 1,500 to 4,500 feet) than above and below these altitudes.

Electricity is considered to be more intense in elevated and open places than in lower and enclosed localities. As the positive state of electricity has been shown to increase with the cold, this condition must prevail most on the mountains. The increased rapidity of evaporation likewise tends to strengthen the source of positive electricity. Moreover, a small portion of the mountain air is supposed to be constantly transformed into ozone.

In the rainy zone (from 1,500 to 5,000 feet), mists and clouds are more frequent than in the plains. In the higher situations (above 5,000 feet), the clear days become more numerous; and all at once a serene sky is often perceived on emerging from the clouds, and all the distant expanse of mountain scenery opened to view.

The light is likewise considered to be more intense on the mountains than in the plains; having to traverse thinner atmospheric strata, it is reflected in a greater proportion than it is absorbed. There is also a more intense exposure to the rays of the sun (insolation), and during a greater part of the day, the sun rising earlier and setting later in high localities.

The lower or sub-Alpine region (from 1,800 to 4,000 or 4,500 feet above the level of the sea) abounds in vegetation. In the true Alpine region (above 4,000 or 4,500 feet) the trees gradually diminish, until we only find shrubs ('Alpenrose'), and higher still only short Alpine grass, interspersed with gentiana, anemone, &c., which often reach to the line of 'perpetual snow.'

Breathing becomes deeper, as already observed, in the higher regions. There is a feeling of greater elasticity and pleasure in the thoracic movements. The contractions of the heart become more frequent.

An early effect of mountain residence is improved digestion. The sensation of gastric pressure and fulness after meals, so distressing to the dyspeptic, soon gives way. But constipation occasionally takes place, and ought to be prevented by carefully regulating the diet. The nervous system is most favourably influenced by mountain air. This is especially evidenced by a more cheerful disposition and greater soundness of sleep. Dr. Weber* mentions the case of a gentleman, deeply engaged in mental occupation, whose only complaint is want of sleep, and who mostly spends his holidays on the Rigi, where he enjoys perfectly sound sleep during his whole stay and for some weeks afterwards. He had previously tried for the same purpose a residence on the borders of the Rhine, on the sea-coast, and even in lower situations of Switzerland, but without avail. He only succeeds in his purpose when he chooses a place above the height of

---

* Notes on the Climate of the Swiss Alps, and some of their Health-resorts and Spas. By Herman Weber, M.D., F.R.C.P., Physician to the German Hospital. Dublin: John Falconer.

3,000 feet. Some persons, however, form an exception to this rule, and are unable to sleep well in high localities. In general, less amount of rest is required than on the plains. Probably this is due to a greater soundness of sleep, which has therefore a more refreshing effect.

The functions of the muscular system appear to be considerably improved by mountain air, as persons under its influence can generally undertake a great deal more of exercise without feeling fatigued than in plains; and when fatigue arises, a shorter rest is required to restore the former vigour.

That the skin is stimulated to greater action may be concluded from the facilitated flow of the blood to the surface, through the diminished pressure of the circumambient air. Though actual perspiration does not frequently happen, this may be due to the greater evaporating influence prevailing in the high mountains, which might quickly disperse the cutaneous exhalations before they can accumulate into actual moisture. The fact of lowlanders affected with atonic ulcers of the skin being cured by a mere resort to the mountain air, without medical treatment, likewise indicates an improved cutaneous function. However, this result might be equally due to a generally ameliorated condition of the blood and to its more intense nutritive properties. The improved cutaneous circulation likewise favours a diminished accumulation of blood in those internal organs so prone to congestion. Hence piles of recent origin sometimes give way after a few weeks' mountain residence. However beneficial the temporary sojourn in Alpine air may prove in general, some constitutions are unfavourably influenced by it, and are affected with feverishness, giddiness, palpitation of the heart, loss of appetite, dryness of the mouth, and constipation, either from debility of the muscular apparatus, or from diminished intestinal secretion.

As regards the diseases prevalent amongst the inhabitants of these high regions, pleuritis, pneumonia, and bronchitis must be enumerated as the most frequent. In some places the deaths from pneumonia form the third part of the whole mortality. Sometimes a malignant form of inflammation of the lungs, or of the pleura, or of both, occurs epidemically (' Alpenstich'), being generally attended with typhoid symptoms, and inclined to terminate fatally.

The various conditions of dyspnœa—understood by the denomination of 'asthma'—are so frequently met with amongst the residents, that the term 'mountain asthma' has been adopted for their designation.

Pulmonary phthisis occurs occasionally in the sub-Alpine, but very rarely in the true Alpine region. It is scarcely ever found amongst those inhabitants of the Upper Engaddin who have not resided abroad; whilst those that bring the affection home from other countries are generally cured by their native air, if the disease has not yet advanced too far. But the altitude at which consumption is rare or absent varies in different latitudes, becoming lower towards the Poles. Whilst in the tropical climate 7,000 feet may be considered the limit, in the warmer temperate zone the disease becomes rare beyond 3,500 to 5,000 feet; and in the colder temperate zone, beyond 1,300 to 3,000 feet. Thus, in the mountains of Thuringia, Silesia, and the Harz (between 50° and 52° N. lat.) the frequency diminishes above 1,200 to 1,400 feet; in the Black Forest (between 47° and 49° N.

lat.), above 2,500 feet; and in Switzerland (between 46° and 48° N. lat.), above 3,000 feet.

Scrofulous diseases are frequent amongst the ill-fed, crowded inhabitants of the confined valleys; cretinism is likewise restricted to the deeper-seated valleys; but goitre is occasionally met with in the highest situations.

Chronic rheumatism, sciatica, and heart-disease are often found in the cold and damp sub-Alpine regions; also hæmorrhages of various organs.

Ague is very rare in the higher localities, except in broad valleys exposed to the overflow of rivers (as the valley of the Rhone). In the latter it is rather frequent, and even appears in the highest situations of the neighbourhood. This may be explained either by the miasma of lower localities having been carried upwards by the mists, or that the germ of the disease may have been imbibed in the marshy plains, and ripened into the complete disease after a lengthy incubation.

From the above observations we may deduce the advantages to be expected in various ailments. The greatest benefit will be produced by a mountain residence in the various forms of indigestion. The atonic diarrhœa, with bloody and mucous evacuations, so prevalent after a sojourn in hot climates, readily yields to the influence of mountain air. The weakness following acute or exhausting diseases, and associated with an impoverished condition of the blood, is greatly counteracted and improved here. Also the anæmia resulting from ague, and frequently combined with enlargement of the spleen. Many patients of this class have not a sufficiently vigorous digestive apparatus to bear steel or quinine, but are apt to regain a healthier condition of their organism by the improved assimilation and nutrition due to a greater freedom of circulation, to more active functions of the muscular apparatus, to an increased elimination of effete tissue by skin and kidneys, which loss has to be replaced by the formation of equal proportions of healthy materials.

Scrofulous diseases, especially in children, experience rapid improvement in the higher mountainous regions; the glandular swellings soon decrease, whilst unhealthy ulcers heal quickly under the influence of the generally ameliorated assimilation.

For incipient tuberculosis, or phthisical tendency, no better remedy can be ordered than systematic climbing, at a certain elevation (above 3,500 in Switzerland), in a dry atmosphere. The lungs get more expanded, the heart strengthened, and organic metamorphosis improved. If tuberculosis has proceeded to a more advanced stage, the true Alpine climate would deteriorate the disease and hasten the fatal issue. Chronic bronchial catarrh, with profuse expectoration, is also improved by the high Alpine regions, especially exposed to the exhalations of pine-forests, which seem to exert a soothing effect on the pulmonary mucous membrane. If, however, great bronchial irritability or inflammatory disposition prevail, the Alpine residence would be contra-indicated. Chronic rheumatism is obviously not adapted for the lower sub-Alpine regions, with their moisture and frequent changes of temperature. But certain kinds of muscular rheumatism, as lumbago and sciatica, are said to have been sometimes cured by the higher Alpine air. Neuralgia, hypochondriasis, and hysteria, based on a vitiated condition of the blood, on miasmatic influences, on depressing mental emotions, or over-exertion, are greatly benefited by the high mountain air. But where there is any real congestion to the head, apoplectic or inflammatory tendency, or great inclination to pulmonary or laryngeal irritation, the Alpine regions are decidedly contra-indicated.

BADEN (Canton Aargau, Switzerland), on the left bank of the Limmat, and on the Aarau-Zurich railway, 13 miles distant from the former and 14 from the latter place. Altitude, 1,179 feet. Population, 2,700. Situation very picturesque. The descent to the large thermal springs on the left shore of the Limmat is covered with vine. A shady walk extends from the baths to the town. The chain of hills connecting the Schlossberg with the Martinsberg is covered with meadows and fruit trees, whilst the Martinsberg abounds with dense foliage. The baths are led into various hotels, as the Staadhof, Schiff, &c. The former offers excellent accommodation and all conveniences desirable for a valetudinarian; the latter is likewise highly recommendable, and will be preferred by those whose means are more limited. The bathing cabinets are spacious and lofty; the corridors leading to them are heated with warm watery vapours. The atmospheric temperature of the baths is somewhat higher than that of the town, which has a more elevated situation; hence a course of bathing may even be pursued in winter.

The springs possess a temperature of 117° to 122° Fahr. The water is clear, colourless, and has a saline taste. There is some smell of sulphuretted hydrogen, but the existence of this gas in the water cannot be demonstrated by chemical analysis. It gets probably developed by the decomposition of the sulphates through the influence of air and light after leaving the depth of the sources. There are 14 springs which seem to possess the same origin. The small spring in the Staadhof contains in 16 ounces:—

Sulphate of soda	2·28
Sulphate of magnesia	2·24
Sulphate of lime	10·8
Chloride of sodium	13·0
Chloride of potassium	0·71
Chloride of magnesium	0·56
Chloride of calcium	0·71
Fluoride of calcium	0·01
Carbonate of magnesia	0·14
Carbonate of lime	2·59
Total	33.05 grains.
Carbonic acid	22· 8 cub. centimetres.
Oxygen	5·91
Nitrogen	125·26

The gas evolved contains in 100 vol. 33·33 of carbonic acid; 66·35 of azote, and 0·32 of oxygen.

The gas is also made use of for inhalations in vapour-baths. The water is allowed to cool to a temperature of 88° to 98° Fahr. before it is used for bathing. After only a few of the baths have been taken, the saliva assumes a saline taste. Baden is recommended in chronic catarrhs of the respiratory organs, and of the intestines, bladder, and vagina, provided they are of an atonic character; in gastric neuralgia, chronic rheumatism, scrophulosis, and cutaneous diseases. The water is also employed internally. In all cases of tendency to congestion of the brain, to hæmorrhages, &c., Baden is contra-indicated.

The duration of the baths must be adapted to the form of disease and to the individuality of the patients; it ranges from 15 minutes to 3 hours. Douches of various kinds are also available. A peculiarity of this spa has to be mentioned—viz., that, after bathing, from half an hour to an hour's rest in bed (without sleeping) is generally enjoined ; further, that generally the baths are administered as cool as possible, and the duration gradually prolonged. This shows the importance of ascertaining the habits of a spa; for in many a health resort, with a lower temperature of the springs, baths are taken so hot as to endanger the welfare of the patients. Whilst here the cure is sought to be obtained by gradual prolongation of contact with the thermal water, there the same end is attained by gradual increase of heat. I have pointed out the danger in speaking of Teplitz. The repose in bed enjoined after bathing (instead of exercise) exerts decidedly a most favourable influence. As reaction is considered the principal curative agent, the horizontal position, and encouragement of cutaneous function (without the necessity of active perspiration) after the direct contact with the spring, certainly assists in producing the favourable effects witnessed in many cases. I found the spa especially useful in persons debilitated by previous illness, and affected with slight rheumatic pains of the muscular system, with catarrhal affection of the uropoietic organs, and in other morbid states where saline waters are indicated, but where any violent inroad into the system would be injurious.

Physicians — Drs. Minnich, senior and junior ; Stephani, Diebold, Schnäbeli, Schmitz.

BADENWEILER (a village in Upper Breisgau, grand duchy of Baden), a league from the *Mühlheim* station of the Freiburg-Basel railway. Altitude, 1,450'. Population, 2,000. A whey establishment exists here, besides a spring of 81° Fahr., and 7½ grains of constituents in 16 ounces (principally sulphate of soda, of potash, and of lime). The bracing air and charming landscape furnished by the neighbouring Black Forest contribute materially to enhance the welfare of the valetudinarians.

Physician—Dr. Siegel.

BAGNÈRES-DE-BIGORRE (*vicus aquensis*), a town of France, dép. Hautes Pyrenées, on the left bank of the Adour, at the entrance of the valley of Campan, 13 miles SSE. of *Tarbes*, 1,900 feet above the level of the sea, may be reached by rail from Bordeaux (which lies 164 miles to the NW.). Population, 9,000. (About two days' journey from London.) The situation is most charming, the landscape variegated and highly picturesque, the climate mild and equable, with excellent accommodation for visitors and multifarious inducements for excursions into the neighbourhood. The mineral springs here are numerous, and enjoy great reputation for restoring the bodily strength and mental vigour of nervous, debilitated, hypochondriacal, and hysterical patients. The bath establishments are beautifully constructed; the *Marie Thérèse*, which is built of Pyrenean marble, contains seven springs, with a temperature ranging from 86° to 119° Fahr.; besides, there are many private baths supplied from smaller springs. The *Source de la Reine* contains in a quart of water $42\frac{1}{2}$ grains of solid ingredients—2 chloride of magnesium; 0·95 chloride of sodium; 25·93 sulphate of lime; 6 sulphate of soda and magnesia; 4 carbonate of lime; 0·68 carbonate of magnesia; 1·23 carbonate of iron; 0·09 fatty matter; 0·09 extractive; silica 0·55.

The *Bains de Santé* contain only $24\frac{1}{3}$ grains in a quart of water (3 grains of chloride of magnesium; 1·1 of chloride of sodium; only $7\frac{3}{4}$ grains of sulphate of lime, and no iron; the other ingredients are similar to the former). One of the springs of *Pinac* is sulphurous, and has a temperature of 68° Fahr. The composition is similar to the first, with the exception of its possessing a grain more of chloride of magnesium, 2 more of chloride of sodium, 4 less of sulphate of lime, 2 less of sulphate of soda and magnesia, rather less iron and rather more carbonate of lime; total, 43 grains. A cold chalybeate spring issues from the side of *Mount Olivet*—la *Fontaine Ferrugineuse*. The sulphates and chlorides contained in the thermal water exert a purging and deobstruent effect when taken internally, whilst the lime and iron admixed in their composition prevent a too lowering action. They are, therefore, highly useful in obstructed abdominal circulation, in disturbed functions of the uterine nervous system, in chronic rheumatism, and some forms of cutaneous diseases. They have altogether a less exciting and milder effect than the neighbouring sulphurous springs, the capacity of the water for absorbing warmth being diminished by the saline ingredients. The climate exerts a soothing effect on persons suffering from pulmonary diseases. Season, from June to September; afterwards such patients generally retire to the milder neighbouring Pau. The baths especially increase diuretic function (like all saline baths, as shown by Dr. Beneke's experiments.)

Physician—Dr. Ganderax.

BAGNÈRES-DE-LUCHON, a town in the south of France, department of the Haute Garonne, in a fertile valley on the banks of the Gave de la Pique (a tributary of the Garonne), east of Barèges, south-east of Bagnères-de-Bigorre, 5 miles from the Spanish frontier, and 22 miles south-south-west of *St. Gaudens* on the Garonne, is connected by diligence with Pau and Tarbes. (About two days' journey from London.) Population above 3,000. Altitude, 2,000 feet. Not only does the town enjoy a most charming situation, but it offers excursions into the surrounding country of surpassing beauty and variety. Season lasts from middle of May to October. Numerous springs issue from the foot of the mountain, called *superbagnères*. The water is clear, colourless, feels saponaceous, and exhibits a disagreeable sulphurous odour and taste. It contains a light flocculent substance resembling scraped lint, and deposits a good deal of sulphur in its course. A quart of water contains only 4·33 grains of solid constituents (viz., 0·47 sulphuret of sodium; 0·03 sulphuret of iron; 0·01 sulphuret of manganese; 1·11 chloride of sodium; 0·07 sulphate of potash; 1 sulphate of soda; 0·61 sulphate of lime; 0·13 silicate of alumina; 0·15 free silica). The various springs slightly differ in their composition, and exhibit a range of temperature from 60° Fahr. (*froide saline*) to 154° (Bayeu); *the average* is 106½° Fahr. By combining springs of different temperature and composition a great variety of baths is administered, and consequently adapted to very different morbid conditions. A similar plan is pursued as regards the internal use of the springs. The spa is in general resorted to for obstinate cutaneous affections; in pseudo-anchylosis resulting from imperfectly healed fractures or dislocations, or from gunshot wounds; in cases of chronic rheumatism and gout with articular deposits; also in bronchial catarrh and in obstructed abdominal circulation. The springs excel all other Pyrenean spas in their quantity of sulphuret of sodium, as they originate from the highest prominence of the Pyrenées. Whilst the sulphurous springs in the east of France and also in Germany seem to receive their gas admixed with carbonic acid in the interior of the earth, or develope sulphuretted hydrogen from the contact of a sulphate of earth with organic substances on issuing into the air; here the sulphuret of sodium is in a constant state of decomposition, and introduces the sulphuretted hydrogen and the alkali at the same time into the organism. Hence the German springs of this class have a less exciting and tumultuous effect, stimulating rather the mucous membranes and the kidneys, whilst the French excite more the venous and cutaneous systems. Greater caution is therefore requisite in the use of these baths. Often the less exciting baths of Bagnères de Bigorre are recommended to precede the use of those of Bagnères de Luchon. Most benefit is derived here by persons of lymphatic and indolent habit affected with rheumatic and nervous complaints. On the other hand, chronic irritation of internal organs, tendency to congestion, inflammation or nervous irritability, contra-indicate the spa. Generally the course commences by five or six baths of the Lasalle or Richard spring, and is then followed by the great baths of the Queen spring. This is done with a view of increasing the strength, but the proceeding is erroneous; for whilst the former continues to maintain its gaseous contents (the original temperature being lower), the latter precipitates part of its sulphur by contact with the atmosphere, becoming first greenish-yellow, then white; hence the bather actually receives a milder bath after a strong one.

Physicians—Drs. Barrie, Pegot, Fontan, Spont.

BARÈGES, a village in the Hautes Pyrenées, on the river Bastan, west of Bagnères-de-Luchon, south of Bagnères-de-Bigorre and of Tarbes (30 miles distant), 5 miles east of *Luz* station, with which it is connected by diligence. It may be reached from *Pau* through the Pass of Pierrefitte and Laredan and the valley of Bastan. With an altitude of 4,000 feet, it is enclosed between river and hill. Avalanches descend in winter and spring from the surrounding steep and barren mountains. The accommodation is pretty good in summer—partly by stone houses and partly by wooden huts erected in summer and taken down after the season is over (September). But, notwithstanding its uninviting aspect, it has acquired the greatest reputation amongst the French sulphurous spas. The springs are nine in number, and range in temperature from 86° to 111° Fahr.:— Barzun, La Chapelle, Genecy, Dassieu, Le Fond, Bain Neuf, Polard, L'Entrée, Le Tambour. The water is clear, transparent, unctuous to the touch, has a disagreeable smell and taste, and deposits a kind of organic matter called *Barégine*. The physical and chemical properties of the different springs are the same, showing a common origin.

A quart of water contains 3·18 grains of solid constituents—viz., 0·64 sulphate of soda; 0·77 sulphuret of sodium; 0·61 chloride of sodium; 1·0 of silica; 0·03 of lime; 0·07 of caustic soda; traces of caustic potash, ammonia, and barégine; 0·24 cubic inch of nitrogen. The following proportions were obtained, according to Gax, as the result of treatment in the military sanitarium erected near the springs:—As regards cutaneous diseases of an herpetic character, 31 were cured out of 51; of a pustular character, 10 out of 20; furfuraceous, 14 from 18; squamous, 7 from 10; syphilitic, 1 from 5; mentagra, 1 from 2; psoric, 1-1. Out of 300 rheumatalgiæ, 125 were cured, 136 improved, 35 unaltered, 3 became worse. Lumbago: 17 cured, 40 improved, 2 were attacked by inflammation of kidneys and bladder in consequence of the douche. Obstinate chronic rheumatism, after every trace of inflammation is removed, has the most chance of being cured here; also mercurialism after syphilis and chronic indolent ulcers. The same contra-indications prevail as in the former spa. Moreover, too much stress cannot be laid on the circumstance that the physical and chemical qualities of the water are not alone to be considered, but the climate, the accommodation, the food—even the beverages that can be obtained—and the journey. Want of comfort, the difficulty of obtaining palatable food, the unpleasantness of a tedious journey, has often destroyed all advantages that were rationally expected from a perfectly well-indicated health-resort.

Physicians—Drs. Pagès, Campas, Lebret.

BATH (*Aquae solis*), on the Avon, capital of the county of Somerset, 12 miles east-south-east of Bristol, and 106 miles west-south-west of Paddington (about three hours' journey). Altitude, 95 feet. Annual rainfall, 38 inches. Population, 52,000. Season, from November to April. The city is sheltered against the east winds prevailing in the neighbourhood, but not against west winds, which impregnate the place with humidity and warmth. The lower part of the town is particularly relaxing and damp, as the ground consists of a dense clayey soil, which impedes the prompt evaporation and percolation of the rain-water, whilst the upper part is more built upon sandy and porous ground, and is therefore less oppressive and humid in summer. The mean annual temperature is 51·19° Fahr. There are four springs, probably arising from the same origin, with a temperature ranging from 117° Fahr. (hot bath) to 109° (the cross bath). Commodious public swimming baths are available on alternate days for the two sexes, and most beautiful and well-appointed private baths in great variety. The waters are principally employed for bathing, and contain nearly 15 grains of solid ingredients in a pint, viz., 2·72 chloride of calcium ; 0·74 chloride of magnesium ; 3·48 sulphate of soda ; 0·60 carbonate of soda ; 6·65 sulphate of lime ; 0·35 silica ; 0·054 carbonate of iron ; loss, 0·34 ; besides an inch of carbonic acid and a large quantity of nitrogen.

The springs being 17 feet higher than the Avon, turned a mill in the time of the Romans, with the stream of hot water proceeding to the river. Through its excessive summer heat, Bath is rather resorted to in winter ; but the effects cannot be as striking as they might be in the more congenial warmth of summer and spring. The great reputation of the spa for chronic rheumatism and gout, for several forms of local paralysis, as the 'dropped hand' of painters, &c., is undoubtedly declining ; and many are the conjectures to account for this diminished fame. But the cause seems to be obvious enough. When the cutaneous function is most disposed to assist in the elimination of morbific materials—that is, in the warm season— the oppressive heat deters visitors from exposing themselves to a relaxing climate, when, by an easy journey abroad, they may obviate this inconvenience ; and, during winter, the average temperature (of $45\frac{1}{4}°$ Fahr. in November, $42\frac{1}{4}°$ in December, $37\frac{3}{4}°$ in January, $41\frac{1}{4}°$ in February, and $44\frac{1}{2}°$ in March) is not sufficiently high to prevent patients from losing the advantages of the course in the intervals of bathing.

The waters are also employed internally in cases of acidity, biliary obstruction, anæmia, and general debility, without any inflammatory symptoms. But before and during the course, aperients are administered if the bowels do not act freely (contrary to the practice prevailing in the German spas). The water is to be swallowed as quickly as possible, to prevent the escape of the gaseous contents and the premature deposit of the iron. Sometimes a kind of lethargic torpor or giddiness ensues at first, which has to be relieved by opening remedies. Great care must be taken against exposure to cold or damp, for a check of perspiration would immediately necessitate a discontinuance of the course. In the King's Bath, and also in the other public baths, there is a subaqueous douche, for causing a stream of water to hit any affected part of the body whilst immersed in water. This is called the *wet douche*, or *wet pump*. Through the cooling process going on, and the spaciousness of the reservoirs, the original temperature of 116° Fahr. is lowered to 98°, especially towards the circumference. In atonic or erratic gout the internal use of the waters proves most efficacious, by bringing on a regular fit in the extremities, and thus relieving the internal organs. The water should never be used till all inflammatory symptoms of the paroxysm have subsided. The debility, loss of appetite, articular swelling and stiffness immediately after the paroxysm, indicate the resort to Bath. But if delayed till chalky deposits have formed in the joints, less effect can be expected. Paraplegia and dyspepsia and many cutaneous diseases are frequently relieved or cured in Bath, the only hot spring of Great Britain.

BUXTON (*Bucostenum*), a market-town of Derbyshire, 31 miles west-north-west of Derby, and 163 miles north-north-west of Euston-square or King's Cross stations (about six hours' journey). Population, 1,800. Altitude, 900 feet. The bracing air of this elevated locality amongst the Derbyshire hills exercises by itself a favourable influence on the debilitated body and depressed nerves of the visitors. Several gravel walks rise one above the other, and serve as exercise for those invalids incapacitated for longer walks. Moreover, a beautiful romantic and shady promenade stretches for nearly a mile on both sides of the lovely Wye, interspersed with numerous serpentine walks. There is a large public bath with a powerful douche, and several private baths, besides a drinking spring. The temperature of the water is 82° at the source, but some degrees are lost before use. A gallon of water contains about $19\frac{1}{2}$ grains of solid constituents—viz., $7\frac{1}{2}$ carbonate of lime; $4\frac{1}{2}$ carbonate of magnesia; $2\frac{1}{2}$ sulphate of lime; $2\frac{1}{4}$ chloride of sodium; $2\frac{1}{2}$ chloride of potassium; traces of silica and of oxide of iron; besides 2·06 cubic inches of nitrogen and 3·47 of carbonic acid gas. The water is clear, tasteless, and inodorous. Some persons, especially of sanguineous habit, find it inconveniently stimulating, and complain of headache, giddiness, &c. Gouty patients have sometimes found a paroxysm occurring a few days after its use. In general it agrees well with the digestive organs. Its undoubted diuretic effect is probably more due to the water itself than to its chemical constituents. It has been remarked that the water passes off less rapidly than a liquid more impregnated with saline particles or with carbonic acid; hence the sense of gastric oppression and cerebral fulness during its stay in the stomach. In gravel and uric acid sediments the water has been found very efficacious. But the principal use is made of the baths, which are generally admitted to be highly restorative and tonic. As they constantly flow in and out, the same intermediate temperature between warm and cold is kept up, neither exhibiting the too exciting influence of heat, nor the too sedative influence of cold. A slight chill is felt on entering, which soon gives way to a gentle glow and feeling of ease. The bath heated to 98° Fahr. gave to Dr. Johnson the sensation of bathing in new milk. He recommends patients with delicate constitutions to commence with baths of 92° Fahr., and only use the natural temperature after some preparation.

The spa is chiefly, and often successfully, employed for chronic gout and rheumatism.

BERG, a quarter of a league from Canstatt (near Stuttgardt, in Würtemberg), on the so-called 'Island,' possesses two springs—the 'Sprudel' (bubbler), with a natural temperature of about 70° Fahr., and the 'Inselquelle,' with a temperature of 66° Fahr. The former contains 33 grains of solid ingredients in 16 ounces—viz, $12\frac{1}{2}$ chloride of sodium; nearly 1 chloride of potassium; $6\frac{3}{4}$ sulphate of lime; $3\frac{3}{4}$ sulphate of magnesia; $\frac{3}{4}$ sulphate of soda; $7\frac{3}{4}$ carbonate of lime; 0·17 carbonate of iron; and $14\frac{1}{2}$ cubic inches of free carbonic acid. The latter contains only 24 grains of solid constituents, and $8\frac{1}{2}$ cubic inches of carbonic acid. The

bassin-baths supplied by the Sprudel with constant influx and efflux have a particularly strengthening effect on persons suffering from indigestion or inactivity of the hepatic system. But, from the lowness of the temperature, only two or three minutes' stay ought to be allowed at first, and gradually prolonged to ten minutes.
Physician—Dr. Härlin.

BERKA, on the Ilm (Thuringia), 5 miles from Weimar station (of the Eisenach-Halle railway), possesses an establishment for pine foliage vapour baths, and in its neighbourhood a sulphurous and chalybeate spring; the former contains $13\frac{1}{2}$ grains of solid constituents in 16 ounces—viz., $5\frac{1}{2}$ sulphate of lime; $4\frac{1}{3}$ carbonate of lime; 1 sulphate of soda; nearly 2 sulphate of magnesia; 0·7 chloride of calcium; some extractive matter; besides 3·4 cub. inches of carbonic acid, and 6·4 of sulphuretted hydrogen with nitrogen. The chalybeate contains $21\frac{1}{2}$ grains of solid constituents in 16 ounces (amongst them $13\frac{1}{2}$ of sulphate of lime; $3\frac{1}{2}$ carbonate of lime; nearly $\frac{1}{2}$ chloride of calcium; $\frac{1}{2}$ chloride of magnesium; $\frac{4}{10}$ carbonate of magnesium; 3 sulphate of magnesia; $\frac{3}{10}$ carbonate of iron). For chronic rheumatism, with anæmia and great debility, the above healing agent cannot fail to prove highly serviceable.
Physician—Dr. Ebert.

BERTRICH, WSW. of Coblenz, in Rhenish Prussia, on the Usebach; 12 miles SW. of Cochem, on the Moselle; 35 miles N. of Treves, with an elevation of 400′ above the level of the sea, and sheltered by surrounding hills against north and east winds. By the Moselle steamer *Alf* may be reached in 8 hours, and thence another hour's omnibus ride westward brings the visitor to the spa. The temperature of the spring, about 90° Fahr., with a constant afflux of thermal water, must give the place a high rank amongst those spas especially resorted to for the cure of chronic rheumatism and gout. Constituents: $13\frac{1}{2}$ grains in 16 ounces—viz., 7 sulphate of soda; $3\frac{1}{3}$ chloride of sodium; $1\frac{4}{10}$ carbonate of soda; $\frac{6}{10}$ carbonate of lime; $\frac{1}{2}$ magnesia; $\frac{3}{10}$ barégine; some alumina, silica, and traces of iron; with $4\frac{1}{2}$ cubic inches of carbonic acid. When excitement of the venous and nervous systems coexists with general atony, and has resulted from diseases due to suppressed cutaneous function, this spa is eminently useful. Without any weakening effect, the skin is gradually improved in its metamorphosis, whilst the saline and alkaline ingredients of the water improve the function of the liver, counteract acidity, and thus help in the removal of effete materials and in restoring a healthy equilibrium.
Physician—Dr. Cüppers.

BEX, a village in the Canton of Vaud (Waadtland), Switzerland, on the right bank of the Rhone, in the charming valley of the Avençon, 1,380′ over the level of the sea, 26 miles SE. of Lausanne (on the Lake of Geneva), from which it may be reached by rail in two hours. It lies on the north-western declivity of the Dent de Morcle (8,400′ high), where the high peaks of the Bernese Alps direct their course towards the cauldron of the Lake of Geneva. Besides its picturesque situation and its most beautiful variegated walks, it is sheltered against violent winds, and enjoys a very mild and bracing climate. Moreover, the exhalations of the salt mines and graduation works impregnate the air with saline particles; hence patients affected with chronic pulmonary catarrh and tuberculous disposition resort to this most favoured locality for an autumn or spring residence. Besides saline baths, the place possesses a spring with a considerable amount of sulphuretted hydrogen, available for internal use as a resolvent and stomachic (Minenquelle containing in 16 ounces $23\frac{1}{2}$ grains of solid constituents—viz., $17\frac{3}{4}$ of chloride of sodium; $3\frac{3}{4}$ of sulphate of soda; $\frac{1}{8}$ of sulphate of lime; nearly 2 of carbonate of lime; 4 cub. inches of carbonic acid gas, and 0·76 of sulphuretted hydrogen). The Inselquelle contains $10\frac{1}{2}$ grains of solid constituents, $\frac{1}{2}$ cub. inch of carbonic acid, and 0·13 of sulphuretted hydrogen, and is principally used for bathing. There are very good *pensions*, where the visitor can be accommodated for the moderate sum of 3 francs (half a crown) a day.

BOTZEN (Bolzano in Italian), a town of Tyrol, at the confluence of the Talfer and the Eisach, 79 miles south of Inspruck, 34 north-north-east of Trient (about two hours' railway journey on the Botzen-Verona line). It is enclosed in a beautiful valley by high mountains; a strong dam, nearly 2 miles in length, protects the place against inundations of the river. In incipient tuberculosis the town is frequented as a most pleasant, mild, and amusing residence. · The higher Upper-Botzen or Ritten offer a pure bracing mountain air for those who wish to escape the oppressive heat prevailing in the Tyrolese valleys during summer.

Notwithstanding the beautiful climate, patients with irritable thoracic organs have to be particularly careful as regards the great contrast of temperature prevailing between sunny and shady places, especially in February, March, and commencement of April (the warmest winter months). They have also to guard against the cold winds often suddenly blowing down from the neighbouring glaciers, whilst a beautiful congenial weather and a clear inviting sky induce lengthy walks in the charming environs.

Physician—Dr. Cazenave.

Hotels—Kaiser-Krone, Europe, and Mezza Lune (Half Moon).

BIARRITZ, sea-bath of the west coast of France, in one of the bays of the inner angles of the Bay of Biscay, between Bayonne (reached in a 20 minutes'' railway ride) and the village of Bidart; 129 miles south-west of Bordeaux. (About 34 hours' journey from London.) Population, 2,700. Mean annual temperature, 56° Fahr.; summer temperature, 70° Fahr. Three bathing places are used—the *Port Vieux*, for the better class of visitors, with more luxurious accommodation; the *Côte des Fous*, where the bathing houses are less elegantly furnished, but where evidently the air is purer and more bracing, and the movement of the waves more energetic; and the *Côte de Busques*, protected against north and north-west winds, and only open towards the south-west; less used on account of the difficulty of access. All the bays offer fine sandy beaches, and are admirably adapted for sea bathing. From the cliffs a splendid view may be obtained of the restless Bay of Biscay, agitated and rendered more turbulent by the slightest increase of wind. The beautiful scenery, the genial climate ($43\frac{1}{2}°$ N. lat.), and the seclusion, render it a most desirable and fashionable sea bath from July to September.

Physicians—Drs. Affre, Chapman, Girdlestone.

The Hôtel de France offers the best accommodation.

BOULOGNE-SUR-MER (Gesoriacum), a fortified seaport town of France, capital of Pas de Calais, at the mouth of the Lianne, on the English Channel; terminus of the Amiens railway (139 miles NNW. of Paris, and 19 miles SW. of Calais; 29 miles from Folkestone, and 112 miles from London). $50\frac{1}{2}°$ N. lat.; $1\frac{1}{3}°$ E. long. Population, 36,000. The upper town is situated on a hill, from which the English coast may be seen; the lower, or new town, extends to the sea. The *Tintelleries*, situated in a valley towards the north, is the favourite resort of the English residents. The baths are most convenient. The chief architectural attraction is the monument—a most beautiful structure intended to commemorate the invasion of England by Napoleon, who is represented by a colossal bronze statue at the top. The jetty, extending about 2,000 feet from the quay, commands an excellent view of the harbour and part of the coast. Charming walks and drives into the environs offer themselves to the visitors. The climate is mild; the average temperature of the sea is about 58° Fahr. (11·7° R.). In a beautiful building near the shore, warm, sea, and douche baths are administered. The bathing ground of the sea is sandy, safe, and free from pebbles, whilst the surrounding downs (100 to 150 feet high) protect the bather against the winds, but do not prevent the congenial influence of the sun from warming the ground mornings and evenings.

BLANKENBERGHE, Belgian sea-bath (prov. West Flanders), 9 miles north-west of Bruges; half an hour's railway journey; equally distant from Ostend. Population, 1,800.

The strand is formed of a fine hard sand, and is especially adapted for sea-bathing, as the coast is gradually and imperceptibly sinking here, leaving about 100 yards free between ebb and flow tide. The downs are about 50 yards wide, and lead to the village by the descent of some steps.

Physician—Dr. Verhaege, of Ostend.

BERWICK (North), a seaport town of Scotland, at the mouth of the Firth of Forth, 22 miles east-north-east of Edinburgh, with which it is connected by railway. About 2 miles from the shore, to the north, the insulated Bass Rock reaches a height of 350 feet, with a circumference of 1 mile. It was formerly used as a state prison. Though the latitude (56° N.) renders it too cold to be recommended as a residence in early summer, the beautiful scenery of the environs, the bracing air, and the mildness of the climate in the hottest summer months, offer many inducements for those who wish to combine sea-bathing with walks and rides in a romantic portion of Scotland. Distance from Euston Square 422 miles (viâ Crewe); about 15 hours' journey.

BLACKPOOL, a village on the western seacoast of England, 4 miles SW. of Poulton, in the County of Lancaster, north of Liverpool, forms a branch of the Preston and Wyre railway. Population, 3,500. Though popularly called the 'Northern Brighton,' its situation three degrees farther to the north than the favoured south-east town points out the greater roughness of the climate. Accommodation for bathers and visitors is, however, perfectly satisfactory.

BOURNEMOUTH, Hampshire, on Poole Bay, 5 miles omnibus ride west of Christchurch (99 miles from Waterloo station); rainfall about 29 inches. It lies at the mouth of the Bourne, on a slope. The Isle of Wight is about 10 miles distant to the east. The valley is sheltered by hills on both sides, and characterised by great luxuriance of vegetation, Deep ravines intersect it at different points; it stretches for about $3\frac{1}{2}$ miles towards the north-west; whilst protected from north and north-east winds. it is left open to the north-west and south-west. Westerly winds are generally the most frequent and violent, but in summer and spring east winds prevail. The rain-clouds are diverted from the town by the hilly Isle of Purbeck. Through the sandy ground the water soon percolates and dries up, so that visitors are not long prevented from their walks in the pleasant promenades even after heavy showers. Mean annual temperature 51° Fahr. (winter, 42°; spring, 49°; summer, 60°; autumn, $51\frac{3}{4}°$). The climate is in winter mild, without being relaxing. The sheltered position prevents many of the injurious vicissitudes of temperature and winds, and it is therefore peculiarly adapted to persons affected with irritable thoracic organs or with incipient tuberculosis. Journey from London about $5\frac{1}{2}$ hours.

BRIGHTON (Brighthelmstone), celebrated sea bath of the south coast of England, on the English Channel, $50\frac{1}{2}$ miles from London (an hour and a half's railway journey). Lat. N. $50\frac{1}{2}°$; long. W. $0·8°$; 28' above the level of the sea. Population increased from 7,000 (in 1801) to 77,000 (in 1861). The town is sheltered by the south downs on the north and the north-east, and stretches for three miles along the coast, having a sea-wall 60 feet high in front, a valley in the centre, and slopes on the east and west. The South Coast Railway connects it with Portsmouth. 44 miles distant to the west; an eastern branch, with Hastings. The most remarkable structure to be noticed is the suspension chain-pier, which extends 1,014 feet into the sea. The manifold amusements, the beauty and variety of the squares and streets, the gaiety of the fashionable world, all tend to stamp it as a most pleasant residence for weak, nervous, hypochondriac patients. The climate in general has a bracing and restorative character, especially the eastern part of the town; but in the west it is more damp and mild. The Steyne is considered the medium between the two varieties. Rainfall only 25·6 inches. Moreover, the nature of the sloping ground favours a speedy disappearance of moisture, as a substratum of chalk lies under the superficial soil. During December, January, and February the climate is pretty equable and mild—more dry and bracing than moist and relaxing. But in spring the prevalence of north and easterly winds ought to prevent persons with delicate respiratory organs from choosing it as a residence. The warmth often prevailing in this season may only expose the invalids more frequently to these irritating blasts. The direct solar influence in heating the body does not produce a universal warm temperature; hence the great difference between sunny and shady places, and the frequent atmospheric vicissitudes in this season. Whilst in summer and autumn it is one of the most charming resorts for sea-bathing and recreation, in winter it ought principally to be selected by persons of strumous, scrofulous, indolent habits, or by those whose power of nutrition and sanguification has been lowered in consequence of tedious exhausting diseases, or through mental over-exertion, or depressing physical influences. Plethoric persons, on the contrary, as well as those affected with indigestion of an irritable character, or with disposition for affections of the pulmonary mucous membrane or tissue, would do better by choosing a milder climate. Delicate individuals generally feel better in the western (moister and milder) part; but where the system is in a relaxed state, the dry and bracing air of the eastern portion agrees best. The Steyne is somewhat sheltered from the cold north-easterly and violent south-westerly winds. In the autumn and early part of winter the Brighton climate is milder and steadier than that of Hastings; whilst in the spring it is rendered harsh, cold, and irritating, by the north-easterly winds, and ought to be avoided by delicate individuals. During autumn and winter it is particularly beneficial to anæmic, chlorotic, and debilitated females suffering from deranged catamenial functions. Relaxed nervous persons feel more energy and vigour here than elsewhere; but individuals of an irritable nervous system, or of a dry irritable skin, or of gastric dyspepsia, are not benefited here—on the contrary, their complaints are often aggravated.

BORDEAUX, capital of the Gironde, in the south-west of France, on the left bank of the Garonne, 60 miles from its mouth in the Atlantic. Lat. N. $44\frac{1}{2}°$; long. W. 0° 34'. Population, 162,000. Its navigable river, 2,600 feet wide and 60 to 90 feet deep, communicates on one side with the Atlantic, and on the other by the Canal du Midi with the Mediterranean. The town is 363 miles distant from Paris (18 hours' railway journey), and also connected by steamers with London. Delicate persons, inclined to pulmonary disease, often resort there for the winter. Its proximity to the Atlantic (33 miles from La Teste, $1\frac{1}{2}$ hour's railway journey), its southern position, and other favourable climatic influences, render the atmosphere mild and soothing in the cold season. With all the comforts of a large seaport town it offers a suitable winter residence as a change. But persons affected with a dry irritable cough and dyspnœa would feel their condition aggravated here by the frequent vicissitudes of temperature.

MONTPELLIER, a French city, capital of the department of Hérault, near the Lez, and on the railway from Nîmes to Cette, 75 miles west-north-west of Marseilles. Population, 51,000. $43\frac{1}{2}°$ N. lat.; 4° E. long. It is situated on the slope of a hill, and is celebrated for the splendid promenade of Peyrou and for the mildness of its climate. Mean temperature of the year, $57\frac{1}{2}°$: winter, $44°$; summer, $71°$. But, notwithstanding its favourable southern position, it has lost its prestige as a resort for consumptive invalids. Predominance of northerly winds during winter and spring, and the dry and variable atmosphere, favour even the development of the disease. In fact, phthisis prevails to a large extent among the inhabitants.

CHARLOTTENBRUNNEN, a village of Silesia, south of Altwasser; 5 miles south-east of Waldeburg station (an hour's drive); south-west of Breslau; upwards of 1,300' over the level of the sea. It is surrounded by beautiful fir forests, in a valley on the eastern declivity of the Schweidnitzer mountain, sheltered by high mountains, and only open to the south. Notwithstanding its high situation, the climate is remarkably mild and bracing. It contains excellent arrangements for whey-cures, besides a mild chalybeate (Charlottenquelle) and an acidulous spring (Elisenquelle). The former contains $5\frac{1}{2}$ grains of solid constituents in 16 ounces : amongst them $\frac{1}{5}$ grain of carbonate of iron ; $1\frac{1}{2}$ carbonate of soda ; $2\frac{1}{3}$ carbonate of lime ; $\frac{1}{2}$ carbonate of magnesia; and 18 cubic inches of carbonic acid. The Elisenquelle contains only 4 grains in 16 ounces ; only a trace of iron, and $17\frac{1}{4}$ inches of carbonic acid. The environs abound in charming landscapes ; amongst them the ruins of the Castle of Kynau, the romantic Schlesier Valley, &c., may be mentioned. The place is mostly resorted to by persons afflicted with chronic pulmonary catarrhs, for the whey-cure, and climatic advantages. Atonic dyspepsia, anæmia, and obstructions of the uterine circulation, are counteracted by the springs.

Physicians—Drs. Neisser and Weiss.

CLARENS, on the north-eastern shore of the Lake of Geneva, an hour's railway journey from Lausanne, south of Vevay (14 minutes' journey), is highly recommended as a climatic health resort for an autumn residence of persons with delicate constitutions or with chronic bronchial catarrhs.

On account of the protection afforded by high mountains and rocks, that part of the shore situated between the 'Bassés' on the north and Veytaux (Chillon) on the south is sheltered against the cold north winds and endowed with a particularly mild climate, whilst the *pensions* afford excellent accommodation. Lausanne and Geneva, however, being devoid of this protection, would be perfectly inappropriate for a winter or autumn residence of invalids. The places particularly selected are, starting *from Lausanne*:—

1. VEVAY, the second town of the canton of Vaud (40 minutes' railway journey). Population, 5,000. It is situated close to the northern shore of the Lake of Geneva, at the mouth of the gorge of Vevayse, with most charming and picturesque scenery. The walks in the neighbourhood are delightful. A promenade on a clear night towards Montreux, when the moon is reflected in the lake on the one side, and the beautiful and variegated mountains rise to view on the other, is one of the most romantic and

pleasant walks that can be pictured by the imagination. Indeed, the remark of an intelligent English traveller is perfectly appropriate—viz., that it is a place particularly suited for a honeymoon sojourn. The Hôtel des Trois Couronnes, especially its beautifully laid-out garden, looking on the green lake, with the numerous pleasure-boats rocking invitingly to and fro, leave impressions on the mind of a most enduring and agreeable character. The place is also used for courses of grape-cure.

Physicians—Drs. de Montet, Churchod, Guisan, Muret, Dor.

2. CLARENS, referred to above.

3. VERNEX (for Montreux), 5 miles' railway journey from Clarens.

4. MONTREUX offers such excellent protection and beautiful views from the eminence on which it is built, that it is even frequently chosen as a pleasant winter residence by persons of delicate build and tuberculous diathesis. Accommodation is likewise excellent, and attracting numerous visitors. The mean winter temperature here and in the southern—Veytaux (6 minutes' journey), (also station for the celebrated solitary castle of Chillon, two miles' distant) approaches that of Venice very nearly. While the temperature of the latter amounts to $2 \cdot 7°$ R. ($37\frac{1}{2}°$ Fahr.) here. in the severe winter of 1854-55 it amounted to $2°$ R. ($36\frac{1}{4}°$ Fahr.), Their being situated so very near the mountains, the shelter against cold winds is proportionally greatest; hence the climate is extremely mild and equable, without being too relaxing.

COLBERG, or KOLBERG, a fortress and seaport town in Prussian Pomerania, 25 miles west of Köslin, on the right shore of the Persante, about one mile distant from its entrance into the Baltic; north-east of Stettin (about $5\frac{1}{2}$ hours' railway journey).* Population, 9,500. Besides the sea-bathing, the saline springs afford opportunities for warm saline douche and vapour-baths. The climate being rough (lat. above 54° N.), the season only lasts from middle of June to October.

Physicians—Drs. von Bünau, Hirschfeld, Behrend, Bodenstein, Neubauer.

CRANZ, or KRANZ, sea-bath on the Baltic, 20 miles north of Königsberg, in the north-eastern portion of Prussia, has a still more northerly situation than Kolberg, but offers likewise arrangements for warm douche and vapour-baths.

Physician—Dr. Thomas.

CUXHAVEN, sea-bath at the western bank of the Elbe and at its mouth into the North Sea. Lat. N. $53\frac{1}{2}°$; long. E. 8° 44'. (Population, 1,100.) Connected by steamers with London. The ground consists of firm sand. The bathing-cars are divided into those destined for flood-baths and those for ebb-baths. The former are more strengthening and stimulating, as the movements of the waves are more energetic, and provoke stronger reaction. Persons of weak constitutions have first to use warm sea-baths, then ebb-baths, and by gradual transition resort to the more exciting flood-baths. According to Neumeister's and Ruge's experiments,

the sea-water had the smallest amount of solid ingredients during ebb tide and under the influence of south-easterly winds (135 grains in 16 ounces); whilst during flow tide and north-westerly winds the amount was the highest (240 grains).
Physicians—Drs. Louis, Schultze, Rönnberg.

CASTELLAMARE, charmingly situated on the south-east side of the Bay of Naples and at the foot of a wooded promontory, a town of 15,000 inhabitants, about 17 miles distant from Naples (by railway). Lat. N. $40\frac{1}{2}°$; long. E. 14°. Galen praised it for the purity of its air. Pliny met his death there, from the eruption of the neighbouring Vesuvius. A most beautiful view of the gulf and of the islands of Ischia, Procida, &c., may be obtained here from several parts of the town and of the adjacent country seats. Sheltered against south winds, but exposed to the north wind blowing over the gulf, it has a somewhat keen winter climate; but in summer the absence of all miasmatic and marshy influences, the refreshing sea-breezes (which assist in keeping the temperature 10 degrees below that of Naples), and the charms of the surrounding scenery, make it one of the healthiest and most pleasant residences in the whole of Italy. The royal palace built here is justly denominated ' Quisisana' (here one recovers); but besides sea-baths, numerous mineral springs are available here for the cure of chronic diseases. *Acqua media* contains 41 grains of solid ingredients in 16 ounces, principally chloride of sodium, chloride of calcium, sulphate and bicarbonate of soda; *acqua sulfurea* contains 58 grains, and $\frac{1}{4}$ cub. inch of sulphuretted hydrogen; *acqua ferrata del Pozillo* contains more carbonic acid than the former, but no sulphuretted hydrogen; *acqua acidola* possesses less ingredients (only 15 grains) and gases, but was already recommended by Pliny against lithiasis and gravel; *acqua del muraglione* contains $70\frac{1}{2}$ grains of solid constituents, but neither iron nor sulphuretted hydrogen. The temperature ranges from 57° to 64°. The springs enjoy a great reputation for the cure of chronic cutaneous diseases, chlorosis, uterine infiltrations, dyspepsia, rheumatism, &c.

Persons of sluggish circulation and feeble power of reaction, with an irritable and debilitated nervous system, should use Castellamare in preference to a more northern locality, especially if sea-bathing is recommended as an after-cure to follow the course of either a chalybeate or of a saline spa. However beneficial the effect of the waves may be in rousing the energy of the nervous and muscular system, such persons frequently lose all the advantages of sea-bathing, and often add injury to the loss, by the exposure to the atmosphere before and after the immersion. Here the equable, mild, and warm air ensures against this risk, besides the many other climatic circumstances of a favourable character.

CAUTERETS, village in the Hautes Pyrenées, South of France, 25 miles SW. of *Tarbes* (with which it is connected by diligences). It stands 3,000 feet above the level of the sea, in a fertile and charming valley running in a direction from north to south, and surrounded by rugged mountains; it is 10 miles NW. of Barèges. The valley is sheltered towards the east and west; rain and morning fogs are frequent. Though the climate is mild it requires great care, especially by persons suffering from thoracic diseases. Season, from June to middle of September. There are 14 springs, with a temperature ranging from 98° to 131° Fahr. They contain under 2 grains of solid ingredients in 16 ounces, more or less sulphuret of sodium, and some nitrogen. The springs resemble those of Bagnères-de-Luchon, containing, however, less sulphuret of sodium, and more silicates and carbonates of alkalies or earths. They contain little sulphuretted hydrogen, and are altogether milder and less exciting. The *Source de Raillère* is particularly recommended for persons affected with chronic laryngitis. *Half-baths* are frequently used here to support the internal treatment, with a view of diverting the circulation from the thoracic to the abdominal and lower portion of the system; besides, *foot-baths* are often taken at the Source d'Espagnols. There are 8 bath establishments. Chronic rheumatism and certain skin diseases are likewise combated by the spa.

Physician—Dr. Dupré.

CAIRO, capital of EGYPT, near the right bank of the Nile, 5 miles from the origin of its Delta, south-east of Alexandria, 130 miles distant (about $6\frac{1}{2}$ hours' railway journey), west of Suez, 90 miles ($4\frac{1}{2}$ hours' railway journey). Lat. N. 30°; long. E. 31°; 40 feet above the level of the sea. Population, including the suburbs of Boulac and Old Cairo, 254,000. Mean temperature of the year 72° Fahr.; of winter $58\frac{1}{2}$° Fahr.; of summer 85° Fahr. Rain only falls for about an hour 10 or 12 times a year. The city is built on a slope of one of the lowest ridges of the chain of Jebel Mokkatam, and has an extent of three square miles. It is surrounded by old walls; a citadel, with the palace of the Viceroy, occupying the highest part of the ridge. A series of gardens and plantations separates the city from its suburbs; a canal of irrigation traverses the town; the streets are unpaved and narrow; the houses gloomy; but many magnificent buildings, mosques, and bazaars interest and amuse the traveller. Shepherd's hotel affords every accommodation of a large town. Access from Trieste by Lloyd's steamers to Alexandria, and thence by rail. The climate is mild, dry, equable, free from piercing winds, from rain and snow, and has a particularly exhilarating effect; as a winter residence for tuberculous patients (especially before the disease has progressed too far), it is annually sought by increasing numbers. Best time of arriving is the middle of October, which offers an ordinary European midsummer climate; November and December are like fine spring and autumn months of the northern countries. The coldest season is from beginning of January to the middle of February, when the temperature sometimes sinks considerably, especially during violent storms from the south—in the mornings to 44° or 46° Fahr., with a rise in the course of the day to 55° Fahr. In the second half of February the warmth increases again; the more so under the prevalence of south winds. May is the most unpleasant month, in consequence of the violent winds sweeping more frequently than usual over the Arabian and Lybian Desert, and sometimes lasting three or four days. In June, north winds prevail. From the middle of June to the end of September the thermometer indicates a heat of 68° in the morning, 95° to 104° in the afternoon (about three), and 91° to 95° at sunset. In January, patients ought to resort to Upper Egypt, especially *Assuan* (a town on the east bank of the Nile, near the borders of Nubia, 110 miles south of Thebes. Lat. N. 24° 5'; long. E. 32½°), where an almost constant summer temperature prevails. Patients are recommended to choose a residence rather outside the gates of Schubra, in one of the country-houses, than in the dusty town hotels, or in a *pension* on the Nile. The advantages of a winter residence here are almost unique, not only for consumptive patients, but also for those who suffer from atonic dyspepsia, hypochondriasis, nervous debility in consequence of mental overwork, &c.

The following table shows the temperature of the usual winter resorts for tuberculous patients (by the *Centigrade** thermometer):—

	Annual	Winter	Spring	Summer	Autumn
Meran	+12·3°	+3°	+13·7°	+21°	+12·3°
Venice	+13·7°	+3·3°	+12·6°	+22·8°	+13·3°
Pisa	+15·8°	+7·8°	+14·8°	+23·2°	+17·3°
Coïmbra	+16·6°	+11·24°	+17·25°	+20·8°	+17·40°
Palermo	+16·7°	+11·3°	+14·7°	+22°	+18·9°
Algiers	+17·8°	+12·4°	+15·5°	+23·6°	+19·9°
Madeira	+19·7°	+17·49°	+18°	+22°	+21·5°
Malaga	+20°	+15·10°	+18·24°	+25°	+21·5°
Cairo	+22·4°	+14·7°	+21·9°	+29·2°	+23·6°

COÏMBRA (Conimbriga), a Portuguese town on the right bank of the Mondego, 110 miles north-north-east of Lisbon. Population, 13,000. Lat. N. above 40°; long. W. about 9°. The west coast of Portugal has shown itself particularly *adapted* to tuberculous patients. The mean annual temperature equals the ordinary northern summer heat. In winter the cold never reaches the freezing point; whilst in the hottest days of summer the atmosphere does not exhibit the oppressive heat of analogous localities. The range between the coldest days (+10·7° Centigrade) and the hottest (20½° Centigrade) amounts only to 9·8° Centigrade, showing an equability of temperature very rare in Europe. Frost and snow occur seldom; but rain is extremely frequent, and more so than at any other winter resort. The prevailing winds blow from the west, south-west, and north-west. Accommodation for visitors is *extremely deficient*, both as regards food and lodging. Thus, notwithstanding all the favourable mention justly due to the climate, the place cannot be recommended as a curative resort. For two conditions are imperative to improve the disturbed health—first, well-built and convenient residences, to ensure an equable temperature *in* the houses when unseasonable weather forbids outdoor exercise; and secondly, good, substantial, and seasonable food to supply the waste constantly occasioned by organic metamorphosis. If, then, patients with pronounced consumptive tendency fly to a warm place

---

* 10 degrees Centigrade are equal to 18 degrees Fahrenheit (the scale commencing from freezing point.)

with the view of benefiting their lungs, and are exposed to draughts and chills indoors from badly-closing windows and doors—being deprived at the same time of their accustomed and easily-digestible food—the morbid tendency must inevitably increase, and, instead of benefit, they will only find aggravation of their bodily ailments as the result of the distant journey.

CHELTENHAM, a fashionable town in the west of ENGLAND, 8 miles east-north-east of Gloucester; 121 miles from Paddington station (about 5 hours' journey). Population, 39,000. Lat. N. about 52°; long. W. 2°. It lies sheltered and level in the valley of the Severn, nearly surrounded by hills of a moderate height and pleasant appearance. Mean annual temperature, $51\frac{1}{2}°$ Fahr. (spring, $50\frac{1}{4}°$; summer, $64\frac{1}{3}°$; autumn, nearly 51°; winter, $40\frac{1}{2}°$). The promenade at the end of the Colonnade is greatly admired, with the magnificent Queen's Hotel, and the charming rides and walks in the neighbourhood. The avenue of elms gives shelter and charm to the visitors, who flock here mostly in summer for the use of the celebrated mineral water (from July to October). Numerous springs arise about Lansdowne Crescent, and are conducted into the various pump-rooms.

The strongest spring of the old *well* contains 118 grains of solid constituents in a pint of water—viz., 47·8 chloride of sodium; 4·29 chloride of calcium; 7·30 chloride of magnesium; 59·2 sulphate of soda; besides 1·16 cubic inch of carbonic acid, and a trace of sulphuretted hydrogen. Temperature of the water, about 50° Fahr. The strong spring of the *Pittville Spa* contains $106\frac{1}{4}$ solid constituents in a pint; rather more chloride of sodium, calcium, and magnesium; less sulphate of soda (only 14 grains), but some sulphate of magnesia (3), iodide of sodium $\frac{1}{4}$ of a grain, and bicarbonate of soda $2\frac{1}{4}$. The *chalybeate saline* contains some iron; the *sulphur saline* some sulphuretted hydrogen. The *original chalybeate*, near the Montpellier Gardens, contains nearly a grain of carbonate of iron in a pint of water, with only 7 grains of saline matter (some muriate of lime and magnesia, sulphate and muriate of soda), besides 3 cubic inches of carbonic acid.

At the opposite side of the town, about half a mile from the Old Wells, the splendid pump-room of the *Pittville waters* is reached, with its gardens, shrubberies, and ponds, crowned by an imposing dome, and bounded by the charming, well-cultivated Cottswold Hills.

The greatest advantage is derived from the springs in functional derangement of the liver and stomach; in the various forms of dyspepsia and constipation, whether arising from deficient muscular action or from morbid secretions. Especially valetudinarians from a tropical climate are often restored to their previous health by drinking first the saline and afterwards the chalybeate springs, and assisting the course occasionally by medicinal aperients. In absolute plethora and general tendency to make blood rapidly, congestion to internal organs may sometimes be *avoided* by combating the torpid action of the liver and kidneys through a course of Cheltenham: in general, however, those persons would derive more benefit by proceeding to pure saline spas. But in *relative plethora*, when a chilly surface, coldness of extremities, feeling of debility, &c., indicate a languid circulation, the large internal blood-vessels have sometimes a too great load thrown upon them, and require derivation and increased function of the emunctories to prevent serious local mischief. In these cases, which might be mistaken by superficial observation for debility, Cheltenham is very beneficial; the secretions become improved, the circulation more equalised, and general tone increased. In many cases, where persons with deranged biliary secretion are affected by consequent anæmia, hypochondriasis, or hysteria, a visit to this charming watering place will prove highly beneficial, offering the additional advantage of easy access. It cannot, however, be denied that the small quantity of carbonic acid renders the water less easily digestible than that of analogous foreign spas endowed with a great amount of carbonic acid. The effect will be less pronounced and decisive in proportion. This is also shown by the mercurial and other purgatives preceding and accompanying the course here; whilst in the continental saline and acidulous spas the springs alone are generally capable of restoring the disturbed equilibrium without any pharmaceutic help.

CLIFTON, a fashionable watering-place in Gloucestershire, about 1 mile west of Bristol; 119½ miles from Paddington Station (4½ hours' journey). It is built on the slopes and summit of a precipitous limestone hill, 460 feet high, and is separated from a similar cliff by the navigable Avon, flowing through a deep chasm. Population, 21,000. Mean temperature—January, 39·3°; July, 62·7°; rainfall, 32 inches; rainy days, 169. The beautiful and charming scenery of the Leigh woods, opposite the town, render it one of the most picturesque and romantic spots in England. The town, extending from the margin of the river to the extreme height of the southern slope of the hill, thereby offers a great variety of situations to the various invalids. The atmosphere is considered as highly elastic, mild, and vivifying. Exposed to the southern and western winds nearly three-fourths of the year; cleansed and braced by the sea breezes sweeping up from the Atlantic Ocean through the whole Severn estuary, and intersected by a navigable river with a tide occasionally rising to thirty feet (being only eight miles distant from the Bristol Channel), Clifton possesses many advantages of a sea-side residence, without the bleakness and roughness sometimes inseparable from the latter. Hence it enjoys great celebrity as a mild winter residence for persons affected with chronic irritation of the pulmonary organs. The lower portion of the town being warm, equable, moist, and more sheltered, has to be selected by persons whose lungs are inclined to be affected; whilst the upper portion, being drier and more exposed, is adapted to persons who require a bracing but mild atmosphere. In summer the lower part is too hot and oppressive for valetudinarians, besides being sometimes inconvenienced by fogs arising from the river. But whilst it is one of the most pleasant and picturesque localities in summer, on account of the variegated and beautiful scenery of the environs, in winter there is little opportunity for outdoor exercise, which is certainly a great bar to its utility as a restorative and invigorating climatic health resort; nevertheless many invalids whose strength has been reduced by long exhausting diseases, and whose thoracic organs, though irritable, are not so seriously affected as to necessitate a tedious journey to a distant southern climate, ought to spend here the severest winter months, instead of travelling abroad. The home comforts and the simple nutritious food of his native country are often longed for in vain by the English valetudinarian abroad, and this want, combined with a relaxing southern climate, often injures the general resisting power of the system, whilst the lungs are momentarily improved. Unfortunately, it is an occurrence so frequently noticed, that patients with tubercular disease of the lungs have passed one or two winters with apparently great benefit in Madeira, and when they remain here the following year, they are not seldom carried off with unusual rapidity. I do not attribute this fatal termination so much to the roughness of the English climate, but to the diminished nutrition and reactive strength of the constitution. The general stamina being lowered, nature has lost the power of assisting in the battle against the inroads of the new disease. Formerly Clifton has been renowned for its tepid spring (of a temperature of 74° Fahr.) called *Hotwells*, at the bottom of St. Vincent's Cliff, near the river; it contains about $4\frac{1}{2}$ grains of solid constituents in 16 ounces, viz. $1\frac{3}{4}$ carbonate of lime, half a grain of chloride of sodium, nearly 1 grain of sulphate of lime, about $\frac{1}{3}$ of a grain of sulphate of soda, about $\frac{1}{5}$ of sulphate of magnesia, about $\frac{1}{4}$ of nitrate of magnesia, $\frac{1}{100}$ of carbonate of iron, and some carbonic acid. It has been highly recommended for dyspepsia, gravel, and other diseases resulting from mal-assimilation; but in latter years the climate has formed the chief attraction for visitors.

DIEPPE, a seaport town of FRANCE, on the English Channel, at the mouth of the Arques, department of Seine Inférieure, 33 miles north of Rouen (2 hours' railway journey). It is the Brighton of the Parisians; 125 miles distant from Paris ($6\frac{1}{4}$ hours' journey), in daily steamboat communication with Newhaven (about 7 hours' sea voyage). Lat. N. $49\frac{1}{2}°$; long. E. 1° 5′. Population, 20,000. The town proper communicates by a flying-bridge with the suburb of Le Pollet. The port is enclosed by two jetties, and bordered by quays. It is much frequented in summer for sea-bathing, the movements of the waves being very strong, and all the arrangements and accommodation most satisfactory. Persons who are very sensitive to cold ought first to use warm, then tepid sea-baths, before immersing into the sea itself. On the other hand, persons endowed with a vigorous circulation will find more benefit from this northern and more exposed French sea-bath than from a milder and more sheltered locality.

DOBERAN, a market town in the grand duchy of MECKLENBURGH-SCHWERIN, 40 miles north-north-east of Schwerin, 10 west of Rostock Station. Lat. N. 54°, long. E. about 12°; situated on a river which falls into the Baltic, $2\frac{1}{2}$ miles below the town, and in a valley surrounded by low woody hills. The coast of the Baltic extends from east to west for several leagues to the north of the town, separated from the sea by a dam (called *Heilige Damm*), from 10 to 16 feet high, and 50 to 200 yards broad. This locality is extremely well adapted for sea-bathing, and communicates with the town of Doberan by shady woods and a good road. The bathing places for the two sexes are sufficiently apart, and possess a very good sandy ground, besides the advantage of the waves being prevented by the sheltering dam from running out freely and thus acting more directly on the bather.

Moreover, there are warm sea-baths and all conveniences for rain and douche-baths, besides a sulphurous chalybeate and saline spring. The sulphurous spring possesses 61 grains of solid constituents in 16 ounces, viz. 40 chloride of sodium, 7 chloride of magnesium, $3\frac{1}{2}$ sulphate of magnesia, &c., and some sulphuretted hydrogen gas. The chalybeate contains 6 grains, and amongst them $\frac{8}{10}$ of carbonate of iron, 2 carbonate of lime, and 1 carbonate of magnesia, with $4\frac{1}{2}$ cub. inches of carbonic acid. The saline spring contains 160 grains, resembling Homburg's Elisabethquelle in its composition, but containing only $3\frac{1}{2}$ cub. inches of carbonic acid.

Physicians—Drs. Döbereiner, Kortüm, and Römer.

DÜRKHEIM (RHENISH BAVARIA), lies at the foot of the Haardt Mountain, on the Isenach, about 358' above the level of the sea, surrounded by vineyards and fruit trees; 18 miles north of Landau, 2 hours' omnibus-ride from Neustadt an der Haardt Station (in the south), not far from Mannheim. The atmosphere exhibits a uniform and equable dryness particularly adapted to scrofulous patients, whilst the open situation freely exposed to the influence of the sun produces a congenial warmth. Seven saline springs arise here of similar composition. The *Virgilius Brunnen* contains 99·7 grains of solid constituents in 16 ounces, viz. 78·9 chloride of sodium, 0·67 chloride of potassium, 13·8 chloride of calcium, 3·78 chloride of magnesium, 0·03 chloride of aluminium, 0·19 bromide of sodium, 0·019 iodide of sodium, 0·16 sulphate of lime, 0·18 bicarbonate of lime, 0·09 bicarbonate of iron, 0·05 bicarbonate of magnesia, 3·98 cub. inches of carbonic acid, 0·64 cub. inches of nitrogen. *Bleichbrunnen* contains 81 grains, rather more iron (0·12), and less bromine and iodine; the *Fitzsche Brunnen* $74\frac{1}{4}$ grains; the *Wiesenbrunnen* 39 grains, with 2·49 cub. inches of nitrogen. A new saline spring has been obtained in 1861 by boring, with 127 grains of solid constituents, amongst them 0·3 grains of chloride of lithium. The mother-lye of this latter spring is particularly distinguished by its quantity of chloride of lithium, 85 grains in 16 ounces, besides $16\frac{1}{2}$ of bromide of potassium, 61 chloride of strontium, 317 chloride magnesium, 123 chloride of potassium, 2,280 chloride of calcium, and 161 chloride of sodium—total, 3,047 grains. In cases of scrofulosis, Dürkheim is frequently resorted to instead of Kreuznach, its climate and environs being so extremely attractive. Persons of anæmic delicate constitutions, requiring the resolvent effects of a saline spa, ought to prefer Dürkheim on account of the iron admixed in some springs preventing a too lowering action of the course.

Moreover, Dürkheim is frequently visited for the employment of the so-called *grape-cure*. After an acute attack of bronchitis, scrofulous individuals are apt to retain thickening of the pulmonary mucous membrane with a tough mucopurulent expectoration impeding the free passage of air in the smaller bronchial tubes. In such cases the grape-cure is often employed with great success, as the juice improves the secretory functions of the mucous membranes, loosens the tough sputa, and thus diminishes the after consequences of the original inflammation.

The grape juice consists of—grape sugar, albumen, gum and dextrine, tartaric acid, malic acid, grape acid, and different salts of phosphate of lime, sulphate of potash, bitartrate of potash, tartrate of lime, chloride of sodium and of calcium, colouring matter, tannin, and in some sorts of grapes an iron salt. The ripe grapes are either eaten fresh, a pound three times a day, and gradually increased to 2 and $2\frac{1}{2}$ pounds for a dose (of course without the skins and husks), or if the teeth become blunt, or erosion of the gums and tongue is apprehended, the fresh juice is taken instead. The cure lasts from four to six weeks, according to the severity of the case. The immediate effect of the large consumption of grapes is at first—gastric oppression and eructation through the development of carbonic acid, increased heat of the skin, greater frequency of the pulse, with a feeling of fulness and heaviness in the head. But after a few hours these symptoms give way, either by the appearance of increased urinary secretion, or of cutaneous perspiration, or of liquid alvine evacuations. In proportion as the organism becomes accustomed to the remedy the disturbance diminishes, so that after a few weeks the patient feels no more inconvenience, but gets daily relieved by two or three liquid intestinal discharges. Nutrition of the body is not impaired by the course, on the contrary, increased weight has been observed in many cases. Diet is adapted to the individuality of each patient. Persons of reduced strength are allowed substantial meat-dishes, whilst plethoric and vigorous individuals are enjoined to eat meat very sparingly, and to restrict themselves to the lighter kinds of food, as the grapes in themselves are considered highly nutritive and would disagree with fatty, salty, and heavy nutriments. For these cures places are chosen which enjoy especial climatic advantages, so as to combine the curative influence of the atmosphere with the solvent effects of the grapes. Besides Dürkheim the following localities are particularly recommendable:—Meran in Tyrol, Neustadt an der Haardt, Gleisweiler (near Landau in Bavaria), Bingen on the Rhine, Montreux, Clarens, and Vernex on the Lake of Geneva, Aigle and Sion in the Valley of the Rhone, &c. According as the requirements of the patient either indicate the desirability of a more mild and sheltered or more bracing atmosphere, one or other of the above places has to be selected.

Physicians of Dürkheim—Drs. Herberger, Kaufmann, Schäfer, Löchner.

DOVER, a seaport on the north-west side of Dover Strait, 88 miles east-south-east of London (about $2\frac{1}{2}$ hours' railway journey); $22\frac{1}{2}$ miles north-west of Calais. Population, 24,000. Lat. N. 51° 7′; long. E. 1° 19′. The chalk downs contain the castle, citadel, and several strong detached forts, besides a harbour of refuge. The Admiralty Pier, the west arm of the harbour of refuge, being thrown out to the extent of 1,200 feet, renders the access of ships always easy. The town lying in a depression of the cliffs, facing the high sea, has sheltered portions, but of limited extent, exposure to high winds being the general character of the place. The climate is, therefore, not suited for persons of delicate constitutions, the sea exposure being very great. The arrangements for visitors and sea-bathers are very good, the town offering beautiful views from its chalky cliffs and ancient castle; but the atmosphere possesses a certain dryness and coolness as the strand is greatly exposed to easterly winds. Persons of a torpid and phlegmatic habit, requiring a bracing climate to assist the advantages of sea-immersions, ought to resort rather to Dover than to a milder sea-bath.

EAUX-BONNES, a hamlet of FRANCE, department of Basses Pyrenées, 22 miles south of Pau, with which it is connected by diligence, west of Barèges (about two days and four hours' journey from London). N. Lat. 43°. It lies embedded in the valley of Ossau, at the foot of the Pic de Gers, above Laruns. The valley is surrounded by mountains 8,000 feet high, and the altitude of the spa itself is 2,100'. The melting snow of the mountains and heavy falls of rain occasionally inundate portions of the valley. The village enjoys a pleasant situation, with its single row of houses for the accommodation of visitors, and some convenient promenades. Charming excursions may be undertaken into the neighbourhood, especially by persons of unimpaired bodily vigour, fond of mountain scenery and pedestrian exercise. Though greatly frequented by persons affected with chronic laryngitis and other affections of the pulmonary mucous membrane, on account of the celebrity of the springs, the climate has many disadvantages. The high surrounding mountains prevent the free entrance of the solar rays; changes of temperature often occur suddenly, so that patients require to use great caution in being well provided with warm clothing, for even in fine summer days the evenings and mornings are often cool, whilst the midday exhibits great heat. If proper means, however, be taken to guard against injuries arising from these vicissitudes, the high and sheltered position of the locality in the most salubrious part of southern France, certainly renders it a most appropriate summer residence for persons affected with bronchial and laryngeal irritation.

Five springs arise here: three warm ones at the foot of the Mount Trésor—*La Buvette*, with a temperature of 91·4° Fahr.; *En Bas*, 89·6° Fahr.; *La Nouvelle*, 87·8° Fahr.; and two colder ones at a little distance from the village, viz. Ortech (73·4°), and *La Froide* (55·4°). A quart of the water only contains 6·8 grains of solid constituents, viz. 2·8 sulphate of lime, 0·3 sulphate of magnesia, 0·11 carbonate of lime, 0·15 oxyde of iron, 0·23 silica, 0·5 hydrochlorate of soda, 0·1 hydrochlorate of magnesia, trace of hydrochlorate of potash, 2·5 organic matter impregnated with sulphur, and 2·6 cubic inches of gaseous ingredients, viz. 1·5 nitrogen, 0·48 carbonic acid, 0·67 sulphuretted hydrogen. The springs are more employed internally than for baths, and enjoy a great reputation in chronic rheumatism and in those affections of the pulmonary organs asso-

ciated with a general laxity of tissue or with a scrofulous diæthesis. Where great debility and deficient sanguification prevail, as in chlorosis, irregularity of catamenia, the colder springs greatly assist in promoting the requisite strength. However useful in chronic inflammatory conditions (being one of the most distinguished thermae of the Pyrenées), it has to be avoided in common with all other health resorts in acute attacks of inflammation, in apoplectic tendency, and in all those conditions of disordered health where prompt remedial measures can alone ensure rapid retrogression of disease. Season lasts from June to middle of September.
Physician—Dr. Pidaux.

EAUX-CHAUDES lies in the western part of the valley of Ossau, and is reached by diligence from Pau, on the same road which leads to the eastern Eaux-bonnes as far as Laruns. Here the road divides and brings the visitors across a splendid marble bridge over the Gave de Gabas to the romantic village of Eaux-chaudes (2 days and 6 hours' journey from London). Though the village is badly built and incapable of extension through the narrow fissure of the enclosed valley, the environs are extremely beautiful and attract many visitors from the distance. Similar vicissitudes of temperature take place as at Eaux-bonnes, requiring similar precautions as regards dress. The springs enjoyed formerly a great reputation for chronic rheumatism and neuralgia, as they all possess a great quantity of the so-called *sulfuraire*, a whitish mucous substance, different from glairine, contained in all sulphurous thermae of the Pyrenées, and analogous to the conferva filiformis sulfurata, found in the Weilbach water. Probably this gelatinous substance exercises a soothing nourishing effect on the cutaneous surface. Six springs arise at the foot of the mountain, with a range of temperature from $96·8°$ (le Clôt) to $51·8°$ (Mainvielle]. They contain only 4·7 grains of solid constituents in a quart of water, viz. 1·7 chloride of sodium, 1·12 sulphuret of sodium, 0·54 carbonate of soda, 0·64 sulphate of soda, 1·59 sulphate of lime, 0·07 silicate of lime, a trace of silicate of magnesia, of silicate of alumina and iodine, and some nitrogen. The above shows great analogy to Wildbad, both as regards temperature and composition, chloride of sodium being the chief ingredient in each, and the temperature very near the natural warmth of the blood. Hence we can readily understand its efficacy in affections of the sero-fibrous tissues. The sulphuret of sodium contained here with the sulphuraire must assist the general effect, and indicates the spa in many obstinate cutaneous diseases, especially when connected with scrofulous cachexia, and with a sluggish, lymphatic habit. The origin of the springs being much higher than the village, the water has to be conducted to the latter in pipes. This must be considered as a certain disadvantage compared with Wildbad.
The springs are employed both internally and externally.

ETRETAT, a maritime village of FRANCE, on the English Channel, 15 miles north-north-east of Havre, south-west of Fécamp Station (population 1,600), offers the advantage of very strong movements of the waves, on account of the precipitous nature of the strand, and is therefore particularly adapted to persons of vigorous constitution, with an unimpaired power of reaction.

Physician—Dr. Miramont.

FÖHR (the island of), five miles from the north-west coast of Schleswig, in the North Sea, lat. N. 54° 4', long. E. 8° 3', with an area of twenty-five square miles. The *Wilhelminen-sea-bath* lies in the village of *Wyck*, in the south-eastern part of the island, west of Flensburg, north-west of *Husum* (two or three hours' sea voyage from the latter place, which may be reached by rail in six hours from Hamburg). The downs of Sylt and Amrum, protecting the island against westerly winds, impart to it a great mildness of climate. But vicissitudes of temperature are frequent, nevertheless, and require corresponding care in being provided with warm clothing. The baths are taken about three-quarters of a mile from Wyck, in the southern part of the island below a raised shore, on a gently sloping fine sandy ground. The protection against the prevailing north-westerly winds causes the baths to have a milder and less exciting effect than those in more exposed localities with stronger waves. On the other hand, a peculiar strength of streaming is produced by the regular ebb and flow between Föhr and the opposite Halligen. Warm sea-baths, as well as rain and douche-baths, are to be had there. Along the houses of the south coast ('Sandwall') a promenade extends, generally used by the visitors, whilst towards the east a friendly plantation of oaks and fir-trees ('Königsgarten'), protected by the dam, is available. Moreover, the different villages of the island serve as points of excursion. The place is to be recommended in cases which require the bracing influence of sea-air, and the stimulating action of sea-baths, without exciting a too violent reaction by strong movement of waves ; for instance, in convalescence after protracted diseases, when a friendly unpretending social watering-place is needed to raise the depressed condition of the mind, as well as the drooping power of the body.

Physicians—Drs. Schjödte, Hitscher.

FÉCAMP, a French sea-bath, on the English Channel, at the mouth of the river Fécamp, on the branch railway from Rouen (about three hours' journey), twenty-one miles north-north-east of Havre (about one hour and three-quarters' railway journey), may be reached from Paris in about five hours and a half. Population 12,000. It offers the advantage of more accommodation and amusement than Etretat, its next neighbour, for those who require relaxation of mind and a greater variety of social amusement for a moderate outlay.

GAIS, in the canton of Appenzell, in Switzerland, south of St. Gallen station (about three hours' diligence ride), and south of Rorschach, on the lake of Constance, about two days' journey from London. Altitude 2,875'. It lies on the southern declivity of the Gabris, in a charming open valley, sheltered by surrounding green hills and mountains. The air is bracing and pure, but keen. It is protected against east and north-east winds, but exposed to the south winds, as the towering mountains lie at a distance of two leagues to the south and south-east. The summer temperature is pretty equable, but evenings and mornings are very cool. Though the moist meadows and peat grounds of the neighbourhood impart a certain humidity to the air, the high and open situation, the absence of forests and foliage, and the nature of the ground, cause a speedy absorption of moisture, and hence an equilibrium results in the atmosphere equally free from oppressive dryness and extreme humidity. But the south-west wind sometime blows with unpleasant violence. Mean barometric pressure $25\frac{1}{2}''$. Mean summer heat 68° Fahr. Epidemic diseases are very rare. Inflammatory, catarrhal, rheumatic, and gastric disorders prevail most among the inhabitants. A small shady walk runs along the back of the houses. Fine views are obtained over the valley of the Rhine at the neighbouring chapel, Am Stoos. Several other charming excursions may be made into the neighbourhood. But for weakly persons the place offers too little opportunity of sheltered promenades. Every morning at six goat-whey is brought warm from the Voralpe (three leagues distant), where it is prepared out of the milk sent down from the high Alps the previous night. The whey varies somewhat according to the conditions of the weather prior to the obtaining of the milk. After a few days' rain the whey tastes grassy and gluey, whilst in fine weather it exhibits a sweet aromatic taste. The following explanation is given by the herdsmen :—In fine weather the goats roam about the highest and most dangerous declivities, to feed upon the aromatic mountain-herbs, abounding in rich juicy ingredients, whilst in rainy weather they are kept near the huts, and are obliged to live upon the grassy, watery herbs of the impoverished soil. More than a hundred years ago Gais has been used for whey-cures in pulmonary diseases, and enjoys still the greatest reputation amongst its numerous competitors. *Whey-cures*, in appropriate, high, bracing, or mild localities, are particularly indicated for bronchial catarrh, after an acute inflammatory process, when the patients possess a weak irritable system and deficient sanguification, so that they could not bear any violent inroads or weakening courses of alkaline mineral waters. Whey contains all materials requisite for a healthy and normal metamorphosis, viz. milk-sugar, and the salts contained in animal food, with the exception of the nitrogeneous plastic constituents. Whenever, therefore, the cure of a disease requires the diminution of the nitrogenous elements of the organism, without altering the normal inorganic constituents, the whey ought to be employed according to Dr. Beneke. It is prepared in the following manner:—The fresh milk is warmed in a large copper cauldron over an open fire. A certain quantity is then taken out and put aside. Then a piece of goat's rennet cut into slices and enclosed in a small linen bag is put into the cauldron. The ' Senne' then observes whether flowers form in the milk. The quantity of rennet and the temperature of the milk must be determined with the greatest nicety ; deficiency of either causes the separated caseine to be soft and spongy, and consequently not completely separated from the whey ; on the other hand, excess of rennet or of heat decomposes different sorts of milk destined to remain in the whey, especially phosphate of lime, imparting a nauseous taste, and diminishing its curative powers. On an average, 1,000 parts of milk coagulate in half an hour from an addition of $\frac{1}{500}$ part of rennet.

The temperature is raised after the addition of the rennet to 133 Fahr. and the coagulated particles of cheese removed. The portion previously put aside is now added and the whole again heated, assuming a whitish-colour, and called cheese-milk (*Käse-milch*), whey-vinegar (*Sur*, whey having become acid, through the admixture of several species of rumex) is then added; the caseine hitherto dissolved now separates and swims like coagulated albumen on the surface. This is taken out, and the clear liquid is poured through a thin cloth into wooden tubs, which are hermetically closed and brought to the different whey establishments. The whey forms a yellow greenish liquid of a sweet aromatic flavour, sometimes slightly opaque from imperfectly separated caseine. Should the latter circumstance cause it to disagree, it might be cleared by adding white of egg. Whey may be prepared from the milk of cows, goats, &c. The following difference of composition prevails according to Valentiner:—

Ewe's Whey contain	Cow's Whey contain	100 *parts of* Goat's Whey contain
91·96	93·26	93·38 of water.
5·07	5·10	4·53 of milk-sugar.
2·13	1·08	1·14 of coagulated albumen.
0·25	0·11	0·37 of fat.
0·58	0·44	0·57 of salts and extracted substances.

This shows ewe's whey to contain almost double the amount of albuminates than cow and goat's whey, the latter containing the smallest amount of milk-sugar. Ewe's whey possesses most phosphate of lime combined with albuminates. Good whey must be almost free from fat and exhibit a neutral or at the utmost a weak acid reaction. The diuretic effect is the most marked, through the milk sugar, and great amount of water. If the sugar is not quickly absorbed it enters the intestinal canal, increases its secretion, and hence acts as a purgative, whilst increased urinary secretion is produced if the sugar becomes absorbed into the blood immediately after ingestion. If constipation arises, whey ought not to be taken fasting, when absorption is most powerful, but a few hours after breakfast. According to the experienced Dr. Heim Gais is particularly useful in nervous debility, in marasmus and emaciation after exhausting diseases, or excessive mental labour. As regards thoracic diseases, it is more indicated, according to Autenrieth, when they are based on nervous debility than on inflammatory irritation. Whey conjoined with the sanative influence of the Alpine air, is considered useful in chronic laryngeal, and bronchial catarrh, hæmoptysis and incipient phthisis due to pulmonary atony, or to suppressed catamenial flow. But the above hints must of course be subordinate to the individuality of the patients. Excellent accommodation is found in the Hotel of the Ochsen.

GREAT BRITAIN offers in its climate three different aspects according to Dr. Jackson; a *moist* aspect at the western side, a *dry* at the eastern, and a *warm* aspect at the southern side. Sudden and violent vicissitudes of temperature are prevented to some extent by its insular position. The mild winter season is principally due to the influence of the *Gulf Stream*, which is said to diffuse so much heat through the Atlantic Ocean, that it would be sufficient to transform the whole temperature of France and Great Britain from the freezing-point to summer heat. The eastern shores of America, lying in the same latitude and bordered by the same ocean, derive comparatively little advantage from it.

Winds prevail here from the south-west, west, or north-west, during nine months in the year. By having traversed a great tract of the ocean before arriving they impart a humid character to the western shores. When the western mountains check the progress of the currents, the atmosphere lowers and its aqueous vapours falls down as rain. Hence an average yearly rainfall of fifty inches and 208 rainy days characterise the western shores. During March, April, and May winds prevail from the north-east and east-north-east, and are chiefly directed to the eastern coast. Having principally travelled over land, these atmospheric currents are comparatively free from moisture, and rather apt to absorb than to give off aqueous vapours. Hence there is considerably less rainfall on the east coast, only 27 inches annually, and no more than 156 rainy days. The mean winter temperature of the east coast is two degrees less (viz. 38·2° Fahr.) than that of the west coast (40·3° Fahr.). There is less difference in the summer temperature, being about 59° in each. The western climate is thus moist, mild, and relaxing, whilst the eastern is more dry and bracing, but unfavourably influenced by easterly winds during spring. Between the two the south coast inclines more to the character of either extreme, according as it approaches more the eastern or western shore, being naturally warmer in consequence of its more southern position.

The climate of *London* is partly influenced by artificial circumstances. The multitude of human beings crowded together and the numerous buildings and manufactories cause a certain degree of warmth to be retained and diffused. Draining and paving produce, on the other hand, a certain dryness of the atmosphere. The mean *annual* temperature of London is therefore one and a half degree higher than that of its environs. But this excess of heat is greater in winter than in summer, attaining its maximum in January, when *London* is 3° warmer than the environs. In spring the temperature is nearly equal, and in May it is lower in London. The excess of winter heat is shown by Mr. Howard to occur principally during the nights, which are $3\frac{1}{10}°$ warmer than in the country. The heat of the day, on the contrary, falls about a third of a degree short of that on the open plain, probably in consequence of the solar rays being intercepted by a constant veil of smoke. The range of temperature between its extremes and the variation of the successive days are likewise considerably less in London than in its environs. London acquires and loses its heat more slowly than the environs. Hence its climate may be considered, according to Sir James Clark, as warmer (in winter), steadier and drier than that of the environs. Especially at night the sensitive valetudinarian experiences the advantage of breathing not only in a warmer and drier, but also in a purer atmosphere than during the day, when the unceasing traffic and the ubiquitous fires load the air with dust and smoke.

London is placed in the western extremity of the valley which forms the estuary of the Thames, and is intersected by the river from west to east. A little below, a smaller plain to the north is supplied with the River Lea, which falls here into the Thames. The sea is distant fifty miles to the south, and separated by rising grounds, and about as far to the east, where the Thames enters. The site is bounded by moderately high hills. The soil, loam and gravel, on a substratum of clay. Though some portions are below the level of highwater, and others covered with woods, through the perfection of the embankment and of the drainage, the climate is dry and healthy. The sun remains with us in the longest days sixteen hours and a half, and in the shortest seven hours and three-quarters (the latitude being 51° 31' N.). The mean temperature of the atmosphere is about $48\frac{1}{2}°$ Fahr., but in the more populous parts it amounts to $50\frac{1}{2}°$ Fahr. The mean temperature of the year varies periodically $4\frac{1}{2}°$ in different years, and the periods seem to be completed in seventeen years. If we assume the cycles to commence by a year of mean temperature, the coldest year occurs at the end of ten years, and the warmest at the end of seven after the coldest. The year 1816 was the coldest of a cycle, and seems to have had its parallels in 1782 and 1799. The range of temperature is 100° Fahr. viz. from the greatest heat (95° Fahr.) to the most intense cold (5° below zero). In general, however, the heat rarely rises above 80 degrees in Great Britain, and then it is often followed by thunderstorms, more or less violent and lasting, according as they fall in the lower or more hilly districts. They mostly arise from the entrance of Atlantic currents, and are therefore followed by rain and diminution of temperature. As regards cold, the average of twenty-four hours is scarcely ever under freezing-point. Continued frost is extremely rare in winter. Only occasionally a very rigorous cold season of a few weeks occurs, and yields, like the great heat, to Atlantic winds. The greatest heat occurs about a month after the summer solstice, and the greatest cold the same period after the winter solstice. The mean temperature is fully developed about a month after each equinox. The following is given as the reason of the temperature being always a month behind the sun, both as regards its increase and decrease in these latitudes. Experiments have shown that in a calm air the direct action of the solar rays will invariably raise the thermometer an equal number of degrees, whatever the temperature or season may be. The accumulated heat *felt* near the surface is obviously due to the stoppage of the rays, and to their multiplied reflections, by which means they are, as it were, absorbed and fixed in the soil and circumambient atmosphere. At the end of winter the earth commences by being gradually heated as the season advances. When the sun declines in autumn, the warmed earth gives out the heat previously received. The thermometer being placed between the sun and its reflector, the earth, the indicated heat is the product of both bodies. If, for instance, a flat screen be suddenly placed before a fire, no heat is reflected till the screen has absorbed a sufficient quantity of rays to get heated itself. The earth must be considered as a screen behind the thermometer. Without this effect the maximum and minimum heat would exist at the solstices, and the mean at the equinoxes; for the quantity of parallel rays falling on a given area is greatest when they are vertical and smallest when they are oblique, and null in a perfectly horizontal position. As the sun declines to the north, we derive increased heat, in proportion to his altitude; but we perceive it less, as a part is absorbed by the earth. But when he declines in the autumn towards the south, we receive less heat, but feel more warmth, on account of a certain quantity given off by the heated earth.

The characteristic of the British climate is its variable temperature, exhibiting very great ranges within a few days. Most of this vicissitude is due to the moon, which disturbs the density of the atmosphere by its gravity, and produces in the temperate latitudes various currents, differing as regards temperature, moisture, and electricity. Thus great variety of weather ensues, modified, however, by the influence of the sun.

The mean height of barometer is 29·8 inches; the average annual rainfall, 24·83 inches. The character of the years corresponds to their mean temperature, the warm ones being uniformly dry, and the cold ones wet. The character of the prevailing winds is westerly; the mean of De Luc's hygrometer for the climate, 66°.

By temperature the winter begins December 7, and lasts 89 days (90 in leap-years); mean temperature, 37·76°; the medium of twenty-four hours ranges from $34\frac{1}{2}°$ to $40°$.

The predominant winds of the season are south-west at the commencement and end, northerly in the middle. Mean height of barometer, 29·80 inches, with a range of 2·25. Mean evaporation, 3·58 inches; this is a third less than in proportion to the mean temperature, showing unusual *dampness* of the air. De Luc's hygrometer averages 78°. Average rainfall, 5·86 inches—greatest at the commencement, and gradually declining.

The actual quantity of atmospheric vapour is now at its lowest proportion, notwithstanding the sensible indications of moisture during the short frosts, and gradually increases with temperature and evaporation. In consequence of this low condition of vapour and the weak electricity, in mild weather the clouds are easily resolved into rain.

Great frosts are preceded here by continued thick mists, through the condensation of the vapour emitted from the rivers and from the moist soil. Still the inhabitants suffer more here from the cold than in higher latitudes, partly from an unequal provision being made against occasional unforeseen severity of weather, and partly from the changes appearing rather suddenly, whilst in continental climates the *gradual* increase of cold prepares the constitution against its baneful influence.

By temperature, Spring commences on March 6, and lasts 93 days, the temperature rising from 40° to 58°; mean, 48·94°. But the increase of temperature effected by the approach of the sun is counteracted in the fore part of the spring by *northerly* and *easterly* winds, but in the latter part it is proportionally promoted by *southerly* winds. Evaporation is vigorous, and often followed by showers (occasionally with thunder and hail). The temperature, therefore, does not steadily rise from day to day, but by sudden starts, when the sunshine breaks up previously cold and cloudy weather. The vapour, abundantly thrown up into colder regions above, decomposes after some time, causing a fresh fall of temperature, amidst wind, showers, and hail, with occasional frosty nights.

Notwithstanding these changes, the heat and vapour accumulate, the barometer averaging 29·83 inches; the extreme elevations and depressions diminish; and by the end of the season the range is limited to $1\frac{1}{2}$ inches; mean range, 1·81. Evaporation, 8·85 inches—about a sixth *more* than indicated by the mean temperature. In correspondence with this state of dryness, De Luc's hygrometer shows 61°. Average rainfall, 4·81 inches. Though rain gradually increases, it is exceeded by the evaporation; hence the soil is uniformly dry. In the commencement of the season the lower atmosphere becomes clear and transparent, but the sunshine is often eclipsed for long periods by a close veil of clouds hanging low in the sky; at other times the easterly or northerly winds drive clouds to the opposite quarters of the horizon with little modification; but towards the latter part of the season clouds connected with variable breezes traverse the sky in succession, and bring on showers of opaque hail or even snow. A snow-storm in this season occasionally proves the forerunner of the first hot weather, developed about ten or fourteen days afterwards. A wet spring does not appear ungenial here, provided it be followed by a warm and dry summer.

On the 7th of June summer begins, *by temperature*, and lasts 93 days. The mean temperature is 60·66° F., or 11·72° above that of spring. The medium of twenty-four hours ranges from 58° to 65°. The mean height of the barometer is 29·87 inches. The atmosphere now acquires the greatest quantity of heat and vapour, and consequently the greatest barometric weight from the vertical rays of the sun. As our pole inclines more towards the sun, the moon becomes depressed as regards our latitude, and consequently the density and temperature of the atmosphere become more equable and uniform. The predominating winds are those which range from west to north. Mean evaporation is 11·58 inches—above a fourth more than indicated by the temperature. De Luc's hygrometer points to 52°. Mean rainfall, 6·68 inches. North-west currents bring us fair weather and sunshine, unless interfered with by southerly currents with an easterly direction, which would most likely mix with the western current, and produce rain and thunder while being decomposed.

Autumn begins, *by temperature*, the 8th of September, and lasts 90 days. Mean temperature, 49·37°, or 11·29° below the summer. Medium of the day declines from 58° to 40°. Mean height of barometer, 29·78 inches— 0·09 below that of summer; prevailing winds are south-west. Evaporation, 6·44 inches—or a sixth part less than indicated by the temperature. De Luc's hygrometer shows 72°. Average rainfall, 7·44 inches. Proportion of rain increases the whole season. The earth now acquires the requisite moisture for its springs and deeply-rooted vegetables. All these changes are due to the return of the sun towards the south. Through the daily declining heat, the accumulated atmospheric vapour becomes decomposed, and its loss is not made up, as in summer, by new vapours. Hence heavy rains, with a lower barometer. The air being more saturated, evaporation falls short of the corresponding temperature. Nevertheless, the fore part of the season is the most delightful in the year here. When the decomposition of the vapours is just commencing, or the atmospheric electricity gives buoyancy to the suspended particles, a pleasant calm sometimes prevails, with perfect sunshine, diffusing a rich tint on the landscape as the day declines. The latter part of autumn and commencement of winter are subject to gales from the south-west, chiefly at night, forming part of a subsiding set of currents. In day time the north-east breezes, the result of sunshine, prevail almost exclusively, and may be considered as ascending currents.

That the westerly gales come from above seems to be shown by their occasional great violence, for the air acquires a westerly momentum in a higher latitude by revolving round its axis in a larger circle, and this momentum it may bring with it when suddenly turned northward. It is even surmised that the sudden depression of the barometer, attaining its minimum during the greatest force of the wind, may be due to the actual momentary loss of atmospheric gravity by the centrifugal force of the air.

The above description of the climate shows that for persons inclined to thoracic diseases it must have many disadvantages, and indeed the mortality from consumption is higher here than in continental localities of the same latitude. Though the cold is more intense there in winter, the temperature increases gradually, and thus prepares the constitution for its severity, and compels the inhabitants to protect themselves by warmer clothing; whilst here the mildness of winter often causes a minor perception of cold, inducing a less warm mode of clothing, and when the sudden vicissitudes into cold or damp weather occur, the body is insufficiently protected against the sudden tide of the circulation towards the central organs. The weakest portion is then liable to be congested, previous bronchial irritation becomes aggravated, or new processes of pulmonary affection are instituted. On the other hand, it must be stated that the British climate possesses a *conservative* character, and nowhere are so many old persons seen with all the vigour of manhood than in this country. Indeed, it is very rare to meet here with aged individuals hobbling along with a bent back and a feeble step. The reasons are obvious. The temperature is never so hot in summer or so cold in winter as to interfere with the performance of the regular functions of the system. The food, simple and substantial, plays likewise an important part, not only in promoting longevity, but in keeping up the vital stamina and youthful vigour for a longer period. The muscular apparatus of the stomach is not weakened and distended, previous to its commencement of work, by the imbibition of a warm liquid with a little nutritive matter in the shape of soup. The palate is not artificially coaxed by numerous culinary contrivances into an undue consumption of made-up dishes. A meal here answers the purpose of supplying the waste which the system has previously undergone. People rise from their meals without oppression, to pursue their ordinary avocations with that unswerving energy inspired and kept up by the frequently uninviting character of the horizon. The average annual mortality of London is reckoned at 25 out of 1,000 inhabitants; that of all England, 22; in the healthiest districts, 16 to 18; in Paris, 33; in Vienna, 39.*

Most inhabitants of this metropolis, especially of the middle class, do not reside in the same houses in which they pursue their daily duties; but they strictly separate private life from business. Whilst the latter is carried on in a central part, the residence is chosen at some distance. This ensures less prolonged working hours, and a greater facility of throwing off business thoughts by the change of scene every evening. In former times, the choice of private habitation was restricted to walking or omnibus distances; but through the spread of railway accommodation, places from six to twenty miles distant are almost considered as suburbs nowadays. But however rational it must be thought to hurry after work to a less noisy and more open locality, the other extreme of selecting greater and greater distances has its decided drawbacks. In fact, a locality too exposed is for many morbid dispositions as injurious as a too confined and close space for others. Nothing is more connected with prevention or production of disease than the private residence, and even more so than if it was constantly inhabited; for in the latter case the constitution would become more readily inured to it. We ought not only to enquire which is in itself the most healthy site, but also what will be the effect of the daily change? Will it be useful, for instance, to delicate individuals, who have breathed a whole winter day the warm air of the confined city, to be suddenly turned out in the evening into a bleak exposed atmosphere of a distant and high suburb? Another point deserving consideration is the mental peculiarity of the traveller. Persons endowed with an easy, calm mental calibre, regular in their habits, and steady in all their pursuits, may be benefited and usefully stimulated by the daily vicissitudes of temperature. On the other hand, nervous, anxiously-disposed and impulsive individuals, who have to undergo the daily hurry and mental worry *antécedent* to the railway journey, will often find *this regular addition* to the other wearing anxiety of the day to play the part of the last straw, which 'breaks the camel's back.' They will *feel* more braced and refreshed when they arrive in town, and be less liable to minor complaints; but causes of severer derangements accumulate in the system, and ultimately lead to severe diseases, or mal-assimilation, *apparently* unconnected with their mode of living.

In selecting a residence, the peculiar individual disposition should, therefore, invariably be taken into account; for it may be predicted with certainty that diseases and mortality would diminish if each family, instead of merely consulting convenience and taste in the choice of a locality, were to ask their medical attendant whether the particular spot chosen is adapted to their constitutions. Whilst, for instance, a high and exposed situation will have a bracing and salutary effect on vigorous individuals, it may prove injurious, especially in the inclement season, to persons affected with a phthisical tendency.

* Annales Hygiène, October 1850, p. 362.

The following short hints on the altitude and soil of the various parts of the metropolis may afford some guidance in this respect.

A line drawn from *Hendon*, in the *north-west*, to *East Wickham*, in the *south-east*, shows us, first, in the western portion of Hendon, an altitude of 220 feet over high-water mark, and a superstratum of gravel over the London clay. The other parts are devoid of gravel. To the left of this line the altitude gradually diminishes, in the direction of the river *Brent*, to 90 feet above *Willesden*, and then increases again to 146 north-east of *Willesden*, 120 east, 158 and 140 south-east. Passing the North-Western Railway, we descend from 120 to 100 feet at the *Paddington* Canal, to 80 at the north, 60 at the south of *Wormwood Scrubs*, then we descend to 40 and 20— all on clay soil. Proceeding still southward, we meet with brick-earth as superstratum, surrounded in the form of an island by a strip of gravel, bordered by Notting Hill on the east (lying mostly on clay), and Hammersmith on the south (built on gravel).

If we take up our original line, and journey from Hendon towards *Hampstead*, the ground (clay) lowers first, and then rises again to 430 feet at Hampstead Hill, which has a superstratum of *Bagshot sand*; we then gradually descend to 80 feet at Hampstead Road, to 60 at Gray's Inn Road, all clay soil, till the line intersects the eastern portion of Holborn Hill, which is built on gravel. The line then passes through Cheapside (48 feet high, built, like the whole city, on brick-earth); crosses St. Paul's Cathedral (412 feet high); and on proceeding to the river passes over gravel soil, which encircles the city, extending on the south to the river, on the east as far as East India Docks, on the north-east along the Mile End Road, not quite to the Regent's Canal (whence a strip of brick-earth stretches as far as Victoria Park); on the north, from Bishopsgate Street (inclusive) to Finsbury, City Road, and Islington ; on the west, not quite to Farringdon Street.

The line now crosses the river (clay soil) obliquely over London Bridge ; proceeds through Bermondsey (below high-water mark, but built on gravel), this side the Greenwich Railway ; then passes through Deptford (gravel), over the river Ravensbourne, and arrives at Greenwich (20 feet high), possessing siliceous sands as far as the Observatory (210 feet high), and pebble beds afterwards; then the line crosses *Blackheath* (130 to 100 feet high), pebble bed ; then passes over clay soil to *Shooter's Hill* (412 feet high, with a superstratum of gravel at the top) ; the line descends then again on clay to 300, 200, 180 feet, and arrives at *East Wickham* (pebble bed, 150 feet high).

All through London the clay rests on a bed of chalk.

Among the suburbs on the north side of the Thames, *Brompton* enjoys the mildest and most equable winter climate. Built on gravel, with a moderate elevation of 20 feet between Chelsea (10 feet) on the south, and Kensington (40 to 60 feet) on the north, it is somewhat protected against north winds, without being so enclosed as to prevent evaporation or free circulation of the atmosphere. Its northern neighbour, *Kensington* (from 40 to 60 feet) has a border of brick-earth on the south ; then clay, more to the north ; then gravel. It has great advantages in the numerous trees and open squares; but as it partly rests on the slope of a hill—for the ground rises towards the north-west (Notting Hill) to 125, and towards the north (Bayswater) to 80 feet—it must be exposed to greater vicissitudes of temperature than Brompton : still it would be a more desirable residence for the whole year, especially the eastern and western part, than Brompton, which is too relaxing in summer.

Bayswater, and particularly that part intersected by Queen's Road, enjoys the advantage of a moderately high elevation (80 feet), and of being partly built on gravel soil. The air is bracing in summer and not too bleak in winter, as the ground, though a little lower on the clayey *Westbourne Grove* (60 feet), exhibits some eminences further north, and higher hills still more northerly. *Regent's Park*, though somewhat more elevated, from 80 feet to 206 (at Primrose Hill), is built on clay, and lying on a declivity of the hill, the moisture will be more apt to be retained on the ground, evaporation being further somewhat impeded through the steep northern hills. The climate will therefore be mild in winter, but somewhat relaxing in summer. *St. John's Wood* (from 140 to 160 feet high), also built on clay, has a bleaker climate in winter, being more exposed to vicissitudes of temperature, with the disadvantage of retaining moisture longer than gravelly soil would; whilst the neighbouring Hampstead heights, on the north-east, afford only partial protection against northerly winds. In summer, however, it is a very desirable residence.

Hampstead Hill (430 feet) and *Highgate Hill* (412 feet high), both having siliceous sands of the Bagshot series as a superstratum, whilst the other gravelly soil mentioned is only composed of *drift, gravel, and sand,* are very bracing, and would be extremely well adapted for sanitaria, to admit convalescents after severe and exhausting diseases. Three or four weeks spent there would probably have a more restorative effect than double the time at the ordinary home. But, of course, for a winter residence both places are too bleak, and might, by the vicissitudes of temperature, produce bronchial and pulmonary as well as rheumatic diseases, whenever a predisposition exists to these ailments.

In the north-east, *Dalston* and the southern part of *Hackney* are built on gravel, and have a moderate elevation of 40 feet; the climate is therefore mild in winter, and somewhat less relaxing in summer than Brompton. That portion of Hackney surrounding London Fields is more humid and relaxing than the eastern and northern part. *Victoria Park*, built on gravel, with the exception of a strip of brick-earth at the south-western termination, is not very elevated, having an altitude of 40' at the western frontier, and of 20' where it approaches *Bow* (built on gravel), at the south-eastern frontier. It is therefore very mild, but too relaxing in hot summers. North of *Kingsland Railway Station*, till very near Stoke Newington, the houses are built on brick-earth, and enjoy an elevation of 60 feet (this includes part of West Hackney). *Stamford Hill* (97 feet high), in the north, to 80 feet towards *Upper Clapton*, is built on gravel, and also the contiguous portion of Lower Clapton. It has a very bracing and salubrious climate. *Stoke Newington* (80 feet), built on clay, lies on a somewhat sloping ground, from west to east, as the north-western Highgate hills gradually descend towards Stoke-Newington. The latter, therefore, shares some of the disadvantages belonging to Regent's Park.

Highbury, situated to the south and west of Stoke Newington, is built on a ground rising to 132 feet (Highbury Place and Hill), with strong clays in the west, and brick-earth in the east: from here the ground gently slants again to 120 and 100 feet. The climate thus partakes of a bracing and mild character, the altitude allowing a free circulation of the atmosphere; and though the ground would absorb moisture more readily if it was gravel, the eminence on which it stands, with the sloping circumference, favours evaporation.

West Ham, east of Bow (built on gravel), borders on a bed of peat and alluvium, which stretches from the north-western part of the River Lea, along the Leyton, Hackney, and Plaistow marshes, and extends beyond Barking Level, with an altitude of only 10 feet in the north, and diminishing towards the south.

Walthamstow, north-east of Stamford Hill, rises from 80 to 100 feet, with clay soil, except the centre, which consists of gravel. *Snaresbrook*, its eastern neighbour, enjoys an altitude of 100 feet, with the advantage of a gravelly soil. The ground slants to the south (80 to 60 feet). *Wanstead, Stratford*, north-east of Bow, with an altitude of 20 to 10 feet; *West Ham* to its south, *Plaistow* to the south of the latter, *East Ham* to the east, and *Barking* still more easterly; all lie on gravel soil, with a low elevation, and exposed somewhat to the neighbouring marshy exhalations. As regards the more distant western suburbs, *Hammersmith* lies partly on gravel, towards the south, and on brick-earth in the northern part (10 feet), which soil extends to *Shepherd's Bush*, and considerably beyond *Uxbridge Road*; *Chiswick*, west of Hammersmith, is built on brick-earth, and likewise *Fulham*. Being contiguous to the Thames, they have a very slight elevation; but the Thames becoming a pure river through the deviation of the sewage by means of the stupendous main drainage works lately accomplished, the freshness imparted to the air by the rapid course of a tidal stream will afford some compensation for the deficient altitude.

South of the Thames we have *Barnes*, built on brick-earth, rising towards the south to 20 feet (gravel soil) on the common. *Putney Heath*, rising towards the south-east to 163 feet, with gravelly soil, surrounded by sandy clays. *Putney*, south of Fulham, gravel soil (20 feet). *Wandsworth*, to the east, same soil, with an altitude rising to 60 feet, intersected by the river *Wandle*; the common to the south-east on gravel soil, surrounded by clay, rising from 40 to 93 feet. *Battersea Fields*, south of Chelsea, on brick-earth. *Clapham*, on gravel soil, rising southward from 20 to 60 feet, and to 93 feet (Clapham Common). *Camberwell*, to the east, gravel soil, 10 to 20 feet, then rising southward on sandy clays to 40, 60, 80, and 130 feet, with *Peckham*, on sand and mottled clay to the east, 20 feet high, separated by shelly clays from the southern *Peckham Rye*, rising from 20 to 40 feet, and possessing soil of *striped sand*, with a southern border of pebble bed; moreover, rising ground toward the east from 60 to 148 feet (*Nunhead, Telegraph Hill, Hatcham* on sandy clay), and toward the south from 60 to 80, 100, and 160 to 284 feet in the south-east (*Forest Hill*) built on clay, and also towards the west, from 60 to 80 feet (*Denmark Hill* rising to 130 feet, with gravel in the centre and clay at the circumference), afford an excellent protection against north-eastern, south-eastern, and south-western winds. This confirms the popular belief in its salubrity for persons affected with bronchial irritation or incipient phthisis. According to the above geological characteristics, it must prove especially useful, as a summer residence, in cases of profuse bronchial secretion, whilst in severe winters, and where the cough exhibits a dry and irritative character, Brompton would deserve the preference. Those who desire further information on the geological condition of London, are referred to the excellent chart of London by R. W. Mylne, Esq. F.R.S. But apart from the natural position and character of a locality, we have to consider its artificial characteristics. For, however favourable the site, its advantages may be diminished by numerous buildings intercepting air and light, with numerous inhabitants contaminating the air and diminishing its health-giving oxygen. Hence a list of the population and mortality, compiled from the pamphlet of Mr. Coke ('Census of the British Empire'), will form an appropriate conclusion of the subject.

	Population	Mortality in 1,000	Average Elevation above Highwater Mark
LONDON	2,582,635	23·6	39
West Districts:			
Kensington	153,233	18·6	44
Chelsea	59,980	24·8	12
St. George's, Hanover Square	80,488	17·1	34
Westminster	66,642	25·1	2
St. Martin's in the Fields	23,638	22·2	35
St. James's, Westminster	35,865	21·5	43
North Districts:			
Marylebone	159,652	22·5	100
Hampstead	15,545	16	350
St. Pancras	182,919	21·7	80
Islington	125,310	19·5	88
Hackney	70,862	18·8	55
Central Districts:			
St. Giles's	54,097	26·7	68
Strand	43,686	23·7	50
Holborn	45,741	25·6	53
Clerkenwell	65,205	21·7	63
St. Luke's	55,526	25·4	48
East London	42,539	24·9	42
West London	27,988	23·5	28
London, City	50,741	20	38
East Districts:			
Shoreditch	119,298	23·1	48
Bethnal Green	97,549	22·2	36
Whitechapel	79,361	27·8	28
St. George's in the East	48,627	27·1	15
Stepney and Mile End	120,203	24	16
Poplar	63,172	22·7	9

	Population	Mortality in 1,000	Average Elevation above Highwater Mark
South Districts:			
St. Saviour's, Southwark	35,878	27·7	2
St. Olave's, Southwark	19,214	27·4	2
Bermondsey	53,241	24·8	0
St. George's, Southwark	53,666	25·8	0
Newington	73,486	22·8	· 2 below
Lambeth	150,666	22·1	3
Wandsworth	60,572	18·8	22
Camberwell	63,078	21·6	4
Rotherhithe	21,152	23·8	0
Greenwich	113,513	24·8	8
Lewisham	50,293	16 8	28

The mortality in London has decreased in the last decennium. Whilst in the ten years from 1840–1849 25·1 died per 1,000 inhabitants; in 1850–1859 the mortality fell to 23·6 per 1,000; so that to 1,000 deaths of the first decennium we had but 946 in the second.

' Our lives are thus preserved from many dire calamities, and our health is mainly under the care and special guidance of this highly educated and scientific class of professional men (medical officers of health), appointed pursuant to the Public Health Act; and it is also ascertained, through the Registrar-General's department, that during the time the Act has been in operation, the death-rate throughout all England has been *reduced* about 0·52 per 1,000 in the year. But we must still look for a greater improvement. In an average of ten years, calculated to the same population, in proportion to

100 deaths in Whitechapel . . there were 58 in Hampstead.
100 ,, St. Saviour's, Southwark . . . . ,, ,, 61 ,, Lewisham.
100 ,, St. Olave's, Southwark . . . . ,, ,, 62 ,, St. George's, Hanover Square.
100 ,, St. George's in the East . . . . ,, ,, 67 ,, Kensington.
100 ,, St. Giles's . . . ,, ,, 70 ,, Hackney.
100 ,, St. George's, Southwark . . . . ,, ,, 73 ,, Wandsworth.
100 ,, Holborn . . . ,, ,, 76 ,, Islington.
100 ,, St. Luke's . . . ,, ,, 79 ,, London, City.
100 ,, Westminster . . ,, ,, 86 ,, St. James's, Westminster.
100 ,, East London . . ,, ,, 87 ,, St. Pancras.
100 ,, Greenwich . . . ,, ,, 88 ,, Clerkenwell.
100 ,, Bermondsey . . ,, ,, 87 ,, Camberwell.
100 ,, Chelsea . . . . ,, ,, 89 ,, Lambeth.
100 ,, Rotherhithe. . . ,, ,, 83 ,, Bethnal Green.
100 ,, Strand . . . . ,, ,, 95 ,, Marylebone.'

INFLUENCE OF HABITUAL RAILWAY TRAVELLING ON PUBLIC HEALTH.

As the *mode of reaching* the various rural spots forms an extremely important link in the chain of sanitary measures, I should think this treatise incomplete without bringing before the reader extracts of the most important points mentioned in the excellent report of the 'Lancet' Sanitary Commission as regards *the influence of railway travelling on public health.**

In the year 1825 there was, in the whole world, only one railway carriage built to convey passengers. It ran on the first railway between Stockton and Darlington, and bore on its panels the motto

'Periculum privatum, publica utilitas.'

Materials and purpose of present enquiry.—Medical men are often asked whether they consider railway travelling prejudicial to health. The very frequency of the interrogation points to the conclusion that a vague dread of certain undefined consequences peculiar to this mode of travelling, has been gradually growing up in the public mind. In his evidence before a Committee of the House of Commons, in 1859, Lord Shaftesbury said, 'The very power of locomotion keeps persons in a state of great nervous excitement, and it is worthy of attention to what an extent this effect prevails. I have ascertained that many persons who have been in the habit of travelling by railway, have been obliged to give it up in consequence of the effect on the nervous system.'

Social changes.—People in the present day do more work with less recreation than at any former time. In the eighteenth century, the previously enjoined public exercises were gradually discontinued. But, even then, a journey by horse or coach had the advantage of affording a period of rest from anxieties whilst on the road, and of physical exercise in the open air; the mind being necessarily diverted by the personal incidents of the journey.

The following remarks are extracted from the communication of Mr. W. Bridges Adams *on the construction of rail and carriage* :—

Ordinary carriages on common roads have flexible springs, and an irregular rough surface to roll over. Railway carriages have very rigid springs, and a regular rough surface to roll over. The *large irregular* concussions of the highway are converted on the railway into a series of *smaller regular concussions.* In most vehicles, there are two varieties of

---

* Hardwicke, 192 Piccadilly, June 1862.

movement—the vibratory and oscillatory. Vehicles *without oscillation* are heavy of draught. The less the amount of oscillation, the more perfect should be the springs, to allow the wheels to yield rapidly.

Why should the railway produce effects which the common road does not? There is but one answer: the *friction* is practically greater in amount on the rail than it is on the road; because, in lieu of four wheels, a pair of garden-rollers are used, the wheel and axle moving solidly together. Now, a garden-roller will only move forward in a straight line. Railways consist of straight lines and curves. But the so-called straight lines are not straight *relatively to the action of the wheels*, but a series of irregular curves.

With ordinary road-wheels, the friction is not incessant, and only takes place when bearing equally over the width. Moreover, the surface on which they roll is more or less yielding, and vibration does not pass unbroken through the wheel to the vehicle. But, as railway wheels bear on a hard surface, the vibration is considerable. The probability is, that from a fourth to a sixth of the whole movement is *sledging*, increasing with the velocity. In this mode a great amount of surplus power is required.

The train is guarded by the action of the side flanges, and not by the tractive power. As the flanges approach the rail, there is a constant succession of blows, analogous to the jerks experienced when a vehicle is driven along the edge of the kerbstones in the streets.

The first thing to do is to settle the quarrel between wheel and rail, which, as Stephenson said, should be as man and wife, but at present are a very ill-assorted couple.

In *passenger-carriages*, the long springs somewhat modify the sensations experienced. But, being very rigid and only slightly curved, they afford relief to a very limited extent.

Effects of railway travelling on healthy persons.

As elucidating the *chilling influence* of railway travelling, Dr. C. J. B. Williams states, *inter alia* :—

' Unquestionably the great charm and superiority of railway travelling is its *speed*; and in this fast age of rapid progress it would be an ungracious task to put a drag upon the wheels, provided that this charming velocity can be maintained without risk to health. To say nothing of the perils from accidents, the velocity of railway travelling may bring with it dangers of another kind. I allude to the injurious influence of the draughts of air. The velocity of a railway train brings it in collision with the air to a degree that amounts to a high wind. In the thirty or forty sultry days which may occur during our summer months, this fine breeze may be all very pleasant; but in the remaining 300 days and upwards, this current is too cold to be borne in safety. The speed of the railway intensifies the cold, and renders the draught of air dangerous, even when its temperature may not be lower than 50° or even 60° Fahr. The disorders which I have found to be most commonly excited by the influence of cold in railway travelling, are the various catarrhal affections of the respiratory organs, sore throats, earache, toothache, pleurisy, pneumonia, and various forms of rheumatism, particularly lumbago and sciatica. It is very remarkable how many cases of serious pulmonary disease in my experience have dated their origin to cold caught in railway travelling. The plurality of English folk prefer being chilled to their notion of being suffocated. Foreigners, on the Continent, commonly go to the opposite extreme. But I am confident that the graver error is on the side of our countrymen. In cold weather and in fast trains, there is vastly more risk of chill from open windows than of suffocation or any other evil from closed ones. In conclusion, I would advert to the *desiccating* effect on the skin and mucous passages produced by long railway journeys, as another result of the operation of the current of air, which may be mitigated by the same means of exclusion and protection; but it is more completely removed by restoring the action of the skin by active exercises or by a warm bath.'

Physiological influence.—Habitual travellers are under the necessity of twice daily ' catching the train,' and to a certain extent all their actions prior to departure in the morning and afternoon are influenced by the pervading sense of this anxiety. Dr. Brown-Séquard observes, that the anxiety is so predominant in many otherwise healthy constitutions that it produces often a practical incapacity for habitual travelling; and must evidently, when it falls short of this, frequently be injurious.

Effects on the muscular system.—The immediate effect of being placed in a vehicle subjected to rapid short vibrations and oscillations, is that a considerable number of muscles are called into action and maintained in a condition of alternating contractile effort throughout the whole journey, and to this constant strain on the muscular system must be ascribed a part of that sense of bodily fatigue, almost amounting to soreness, which is felt after a long journey.

Influence on the cerebral and spinal centres.—The hollow cavities of the spine and cranium, thus partially steadied by the muscles attached to them, contain the great nervous centres, to which concussion of any kind is so peculiarly hurtful that they are naturally cushioned on exquisitely-devised water beds, or are slung by fibrous ligaments, which have the effect of deadening the shocks of ordinary movements. The jolting of a railway carriage is a series of small and rapid concussions, and it is worthy to be noted that these increase in proportion to the rate of speed, and that most of the trains by which season ticket-holders travel are express.

The seats of carriages.—The well-padded and springy seats of first-class carriages do much to obviate the mischief of these concussions. In condemning the third-class passengers to sit on hard wooden benches, which transmit without mitigation the shocks incidental to the movement of the carriage, the railway companies submit them unnecessarily to one acknowledged source of evil influence on health.

Of mental influences.—The mental condition of passengers by train is commonly, perhaps, sufficiently placid and unconcerned, but several eminently careful observers have alluded to an often experienced condition of uneasiness, scarcely amounting to actual fear, which pervades the generality of travellers by rail. The possibility of collision is constantly present to such persons. So, too, the frequent lateness of trains, and the bad time which they keep, are causes of anxiety.

Effects on the eye.—Objects on the road are passed with such velocity that they only produce momentary impressions on the retina, and thus the visual powers are severely tried. The rapidity with which the brain is necessitated to take cognizance of the retinal images taxes it also more or less heavily. When the traveller sets himself to read, he imposes yet further labour on the eye in tracing the shifting characters of his book or newspaper, and also on the brain.

Impressions through the ear.—The rattle and noise which accompany the progress of the train create an incessant vibration on the tympanum, and thus influence the brain through the nerve of hearing. Assailed through the avenues of the eye and ear, and subject to concussions due to vertical movement and lateral oscillation communicated through the trunk, and actually transmitted by the bony walls of the head when it rests against the back of the carriage, the brain is apt to suffer certain physiological changes. Amongst the well-known effects are occasional dizziness, headache, sickness, and mental fatigue.

Rapid ageing of season ticket-holders.—One of the leading physicians of the metropolis says, ' Travelling a few years since on the Brighton line very frequently, I became familiar with the faces of a number of the regular passengers on that line. Recently I had again occasion to travel several times on the same line. I know well how to allow for gradual deterioration by age and care; but I have never seen any set of men so *rapidly aged* as these seem to me to have been in the course of those few years. It is idle to say that journeys from one end of London to the other occupy as long or a longer period of time, for the hurry, anxiety, rapid movement, noise, and other physical disadvantages of railway travelling, are peculiar to that method of conveyance, and a railway journey of an hour, at the rate of fifty miles, is almost as fatiguing as half a day's journey on the road.'

Diminution in number of season ticket-holders.—It is the inconvenience so endured that may probably have produced the remarkable falling off in the number of season tickets issued to the public, as shown by the Government returns. The number of season ticket-holders in England and Wales in 1859 was 35,322; in 1860, it had fallen to 30,500.

Question of Life Assurance.—A physician, who has studied the subject of the duration of life in relation to insurance states, that he makes a rule of inquiring of intending assurers whether they are in the habit of taking such long journeys, not with an eye to the probabilities of accident, but in the conviction that the health is likely in the end to be impaired by them, and any tendency to disease to be fostered and exaggerated.

The relations of railway travelling to disease.—Much evidence has been adduced to show that, *where predisposition exists*, railway travelling may become the exciting cause of cerebral disease. The first and most common symptom of disturbance thus produced is *sleeplessness*, with noise and singing in the ears. This is the earliest troublesome symptom of over-work amongst the experienced engine-drivers and guards.

Apoplexy.—Where there is any reason to suspect a tendency to apoplexy, railway travelling should unquestionably be considered as an element of danger. The sudden death of Lord Canterbury in a railway carriage caused the subject to be much discussed some few years since. In a communication from Dr. W. Rogers, Winslow, Bucks, fourteen years surgeon to the railway works at Wolverton, he mentions having been called to several cases in which persons had been seized with apoplexy while travelling.

Where disease of the bones of the spine exists there is an obvious unfitness for habitual railway travelling.

As regards *diseases of the ear*, Mr. Harvey mentions having recently had under his notice two persons, in whom headache, accompanied by deafness and incessant noises in the ears, was a prominent symptom, regularly produced by railway journeys taken to and from Brighton daily. These cases, and others in the same way, resisted all kinds of treatment, until the vibrations and travelling were relinquished.

Some individuals suffer from vertigo, faintness, and nausea, on riding backwards in any close carriage. Dr. Williams inclines to think that this is caused by some disorder of the cerebral circulation, in a manner similar to sea-sickness. The backward motion promotes the afflux of blood to the anterior lobes of the brain with a corresponding privation of it in the cerebellum and medulla, and disturbance of the functions of the trisplanchnic and associated nerves.

Retention of the secretions.— Habitual suppression of the desire for micturition is not only a cause of inflammatory affections of the bladder, but has induced reflex paralysis of the lower extremities.

Influence on diseases of the abdominal viscera.—Dr. Brinton regards the marked influence of railway travelling in provoking hæmorrhage as specific in persons predisposed to such bleedings; and he has frequently traced epistaxis, hæmoptysis, and hæmorrhoidal bleedings to this exciting cause.

Precautions and improvements suggested—parliamentary interference. —If there has been culpable heedlessness as to the welfare of the millions of lives yearly intrusted to the charge of railway companies, it might be supposed that stringent enactments would soon be introduced bristling with penal clauses; and that the Statute Book which throws its ægis round pheasants and partridges, would also contain laws for the better protection of railway passengers.

How not to do it.—In the House of Commons, Mr. Bentinck asked the President of the Board of Trade whether, in consequence of railway accidents, it was the intention of Her Majesty's Government to introduce any measures founded on the report of the Committee on railway accidents? Mr. M. Gibson said, it did not appear, from the reports made by the inspectors to the Board of Trade, that any new circumstances had lately arisen to render desirable the interference of Government in the management of railways.

True cause of collisions.—Careful investigations led to startling revelations of the manner in which railway employés are kept at work for many hours beyond the time that their faculties remain equal to the imposed strain, and thus the lives of passengers are continually endangered.

Their prevention.—The Commission having at once directed attention to this unrecognised source of danger, an edict was shortly afterwards issued *in France*, reducing the working time of railway employés from thirteen to eight hours per day; and woe be to the company who shall disregard the Imperial mandate! But as the only despotic power in this country appears to be that of 'the railway interest,' it will, it is feared, be very long before any similar restriction becomes law among us.

Signals should be uniform on all lines, because the signal men occasionally change from one company to another, and may confuse the old and new regulations with disastrous results.

Use of colour-signals.—*Colour-blindness* exists among some men, with consequent inability to distinguish red (danger) from green (caution). Moreover, when an engine is travelling at high speed in the teeth of a sharp wind or through rain or fog, it is difficult for the best eyes to distinguish the colour of a signal, especially if suddenly exhibited.

Other causes of preventable accidents are inefficient amount and action of break-power, and a want of means of communication between guards and drivers. The Committee of 1857 recommended both these subjects as requiring attention, but in vain.

The pace.—The high rate of speed now maintained on all railways is unnecessary; whilst the increased motion it produces, and the enormous wear and tear it causes, are absolutely injurious. Its diminution would increase the safety of travellers, and was one of the many important suggestions made in the report of the Parliamentary Committee, not one of which has yet been carried into effect.

Long carriages.—According to the plan which obtains on the other side of the Atlantic, the whole length of each carriage would be open, with a passage in the centre, and a platform at each end for exit or entrance. The objection to such an innovation as being opposed to our national prejudices, is too trivial to need refutation. Indeed, it may be doubted whether that conceited spirit of exclusiveness, that *unwholesome mistrust* of our neighbours, peculiar to the travelling Englishman, is ever a healthy feeling to foster or encourage.

Safety.—Such an arrangement would afford to timid persons that sense of security which they always derive from the presence of numbers, and would prevent the distressing effects of retention, since there could be conveniences fitted at the end of each carriage. Moreover, in case of the engine leaving the rail, carriages of such length would be far less likely to follow than the short-bodied vehicles which now fly over so readily. Experiments have already proved that carriages of this length are more free from both vibration and oscillation than those in ordinary use.

Temperature.—There are probably more colds caught at railway-stations than in any other buildings. After becoming heated by previous sharp walking, travellers loiter on the platform, oftentimes in a cutting wind, to wait for the train. There is no reason why a fixed time, say two minutes, should not be allowed at every station to prevent unnecessary hurry.

From the above report it might be inferred that if small *regular* journeys are fraught with so much hidden danger, long railway journeys must be absolutely injurious. This deduction would be perfectly erroneous. In travelling great distances, the journey is the business of the day—the mind has no other task, no other difficulty, no other disturbing anxiety. It is true the concussions are rather more wearying than on the common road, but then the traveller looks forward to the pleasant prospect he will have at the termination. The elasticity of body and mind, the change of scenery, and the expulsion of business thoughts, soon wipe off the effects of the fatigue, and restore the former equilibrium. A similar effect follows *occasional* journeys. But *habitual* railway travelling has quite peculiar effects of its own.

The transition from a night's rest to the next day's work ought to be *gradual*; rising, dressing, early meal, all ought to be attended to without hurry or mental agitation, as a proper preparation for the exciting labour which has to follow. If instead of this the rest is *suddenly* interrupted and the day *commenced* with hurry and fretting, and all preparatory functions performed under the dread of missing the train, *as evidenced by the constant study of the watch*, and if the same process of mental anxiety is undergone at the *termination* of the day's work, this daily *addition* to the already excessive mental wear and tear must *ultimately* impair the stamina, resisting power and nutrition of the organism. Hence habitual railway travellers are, as a rule, free from *small* complaints, and apparently healthier and more vigorous the first years of the change than formerly, but in later periods they become more subject to *severe* ailments, based on mal-assimilation and on affections of the nervous centres.

Yet as the constant increase of the population *compels* frequent resort to distant railway residences, how can the benefit of a beautiful rural spot be enjoyed without detriment to health? Simply by *ignoring the time-table, and never hurrying to catch a train*. Let the traveller take his chance, as in former omnibus times, and rather wait inside the station till he can proceed to his business or his home by the next train. But if he neglects this certainly difficult rule, and persists in hurrying daily from rest to work and from work to rest, with a great amount of mental labour compressed between these two exciting journeys, he can as surely reckon on an eventual injury of some vital organ as he witnesses the effects of drops of water constanly falling on a solid rock. Whilst unmoved by the most violent torrent, its resisting mass gradually yielded to the incessant dropping, and became at last hollowed out at its most exposed position.

HEIDEN, the most celebrated whey establishment of Appenzell (after Gais), at the north-eastern border of the Appenzell Mountains, 2,424′ over the level of the sea (1,200′ over that of the Lake of Constance). The upper part of the village is built on a plateau, which affords a charming view of the Lake of Constance (1½ leagues distant), and of the Bregenz, Bavarian, and Suabian Mountains. It is enclosed by the promontories of the mountain chain; the lower older portion is situated in a pleasant valley called Bissau, bordered at the background by the Bischofsberg, Kaien, and other mountains, which offer the most beautiful views of the Lake, of Thurgau, of the Rhine valley, of the Bregenz and Tyrolese Mountains, of the Rigi, and of the green meadows and villages studding the distant hills. The climate is mild and bracing, but unfortunately the place is mercilessly exposed to the sun, through the absence of shady walks, though most charming excursions may be made into the neighbourhood. Its distance from Rheineck station (to the east) is one league; from St. Gallen (to the west) three. *Physicians*—Drs. Küng, Beck, and Benzinger, of Altstätden.

Heiden offers the further advantage of possessing a bathing establishment *im Werd*, fed by a chalybeate spring, with some smell of sulphuretted hydrogen. The visitors enjoy a more sheltered climate than at Gais, and a greater variety of residence. For besides the beautiful ' Freyhof, ' built on the southern declivity of the plateau, in the midst of the village, with its open balcony and well-cultivated garden, accommodation may be had at the ' Löwe,' and at some commodious private houses. The population numbers 2,500. Opposite the Freyhof large farm-buildings have been erected, with a capacious square saloon, and with some chambers situated immediately over cow-stalls, and used for cases in which the exhalations of the stables are considered useful to soothe bronchial irritation and dyspnœa. The two buildings are connected by a tasteful garden and a large covered hall, 90 feet long, used for bowling and walking in unfavourable weather. Moreover, douche, river, and wave baths have been erected by Dr. Küng, on his own grounds, near a brook running through a wild ravine. A shady foot-path leads from this establishment to the neighbouring village of Wolfhalden. Cows', ewes', and asses' milk, as well as herb juices and the most important mineral waters, are obtainable here. No wonder, then, that many varieties of ailments are counteracted by a use of the various remedial measures available; chronic, bronchial, or laryngeal irritation, tendency to tuberculosis, dyspepsia, gastric oppression, sluggish action or impaired circulation of the liver, neuralgic or rheumatic pains of the joints or muscles without exudation or organic changes, more due to deficient nutrition than to real rheumatism; chlorosis, nervous giddiness, emaciation of young persons through too sudden growth, where the development of vital organs cannot keep pace with the rapid stretch of the muscular and osseous systems; in fact, whenever a disproportion arises between the albuminates and non-nitrogenous constituents of the blood, especially in persons of phlegmatic spare habits, whey-cures will assist in eliminating the obstructive portions of plastic elements. Though apparently weakening, they will ultimately infuse new strength and gain to the organism, because new and healthy tissue will fill up the vacancy produced by the increased renal, cutaneous, and intestinal secretions. Nevertheless it must be admitted that if by a miracle the best Alpine whey could be brought to the valetudinarian's bedside at home we should not observe the beneficial results described. A great portion of the improvement is certainly due to the exhilarating mountain atmosphere, provoking increased muscular exercise, and to the purer and thinner air stimulating the lungs to inhale greater quantities than usual, in order to obtain the requisite amount of oxygen for the decarbonisation of the blood. The chest thus becomes more expanded, the head more raised, and the muscular apparatus better developed. The regular walks not only serve as derivatives by drawing the blood from the internal organs to the extremities and surface, diminishing the tendency to internal congestions and to injurious plastic changes, but they lighten the burden of the smaller capillaries. The muscular movements induce constant waste of tissue; the effete particles thus eliminated, either in a gaseous form (by skin and lungs) or in liquid and solid form (by the renal and other emunctories) have to be replaced by the blood, newly formed out of food. The diminished blood naturally flows more freely through the smaller vessels, and returns more easily to the centre of circulation. This facilitated reflux of venous blood prevents many of those numerous diseases due to the so-called 'torpid liver.'

But the visitors must guard against the other extreme, of being enticed to excessive pedestrian exercise. This would prove more injurious than complete rest. For all the benefits ascribed to quiet, moderate and regular walking would be lost by overstraining the muscular and nervous systems. Pains and other signs of nervous over-exertion would ensue and be transmitted to the central nervous system. A feeling of general exhaustion and debility would naturally follow and impede the regular functions of the various organs of reproduction. Many diseases have been aggravated, and dangerous results produced by such inconsiderate excess. The proper measure to be observed by every valetudinarian is this—there must be a feeling of comfort and pleasant languor after the walk, so that rest becomes refreshing. But if the slightest exhaustion or pain is felt, even some time *after* resting, the pedestrian has decidedly overstepped the bounds of healthy exercise.

HEINRICHSBAD, Swiss whey establishment, in the Canton of Appenzell-Ausserrhoden, two miles north-east of Herisau, half a mile from *Winkeln Station*, south of St. Gallen, and west of Gais, at an altitude of 2410' over the level of the sea, enjoys a beautiful situation. A large Curhaus is erected here to accommodate about 120 guests. It is protected against violent winds, and has altogether a more sheltered position than Gais and Gonten, the air being somewhat milder and moister on account of the peat-ground covering some portions of the neighbourhood. Two chalybeate springs arise in the vicinity, and are employed for drinking and bathing, to assist the whey-cure in cases of great anæmia and debility, in 'renal and vesical pains,' &c. The goat whey is prepared on the Santis; cow's whey, for baths, at the establishment.

Physicians—Drs. Fisch and Tobler.

WEISSBAD, whey establishment, two miles south-east of Appenzell, 2,524' over the level of the sea, south of Trogen and of Gais, the most sheltered of the group, being surrounded by the promontories of the high Alps, and situated in a section of a narrow, deep meadow-valley replete with foliage. Fine shady walks from the cur-haus along the three brooks, which join here to form the Sitter, afford exercise and shelter against the heat of the sun. Further walks on the shore of the Sitter to Appenzell, and along the Schwendibach to the Alp, and to the village of Schwendi, can be made on an even but not shady road. As only 130 to 140 visitors can be accommodated at the establishment, it is advisable to bespeak rooms before arrival. The climate is not only milder than that of Gais, on account of the more thorough protection against all winds, but also moister, the air being more saturated with watery vapour, partly from the rapidly flowing rivers, and partly from its greater proximity to the Alps, by ascending fogs from the valleys. When Gais is only cloudy, Weissbad is generally treated with rain. When clouds and fogs have been long expelled from Gais by the sun after a storm, they are still often hovering densely over Weissbad. While thus patients may be sent here, even in a more advanced state of phthisis, for whom the protection of Gais and even of Heiden would be insufficient, the climate is, on the other hand, too relaxing, and in the clear sunny days the heat too oppressive, for torpid and phlegmatic habits, and for those who are only affected with atony of the thoracic organs or with incipient phthisis.

Physicians—Dr. Hersche, of Appenzell, and Dr. Zellweger, of Trogen.

HELIGOLAND, an island under 'British possession, lies free in the North Sea, under a latitude N. of 54°, and a longitude E. of $6\frac{1}{3}$°. It is nearly equidistant of the mouths of the Elbe and Weser, and consists of an almost perpendicular rock of variegated sandstone 206 feet high, with a length of 2,200 yards and a width of 650, the whole circumference amounting to about 13,800 feet. It may be reached from Hamburg by steamer in eight to twelve hours. A flat triangular foreland spreads to the northern declivity of the island, and about a mile to its east, sparingly cultivated. Downs rise to a height of about 80 feet, and serve as a bathing-place with their firm sandy ground. But as the passage to the downs is often prevented by stormy weather, or causes sea-sickness to sensitive persons, places have been erected on the strand of the island, where the different sexes bathe at various hours. The little town possesses about 4,000 inhabitants. From the foreland, about 200 steps lead to the so-called 'Oberland,' where numerous excellent hotels and private residences are found capable of accommodating about 1,500 visitors at a time. Sea excursions round the island are sometimes made at night with torchlights. Balls and concerts at the conversation-house are frequently given for the amusement of the visitors. Heligoland possesses the advantage of a pure, bracing, and stimulating maritime climate, without any disturbing influence, and is peculiarly adapted for vigorous persons requiring sea-baths with strong movements of waves. Weakly or sensitive individuals are not to be advised to resort here, as nervous excitement with feverish irritability, giddiness, and subsequent languor and relaxation, generally ensue the first few days, but gradually subside, as the system gets acclimatised. Moreover, absence of shady walks causes too strong a reflex of light, and must be particularly injurious to persons affected with sensitive or irritable sight.

Physician—Dr. von Aschen.

HERINGSDORF, Baltic sea-bath, 5 miles north-west of Swinemünde, between Rostock and Colberg, 40 miles north of Stettin, lat. N. 54°, and about 13° long. E. lies on a mountainous ridge (150' high) of the island of Usedom, formed by the rivers Peene and Swine. Shady pine-foliage abounds in the village. The temperature is equable during June, July, and August, rarely disturbed by rain. Mean temperature of summer, $63\frac{1}{2}°$ Fahr., and of the sea, $63\frac{1}{2}$ to $65\frac{3}{4}°$ Fahr. North and north-west sea-winds predominate. The bathing-places have a smooth, firm, and even sand, and are protected against the land winds by the high shore and its abundant forests, whilst the open space towards the north, east, and west, allows a free breaking of waves against the strand. The residences offer a fine prospect of the sea. The pleasant situation and rural aspect of the social little village, give it a great preference over more noisy and fashionable watering-places, especially in convalescence after prolonged diseases, when the mind requires freedom of conventional traffic to regain its former elasticity and vigour. . In an hour's ride, the place is reached from Swinemünde, which stands in constant steam communication with Stettin (time of journey about six hours). Season from middle of June to September.

Physicians—Drs. Smege, von Wallenstedt.

HAVRE DE GRACE, French sea-bath on the Channel, just opposite Brighton, at the mouth of the Seine, a thriving town with 21,000 inhabitants and many well laid out gardens and promenades, may be reached by rail from Paris in six and a half hours, and by steamers from London or Brighton. The town is divided into the old portion, and the more northerly newer part called *Ingouville*, which lies on a rising ground, extending from east to west as far as the neat village of *Sanvic*, studded with beautiful houses and luxuriant well-arranged gardens. The neighbouring charming village of *St. Addresse* is laid out with great taste, and covered with fine villas and abundant foilage. The sea-bathing is excellent here, and offers the advantage of the flood-tide remaining in about three hours daily. Thus the visitors save the tedious road over an extensive strand, and may enjoy a bath that has been unusually long exposed and agitated by the sea-winds. It has, therefore, very bracing properties, and deserves the preference when amusement and social intercourse are sought to be combined with the restorative influence of sea-bathing.

Physicians—Drs. Launay, Lecadre, Lefebure. *English physician*—Dr. Tarrel.

TROUVILLE, a small rural sea-bath, near Havre, lying on the southern arm of the bay formed by the mouth of the Seine, whilst Havre occupies the end of the northern arm. The situation is thus more sheltered against bleak sea-winds, and the force of the waves somewhat broken, whilst it possesses a fine firm sandy ground for bathing. Persons inclined to irritation of thoracic organs, or to affections of the nervous system, will find this a more congenial and suitable summer residence than the neighbouring Havre. Accommodation satisfactory. But the visitors must

guard against dangerous *quicksands*, and should on no account bathe in the sea without guides, as only two years ago a whole family perished from this cause in trying to save each other.
Physicians—Dr. Allies, Dr. Roccas.

HYERES, a town in Provence, department of the Var, in the south-eastern portion of France, 11 miles east of *Toulon*, with which it is connected by rail and by diligence. The station is about three miles distant; the Mediterranean sea two and a half miles. Lat. N. 43°, long. E. about 6°. It lies on the southern slope of a hill, surrounded by mountains, which close it in and protect it completely towards the north only, whilst the west and north-west winds are not fully intercepted. The *mistral* (north-west wind) sometimes penetrates with great violence through a deep indent of the valley, and produces sudden coolness. In the mornings and evenings especially, vicissitudes of temperature occur through the changes of land and sea winds. The air is, however, in general more mild, and the climate more equable than at Nice, on account of the radiation and reflexion of the solar rays, produced by the amphitheatre-like enclosure of the surrounding heights; whilst, on the other hand, the chilling Alpine ranges lie somewhat farther off. The annual number of rainy days only amounts to forty, and these generally occur in October and November. Winter and spring sometimes offer an uninterrupted number of fine clear days. But the noxious and cold north-north-east wind occasionally prevails in winter, and counteracts by its passage over the ice-clad Alps the milder and humid winds coming from the Mediterranean. Vegetation is extremely luxurious, and almost tropical, and the environs charming. It is adapted as a winter residence for persons affected with chronic pulmonary ailments or incipient phthisis, if there is more atony and torpor in the constitution than inflammatory or congestive tendency. Season from December to May. The eastern part of the town and basin is the most protected against the north winds, and the temperature therefore less variable there. Patients of an irritable, nervous, or vascular system, are recommended to reside at *Costebelle*, lying about two miles from the town on the southern declivity of a hill. On the high road to Toulon, a beautiful and commodious hotel (Les Iles d'Or) is erected on the slope of the charming Schlossberg, with various buildings attached for private residences and pensions. It contains a sunny pavilion, covered with glass, and capable of being heated in cold winter days. Its terraces afford a beautiful view of the sea. But it is necessary to mention that, however favourable the climate in some winters, the cold of one night was sufficiently intense to destroy all the orange trees. Though vines and olive trees cover the bases of the hills, while evergreen shrubs abound at their tops with an abundance of rosemary, lavender, and other aromatic plants, the occasional blowing of the mistral counteracts a great portion of these advantages. Consumptive patients especially ought to remain confined to their rooms during its prevalence. But, with proper precautions, it is one of the mildest climates in the Provence. Population of the town, above 9,000. Most frequented hotel: Hôtel des Ambassadeurs.
Physicians—Drs. Allegre, Honoraty, Chassinat, Verignon.

CANNES, a French town in the department of the Var, on the bay of Cannes, station of the Toulon-Nice Railway, 21 miles south-south-west of Nice (an hour's ride); five hours' ride from Toulon; most charmingly situated in a valley, completely protected by the high Estérel Mountains towards west and north, whilst the sea-winds are freely admitted from the south. Lower mountain ridges take their course towards east and north-east, and intercept the lower aerial currents. A beautiful view of the environs may be obtained on the summit of Mount Chevalier. Wooded rising ground at the back, and the *Lerin* islands in front, with the delightful walks amongst the valleys and mountains of the neighbourhood, present it as one of the most picturesque spots in the south of France. South-south-east and north-east winds mostly prevail in the cold season. The climate greatly resembles that of Hyères. Mean annual temperature, 61° Fahr.; winter, 51° Fahr.; spring, 65° Fahr.; autumn, 57° Fahr. Annual rainy days, fifty-two. The climate is milder than that of Nice, less humid and relaxing than that of Pau, and would therefore suit many persons with chronic, laryngeal, or bronchial catarrhs, for whom Nice would be too irritating. Social life is, in general, more pleasant, and accommodation considerably greater and more varied than in the Riviera. Besides the Grand Hôtel de Cannes, Gray's Family Hotel, Bellevue, &c., there are numerous villas and pensions on the road to Toulon, lying in a well-protected situation, and affording ample accommodation. The easy access by steamer from Marseilles, as well as by rail, is another recommendation. Population, 5,800.
Physicians—Drs. Seve and Whitley.

HARROGATE, in the west riding of Yorkshire, 210 miles north-west of King's Cross or Euston Square Station (seven hours' railway journey), 18 miles north of Leeds, is beautifully situated on high tableland with cultivated grounds and blooming heaths, and exposed to the bracing winds and exhilarating atmosphere of an open and hilly country. It contains nearly 100 mineral springs, which have been divided into four classes, viz. *sulphurous saline, saline chalybeate, pure chalybeate, and earthy.* Population, nearly 5,000.

The *Old Sulphur Well* contains in sixteen ounces 68 grains of chloride of sodium, 6·4 of chloride of potassium, 5·5 chloride of magnesium, 8·1 chloride of calcium, 1·5 sulphuret of sodium, 1·2 carbonate of lime; traces of bromide of sodium, of iodide of sodium, of fluoride of calcium, of carbonate of iron and of manganese; of organic matter and some silica, $109\frac{1}{2}$ grains altogether; gaseous contents, $5\frac{1}{2}$ cubic inches, viz. $2\frac{1}{4}$ carbonic acid, $\frac{1}{2}$ carburetted hydrogen, $2\frac{1}{2}$ sulphuretted hydrogen, about $\frac{1}{3}$ nitrogen. Dr. James Johnson describes the quality of the water thus:—'If a venerable and rusty gun-barrel which had not been fired since the Spanish Armada were well scoured out with boiling sea-water—and if to these washings were added a few stale or rotten eggs — and finally, if a stream of sulphuretted and carburetted hydrogen from one of the main gas-pipes in Regent-street were directed through this witch's caudle, till it was supersaturated, then we should have a perfect imitation of Aix-la-Chapelle, Leamington, and Harrogate. Indeed, the Fontaine-Elisée 'itself at Aix is little better than milk and water, compared with this Yorkshire stingo.' Not far from the old well, the *Montpellier Springs* arise; 1, the *strong sulphur-well*, containing 96 grains of solid and $4\frac{1}{2}$ cubic inches of gaseous contents—viz., less chlorides, some more sulphate of lime, and rather less carbonic acid than the old well; 2, the *mild sulphur-well*, containing only 29 grains of solid ingredients (less chlorides, less sulphuret of sodium, and more carbonate of lime), and $2\frac{3}{4}$ cubic inches of gaseous contents. At a distance of about two or three hundred yards, the *Royal Promenade*, or *Cheltenham Pumproom*, encloses the so-called *Cheltenham saline spring*, in a beautiful temple-like structure, with extensive gardens and walks at the back. It contains $28\frac{1}{2}$ grains of solid and $2\frac{1}{2}$ cubic inches of gaseous constituents in 16 ounces. It possesses no sulphuretted hydrogen, half a cubic inch of carburetted hydrogen, and nearly two cubic inches of carbonic acid. It contains, moreover, nearly half a grain of carbonate of iron, less chloride of sodium and carbonate of lime than the Montpellier mild-well, to which its composition is otherwise analogous. About a quarter of a mile from the lower village, to the eastern extremity of the Common, in a marshy spot, a pure chalybeate, called '*Tewitt-well*,' issues, containing about one-eighth of a grain of carbonate of iron, about one cubic inch of carbonic acid and one-half of nitrogen, with only one grain of solid ingredients. At the top of the Common, nearly opposite the Granby Hotel, *the Sweet Spa*, one of the oldest springs, is found enclosed in a small circular building. It contains a little more carbonic acid and nitrogen (but only half the quantity of iron) than the Tewitt, with which it is otherwise analogous. It is, therefore, likewise a pure chalybeate. Then there is the *Starbeck* sulphur, the *Knaresborough* chalybeate spring, and many others of varying strength, allowing a great variety for selection in accordance with the more or less stimulation requisite in each individual case. In cutaneous diseases, especially of the order of squamæ, as psoriasis, lepra ; in herpes, impetigo, chronic ulcers, particularly if connected with dyspepsia, Harrogate has been found very useful ; also in cases of debility, anæmia, irregular menses, in torpidity of the liver, and of other abdominal organs, &c. Bathing is likewise employed to assist the internal treatment. But care must be taken to prepare the patient by aperients before the commencement of the course, if there is any local congestion, distention of the vena portarum, or deficient secretion of bile. The season lasts from July to October. Looking at the great variety of the springs, many ailments based on malassimilation and deficient sanguification, especially if resulting from excessive indulgence in high living or from sedentary habits, must find their cure here. But a certain vigour of the constitution is required to reap all the benefits offered. Persons inclined to pulmonary or bronchial irritation might be injured by the bleakness of the climate incidental to its northern and exposed situation. On the other hand, in many instances in which patients do not require the more intense action of sulphuretted hydrogen (as obtainable in those foreign spas produced by subterraneous volcanic action), and where the saline ingredients so abundant in the principal sulphur-well are useful in stimulating the renal, cutaneous and alvine secretion ; in fact, when stimulation and increased function of the emunctories are more called for than a thorough alterative action, Harrogate will be found extremely efficacious. The tonic and exhilarating properties of the northern atmosphere will counteract to a great extent the weakening effect of the depurating and relaxing sulphurous waters.

HASTINGS, a friendly town in the east of Sussex, on the south coast of England, seventy-four miles south-east of London (about two and a half hours' railway journey), between Brighton and Folkestone, is protected by the high cliffs at the back against northerly winds; but being open towards the south, the mildness of the air is often disturbed in winter by violent south-westerly winds. The northerly shelter differs in various parts of the town. The lower situations, opposite the beach, are particularly guarded by cliffs, almost rising perpendicularly behind them; the higher portions are rather more exposed. There is a deficiency of sheltered ground for promenades in windy weather. During January and December, and during spring, the climate is milder here, and affords greater protection against north and north-east winds, than its neighbouring resorts, and is therefore particularly recommended for persons suffering with chronic pulmonary diseases. The lower situation of the encircling cliffs causes the air to be more thoroughly impregnated by the marine exhalations than at more open or higher localities. For the same reason it must be considered unfavourable in nervous diseases, especially in headaches resulting from impaired digestion, and also in a disposition to congestion of the brain or to apoplexy. The higher portions of the town would be less obnoxious for such persons. In general, the place is more adapted for sensitive and delicate persons, as the air has a moist sedative character. For a summer residence, the higher part of the town ought to be selected, as more bracing and cooler. It is a charming town, with many fine walks and terraces for pedestrian exercise in fine weather; and even after rain the ground soon becomes dry, as the clayey soil is overlaid with sand, allowing a speedy percolation of the rain-water, though the annual rainfall amounts to $28\frac{1}{3}$ inches. The mean annual temperature is 50·4° F.: winter, 29°; spring, $47\frac{1}{2}°$; summer, $61\frac{3}{4}°$; autumn, $52\frac{1}{5}°$. It is a favourite sea-bath in summer and autumn, and ought to be selected by those who possess a languid sluggish circulation, but an irritable nervous system, or who may be easily affected by vicissitudes of temperature, or in convalescence after protracted disease. On the other hand, more bracing localities should be chosen by persons in full health, or families resorting to the sea-side to strengthen the constitution and to diminish its liability to disease *afterwards*—a preventive measure peculiar to this country, which cannot be too highly extolled, and deserves adoption on the Continent.

ST. LEONARDS, about a mile west of Hastings, on the Sussex coast, has a broad esplanade and carriage-road in front, and a range of cliffs at the background, somewhat lower than those at Hastings. Though protected against northerly winds, the atmosphere is less exposed to countercurrents and draughts from above, as it is not so closely hemmed in. The colonnades for walking exercise, in unfavourable weather, afford also a great advantage; but it is more open to the south-west and to easterly winds, hence more liable to vicissitudes of weather: otherwise, the ground partakes of the same dry and bibulous character as that of Hastings. Possessing better accommodation and more modern buildings, it deserves the preference whenever the bracing influence of sea-air is sought to be combined with a sheltering position, as it possesses an intermediate character between the mild and humid climate of Hastings and the more bracing one of Brighton. Season, from November to the end of February. Though ague is not unfrequent in the neighbourhood, no visitor is said to have ever been attacked by it.

THE VALE OF GINSENG, between Hastings and St. Leonards, affords, according to Sir James Clark, a site superior to either of the above. Though open to the sea, it is somewhat retired from the beach, and sheltered by rising ground on each side, not only against north-easterly winds, but also to a considerable degree against the south-west gales.

THE CAPE OF GOOD HOPE, a British colony at the southern termination of Africa, between 26° and 34° S. latitude, and 16° and 28° E. longitude, has an extent of 900 miles from east to west, and an average breadth of 400 miles. From south to north, terraces rise over terraces. Several large bays indent the coast. The rivers are mostly rapid in winter, and dried up in summer, producing an appearance of barrenness and dryness. The seasons are the reverse of ours—viz., December, January, and February, constitute the *summer*; March, April, and May, *autumn*; June, July, and August, *winter*; and September, October, and November, *spring*. The mean temperature of the year is $68\frac{1}{4}°$; of summer, 74° Fahrenheit; autumn, $74\frac{1}{10}°$; winter, $62\frac{1}{3}°$; spring, 63°. The scarcity of rain is more experienced in the interior than in the Cape district. The number of annual rainy days amounts to 75, and the quantity of rain to 41 inches. South-east wind prevails in Cape Town during summer, and exhibits a sultry relaxing character as it passes over the sandy flats between the town and Simon's Bay; but in winter a cold chilly sea breeze from the *north-west* predominates, and is often the precursor of violent gales and heavy rains. In spring and autumn, south-westerly winds are most frequent, generally loaded with humidity, from their passage across the ocean, covering the mountain tops with fogs, which often descend in tempests, and render the atmosphere suddenly cold and raw. They are sometimes also accompanied by a mild rain. The climate was found favourable to the troops stationed there. Deaths from consumption are rarer than at other stations. Fevers of intermittent or remittent character are also very rare; but rheumatism prevails to a greater extent than at home. The *western* province enjoys a more favourable climate in summer, being less liable to stormy winds and violent rainfalls. In winter the *eastern* division is preferable, the atmosphere being clear and bracing, and less liable to violent vicissitudes. The climate of the Cape is considered much more favourable than that of Great Britain, pneumonia, tuberculosis, and fever being very rare. Invalids generally resort to Rondebosch, about five miles from Cape

Town, or to Wynberg, about eight miles distant. As these places are open to the south-east winds, they are cooler than Cape Town; they are also provided with shady walks and rides, and comfortable private and boarding-houses. In a sitting-room at Rondebosch, not much exposed to the sun, the door and windows being left open, the temperature was observed by the late Rev. Mr. Ash to range as follows:—In summer, from December 17th to December 31st, $65\frac{1}{4}°$ to $69°$; during January, $67\frac{1}{4}°$ to $70\frac{3}{4}°$; February, $67\frac{1}{3}°$ to $71\frac{3}{4}°$; March, $65\frac{2}{3}°$ to $69\frac{1}{4}°$. Rain fell during this period on 23 days. In general, north-west winds prevail during the winter; and as they pass over the hot and dry plains of the interior, their searching sharpness is mitigated before arriving at the colony. In summer, the south-east winds prevail, and sometimes blow with considerable violence, bringing moisture and coolness from their passage across the Antarctic ocean. The inhabitants of the sea-side are less affected by hot winds than those residing in the interior. South-westerly winds generally predominate in spring and autumn; they are often charged with humidity, bringing cold fogs and heavy rains. Earthquakes also occur occasionally, but rarely of a serious character. Thunderstorms become more frequent and violent in proportion to the nearer approach towards the tropics. The mean annual barometric pressure ranges from 29·70 to 30·33; the mean annual temperature, from 54·7° to 68·8°. According to the 'Army Medical Report,' the climate must be considered very salubrious, for the mortality in the Eastern province only amounted to 9 out of 1,000; in the Western, to 13; whilst in Nova Scotia and New Brunswick it amounts to 14; in Malta and Canada, to 16; in Gibraltar, to 21; in St. Helena, to 25; in the Mauritius, to 27; in Bermuda, to 28; in the Madras Presidency, to 28; in West Indies generally, to 78; in Jamaica, to 121; and in Sierra Leone, to 480 out of 1,000! Though the country is exempt from epidemics, great age is comparatively rare among the inhabitants. New-comers are often attacked by dysentery if they do not exercise great caution in their dress and habit of living.

ILMENAU, in the valley of the Ilm (THURINGIA), beautifully situated at an altitude of 1,415 feet over the level of the sea, possesses baths of pine foliage and an hydropathic establishment.

Physicians—Drs. Schwabe, Fitzler, Baumbach, Preller.

IMNAU, in the Hohenzollerian possession of PRUSSIA, a village five leagues south of Tübingen, three leagues north of Hechingen, twelve south of Stuttgart, lies in a friendly meadow valley, on the plateau which connects the Rauhe Alp with the Black Forest, 1,241 feet over the level of the sea. It contains chalybeate springs with a great amount of carbonic acid, and with various proportions of iron. The *Fürstenquelle*, or *Oberequelle*, is the weakest, containing, however, more chloride of sodium than the others. In 16 ounces it contains $11\frac{1}{2}$ grains of solid constituents —viz., $\frac{1}{2}$ grain of carbonate of iron, 1 chloride of sodium, $\frac{1}{3}$ chloride of magnesium, 1 carbonate of magnesia, $6\frac{3}{4}$ carbonate of lime, $\frac{1}{5}$ sulphate of lime, 1 silica, $1\frac{1}{3}$ organic matter, and 30 cubic inches of carbonic acid gas. As regards the other springs, Nos. 1 and 3 contain less iron, 2 and

4 considerably more; hence a choice may be made according to the individuality of the patient. The Fürstenquelle is generally easily elaborated, on account of its great amount of carbonic acid, and its small quantity of sulphate of lime. In cases of great excitability of the vascular system, or in weakness combined with bronchial irritation and profuse secretion of mucus, the spring No. 5, which contains no iron, is often taken with goat's milk or whey. When the pulmonary organs become healthier, gradually the stronger springs are resorted to. The springs would be injurious in tuberculosis, as the great amount of carbonic acid might produce irritation and congestion of the lungs.

Physicians—Dr. Rehman, Dr. Wern.

INTERLAKEN (SWITZERLAND), between the Lakes of Thun and of Brienz ('inter lacus'), south of Bern, lies beautifully in a valley, surrounded by high mountains, at an altitude of 1,712 feet. The climate is extremely mild, being sheltered against cold winds by the surrounding Alps, whilst the neighbouring lakes deprive the extreme summer heat of its oppressive character. The whole valley is intersected by the Aar, which leaves the Lake of Brienz to fall into that of Thun. The temperature is higher in summer during the day than on the plateaus of the Appenzeller mountains. The morning temperature being the lowest, there is generally a wider range between morning and afternoon than between afternoon and evening. Generally towards 2 P.M. the warmth increases pretty rapidly, remains rather constant till sunset, and then sinks again a few degrees somewhat suddenly. Mean annual temperature, 50·9° Fahr.; mean temperature of May, 62·6°; of June, 65·3°; of July, 69·3°; of August, 69·5°; of September, 64·1°. It is greatly resorted to by persons suffering from obstinate bronchial catarrh, to drink the whey, which is prepared in an establishment between Belvedere and Schweizerhof, where the valetudinarians may avail themselves of a hall 120 feet long, for walking exercise, in unfavourable weather. Numerous pensions and hotels are spread about the valley for the accommodation of visitors. Those who wish to combine economy with seclusion may reside at the charming village of *Bönigen*, half a league to the east of Interlaken, on the Lake of Brienz, where they may enjoy a view of the whole right shore of the lake, and also of the pointed Augstmalthorn, and of the so-called Hardermannli—a configuration of rocks on the Harder, having some resemblance to the human head. Notwithstanding the great charms and variety of the landscapes, it is necessary to mention a great defect incidental to the place, viz., a deficiency of good spring-water. The whole journey may be accomplished from London in less than two days, by steam and rail, over Basel and Bern. Only two principal winds prevail in the valley of Interlaken, one descending and the other ascending. The ascending current prevails about nine months in the year, and assumes either a west-north-westerly or south-westerly direction, the latter generally being a harbinger of rain. The south wind (*Föhn*), which penetrates these valleys from the chain of the high Alps, often assumes great violence, especially in the valleys nearer to the Alps, as in those of Hasli and Grindelwald. Lower down, the force gradually abates; so that it is often scarcely perceived at Interlaken when it blows still violently at Brienz (three leagues to the northeast), whilst it is not felt at all at Thun, lying four leagues lower down the valley, at the north-west. The Föhn invariably brings a high temperature, often melting in one spring-night layers of snow which would have required weeks of solar influence to be got rid of. In high summer it often causes inundations, through raising the temperature of the high mountains, especially after continuous rains. The *Bise* (north-east or east wind) occurs very rarely, through the mountainous protection. Besides these principal winds, the regular ascending and descending currents of air occur here, as in most of the valleys of the central Alps—viz., during the day the warmer air ascends, causing a 'Thal-wind' (valley-wind), and during the night the cooler air descends from the heights, as 'Berg-wind' (mountain-wind). These regular currents are considered to be the principal cause of the purity of air enjoyed by these localities. According to Dr. Strasser, not one case of scarlatina occurred at Interlaken in seven years, though frequent at a distance of three leagues. Hooping-cough sometimes occurs epidemically. Intermittents occasionally appear in some neighbouring localities, but are rare here. Goître, varicose swellings, ruptures, scrofulosis, and cretinism are frequently met with among the poorer inhabitants. Tuberculosis is not frequent, but principally attacks weavers and wood-carvers, who are generally ill-fed and poorly housed, and lead a sedentary life; but these are generally cured by a sojourn in a higher warm alpine region, if resorted to at the beginning. Pneumonia, bronchitis, and inflammatory catarrhs occur frequently; acute rheumatism rarely; croup occasionally. Interlaken is specially recommended for persons suffering from nervous debility, hypochondriasis, &c., particularly after tedious or exhausting diseases, but for those affected with a rheumatic tendency the place is less adapted, as, through the moist, warm climate, the slumbering evil might be provoked, especially in very wet summers. Children that have become anæmic or feeble by a too sedentary life, or by a too rapid bodily development, are greatly improved here through the influence of the air alone. As regards tuberculosis, Dr. Strasser considers the place indicated for those cases which are intermediate between the erethic and torpid form, where there is no hereditary tendency, and the evil becomes developed, not in early youth or manhood, but in a later period of life. For those who suffer with profuse bronchial secretion, or with an advanced stage of the disease, the place is not suited. If the summer heat becomes very oppressive, so as to cause muscular debility and mental depression, the visitors are recommended either to seek higher localities, or pensions situated on the lakes of Eastern Switzerland, where the evaporation of a greater body of water exerts a cooling effect on the temperature, as *Thun* (on the Lake of Thun, connected by railway with Bern and Basel); *Wäggis*, on the northern shore of the *Vierwaldstädter Lake*, east of Luzern, south of the Zuger Lake; *Beckenried*, on the southern shore of the Vierwaldstädter Lake, east of Stanz, in Unterwalden; or *Brunnen*, on the north-eastern bend of the same lake, south-west of Schwyz, north of Flüelen. In the erethic form of scrofulosis of children, great and rapid improvement is observed here from the whey cure. Chronic bronchial catarrh, especially if the consequence of influenza, or the residuum of measles or of scarlatina, is also improved here. When the cough is connected with tuberculosis, less benefit will be derived—at least, such patients must be particularly careful as regards excursions into the side valleys nearer the mountains, as they are mostly draughty, and often bring on severe relapses. Chronic laryngeal catarrh is very frequently cured by the whey and climate. Another additional curative agent is found in the lake and river-baths. The former are taken at the beautiful village of Bönigen, and the Aare baths, not far from the pensions. The temperature of the river is rather lower here than that of the Lake of Brienz (which ranges from 52° to 65¾° Fahr. in summer). The temperature of the Lake of Thun is higher than either of the above, as it receives no glacier water, but only that furnished by the river Aare; hence, bathers are recommended to use first Thun Lake baths before resorting to Aare-River or Brienz-Lake baths. The Aare baths are particularly useful in uterine atony with irregular catamenia. *Strawberry cures* are also employed here in cases of gout or abdominal plethora. But even without curative objects, this charming and picturesque place is often visited for recreation's sake. The unique views and landscapes offered by Interlaken itself, and by the neighbouring celebrated Bernese Upper Land, are extremely attractive; the excursions to Giessbach, to Reichenbach and the Rosenaui glacier, to the Grindelwald glaciers, to Thun, to Heustrich, to Weissenberg, &c., will all leave lasting impressions of a most pleasurable kind.

Physician—Dr. Strasser.

GIESSBACH (Hotel), on the Lake of Brienz, a charming establishment, with an altitude of 2,400 feet, is situated in a valley gently sloping towards the south-west, surrounded by luxurious forests. Protected against winds, the atmosphere is somewhat cooled and refreshed in summer by the rapid movements of the Giessbach. It may be considered as one of the most picturesque and romantic whey-cure establishments in the world, especially adapted for those who wish to contemplate the beauties of nature in all its vastness, apart from the noise and traffic of the outside world. The whey is brought fresh twice daily in summer from the Achs-Alp, two leagues distant. It may be reached from London in less than two days—by rail as far as *Thun*, steamer across the Lake of Thun to Interlaken, and thence steamboats make the journey three times daily to the celebrated Giessbach, on the southern shore of the Lake of Brienz. This lake, which forms the principal purificator of the River Aare, 1,736 feet over the level of the sea, is surrounded by rocky mountain chains, which descend abruptly to the lake basin. It is almost three leagues (nine miles) long, and one league broad between Ebligen and the Giessbach—thus, on the whole, smaller than its neighbour, the Lake of Thun—but in depth (2,000 feet) it is said to excel all the lakes this side the Alps. The Föhn sometimes sweeps over it with extreme fury, when it breaks forth out of the south-eastern narrow grounds of the Hasli valley; but no misfortune ever happened in consequence. The lake is never frozen over. The Aare, which enters at the broad eastern marshy Delta in a muddy and grey condition, runs through the whole length of the lake, and issues clear and purified at the western extremity, near Interlaken. The Giessbach is principally renowned for its seven waterfall stages, grouped over each other, and foaming down through beautiful rocky formations, covered with luxurious foliage, from a height of 1,100 feet. About forty years ago, the schoolmaster Kehrli made the falls accessible to travellers. In 1853 convenient walks were constructed by the proprietors, Von Rappard, for visiting all the falls, from the highest to the lowest. Every night during the season *illumination* of the cascades by coloured Bengal lights takes place, and attracts numerous visitors; the view is then one of the most wonderful and striking that can be imagined. After a signal, darkness is transformed into lights of various colours, through which the water is seen precipitating over the rocks, and forming the most curious and pleasing groups. The illumination over, the sight-seers, who hired boats for the purpose, leave for Brienz, while the residents are summoned to the excellent and unsurpassed table of *Mr. Schmidlin*, at the restaurant, just opposite the waterfalls. A difficult path leads along the waterfalls to the Faulhorn, after about seven or eight hours' good walking. A beautiful shady forest walk conducts from Giessbach, through the so-called *Enge*, into the Hasli valley, round the head of the lake, to Brienz (two leagues). A very interesting pedestrian tour is the path to Interlaken, over Jseltwald (one and a half league), Sengg (half a league), Ehrschwand (half a league), Bönigen (half a league), and Interlaken (half a league). The village of Ebligen lies opposite Giessbach, under the Tannhorn, which towers to a height of 6,531 feet.

MEYRINGEN, three leagues to the south-east of Brienz, reached by diligence on a good road, is frequently visited as a climatic health-resort. The village lies in the upper part of the Aar valley, on the right shore of the Aare, upwards of 1,800 feet over the level of the sea, surrounded by high mountains. There is nothing remarkable in the place itself, but the environs are most romantic. As the crossing of many Alpine roads, it contains invariably a great concourse of tourists.

GRINDELWALD, or rather, *Gydisdorf* (Grindelwald being the name of the whole valley), four and three-quarter leagues south-east of Interlaken, 3,150 feet over the level of the sea, hitherto only visited on account of the two Grindelwald glaciers to its south, and the mountain passes to the *Rosenlaui* valley (Scheideck), and to the *Lauterbrunnen* valley (Wengernalp). But the climate is so healthy that it deserves to be resorted to more frequently by valetudinarians. The atmosphere is cooler here in summer than in the neighbouring plains. Typhus never appears here, phthisis very rarely; but pneumonia occurs frequently in winter, and chronic catarrhs, with emphysema and heart disease, often affect old people. The place is particularly recommended in cases of nervous debility and hypochondriasis, where pure air, a serene sky, and beautiful mountain scenery are required to raise mental and nervous power. The route from Meyringen to Grindelwald (twenty-one miles) may be accomplished in about eight hours.

ISCHIA, island of SOUTH ITALY, in the Mediterranean, eight miles southwest of Cape Misene, from which it is separated by a channel; twenty miles from Naples (three hours' steam voyage). Population 21,000. The surface is mountainous. Mount Epomeo rises to a height of 2,513 feet, and affords an excellent view of the beautiful bay. Lat. N. $41\frac{1}{2}°$; long. E. $12\frac{1}{2}°$. It is more resorted to in summer, on account of its hot mineral springs, than in winter. In the latter season a cold wind visits the northern coast; moreover, the humidity resulting from its luxuriant vegetation and configuration of the soil acts unfavourably on invalids. On the east and west sides of the coast intense heat is produced in summer by southerly winds, but the northern coast is then cool and refreshing. Dr. Jackson recommends the climate for persons affected with nervous debility, but the stay should not be too prolonged. The springs have all a high temperature, and require an admixture of cold water before being used. Hot-air, vapour, and sand baths are likewise in use here. Ischia probably resting on a still glowing volcano, hot springs issue from numerous rocky fissures; but the chief springs lie in the valle Ombrasco, near the village of Casamicciola, at the foot of the Mount Epomeo. The *Gurgitello* (principal spring) has a temperature of 158° F., and contains principally carbonate and muriate of soda, and a considerable quantity of carbonic acid gas. *Acqua di Cappone* has a temperature of 98° F. *Acqua di bagno Fresco*, or *del Occhio*, is used in ophthalmic affections. The temperature of the *Acqua di Tamburo* ranges between 155° and 210° F.; it derives its name from the drum-like noise produced by the escape of its carbonic acid gas. The springs contain principally carbonate and muriate of soda, with some iron and lime, and a small quantity of sulphuretted hydrogen and carbonic acid. The spa enjoys a particular reputation for the cure of mercurial cachexia after syphilis, with remnants of the original disease, such as cutaneous diseases and affections of the osseous system; ulcerations are less benefited there. The water is used internally and externally. Abdominal fulness, dyspepsia, gastric catarrh, nervous debility, rheumatic and neuralgic pains, paralysis, scars of wounds badly healed, &c., are considered adapted to this spa; but great care is necessary, on account of the high temperature of the water. Many cures are, no doubt, due to the excellent climate, especially in spring, when the equable beneficent warmth of the air is tempered by refreshing sea winds. Colds and draughts are, however, not unfrequent, on account of the variegated ground, being alternately hilly and deep. Besides the hot saline springs, natural vapour baths (stuves) are administered from the natural hot air issuing out of rocky fissures. Bathing cabinets are constructed over these exhalations, which do not appear to possess any medicinal ingredients, but simply hot air with more or less watery vapour, according to previous rain or dryness. These must be particularly avoided in states of congestion, inflammation, feverish condition, palpitation of the heart, or tendency to fainting. The bath arrangements are not as complete as in those countries in which warm springs are rarer. Probably because so many opportunities of bathing are available in Italy, the single baths do not receive the attention they deserve, both as regards analysis and accommodation. Thus the principal spring, Acqua del Gurgitello, is mentioned as possessing 135 grains of solid constituents in 16 ounces; among these, 58 grains of chloride of sodium, and 54 of carbonate of soda. According to others, it is maintained to possess three times the above quantity. The island is also resorted to for sea-bathing.

ITALY extends from the extremity of Sicily (lat. N. 36° 35') to the Rhœtian Alps (lat. N. 46° 37'), and from the west point of the Cottian Alps (long. E. 6° 35') to the east extremity of Terro d'Otranto (long. E. 18° 35'). The Alps and the sea are its natural boundaries. The Alps divide the more severe northern climate from the basin of the Po, with its fertile plains (prolongation of the basin of the Adriatic), the surface of which gradually rises towards Piedmont, in the north-west. The true peninsula is mountainous or hilly, traversed throughout its whole length by the *Apennines*, from north-west to south-east, in a line with the adjacent coast. The western part of these mountains slope down *gradually*, and often end in flat plains, which impede the onward course of the mountain streams, and thus favour the formation of marshes. Amongst the most unhealthy swamps, the *Maremma* of Tuscany must be reckoned, which hitherto resisted all sanitary efforts. The descent of the eastern side is steeper, and thus the coast is freer from these marshes. The shore is generally higher on the western than on the eastern side, except in the Maremma, at the mouths of the Arno, and in the Pontine marshes. Great protection is afforded to the climate by the extensive coast, and the numerous and large gulfs and bays. These great advantages, with the charming aspects and beauties of the landscapes, are counterbalanced by the numerous barren and marshy tracts of land, disseminating malaria and producing sickness. These are more frequent in the western portion, between the Mediterranean and the flat base of the Apennines; also in some valleys enclosed between mountain summits. From Nice, along the gulf of Genoa, to the gulf of Spezzia, the coast is free from malaria; but as the more southern latitude of Leghorn is reached, the injurious influence of malaria becomes more and more marked. From here (lat. N. 43°) to Gaeta (lat. N. 41°) this fever poison reigns supreme; after this the district becomes more healthy, as far as the southern portion of the gulf of Salerno. Here ($40\frac{1}{2}$° N. lat.), at the ruins of Præstum, south of the river Sele, the poison attains its sway again. Farther south, at the coast of Calabria, which has a high position, malaria is almost absent, with the exception of the bay of *St. Eufemia* (lat. N. $38\frac{3}{4}$°). On the eastern shore, along the Adriatic, there are likewise alternations of malaria and healthy districts; but from the abruptness of the mountain declivities, the water can run more freely into the sea: hence these insalubrious marshy plains are less prominent. In Sicily, the plains of *Catania*, south of Etna, on the eastern shore (lat. N. 37°), are affected with malaria. As regards the inland, this evil genius reigns in the flat plains of *Apulia*; in the undulating *Campagna di Roma*, and still more in the Pontine marshes (lat. N. 41°), and in those near Viareggio, Mantua (lat. N. 45°), to the north of Lake Como (lat. N. 46¼°); in the environs of *Venice* (lat. N. 45½°); in the valley of the Po, which pursues a serpentine course from west to east along the latitude of 45° N.; and in the neighbourhood of *Comacchio* (lat. N. 44¾°), not far from the eastern shore. Among the most insalubrious valleys must be reckoned those of *Cecine* (west of Siena) and of Ombrone (east of Siena) in Tuscany, and the valley of Diano in Calabria (lat. N. 39°). From June to October these marshes display the most injurious effects, and cause all those who possess means to resort to cooler districts. The great advantage of Italy in possessing numerous rivers and lakes, beside the sea, has the drawback of engendering heavy dews after sunset, requiring extra protection and care on the part of delicate persons. The rainfall is considerably greater in the continental portion of Italy than in the peninsula, the last months of the year being the wettest in both. Whilst 39·8 inches of rain fall annually on the continental part, 5·4 inches being the proportion for winter, and 13·7 for autumn, in the peninsula (31·7 inches annually) 7·6 inches fall in winter, and 11·3 in autumn. The brilliancy and transparency of the Italian atmosphere increases gradually towards the south; they are especially due to the northerly wind, *tramontana* (coming from the other side of the mountains). Northerly winds generally lower the temperature here, whilst those coming from the south bring warmth, moisture, and clouds. The most important southerly winds are the *sirocco*, coming from the south-east, hot, oppressive, and moist; the *mezzo-giorno* (mid-day), similar to the former, but less severe in character. The *libeccio*, or *south-west*, is usually tempestuous, cloudy, and the forerunner of storms. The *west* wind, *ponente* (sunset), and *east* wind, *levante* (sunrise), are usually mild, and alleviate the severity of the seasons. As regards the northerly winds, the *tramontana*, already mentioned, passing over the northern mountains, and giving up any moisture previously imbibed, is cold and dry, and chases away the clouds formed by southerly winds; violent storms sometimes ensue in summer by its contact with antagonistic currents. The *north-west*, or *mistral*, so injurious in the *Provence*, displays here likewise its character as a cold, impetuous, withering wind, with its clouds of irritating dust, depressing the healthy and enfeebling the delicate. In the peninsula the dust is somewhat allayed by the passage across the sea. The *north-east* wind, or *greco*, is variable—sometimes vehement, usually dry. The sirocco was found by Dr. Jackson to be less disagreeable on the southern side of the Mediterranean than on the northern. In the former situation it was hot and parching, filling every available nook and crevice with grits of sand, and causing unpleasant feverishness; but, withal, it roused the traveller's energies for the purpose of overcoming its evil effects, at least in the desert. But on this side of the Mediterranean it usually produces utter prostration both of mind and body; under its influence the strong man and the invalid both are bowed down—their bodies refuse to act, and their minds to will. When arriving at some portions of Italy, at *Nice* especially, the wind has lost much of its severity, and acts as 'balmy air,' moderating the heat of summer and the coldness of winter. With reference to the temperature of the various parts of Italy, the following table will give some useful comparisons :—

Venice (on the eastern shore) has a mean annual temperature of 55° 4′: winter, 38°; spring, 54¾°; summer, 73°; autumn, 55¾°.

Genoa (on the western shore).—Mean annual temperature, 61°: winter, 47⅓°; spring, 58¾°; summer, 75°; autumn, nearly 63°.

Florence.—Mean annual temperature, 59¼°: winter, 43¾°; spring, 58½°; summer, 74½°; autumn, almost 60°.

Rome.—Mean annual temperature, 60½°: winter, 46¾°; spring, 58¼°; summer, 74¼°; autumn, 62¾°.

Naples.—Mean annual temperature, 60¼°: winter, 47½°; spring, 57½; summer, 74⅓; autumn, 61½°.

Palermo (North Sicily).—Mean annual temperature, 63°: winter, 52½°; spring, 59°; summer, 74·4°; autumn, 66⅓°.

Edinburgh.—Mean annual temperature, 47·13°: winter, 38·45°; spring, 45°; summer, 57·17°; autumn, 47·89°.

Dublin.—Mean annual temperature, 50°: winter, 40·67°; spring, 48½°; summer, 61°; autumn, 50°.

London.—Mean annual temperature, 50·83°: winter, 39½°; spring, 49°; summer, 62·93°; autumn, 51·83°.

Penzance.—Mean annual temperature, 51¾°: winter, 44¼°; spring, 49⅓°; summer, 60·91°; autumn, 52·07°.

Brussels.—Mean annual temperature, 50·68°: winter, 38°; spring, 49°; summer, 64°; autumn, 51·6°.

Paris.—Mean annual temperature, 51·31°: winter, 37·85°; spring, 50·6°; summer, 64½°; autumn 52½°.

As regards snowy days in Italy, they increase from south to north, but not in a regular manner: thus Palermo has two and a half annually; Rome, one and a half; Florence, one and a third; Venice, five and a half; and Milan, ten. The climate of Italy offers great advantages to the valetudinarian requiring change of scene and recreation from mental work; but as a winter resort for consumptive patients, great care is requisite, both concerning choice of locality and the proper way of using the advantages and guarding against the dangers of the country. Though the greatest benefit to be expected is a more unrestrained amount of out-door exercise than he can obtain at home, still he must abstain most carefully from imprudent exposure, from leaving home on wet days, in cool evenings and mornings. When walking in the sun, especially during spring days, he ought not to cross into the much colder shade, for the heat is more due to the direct solar influence than to the warmth of the atmosphere. The visiting of cold churches, bleak ruins, or cold picture galleries, is likewise attended with danger. The invalid is recommended to choose apartments with a southern aspect; to have fires in the cool mornings and evenings, attending to a proper ventilation, and consulting a thermometer exposed to the air, in a shady position, with reference to the amount of clothing necessary before starting.

FLORENCE (Ital. *Firenze*), intersected by the river Arno in its course from east to west, is situated at the foot of the Apennines, in a plain, at a height of 134 feet over the level of the sea. Latitude N. 43° 46'; longitude E. 11° 15'. 146 miles north-north-west of Rome. Population, 114,000. It is connected by railway with Pisa, Leghorn, Milan, Turin, &c. Its attractions, both natural and artificial, are varied and numerous. The surrounding snow-covered mountain tops lower the winter temperature, and render the spring months extremely variable. In summer the heat becomes very oppressive, from the absence of cool currents of air. The tramontana is very severe in January and February. In spring the east wind prevails, and exercises a withering influence. In April and May, when the sun commences to exercise its sway, the shady sides of the streets are still intensely cold. During June, July, and August, it is scarcely fit to be inhabited; after this period, the climate becomes agreeable. The mean annual temperature is $59\frac{1}{4}°$: winter, $43\frac{3}{4}°$; spring, $58\frac{1}{2}°$; summer, $74\frac{1}{2}$; autumn, 59·96°. Annual rainfall, thirty-two inches, most of which occurs during the end of autumn and commencement of winter, when moisture and fogs are not rare. The wet gets soon absorbed, or drained into the Arno. One hundred and nine is the mean annual number of rainy days. Notwithstanding its great beauty and apparently favourable position, Florence is unfit as a residence for consumptive patients. Miliary fever reigns here, but does not attack strangers; inflammatory diseases of the chest, however, are frequent here, and often fatal; but persons of a weakly nervous system, or such as are affected with gout, scrofula, &c., may derive benefit from a short sojourn during winter.

GENOA (Ital. *Genova*), a fortified seaport at the head of the Gulf of Genoa, on the Mediterranean, 79 miles south-east of Turin (with which it is connected by railway). Latitude N. 44° 24'; longitude E. 8° 54'. Population, 128,000. The port is protected by moles towards the sea, and towards the land by the city, which rises like an amphitheatre out of the water, situated on the ridges of hills, and enclosed by two series of walls; the whole embraced by a line of detached forts and outworks, crowning the hills for a circuit of about seven miles. Being bounded by high mountains at the back and by the sea in front, it might be thought to be a most salubrious city for invalids; but the contrary is the case. The vicissitudes of temperature are most frequent and trying. The cold, piercing tramontana is not sufficiently prevented by the mountains from entering the city. Besides this wind, the warm, moist, enervating *sirocco* (south-east) frequently appears, leaving behind an unpleasant lowering fog, named *cuin*. The mistral (or north-west) likewise often exercises its injurious influence. The east and west winds are more pleasant; the latter are pretty constant in summer. The libeccio (south-west) is sometimes very violent. Mean annual temperature, 61°: winter, 47°; spring, 58°; summer, 75°; autumn, 62·9°. Pulmonary affections are very frequent here, also scrofula and rheumatism. It is unfit as a winter resort for invalids, on account of its unsteady temperature, but may be visited for change of scenery; it has also been recommended in some cases of dyspepsia and in certain forms of threatening paralysis.

APPENDIX.

MILAN, a city of NORTH ITALY, situated in a wide fertile plain between the rivers Olona and Saveso. Latitude N. 45¼°; longitude E. 9⅛°. Altitude, 483 feet. The town is nearly circular, enclosed by a wall on three sides, and surrounded by broad ramparts and a strong castle. A canal, nearly eight miles in circumference, encloses the centre. Population, 196,000. Eighty-nine miles north-east of Turin (about three and a half hours' railway journey). An hour's railway ride from the town of Como (the southern termination of the charming Lake of Como). It has little recommendation for invalids, as it lies exposed to all winds, and is therefore liable to great vicissitudes of temperature. The winds which arrive from the Adriatic pass unchecked from north to south east; those that come from the south are but slightly prevented from entering, after crossing the Apennines. The cold winds from the north have the preponderance; hence the mean annual temperature is only 54·9°—viz., winter, 36°; spring, 54·8°; summer, 72·8°; autumn 55·9°. Lymphatic diseases prevail among the inhabitants, in consequence of sudden and frequent transitions from cold and dry to warm and moist air. It is the abode of *pellagra*, or Italian leprosy. The Hospidale Maggiore, founded by Francesco Sforza in 1456, is a grand and imposing establishment, but with the great defect of being too crowded, some wards having three rows of beds running parallel the whole length, and being mostly occupied. The hospital is said to possess six millions of francs as an annual income, but, with all its riches, the great desideratum of free air is curtailed by the surrounding buildings, not even a garden being available as exercise ground for convalescents. Though, on the whole, Milan cannot be ranked as a health-resort, a tour to the Italian lakes and a visit to this beautiful city will in many instances prove a greater restorative of mental equilibrium to the overworked brain than a mere sojourn in the country. The charming scenery afforded by the journey from Milan to the Lakes of Como, Maggiore, Garda, and Lugarno, all accessible by rail, well repays a visit.

NAPLES (Ital. *Napoli*), on the north shore of the Bay of Naples, near the foot of Mount Vesuvius, is 162½ miles south-east of Rome (about eight hours' railway journey). Lat. N. 40⅙°; long. E. 14° 15'. Population, 447,000. It is built in the form of an amphitheatre, on the slope of a range of hills, divided by a ridge into two natural crescents—the eastern containing the largest and most ancient portion of the town; the western, the modern city, called the *Chiaja*. Of the five principal entrances, that by the Bridge de la Madeleine is the most striking. There are few spacious squares, with the exception of the Largo del Castello (in which the palace and the theatre of San Carlo are situated, and in front of the Church of S. Giovanni Paulo). The beauty of the environs is unique, besides affording many extremely interesting classic reminiscences. The ruins of Pozzuoli, to the west; the tomb of Virgil, in the stupendous grotto of Pausilippo, in the island of Capri, to the south; Lake Avernus, the shores of Bajæ, the coast of Castellamare, the orange-groves of Sorrento, the fields of lava, the excavated Pompeii and Herculaneum,—all tend to recall periods of interesting antiquity. The western town forms a beautiful promenade, having the hill of Vomero at the back and the sea in front. Fort St. Elmo overlooks the town on the ridge. Naples lies in the depression between this hill and the headland of Pizzofalcone. It is four miles long from west to east, and two and a half wide. Mean annual temperature, $60\frac{1}{4}°$: winter, $47·6$; spring, $57\frac{1}{2}°$; summer, $74\frac{1}{3}°$; autumn, $61\frac{1}{2}°$. The town is fully exposed to the south-west and west winds from the sea, and not sufficiently protected against north winds by the hills at the rear. If the north-west wind has once crossed the hill of Posilipo (which keeps off the due north wind), it blows unchecked through the whole western portion. Against direct east wind, shelter is afforded by the Somma; but the north-east wind enters between Capo di Monte and Capo di Chino. The south and south-east winds visit the town after passing over the mountains of Castellamare and Sorrento. The moist southerly winds predominate. The south-east wind (sirocco) has a greatly depressing influence; the north-west (mistral) is cold and moist, and so severe that the part generally affected by it has been nicknamed 'Siberia.' Rain mostly falls in October and November. The mean annual amount is between twenty-nine and thirty-seven inches. Snow is very rare, but it sometimes covers the surrounding hills, and imparts intense cold through the winds which pass over the town. The climate is too treacherous to be used for pulmonary diseases. The direct solar heat sometimes masks the variable character of the winds in spring; the sirocco and the marshy exhalations to the east of the town render autumn unhealthy, whilst summer heat becomes tempered through cooling sea breezes. Catarrhal and inflammatory diseases of the lungs are frequent here, especially during the predominance of the mistral. Rheumatism, ophthalmia, and, in the eastern suburbs, intermittent fevers, are not rare. Naples is recommended as a winter resort for cases of general and nervous depression, melancholia, and hysterics, where a bracing climate and the charming scenery may contribute to raise the mental powers. But there must be no disposition to thoracic disease, for the most habitable portion of the town (the western) is the most exposed. September and the commencement of October offer the most pleasant temperature—cheerful days, with moderate heat; small showers, with a quickly-following serene sky. In March the weather is inconstant. On the whole, the climate may be considered as salubrious, as the alternating sea and land winds moderate the temperature, and contribute to purify the air. In the neighbourhood, *Corpo di Cava*, south-east of Naples, surrounded by beautiful foliage and highly situated, offers peculiar advantages as a summer residence for consumptive patients, and also the Convent of Trinita; for the same purpose may be recommended *Castellamare*, south of Naples, on the western shore of the bay (reached by rail within an hour), and the charming and picturesque *Sorrento*, on the south-western portion of the bay (reached in an hour and a half by sea, and in two and a half by land). From middle of May till middle of October, people generally resort to the country.

POZZUOLI, a suburb of Naples, lying on the sea towards the west, is supposed to be more favourable for consumptive patients, the climate being milder than that of Naples. The sulphur vapours diffused through the warm air are considered by some physicians to act soothingly on the pulmonary mucous membrane. Some mineral springs in the neighbourhood, hot (106° Fahr.) and cold, are used for gout, rheumatism, and cutaneous and scrofulous diseases. They contain soda, magnesia, lime, iron, and alumina. But the place does not enjoy as good a reputation as formerly for sanitary purposes.

PISA, a walled city on the eastern shore of the river Arno, in a fertile but marshy plain of Tuscany, seven miles from its mouth, twelve miles north-north-east of Leghorn (half an hour's railway journey); forty-eight miles west of Florence (two and a half hours' railway journey). Lat. N. 43° 43'; long. E. $10\frac{1}{4}°$. Population, 51,000; circumference, five miles. It was formerly one of the most celebrated and thriving towns in Italy. It is the birthplace of Galileo. It owes its mild temperature to the Tuscan hills (3,000 feet high) encircling the landscape from north-west to south-east, thus completely sheltering the valley against north winds, and partially against north-west and south-east winds. But being fully exposed towards the south and south-west, the currents arriving from Livorno and the sea have free access. *Lung Arno*, that part of the town stretching towards the north, and having a southern aspect, is more protected against northern winds than the other parts, by the walls and the height of the buildings; but this very circumstance impedes the free circulation of the atmosphere, the streets being rendered narrow, dark, and damp, whilst the sluggish Arno sometimes emits exhalations not very favourable to the promotion of health and vigour. The climate is, on the whole, mild, relaxing, damp, and depressing. Mean annual temperature, 59·45°: winter, 44·83°; spring, 57·81°; summer, $73\frac{3}{4}°$; autumn, $61\frac{1}{2}°$. December and January are the coldest months; October, November, March, and April, extremely mild. Towards the evening, the temperature generally lowers considerably. The air is much moister than at Nice. The climate, no doubt, soothes the irritation of the pulmonary mucous membrane, and diminishes vascular excitement in general; but as this advantage is counterbalanced by the depressing and lowering character of the atmosphere, consumptive patients ought not to choose it as a winter resort.

ROME is situated on the *Tiber*, seventeen miles north-east of its entrance into the Mediterranean. Lat. N. 41° 53'; long. E. 12° 28'. Altitude, under the Ælian-bridge, twenty feet. Population, 197,000. It is built on marshy ground, at the foot of a range of low hills, in the midst of the undulating flat *Campagna di Roma*. The Tiber separates the town into two unequal portions, which are divided into fourteen *Rioni*, or quarters; twelve of these are Rome proper, on the left shore of the Tiber, containing the Vatican and the Castle of St. Angelo, and only two are on the right bank. Its walls are twelve miles in circumference. The lower parts of the city are often inundated, especially after severe rains. The streets of the modern city are spacious, but badly kept, and winding. The mean annual temperature is $60\frac{1}{2}°$—viz., winter, $46\frac{3}{4}°$; spring, $58\frac{1}{4}°$; summer,

74¼°; autumn, 62¾°. Being exposed to the cold north-east winds as well as to the warm moist south-west winds, violent changes of temperature often occur suddenly. Generally, however, southerly winds prevail during the day, and render the climate soft and relaxing. In the mornings and evenings, northerly winds generally predominate. The west wind, coming from the sea, has ordinarily a refreshing character. The sirocco, or south-east, is mostly dry, and sometimes moist, but always lowering, especially to persons of full habit. The tramontana, so frequent in winter and spring, generally produces a severe piercing cold, and is much dreaded. Snow is very rare; frosts very short. Rainfall about thirty inches; rainy days, 114. The most pleasant month is October, after the mild September rains. November is also favourable; but in the following months, cold northerly winds appear, with winter rains. From the end of May, Rome commences to become more and more unhealthy, fever being generated in June, July, and August. Many inflammatory diseases of the chest prevail in winter, and malaria fever in summer. Rome is considered useful in soothing bronchial irritation. As regards steadiness of temperature, it is superior to Naples and Pisa, but inferior to Nice. According to Sir James Clark, the peculiar *stillness* of the atmosphere is considered as a particular recommendation for pulmonary invalids. Rome is positively injurious to persons inclined to apoplexy or to paralysis, to hæmorrhages or to hypochondriasis. Such streets are to be selected for residence as have an easterly and westerly direction; their houses are freer from currents of cold air. Whilst invalids should avail themselves of the great facilities for outdoor exercise, they ought to guard against visiting cold churches and galleries when in a heated state. In all erethic forms of pulmonary disease the climate is injurious, as it is inclined to produce congestion. The best time of arrival for invalids is October or November. December is exposed to more vicissitudes of temperature, on account of the frequent antagonism between north and south winds. Spring commences early, and brings a more mild and equable temperature. Those who wish to remain in the neighbourhood during the summer may avail themselves of the beautiful neighbouring *Albano*, to the south-east, or *Frascati*, to the east.

PALERMO, a fortified city on the northern shore of SICILY, in a fertile valley on the slope of the bay. Lat. N. 38° 8'; long. E. 13° 22'. Population, 220,000. The climate is the most delightful in Europe. Mean annual temperature, 64°: winter, 52°; summer, 74°. Annual rainfall, 22 inches. On three sides it is enclosed by mountains, being open to the sea in the north. The houses have balconies with glass doors instead of windows, and are flat-topped. The place abounds in fine walks. Steam communication with Messina in the east, with Naples in the north, and with Malta, Marseilles, and Liverpool. The winter temperature is equable, mild, and moderately moist:—October, 66·8°; November, 59·7°; December, 54·1°; January, 51·5°; February, 51·8°; March, 54°; April, 58½°; May, 65°. From June to September it ranges from 71° to 76°; 78° in August, and 73° in September. Through its insular position, the heat is more equably divided between the different months, than at the other Mediterranean health-resorts; it is, therefore, well adapted for consumptive patients. But sharp north winds sometimes appear in February and March, which ought to keep the invalids in their homes, and induce them to order firing during the short prevalence of the cold. In March, rain falls frequently, but in April the temperature becomes extremely pleasant. Those who require a more bracing air are recommended to reside at the hotel of *Trinacria*, situated near the sea, with charming views; but, for invalids requiring a somewhat warmer and more sheltered locality, the Hôtel de France, in the middle of the town, is preferable. Villas, in the so-called *Olmuzza*, are also available for invalids, but, from its low situation, the air is somewhat damp. The season lasts from November till May (inclusive). Dr. Moscuzza and Professor Cervello are recommended as physicians.

VENICE (Ital. *Venezia*), a fortified city lying in the lagoons, a sort of lake, separated from the Adriatic by a belt of low land, which is intersected by six channels, between the Piave in the north and the Adige in the south. The principal of these is the *Porto di Lido*, connected with the island di Lido, two miles southward, by an immense bridge of 222 arches, over which the Padua railway passes. Lat. N. $45\frac{1}{4}°$; long. E. $12\frac{1}{2}°$. Population, 118,000. The town is entirely built on piles, occupying seventy or eighty small islands, separated by canals, and provided with 306 bridges. The Grand Canal divides the city into nearly two equal portions, connected by the white marble bridge of the Rialto. The island of Rialto is the spot on which the city first existed. The streets being too narrow and intricate for carriages, the chief traffic is carried on by *gondolas*, on the canals. The square of St. Mark and the public gardens, nearly surrounded by the sea, offer an admirable sight. It is a magnificent city, full of palaces and objects of interest. It is connected by railway with Padua, Milan, Vienna, Trieste, &c. (with the latter also by steamers; eight hours' sea voyage.) The shallow lake on which the city is built owes its origin to alluvial deposits of the rivers in their descent towards the sea. The piercing north-east wind is dry and cold, but has the advantage of driving off the exhalations of the lagoons. When a warm and moist southerly wind comes in antagonism with it, snow sometimes results in winter, and storms in summer. The Alps to the north of Venice greatly mitigate the violence of the northern currents. West and south-west winds are somewhat tempered by a branch of Lombardian mountains; but direct east and south-east (sirocco) enter without restraint. Mean annual temperature, $55·8°$: winter, $38°$; spring, $54\frac{3}{4}°$; summer, $73°$; autumn, $58\frac{3}{4}°$. Snowfall, $5\frac{1}{2}$ days; rainy days, 75; annual rainfall, notwithstanding the surrounding marshes, only $36\frac{1}{4}$ inches. The climate is mild, equable, soft, and sedative. Venice is therefore useful in chronic bronchial irritation and commencing tuberculosis; but it is not adapted for torpid, lymphatic, and atonic individuals. The climate is subject to less variations than in any other part of Italy, the transitions of temperature being generally slow and gradual. The air was ascertained to be largely impregnated with bromine and iodine. From the marshy environs, one might think the town subject to intermittent fever or malaria; but, probably in consequence of the northern winds, and the ebb and flow of the sea occurring daily through the channels, the air becomes divested of the vapours emanating from the soil. But day and night temperature sometimes differs considerably, especially in spring and autumn ; also sunny and shady places occasionally exhibit such differences of temperature as to produce serious cases of catarrh and rheumatism, by invalids suddenly passing from the former to the latter places. The want of distant promenades for pedestrian exercise is a serious drawback, rendering the sojourn rather monotonous. Season, from September to May.

JERSEY (*Cæsarea*), the largest of the so-called Channel Islands, and the most southern (opposite Weymouth), fifteen miles west of the coast of France (Cotentin), and eighty-eight miles south-south-east of Portland Bill. Latitude N. of the capital (St. Helier), 49° 11'; long. W. 2° 7'. Length of island, eleven miles; breadth, five miles. Population, 54,020 (in 1851); 57,060 (in 1861). St. Helier lies at the eastern extremity of St. Aubyn's Bay, in an open and picturesque valley. The surface is undulating ; hill ranges run from north to south, and enclose several fertile plains. The whole island appears like a continuation of orchards, with alternating hills and dales. Rainfall 27 inches. Reached by steamer from Weymouth in nine hours (Guernsey in six). There is likewise steam communication with Southampton and St. Malo. The inhabitants speak a kind of French patois, as the islands formerly belonged to Normandy, but have been attached to England since the conquest. The island undulates downwards from the rocky north coast to the sandy south coast. The soil consists of a sandy loam, with a subsoil of red clay on a foundation of granite rock. The water is soft in the higher parts and hard in the lower. Mean annual temperature, 53° : spring, 50·97°; summer, 62·84°; autumn, 54·63°; winter, 43·82°. Lying in the current of the English Channel, it is exposed to all winds, and has, therefore, seldom a perfectly calm day. The western breezes prevail for about eight months. In the spring months, the north-east wind sometimes blows for a considerable time. The island enjoys an early spring and a protracted autumn. Vegetation commences early, and the landscape appears green and fresh even in December. Winter is very mild there, with scarcely any frost or snow. In May, the temperature is particularly unsteady, whilst March and October are peculiarly equable and mild. The most salubrious situations of Jersey are on the south-west side of St. Helier's parish. St. Helier itself is very subject to rain and fogs, and is comparatively deficient in opportunities for pedestrian exercise. *St. Aubyn's*, three miles to the west, is considered more suitable for invalids. Chronic rheumatism prevails among the inhabitants to a considerable degree ; also diseases of the liver, scrofula, and remittent fevers; but ague and lithiasis are rare. Inflammatory diseases generally exhibit a mild character. The climate of the Channel Islands resembles that of Penzance, on the south-west coast, as regards equability of temperature, and humidity ; high winds during the winter and cold north-east winds during the spring. Dr. Scholefield considers it probable that the clouds and vapours are attracted by the meridian sun, and partly intercepted at the shore by the lofty forts that block up the town towards the sea; thus materially obstructing the free transmission of air, and the dissipation of noxious vapours and fogs. Mildness and moisture are the great characteristics of the climate. The roads dry very rapidly after rain; but a heavy dew falls at night, very beneficent in summer, and without producing that evening chilliness which often follows a hot day in England. Consumption is comparatively rare here; the place is therefore often recommended as a winter resort for tuberculous patients. But it could only suit those cases in which the malady has not reached an advanced stage, and where the constitution possesses a certain degree of vigour. The action of the climate is soothing and relaxing, and therefore unadapted to weak leuco-phlegmatic individuals.

KIEL, a seaport town in the Duchy of HOLSTEIN, on a fine bay of the Baltic, fifty-three miles north-north-east of Hamburg, at the terminus of the railway from Altona (three hours' journey). Population, 17,000. Lat. N. $54\frac{1}{2}°$; long. E. $10°·$ It possesses an elegant and beautifully situated bathing establishment on the western side of the bay, near the Diester-brooker Wood, a quarter of a league from the town. The climate is mild, and sheltered against winds; the ground gently sloping, and covered with soft white sand. Season, from the end of June to end of September. There is ample accommodation in the bath establishment and in the surrounding garden-houses. The environs are very pleasant.
Physician—Dr. Steindorff.

KÖSEN, in the Prussian province of SAXONY, a station of the Thuringian railroad, between Naumburg and Sulza, south-west of Leipzig, twenty-two miles north-east of Weimar, a mile and a half from the celebrated *Schulpforte*, lies in a charming valley, intersected by the Saale; protected by the surrounding heights against severe north and north-east winds. The saline springs contain 380 grains of solid constituents in 16 ounces—viz., 335 chloride of sodium; 2·2 sulphate of soda; 2·4 sulphate of potash; $33\frac{1}{2}$ sulphate of lime; 1 carbonate of lime; 7·9 sulphate of magnesia; 0·1 oxyde of iron. Temperature, 65°. The water is diluted with common water, and warmed by hot vapour from below for the baths. There is also an apparatus for impregnating the liquid with carbonic acid gas. In cases of bronchial irritation, the walks along the graduation works, and the inhalation of the saline particles floating in the air, is very useful. In cases of scrophulosis the baths are employed with advantage.
Physicians—Drs. Rosenberger and Groddeck.

KÖNIGSDORFF-IASTRZEMB, in the Rybniker district, in Upper Silesia, one hundred and thirty miles south of Breslau, an *ioduretted* spa, lately used for therapeutical purposes. The springs contain, in 16 ounces, 96 grains of solid constituents—viz., 87·9 chloride of sodium; $\frac{1}{2}$ chloride of potassium; $4\frac{1}{2}$ chloride of calcium; 2·6 chloride of magnesium; 0·04 iodide of

EUROPEAN SPAS AND CLIMATIC HEALTH-RESORTS. 357

magnesium; 0·22 bromide of magnesium; ⅓ carbonate of lime; 0·01 carbonate of magnesia; 0·03 carbonate of iron; sulphate of lime, 0·08. From Breslau the rail takes the valetudinarian to *Oderberg*, in the south, and thence the Ferdinands (North) Railway to *Petrowitz*, in Austrian Silesia (towards the east,) where an omnibus expects the traveller, and brings him in half an hour to the new spa, which promises to be greatly resorted to on account of its combination of chlorides and iodides ready for use, in cases of glandular enlargement, without any dilution. The new cure-house has sufficient accommodation for 400 or 500 visitors.

Physicians—Drs. Faupel, Lubowski, Freund.

KRANKENHEIL, on the left shore of the Isar (in BAVARIA), one league east of Tölz, one and a half league north-east of Heilbrunn, eleven and a half leagues south of Munich, on the north-eastern declivity of the Blomberg (3,452 ft. high); 2,467 ft. over the level of the sea; three and a half leagues south-west of *Holzkirchen* station of the Munich-Rosenheim Railroad. The air is pure, bracing, and mild; there are no houses near the springs. On the most picturesque road towards Tölz, the charmingly situated Custom-house is reached in three-quarters of an hour, in which lodgings may be obtained. A quarter of a league farther, Tölz lies in a most beautiful landscape, the proper residence of the cure-guests. Population, 3,000. A diligence goes twice daily from the station to Tölz (in two hours and a quarter). The springs are particularly efficacious in scrofulous diseases of the skin, the principal action being antiplastic and alterative; as they contain only a small quantity of solid ingredients,* they

* INGREDIENTS CONTAINED IN SIXTEEN OUNCES OF THE WATER.

	Iodide of Sodium Spring (Johann-Georgen Spring)	Sulphuretted Iodide of Sodium Spring (Bernhard Spring)	Sulphuretted Spring (Anna Spring)
	Grains	Grains	Grains
Sulphate of potash	0·09	0 07	0·15
,, soda	0·09	0·03	2·25
Chloride of sodium	1·79	2·27	0·23
Iodide of sodium	0·01	0·01	—
Bicarbonate of soda	2·48	2·56	1·49
,, lime	0·70	0·78	1·91
,, magnesia	0·22	0.22	—
,, iron	—	—	—
,, manganese	—	—	—
Silicate of alumina	0·02	0·01	1·84
Silicic acid	0·06	0·07	0·03
Total	5·50	5·07	7·98
	Cubic inches	Cubic inches	Cubic inches
Free carbonic acid	0·32	0·23	0·63
Sulphuretted hydrogen	0·05	0·07	0·23

agree even with very irritable persons. The *iodide of sodium* spring, the *sulphuretted iodide of sodium*, and the *Anna* spring, are used internally. The former (weaker) one is more adapted for delicate persons. The second, which contains a considerable quantity of sulphuretted hydrogen, exercises a more energetic effect on the cutaneous system, and is fitted for the use of robust persons. The *Annaquelle*, the most powerful and abundant, is used in the most intractable cases.

The water is either imbibed pure or mixed with whey. Baths are used tepid or warm. By evaporating the water, the so-called 'quell-salz' (spring salt) is obtained, which is employed either internally in a diluted form, or externally as fomentation over glandular swellings and ovarian enlargements. It is also used for the formation of soaps with fat, and employed in chronic cutaneous diseases with great advantage. The distinctive characteristic of the spa is to be sought in the happy combination of sulphur and iodine.

Physicians—Drs. Höfler and Jungmayer.

KRONTHAL, on the southern declivity of the Taunus, two and a half leagues north-west of Frankfort-on-the-Main, half a league north-west of Soden, 512 feet over the level of the sea, lies in a charming wide valley, only open towards the south. The climate is therefore extremely mild, and well adapted for persons affected with bronchial catarrhs. The springs contain in 16 ounces:—

	Wilhelms Spring	The former Stool Spring
	Grains	Grains
Chloride of sodium	27·20	22·27
„ potassium	0·67	0·77
„ ammonium	0.04	0·07
„ calcium	0·16	0·07
„ magnesium	0·47	0·04
Carbonate of lime	5·10	4·17
Sulphate of lime	0·23	0·21
Phosphate of lime	0·01	0·02
Arsenate of lime	—	—
Carbonate of magnesia	0·72	0·72
„ soda	—	0·18
„ manganese	0·01	0·02
„ iron	0·10	0·05
Hydrate of silica	0·55	0·66
Silicate of alumina	—	—
„ soda	0·41	0·18
Organic matter	0·01	0·11
Free carbonic acid	17·79	20·57
Total	53·55	49·84
Temperature	61°	57° F.

Physician—Dr. Küster.

LABASSÈRE, a *sulphurous* spring five miles from Bagnères-de-Bigorre, is extremely useful in bronchial and laryngeal catarrh. Its temperature ranges from 54° to 57°. It only contains 3·68 grains of solid constituents in 16 ounces—viz., sulphuret of sodium, 0·35; chloride of sodium, 1·58; chloride of potassium, 0·02; carbonate of soda, 0·17; silicate of lime, 0·33; silicate of magnesia, 0·07; alum in excess, 0·01; iodine, traces; organic matter, 1·11. The water is only used internally, and is extremely well adapted for transport.
Physicians—Dr. Labayle, Dr. Verdoux.

LANDECK, in SILESIA, near the town of Landeck, fifteen miles south-east of Glatz, lies in a beautiful mountain valley, permeated by the Biela, and surrounded from the east, south, and west by high mountains; altitude, 1,398′. It is connected by diligence with the *Frankenstein* station of the Breslau-Schweidnitz Railroad (fifteen miles to the north), and with the *Neisse* station of the Breslau-Brieg railway (twenty-three miles to the east). Six springs issue here out of gneiss, with pretty similar composition, but with varying temperature—from 48° (St. Georgebrunnen) to 64° (Mühlquelle.) Analysis according to Fischer : Sulphate of soda, 0·24 grains; crenate of soda, 0·28; chloride of potassium, 0·16; phosphate of lime, 0·04; sulphate of lime, 0·00; carbonate of lime, 0·08; phosphate of alumina, iron, and manganese, 0·01; silica, 0·27—total, 1·12 grains; carbonic acid, 0·26 inch; nitrogen, 0·62; sulphuretted hydrogen, traces. The Wiesenquelle and Marienbrunnen are used for drinking, the others for bathing. Sometimes whey is mixed with the water. By its lower temperature, Landeck is inferior to the others of the so-called indifferent thermæ, but has the advantage of possessing some sulphuretted hydrogen. Moreover, the moor-baths assist the cure in rheumatic and arthritic swellings, and in uterine enlargements resulting from chronic inflammation. The air is very bracing, and at the same time sheltered by the encircling mountains against north and east winds. In chronic bronchial catarrhs, inhalations of the gaseous vapours are used with advantage.
Physicians—Drs. Langner, Adamczik, Wehse.

LANGENBRÜCKEN, in the Grand Duchy of BADEN, on the railway beween Heidelberg and Bruchsal, lies in a charming valley, 440 feet above the level of the sea, on the declivity of the mountain ranges which connect the Odenwald with the Black Forest. Vegetation and foliage are luxurious in the whole valley. Fourteen sulphurous springs issue here—some spontaneously, others through artesian wells. The *Trink-quelle* (drinking-spring) contains 3¾ grains of solid constituents in 16 ounces—viz., sulphate of soda, ¼; sulphate of lime, ½; sulphate of potash, 0·15; chloride of sodium, 0·08; carbonate of lime, 2·12; carbonate of magnesia, 0·35; carbonate of iron, 0·07; silica, 0·01; sulphuretted hydrogen, 0·10 cubic inches; carbonic acid, 27·98 cubic inches. Temperature, 52°. The *Wald-quelle* contains 11¾ grains—viz., sulphate of soda, 1·63; sulphate of magnesia, 3·88; sulphate of lime, 2·41; phosphate of lime, 0·16; sulphate of potash, 0·15; sulphuret of calcium, 0·04; chloride of potassium, 0·10;

carbonate of lime, 1·81; carbonate of magnesia, 1·84; sulphuret of iron, 0·03; alumina, 0·03; silica, 0·13; sulphuretted hydrogen, 0·15 cubic inches; carbonic acid, 3·09. Temperature, 57° Fahr. Gas, douche, vapour, and drop baths are employed besides. The spa has shown itself very serviceable in chronic *catarrh of the bladder*, in rheumatism, and in bronchial irritation; also in certain cutaneous diseases. Through the mildness of the climate, the season commences early in spring, and extends to the end of autumn.

Physician—Dr. Eimer.

LEUK (Loèche, *Canton Wallis*) lies in a remarkably picturesque Alpine valley, on the southern (almost perpendicular) declivity of the *Gemmi*, between fine luxurious meadows; 4,351 feet over the level of the sea. The valley is four leagues long, half a league wide, and only open to the south. Gigantic snow-covered rocks encircle the green valley; the foaming Dala rushes through the place previous to its fall into the Rhone. The village (*Leuker-Bad*) is about two and a half leagues distant from the southern borough of Leuk (on the right shore of the Rhone). The Lausanne railroad carries the traveller as far as Sitten (Sion), south-west; thence the diligence continues the route, with a frequent view of the beautiful precipitous *Rhone*, and completes it in about nine hours. Those who come from Bern or Luzern may take the rail as far as Thun, then drive to Kandersteg (3,600 feet high), and from there ride on mules over the Gemmi Pass (7,000 feet high), unless they prefer to undertake the six hours' walk on foot. The road from the height to the spa is much steeper, and ought to be passed either on foot or in a portechaise. More than twenty springs issue here in a small space. The water is perfectly clear, and inodorous. Occasionally, after heavy rains or extensive melting of snow, it becomes turbid. The principal springs are:—1. The Lorenz spring (temperature 124°), the most abundant; used for drinking and bathing. 2. The springs of the Armen bath (temperature, 116°). 3. The Heilbad springs (temperature, 118°), supplying the Alpine-bad. 4. The Hügel springs (temperature, 118 to 122°). 5. The springs on the Dala (93° to 104°).

The Lorenz spring contains $14\frac{1}{2}$ grains of solid constituents in 16 ounces, viz.:—

Sulphate of lime	10·67 grains
Sulphate of magnesia	2·36 ,,
Sulphate of soda	0·39 ,,
Sulphate of potash	0·29 ,,
Sulphate of strontia	0·03 ,,
Chloride of potassium	0·05 ,,
Carbonate of lime	0·03 ,,
Carbonate of magnesia	0.07 ,,
Carbonate of iron	0·07 ,,
Silica	0·27 ,,
Alumina	traces
Total	14·30 ,,
Carbonic acid	0·12 cubic inches
Oxygen	0·05 ,,
Nitrogen	0·58 ,,

In all the baths, large basins serve for both sexes, who are in the habit of bathing together, invested with thick bathing-dresses; but separate baths may be had for those who prefer them. As the temperature of the water is too high for immediate use, the baths are filled in the evening, and then have the proper heat next morning. They exercise a stimulating effect on the skin, and a diuretic effect on the kidneys. They are recommended in chronic swellings of the glandular and lymphatic system, in inveterate catarrhs, in *catarrhal hoarseness*, chronic rheumatism, gout, paralytic gout, eczema, and herpes. The climate is rough, but very bracing. The mixed bathing of the sexes, which may be thought highly objectionable, has in reality no offensive feature. The authorities attempted to abolish the custom several times, but the guests insisted on their right. If it is remembered that the patients remain in the water from half an hour to two, three, or four hours, with every part as completely enveloped as in a drawing-room, the tedium of a solitary sojourn seems to them too great, and hence breakfast is often taken in the bath; ladies work, and gentlemen read there; general conversation proceeds, and time passes more rapidly and pleasantly. The long maceration of the skin in a warm liquid impregnated with a certain proportion of gypsum and of free nitrogen, cannot fail to have a powerfully alterative effect on the morbidly altered function of the skin and the subcutaneous nervous system. The spa is contra-indicated in all active congestions and inflammatory conditions.*

Physicians—Drs. Bouvin, Brunner, Grillet, Loretan, Mengis.

LIEBENZELL, WURTEMBERG, 24 miles west of Stuttgardt, in a romantic valley of the Black Forest, on the Nagold, 995 feet over the level of the sea, surrounded by steep mountains; one and a half league from the Pforzheim station of the Stuttgardt-Carlsruhe Railroad. The thermal water feels soft and fatty; temperature varying in the lower bath from 75° to 77°; in the upper, from 71° to 74°; constituents, 7¾ grains in 16 ounces—chloride of sodium, with traces of chloride of magnesium, 5·14; carbonate of soda, 0·8; sulphate of soda, 0·6; carbonate of lime, 0·8; oxide of iron, 0·1, silica, 0·4. Gases in 100 parts—72·5 carbonic acid; 24·4 nitrogen; 3 oxygen. It is particularly recommended in chronic metritis, especially if the uterine hyperæmia is the result of abdominal plethora.

Physicians—Dr. Hartmann, Dr. Müller of Calw (five miles to the south).

LIPPIK, *ioduretted saline thermal spring* of HUNGARY, on the *Pakra* river, in south-western Slavonia, about a mile and a quarter from the borough of *Pakraz*, near the so-called military boundary below 46° N. lat., seventy miles east-south-east of *Agram* (station), north of Gradiska on the Save, enjoys a great reputation in enlargements and indurations of the womb. The *Klein-bad-quelle* contains 20 grains of solid constituents in 16 ounces—viz., sulphate of soda, 5¼; chloride of sodium, 4⅔; chloride of calcium, ¾; iodide of calcium, ⅕; carbonate of soda, 9½; carbonate of

* The Hotels des Alpes and de France offer excellent accommodation.

magnesia, nearly ¾; carbonate of lime, 1⅓; phosphate of alumina, 0·02; silica, 0·08. 100 volumes of gas consist of—28·5 of carbonic acid, and 71·4 of nitrogen. Temperature, 111° Fahr. The *Bischofsquelle* is similarly composed, with a temperature of 115°.

Physician—Dr. Mark, of Pakraz.

LIPPSPRINGE, in the province of Westphalia, 378 feet over the level of the sea, five miles north-east of *Paderborn* (station), on the high road from Paderborn to Detmold (52° N. lat.), north-west of Driburg, south-west of Pyrmont. Notwithstanding its northern situation, the climate is mild, partly from its small elevation, and partly from the shelter afforded by the neighbouring Teutoburg Forest against north and north-east winds. The sandy soil, with a depth of six to twelve feet, also contributes in rendering the climate equable, by its power of absorbing the scorching rays of the sun in hot days, and emitting the heat in colder days. At the same time, the atmosphere is charged with humidity by the abundant flow of the Lippe and Jordan springs, in the immediate neighbourhood of the promenade and cure-house. The climate is therefore calming and antiphlogistic. In June, July, and August, the temperature is most equable. The *Arminius-quelle* contains 19½ grains of solid constituents in 16 ounces —viz., 5¼ sulphate of soda, 4¼ sulphate of lime, ⅞ sulphate of magnesia, 5¼ carbonate of lime, ⅔ carbonate of magnesia, 0·14 carbonate of iron, 0·86 chloride of sodium, 1·6 bicarbonate of soda, traces of iodides.. 100 volumes of free gases contain 83¼ of carbonic acid, 15¼ of nitrogen, and 1½ of oxygen. As regards combined gases, there are, in 100 cubic inches, 16·17 of carbonic acid, 4·40 of nitrogen, 0·55 of oxygen. Temperature, 70° Fahr. The spa has latterly gained a high reputation for cases of hereditary phthisical diathesis and incipient tuberculosis, especially if combined with inflammatory bronchial irritation and a generally excitable vascular system, the spring on the island particularly, in the latter instance. In florid forms, the *baths* are contra-indicated, but extremely useful in prevailing venosity and laxity of fibre; also in cases combined with scrofula. If a favourable result is to be expected, the course is not to be confined to four or six weeks; but usually a pause of a few weeks is made after drinking the water for some time, and employed as a whey cure, and then a second course is gone through. Inhalations are also made in an extremely well-ventilated saloon, receiving the gases direct from the source. The baths are connected with a colonnade, to protect the invalids against the vicissitudes of temperature. Beautiful walks and parks give ample opportunity for pedestrian exercise. The inhalations have been found very calming in *palpitations of the heart*, not only of a nervous character, but even when based on morbid function of the organ. Erethic individuals find great relief from them. They are able to breathe deeper and more freely. But weakly, leuco-phlegmatic, and nervous persons are not benefited by them, nor cases in which the lungs are partially destroyed or impassable. Besides the *Arminius-quelle*, which is considered as a *lime spring*, there is a cold *sulphur spring*, with 19¼ grains of solid constituents (13 of gypsum), 1·12 cubic inch of carbonic acid, and 2·32 cubic inches of sulphuretted hydrogen. Whilst in the sulphur spring the hepatic gas is intimately combined with the water, in the Arminius-Quelle the carbonic acid is more firmly attached to the water than the nitrogen; hence the great proportion of the latter (82 in 100) amongst the free gaseous emanations. Young phthisical subjects, disposed to frequent bronchial inflammations, are most benefited by Lippspringe. Cough and bloody expectoration soon give way. The capacity of the lung for air increases through the diminished hyperæmia. Emphysema and bronchial blennorrhœa become aggravated here.

Physicians—Dr. Fischer, Dr. Weber, Dr. Quicken.

OTTILIENQUELLE (the spring on the island), half a mile from Paderborn, contains less iron and carbonic acid, but twice as much nitrogen, and agrees well even with the most delicate excitable individuals, with the greatest disposition to hæmoptysis. It contains 12 grains of solid constituents—viz., $2\frac{1}{2}$ of carbonate of lime, 0·05 of carbonate of iron, $6\frac{3}{4}$ of chloride of sodium, $\frac{1}{2}$ sulphate of lime, $\frac{1}{2}$ chloride of calcium, $\frac{1}{4}$ chloride of magnesium, traces of iodine and bromine. Gases combined with the water in 100 cubic inches—2·34 carbonic acid, 8·98 nitrogen, 1·17 oxygen. Gases freely evolved in 100 volumes—3 carbonic acid, 97 nitrogen. In cases of great emaciation, when retarded metamorphosis becomes desirable, *inhalations* alone are recommended. Not far from the Ottilien spring, a chalybeate has been lately discovered (*Marienquelle*), with $4\frac{3}{4}$ grains of solid constituents—$1\frac{3}{4}$ carbonate of lime, 0·45 bicarbonate of iron. If tuberculosis has already made great progress and produced cavernæ, extensive condensation, and great prostration, the journey to this or any other spa will only hasten the fatal issue. Such patients are to be left amongst the comforts of home, whilst their complaint is being soothed, their strength supported, their diet carefully regulated, and their minds and bodies kept free from any exciting cause. But their digestion demands the greatest attention; for over-filling of the abdominal venous vessels produces the same condition in the pulmonary circulation, and often engenders violent paroxysms of the disease. If with these measures as much out-door exercise is combined as the patient can take without exhaustion and risk, more benefit will be derived than from a distant journey, which in itself may exhaust his remaining feeble powers, and turn the scale irrevocably against him.

Physician of Ottilienquelle—Dr. Hörling.

LUHATSCHOWITZ, in the Olmützer district of MORAVIA, 1,600 feet over the level of the sea, two leagues north-east of the beautiful little town of *Ungarisch-Brod*, five leagues east of the *Hradisch* station of the Prag Olmütz Railroad, 105 miles north-east of Vienna; about 49° lat. N., and 18° long. E., lies in a charming valley of the Carpathian Mountains, between the rivers March and Naag, surrounded by meadows, forests, and mountains, which serve as a shelter towards the north and north-east. The cure-place, called 'Salzbad,' in the neighbourhood, is about a quarter of a league distant from the village. For the accommodation of visitors, neat Swiss cottages and large hotels are available. The climate is mild, but rather moist. Walks of great variety and beauty abound here, and every effort is made for the amusement of the visitors. A whey establishment has lately been added to the curative means.

ANALYSIS OF THE SPRINGS.

	Vincenz-brunnen	Amand-brunnen	Johann-brunnen	Luisen-quelle	Badewasser
Chloride of potassium	1·79	1·59	2·14	1·61	1·85
,, sodium	23·35	25·75	27·88	33·47	20·87
Bromide of sodium	0·25	0·10	0·07	0·08	0·11
Iodide of sodium	0·13	0·12	0·17	0·18	0·35
Carbonate of soda	23·26	36·03	44·21	43·21	24·13
,, lithia	—	0·01	0·01	0·01	—
,, magnes.	0·42	0·56	0·55	0·51	0·42
,, baryta	0·07	0·06	0·04	0·06	—
,, lime	4·63	4·81	4·89	4·40	4·79
,, strontia	0·09	0·11	0·07	0·12	—
,, iron	0·11	0·13	0·09	0·18	0·15
Silica	0·39	0·10	0·41	0·47	0·14
Total	54·85	69·5	80·7	84·4	59·7
Carbonic acid	50 cub. in.	29 cub. in.	16 cub. in.	27·6 cub. in.	28 cub. in.

Whilst the great quantity of chloride of sodium (from 20 to 30 grains) and of carbonic acid (from 16 to 50 cubic inches) promotes the functions of the intestinal canal, the large amount of carbonate of soda (from 23 to 44 grains) exercises its solvent power on albuminous and fibrinous tissues, and vigorously assists in the elimination of morbid secretions. Moreover, the iodides and bromides, with their power of increasing the functions of the glandular and lymphatic system, and of promoting absorption of morbid enlargements, add another potent curative agent, and it is therefore not to be wondered at that the happy union of these various agents indicates the spa in *chronic bronchial, gastric, uterine*, and *vaginal catarrhs*, especially if combined with scrofulosis. Congestion of liver, hæmorrhoidal derangement, and morbid biliary secretion, especially if the results of sedentary habits or of too luxurious living, are greatly improved here; also *chronic metritis*, with irregular catamenia, morbid exudations of the pleura, peritoneum, and of the glandular system. The springs have most analogy in their composition to the Adelheidsquelle, but surpass it in their great amount of carbonate of soda. The small quantity of iron prevents the lowering effects of the solvents to some extent. If we consider the combined advantages of a high position, charming landscape and environs, and good accommodation, with the rare composition of the ingredients, we must look upon the spa as unique, and well deserving to be more

known and resorted to for the various diseases in which chlorides, iodides, and alkaline spas are indicated.
Physicians—Dr. Küchler, Dr. Zimmermann.
Enquiries about the requisite accommodation might be made before the journey to the 'Brunnen-Direction of Count Serényi, in Luhatschowitz, near Ungarisch-Hradisch.'

LEGHORN (Livorno), a seaport on the Mediterranean, 48 miles west-south-west of Florence, south of Pisa (connected by railway with both these towns). Lat. N. $43\frac{1}{3}°$; long. E. $10\frac{1}{6}°$. It is surrounded by walls and intersected by canals. Population, 96,000. The flat and humid environs render the residence unhealthy; but there are beautiful arrangements for sea-bathing, either in commodious small cabinets, enclosed in a court-like building, or in the open sea. Tubes are adapted to the bathing cabinets, through which hot, warm, or cold blasts are directed by bellows to different parts of the body. A bath with these douches is called an Æolus-bath.

LUCCA, a city of ITALY, on the Serchio, 11 miles north-east of Pisa (with which it is connected by railroad). Lat. N. $43\frac{1}{2}°$; long. E. $10\frac{1}{8}$. About 15 miles north of the town are the baths of Lucca, which are reached by a beautiful road, passing near hills and mountains, covered with olives, vines, and chestnuts. In the hot season the coolness of the deep valley is found very refreshing. Midway between the Bagni Caldi and Bagni alla Villa, the Ponte a Seraglio is generally selected as a residence. The lodging-houses of the Bagni Caldi are drier and cooler than those of the Bagni alla Villa. There are bath establishments of springs, the temperature of which ranges from $87\frac{3}{4}°$ to $132\frac{3}{4}°$ Fahr. They contain sulphates of lime, of magnesia, chloride of sodium, and iron. They are employed externally and internally for cutaneous diseases, chronic rheumatism, &c. But the visitors principally resort to this healthy valley in June, July, and August, on account of its lovely climate.

LEAMINGTON, on the Leam, $2\frac{1}{2}$ miles north-east of Warwick, 89 miles from Euston Square station (3 hours' journey). Population, 17,000. Lat. N. $52\frac{1}{2}°$; long. W. $1\frac{1}{2}°$. The spa possesses twelve springs, at a short distance from the Leambridge. They are divided into saline, chalybeate, and sulphurous. The saline contain 105 grains of solid constituents in a pint of water—viz., $40\frac{1}{3}$ sulphate of soda, $40\frac{3}{4}$ chloride of sodium, $20\frac{1}{2}$ chloride of calcium, $3\frac{1}{4}$ chloride of magnesium, with a trace of iron, iodine and bromine; besides $\frac{1}{2}$ cubic inch of nitrogen and 2 cubic inches of carbonic acid.

The saline chalybeate contains 132 grains—viz., 32 sulphate of soda, 67 chloride of sodium, 20 chloride of calcium, 12 chloride of magnesium, 1 oxide of iron, and 3 cubic inches of carbonic acid.

The sulphuretted saline contains 77 grains—viz., 28 sulphate of soda, 25 chloride of sodium, 15 chloride of calcium, 9 chloride of magnesium, 3 cub. inches of carbonic acid, and 1 of sulphuretted hydrogen.

The town is divided into two parts by the Leam, which runs sluggishly in its course towards the Avon. The saline springs have an alterative and purgative action, and are employed for deranged digestion and defective biliary functions in lithiasis and chronic gout; the sulphurous in certain cutaneous diseases; and the chalybeate in general atony and anæmia. The climate is bracing and cool in summer, but too variable and bleak in winter. Season, from May to October. The town has many bathing establishments, and offers every accommodation, besides numerous walks and interesting excursions to the neighbourhood.

LOWESTOFT, County Suffolk, on the North Sea, 20 miles ESE. of Norwich, at a terminus of the Great Eastern Railway (117 miles viâ Woodbridge; 4 hours' journey). Population nearly 10,000. Lat. N. $52\frac{1}{2}°$; long. E. $1\frac{1}{2}°$. The town is situated west of *Lowestoft Ness*, the most easterly land of England; 119 feet above the level of the sea. It has good accommodation for sea-bathing, and is rising in public favour. The climate is more bracing and restorative than that of the south coast, and especially suitable to vigorous persons in convalescence from acute inflammation of the lungs, or of other internal organs.

LYMINGTON, a seaport town in the county of Hants, in the New Forest, on the navigable river of Lymington, close to its mouth in the English Channel, 12 miles south-west of Southampton. Population, 2,600. It is built on a steep declivity, has good accommodation for sea-bathing, and may be reached from London in $3\frac{1}{4}$ hours (distance, 100 miles from Waterloo station) It is connected by steamers with Portsmouth and Isle of Wight. Considering its sheltered position and its southern situation, it deserves to be more resorted to than has hitherto been the case. The saltworks might also be made available for sanitary purposes, as is done in many parts of the Continent.

MADEIRA ISLANDS, in the Atlantic Ocean, are 660 miles distant south-west from Portugal, to which country they belong. They consist of Madeira, Porto Santo, and the Islets of Casertas. Lat. N. between 32° 23' and 33° 7'; long. W. between 13° 30' and 17° 16'. Population of the whole group, 104,000. Madeira is the largest, 31 miles long and 12 miles broad; capital, *Funchal*, on the south coast. Lat. N. 32° 37'; long. W. 16° 54'. Population, 29,700. The island consists of a mass of volcanic rocks, which rise to 6,065 feet in Pico Ruivo. From the central mass deep ridges extend to the coast, where they form precipices 1,000 to 2,000 feet high; only on the west coast some plains exist, besides the table land of Paul de Serra, in the interior. The 'Curral' valley is 2,000 feet deep; the roads are unfit for carriages from their steepness, ponies are therefore used for travelling. The chain of mountains running in an easterly and westerly direction prevents the full effects of the various winds—the north side being sheltered from the scorching south winds, and Funchal from cold northerly winds; but east and west winds have a rather free access. South and west winds generally prevail about Funchal. A regular interchange of land and sea breezes takes place in summer from the north-north-east and south-south-west. The atmosphere, though free from high winds, is never quite calm, but invariably moved by a gentle breeze. The most injurious wind is the *Leste*, coming from east-south-east, and producing great heat and dryness; this unfavourable character may be due to its crossing the African desert. The Leste is not depressing, but stimulating, and sometimes very irritating to phthisical patients on account of its being charged with dust occasionally. It generally occurs three or four times a year, and lasts two or three days, mostly followed by rain. The great advantage of the climate consists in its extreme mildness and equability, there being only a mean annual range of 14°. The steadiness of temperature from day to day also surpasses that of most Italian winter resorts. Whilst a variation of 4° takes place in London, of 2·80° at Rome, of 2·33° at Nice, it only amounts to 1·11° here. Rainy days 70, mostly in autumn, leaving a clear and dry air afterwards ;. but moisture nearly always saturates the atmosphere, so that a small degree of diminished heat produces rainfall. Even in summer the heat is not oppressive. The inhabitants are generally robust, but lepra, elephantiasis, apoplexy, dysentery, and even consumption often occur among them; many of these diseases, however, are to be attributed to their being ill-fed, clothed, and housed. The mean annual temperature is 64·96°: winter, 60·60°; spring, 62·36°; summer, 69·56°; autumn, 67·30°; mean barometric height, 29·86°; rainfall, 29·23 inches. For persons suffering from incipient tubercular consumption, Madeira stands unique as a winter resort. 'There is no occasion,' says Dr. Heineken, 'for a person throughout the winter in Funchal to breathe night or day within doors an atmosphere below 64°, or in the country, and at such a height as to ensure dryness, above 74°; that he may during the summer take abundant exercise without exposing himself to oppressive heat (by choosing his hours), and that in the winter he need not be confined to the house the whole day, either by wet or cold, more perhaps than a score of times.' On the north side of the island, in the parish of *St. Ann*, a summer residence may be advantageously taken by those who have to pass several winters in Madeira, the north-east trade-wind blowing during the day and a cool mountain breeze during the night; moreover, it possesses shaded roads and walks for exercise. This district abounds in plantations, gardens, and vineyards; some of the finest scenery of the island being found between Funchal and St. Ann. Invalids should arrive here in the commencement of October, and remain till beginning of June. Steam-vessels make the passage in six, sailing-vessels in ten to fifteen days. The latter deserve the preference in many instances, as the valetudinarian enters the warmer climate more gradually, besides having the benefit of a longer exposure to the open sea air. Young persons subject to frequent inflammatory diseases of the chest, having overgrown their strength by too rapid development of the frame, and having an hereditary or acquired phthisical tendency, are most benefited by the journey; but where the disease has already made considerable progress, if destruction of portions of the lungs has already taken place, with great emaciation, debility, or fever, the visit to Madeira or any other distant health-resort is decidedly irrational; for it must be remembered that the climate does not actually *heal* the morbid organs—the effects are only negative. The lungs do *not* get so frequently irritated here by vicissitudes of temperature as they would at home; the patients, therefore, can more freely enjoy the advantages of open-air exercise. This is most important in the commencement of the disease, when the system is still in full vigour; but for patients of advanced phthisis, the comforts of home, and the soothing care of relatives and friends, are of more advantage. It is actually found that such sufferers only hasten the dreaded end by the very sojourn in this beautiful southern island. Progressive destruction proceeds more rapidly here than in their own more fitful but conservative climate. Dr. Lund, who still practises in Madeira, has observed cases of tuberculous patients who lived 10, 15, and 20 years on the island, one even 25, all whose brothers and sisters had died of consumption in their native country. Dr. Renton's tables show that—1. Out of 47 cases of *developed phthisis*, 32 died within the first 6 months; 6 died after leaving the island; 3 died probably (altogether 41 deaths). 2. Of 35 with *incipient phthisis*, 26 were considerably and permanently improved; 5 improved (the future progress not ascertained); 4 died subsequently. 3. Of 108 cases of *tuberculous diathesis*, 93 remained perfectly free from any symptom of the disease; 15 were subsequently attacked by it. In *White's* table of 100 cases, 48 had not yet passed over the first stage—in 37 of these the disease was arrested; of 24 cases in the second stage, the malady was prevented from further development in 5; of 28 cases in the third stage, also in 5— one of these latter survived 11 years in the island, two 8 years, and two left the island after 3 years. Accommodation and provisions are excellent in Funchal, as well in hotels as in private boarding-houses; besides, the ordinary comforts of a large and civilized town are available to the visitors.

MALAGA, a seaport town in the south of SPAIN, on a bay of the Mediterranean, 65 miles east-north-east of Gibraltar. Lat. N. 36° 34'; long. W. 4°. Population, 113,000. It is built near the base of a mountain range, in the form of an amphitheatre, and is commanded by an old Moorish castle perched on a rock, and called the Gibralfaro. In 1803-4 the population was decimated by yellow fever. The climate is warm and equable, with very small variations in the single days, and from one day to the other. Winter scarcely exists, but an uninterrupted spring, in which the tropic vegetation continues. Towards north and west, mountain ranges of a height of nearly 3,000 feet are spread one or two leagues from the town, and behind these the still higher Sierra rises. The cold winds are thus kept off from the inner mountains; a branch of vine-covered hills passes towards the shore, and affords some protection against easterly winds. The western mountains, though affording a good shelter against violent atmospheric currents, are still far enough not to prevent the genial entrance of the sun; but the river *Gualdalhorce* passes through a depression of the mountains in the north-west, and admits certain noxious winds into the town. Malaga is divided into an old and new town; the former rests on an acclivity extending towards the old Moorish castle, and consists of narrow dirty streets with lofty houses. The new town is built on sandy level ground, formerly occupied by the sea, and now gradually receding from it. The principal promenade, the *Alameda*, intersects the town, ornamented with statues and fountains. The fertile *Vega* joins the town in the south-east, gradually rising towards the mountains ; an uninterrupted garden of orange groves, of palm, almond, fig, and olive trees, meets the eye. Mean annual temperature, 66° : winter, 56° ; spring, 62·35° ; summer, 76·82° ; autumn, 69° ; snow and ice are very rare. Annual rainfall, 16½ inches ; rainy days about 40, mostly occurring in May, and the rest during autumn and winter. Southerly winds enter freely from the sea ; the south-west, coming from the direction of Gibraltar, is cold, moist, and the forerunner of storms in winter, whilst it is a light sea-breeze only in summer. The sirocco (due south wind) loses most of its African violence by passing across the Mediterranean; the south-east and east winds are mostly charged with moisture, refreshing in summer, and chilling in winter ; west wind coming from inland is dry and warm in summer, and cold in winter; sea winds prevail in spring and summer, land winds in winter ; most of the latter are kept off by the mountains, except the north-west (terral), which enters through the depression by which the river passes, and is hot and dry in summer, and cold and dry in winter. It is maintained of this wind that under its depressing influence criminal offences increase considerably. The inhabitants are remarkably healthy ; nevertheless, phthisis and chronic diseases of the chest constitute about the ninth part of the mortality in the town and hospital. April and May are the healthiest months ; in December and January most illness prevails. The climate of Malaga, though warm, is not relaxing, on account of the small quantity of humidity ; it is mildly stimulating and strengthening, and at the same time soothing from its great steadiness and equability. The mean annual temperature is 2° higher than that of Madeira ; 9° higher than that of Nice ; 12° higher than Venice ; 20° higher than Pau ; but it is 2° lower than Malta, and 4° lower than Cairo. This is partly due to an intense summer heat, but principally to an increased warmth of winter. Barometric pressure is equally steady, sometimes remaining unchanged for twenty days together. The climate resembles that of Cannes, and stands intermediate between the soft relaxing Madeira and the more dry and stimulating Nice, being more inclined to the latter without its noxious properties; it is therefore more adapted to those cases of incipient consumption in which the disease pursues a slow course with abundant expectoration. On the other hand, it is unsuitable where there is any tendency to hæmoptysis or to inflammatory processes of the lungs or pleura.

MENTONE, a small town on the Mediterranean, in a valley of La Riviera, 12 miles east-north-east of Nice (3½ hours' diligence ride). Lat. N. 43¾° ; long. E. 6½°. Population, 4,900. It is the largest town of the principality of *Monaco*, lately ceded to France ; situated on a slope of an Alpine range extending to the sea, and dividing the bay into two parts of unequal size. The neighbourhood abounds in the most variegated vegetation ; sheltering groves of lemon trees in its sunny slopes and ravines.

The towering mountains in the background offer effectual protection against cold winds; pines and olive trees cover the lower hills, whilst orange groves spread their delicious odour along the high road. The north, north-east, and north-west winds (mistral) are kept off by the Alps; the south-west (libeccio) occasions no inconvenience; but the south and south-east (sirocco) enter freely. The north wind, which bounds from the mountain-tops into the sea at a considerable distance from the shore, scarcely touches the town. Rainfall, $23\frac{1}{2}$ inches during the winter. The climate is extremely mild, equable, and greatly superior to that of Nice, as is proved by the numerous lemon trees in constant bloom in open fields, whilst very few of them are found at Nice in very sheltered positions; moreover, the air is moister here, and free from the troublesome and noxious dust of Nice; it is the most favourable Italian winter resort for consumptive invalids. The change of sea and land winds is certainly felt here, but not in such a marked degree as at Nice. The visitors are also particularly recommended to bear in mind that the warmth is due to the direct solar influence, so that transitions from sunshine to shade must be carefully avoided. The abundance and beauty of shaded walks in the mountain valleys contribute greatly to render the residence cheerful and salubrious.

NICE, a seaport town of FRANCE (formerly of Italy), on the Mediterranean, 98 miles south-west of Turin, connected by railway with Toulon (six hours' journey), and with Marseilles (eight hours' journey). Population, 50,000. Lat. N. 43° 43'; long. E. about 7°. It is divided by the Paglione into two equal halves, the old city lying on the left shore, the newer city on the right. Situated in a plain, it leans towards the east on a steep rock rising from the sea, and stretches with its suburbs in a fertile and well-cultivated valley towards north and west. A range of green hills rises over this valley, surrounded by a circle of higher mountains. At a greater distance, snow-clad Alps enclose the whole landscape from the north and north-east, sheltering the town against cold winds, and favouring the luxuriant southern vegetation. Hence the climate is milder than many localities situated farther to the south. Olives, figs, oranges, and palms thrive here. The schlossberg prevents eastern droughts. The temperature from October to April is extremely pleasant and mild. November and the first half of December are generally warm, dry, and clear; but in the second half of December rain falls, and the air often becomes bleaker. January, February, and March are mostly fine: towards the middle of March adverse winds ordinarily prevail till the end of the month, from nine in the morning till five in the afternoon; during these hours the patients must keep their rooms, but may take their walks before or afterwards. Considerable and rapid vicissitudes of temperature often occur in the same day; a great difference is therefore frequently felt by stepping suddenly from the sun into the shade. After sunset the atmosphere becomes frequently charged with moisture, and covers the housetops with dew. Rain falls rarely, and little at a time, but occasionally showers appear. Annual rainfall, 26 inches (Rome, 29; Venice, 25; Algiers, 36). Snow is rare. The mean annual temperature is 58·9°: winter, $46\frac{1}{3}°$; spring, 55·9°; summer,

71·1°; autumn, 61½°. During the night, cold and dry land winds prevail; during day, mild and more humid sea breezes. Nice enjoyed formerly a great reputation for its extreme mildness, in consequence of the apparent thorough protection afforded by the mountain circle. Experience has, however, taught that various winds overcome the obstacle, perhaps through some breaches, and sweep along with vehemence. The north-west wind (a mistral) occasionally penetrates, and lasts sometimes several days. The easterly wind generally commences in March, and exercises a very unpleasant effect on invalids. The southern winds are mostly mild and humid, with the exception of the south-west (libeccio), which often appears with great severity. The south-south-east wind has likewise an injurious effect, especially on nervous and delicate females. The sirocco is considerably modified. The climate of Nice is consequently injurious to irritable constitutions, but more suitable for lymphatic scrofulous patients with profuse bronchial expectoration. In many cases of bronchial catarrh with atony, the warm sea-baths prove very efficacious, especially in early life.

MERAN, in SOUTH TYROL, on the southern declivity of the Tyrolese Alps, 881' over the level of the Adriatic, lies in a most fertile and charming valley between the river Etsch (coming from the western Vinschgau) and the river Passer (rushing down from the north-eastern Passeier Valley). It is completely protected against northern storms by an almost perpendicular mountain-wall, and against north-east, east, west, and north-west winds by mountain-chains of a height of 5,000' to 8,000'. Only open to the south, it enjoys an equable, calm, and somewhat moist atmosphere, with very slight variations of temperature between day and night. Lat. N. 47°; long. E. about 10½°. It lies south of Insbruck, and 20 miles north-west of Botzen (station). October, November, March, April, and May are distinguished by mild temperature, a great number of clear serene days, and almost complete absence of snow. Mean annual temperature, 54½° (Munich, 45°; Berlin, 47½°). Within twenty years (from 1825–44) the thermometer fell only five times below zero in the months of January and February. The summer temperature is lower than in all other towns of South Tyrol and Upper Italy. Autumn and spring are the best seasons for persons suffering from chronic pulmonary catarrh or from incipient phthisis. But if inflammatory tendency or great irritability exist, Meran would be hurtful. Several commodious buildings have been erected here lately for the reception of visitors, and also in the picturesque *Obermais*, on the left shore of the Passer. The latter charming locality, having a higher situation, offers less protection against severe atmospheric currents coming from the Passeier Valley. But the village of *Gratsch*, half a league to the west of Meran (Pension Maurer), at the foot of the *Küchelberg*, is the warmest and most sheltered spot of the whole neighbourhood. The valley of the Etsch and Passeier belong to the most picturesque and beautiful parts of the Alpine regions.

Physicians—Drs. Tappeiner, Theiner, Pirger, Mazegger, and Kleinhaus.

MERGENTHEIM, on the Tauber, a town in the most northern corner of Würtemberg, 591 feet over the level of the sea; 87 miles north-north-east of Stuttgart, 27 miles south of *Würzburg* station. From the latter place the diligence reaches the spa in six hours. It has a population of 2,600, and lies in a charming valley surrounded by vineyards, with a very mild climate; mean annual temperature being 51°; summer temperature, 64°. The principal spring (Quelle im Carlsbad) contains 107 grains of solid ingredients in 16 ounces, viz.:—

Chloride of sodium	51¼
Chloride of potassium	0·78
Chloride of lithium	0·01
Bromide of sodium	0·07
Bromide of magnesium	—
Sulphate of soda	21·89
Sulphate of magnesia	15·88
Sulphate of lime	9·86
Carbonate of magnesia	1·40
Carbonate of lime	5·45
Carbonate of iron	0·05
Silica	0·45
	107·16

Carbonic acid, 7½ cub. inches.

The gases issuing from the spring contain in 100 volumes 27·73 carbonic acid, 71·83 nitrogen, and 01·44 oxygen. The water is used, internally and externally, against derangements of the abdominal organs, as biliary obstruction, hæmorrhoidal and menstrual irregularities, lithiasis. The concentrated bitter water contains 235 grains in sixteen ounces, and has a considerably stronger effect.

Physicians—Drs. Krauss, Höring senior, and Ellinger.

MISDROY, a village on the north-west coast of the Prussian island of *Wollin*, in the district of Stettin, 8 miles east of Swinemünde, 10 miles north-west of Wollin; lat. N. 54°, long. E. 14½°; protected by a woody mountain-ridge, and a large forest. Hence the climate is milder than might be expected from its northern situation. The bathing strand is even, and covered with a fine thick sand; the sea-ground is firm and smooth. Accommodation tolerably good. The railway takes the traveller as far as Stettin, thence the steamer proceeds to Wollin in four hours, and the diligence closes the journey.

Physician—Dr. Oswald.

MONDORF, in the south-eastern portion of the Grand Duchy of Luxemburg, near the French frontier, half a league from the village of the same name; 10 miles south-east of Luxemburg; 5 miles west of Remich, on the Moselle. The spa lies in an extensive plateau, intersected in the west by a mountain-chain running from south-west to north-east. The spring is enclosed by a magnificent tower-like building, and surrounded by beautiful shady walks. The spring contains 110 grains of solid constituents in sixteen ounces, viz.:—

Chloride of sodium	66·98
Chloride of calcium	1·58
Chloride of potassium	24·31
Chloride of magnesium	3·25
Bromide of magnesium	0·76
Iodide of magnesium	0·00
Sulphate of lime	12·61
Carbonate of magnesia	0·05
Carbonate of iron	0·22
Silica	0·05
Arsenic acid	0·001

Free carbonic acid, 1·06 cubic inches.
Nitrogen, . . . 0·47 ,,
Temperature, 77° to 79° Fahr.

By possessing such a great amount of chloride of sodium and bromide of magnesium, the springs belong to the most powerful saline thermæ, whilst the iron improves sanguification and the tone of the whole economy. The nitrogen at the same time soothes the heightened nervous sensibility. They are, therefore, extremely useful in hyperæmic conditions of the respiratory or intestinal mucous membranes, especially if occurring in weakly, leuco-phlegmatic, anæmic individuals.

Physician—Dr. Schmit.

MALVERN (GREAT), on the eastern declivity of the Malvern Hills (128¾ miles from Paddington station, about 4 hours' journey), with a population of 6,000, is one of the finest and most salubrious spots of Great Britain. The Malvern Hills run almost 9 miles in a direction from north to south, attaining a height of 1,400 to 1,500 feet, rising up in a conical form in some places, and running along in narrow undulating ridges in others, the sides sloping down in a broken and precipitous descent, whilst deep ravines frequently intersect the mountain chains, and present a romantic appearance when suddenly bursting upon the view. 'Nature,' Dr. Anderson says, 'seems to have unfolded her choicest beauties in the surrounding scenery, and to have collected here everything that can delight the eye or engage the imagination. The air has always been justly celebrated for its great purity and invigorating quality, whilst its salutary and wholesome water holds out a paramount inducement to those who are suffering from a bodily infirmity. There are two wells here frequented by invalids—the *St. Ann's Well*, which is a little distance above the village of Great Malvern; the other, or the *Holy Well*, is nearly 1½ mile upon the road towards Little Malvern (3 miles distant); and Ledbury, where are a number of genteel residences, and some boarding-houses for the accommodation of visitors. Both these springs are on the eastern side of the range, and, being situated some distance up the ascent of the hill, are removed from the influence of decaying vegetable or animal matters.' The highest point of the Worcestershire beacon (rising to 1,300 feet) offers a most extensive and charming view of the surrounding landscapes, of the vale of Evesham lying below, and of the neighbouring city of Worcester (8 miles distant). On account of its beautiful position and purity and coolness of atmosphere, Malvern is often selected as a summer residence; but the sun exercises a powerful sway in the middle of the day from deficiency of shade, whilst his early retiring behind the hills renders the afternoons and evenings somewhat cool. The houses offer a cheerful look from being built in a villa style, and interspersed among plantations and gardens. The more ancient portion is round Mount Pleasant, a terrace overlooking the Abbey, and containing the Bellevue Hotel, Graefenberg House, &c. The springs do not contain more than a grain of solid ingredients in a pint of water; nevertheless, they occasionally produce nausea, giddiness, and headache, in fact, a kind of temporary plethora, ascribed by the late Dr. Wall to their rapid entrance into the absorbent vessels, in consequence of their great purity. These symptoms soon subside, or may be removed by a mild aperient. The external application of the water is considered useful in scrofulous ulcers, painful fissures of the skin, &c. Mr. Grant considers the qualities of the air peculiarly grateful and invigorating. 'It is so different,' he says, 'from what we are accustomed to breathe in other parts of England: there is something so joyous, so exhilarating in the atmosphere of Great Malvern, that the visitor feels as if he had been transported to some healthier and happier planet.'

As on the Continent the most interesting and salubrious localities are selected for hydropathic establishments, Malvern enjoys a similar distinction here, and may even be considered as the head-quarters of *hydropathy*. *Priesnitz*, a peasant of Graefenberg, in Silesia, was the first to inculcate and to practise the ingurgitation of enormous quantities of cold water with sweating and subsequent cold plunging for the cure of disease.

When a patient drenches the digestive organs and swells the torrent of circulation with blood and water, the secreting and excreting glands are called upon to perform double or triple work, putting the whole organism into peril, especially if there is any inflammatory process going forward in some part of the economy. In chronic diseases, sudden, open injury may not arise, but the blood will experience deterioration in a slow, insidious, and marked manner. Dropsy, carbuncular boils, shifting of an external rheumatic, gouty, or neuralgic affection to some internal organ, as to the heart, liver, or brain, occasionally happen after apparently successful water-cures. Nature often guards vital parts by throwing the morbid element to some distant external tissue. If we thwart these salutary efforts by *violently* repelling the gouty pain, swelling, and stiffness, for instance, through heroic applications of cold, we lay the foundation for grave internal maladies. Those persons, however, who suffer from no real disease, but only labour under some temporary functional derangement of the digestive, biliary, or nervous apparatus, may greatly benefit by the regular mode of living, the pedestrian exercise in the charming and exhilarating open country, and a *moderate* use of cold water internally and externally.

MATLOCK BATH, a watering place in Derbyshire ($143\frac{1}{2}$ miles from

King's Cross station, 4 to 5 hours' journey), the 'Anglo-Saxon Switzerland' according to Dr. Johnson, possesses a pure highly attenuated mineral water, recommended in dyspeptic complaints, gravel, &c. It is beautifully clear, and contains a minute portion of carbonic acid, though it does not sparkle. Incrustations, however, are produced by it on the surfaces of dead substances. The village, with a population of 4,000, is pleasantly built at the bottom and on the slope of the extremely picturesque vale of the Derwent, which is here crossed by a stone bridge. *Matlock Dale*, which encloses the village, extends for 2 miles north and south, bounded on each side by steep rocks, rising to a height of 300 feet. The shores of the Derwent are lined with trees, except where the rocks rise almost perpendicularly out of the water. The high Tor is the most striking of these. The Masson opposite attains a greater elevation, but exhibits a less picturesque appearance. The buildings are grouped in a singular manner up the mountain side. The usual amusement of visitors consists in exploring the caverns, the petrifying wells, and the rocks. The Rutland cavern displays a magnificent view when lighted up. The 'Romantic Rocks' are a series of masses and fragments, apparently torn asunder, with corresponding angles, as if they would exactly fit into each other by being moved back. The springs issue from the rock about 20 yards above the surface of the river. They have a temperature of 68° Fahr., but scarcely differ from spring water in composition. Two large swimming baths in the *North Parade* exhibit the water at its natural temperature. Baths with a higher temperature may be obtained at the hotels (New Bath-house, Temple Hotel, raised above the road, with a terrace in front, &c.). The following poetic effusion, from Jewitt's 'Nooks of Derbyshire,' will show the enthusiasm created by this charming health-resort: 'The drive from the village from any side is striking. The valley, here narrowed almost into a ravine, walled with rich verdure and rough projecting rocks; the high Tor, like some huge bastion, lifting its grey head to the sky; the silver Derwent, making sweet music as it flows, and the Swiss-like cottages peering out of green clusters, or crowning craggy steeps, give to the place an air, if not of romance, at least of genuine picturesqueness. Under the frown of the Tor runs a street with hotels, and above and around, tier upon tier, rise cottages of every form and material, clothed with evergreen and flanked by smiling gardens. The stream as it slowly sweeps round the wooded hill in front of the museum sparkles with the vivid reflection of the white houses and the lofty trees that here adorn its banks. Rising abruptly above the Museum-parade, the pine-covered heights of Abraham, studded here and there with fantastically-built villas, relieving the sombre mass of foliage with which it is covered, and surrounded by a lofty prospect tower; and beyond this again is the summit of the glorious hill Masson, towering over the landscape in infinite majesty.' A large hydropathic establishment exists within a short distance of the bath. The climate must prove singularly restorative as a summer residence in convalescence from protracted fevers, especially after a sojourn in the East. The bracing and exhilarating atmosphere, the variegated natural objects of attraction, the profusion of wood among and above the rocks, with numerous charming villas peeping out from ledges of rock, some of them more than a thousand feet above the level of the Derwent (Abraham's heights)—all this must impart vigour and fresh elasticity to a depressed or shattered nervous system, and to the torpid, languidly-moving circulating fluids of the human machine.

MARGATE, a seaport and watering-place, county Kent, in the Isle of Thanet, on the North Sea, about 3 miles west-north-west of the North Foreland, 15½ miles north-east of Canterbury, 3 miles north-west of Ramsgate, 101 miles from London Bridge station (about 3½ hours' journey), and 73¾ miles from Ludgate Hill station (about 2½ hours' journey). Population, 10,000. It lies in the hollow and on the slopes of two chalk hills. A curved stone pier, with a lighthouse, forms the harbour (lat. N. 51° 24'; long. E. 1° 23'), with eight to thirteen feet at high-water, but dry at low tide. Being exposed to the east wind, the atmosphere is cool, dry, and bracing, and very useful to nervous, torpid individuals. It is greatly resorted to for sea-bathing in summer and autumn. The ground is firm and sandy. Accommodation ample.

RAMSGATE, a seaport town on the east coast of the Isle of Thanet, 15 miles east-north-east of Canterbury, south-west of the North Foreland; 97 miles from London, viâ South-Eastern Railway (about 3½ hours' journey); and 79 miles, viâ London, Chatham, and Dover Railway (about 2¼ hours' journey). Population, 11,800. The town is built on the declivity and summits of two hills, and on the interval, or gate, between them. Its harbour is the largest artificial haven in England, being formed by two stone piers, projecting from 1,500 to 2,000 feet into the sea, and enclosing an inner basin. It is provided with a lighthouse, and protected by batteries. Sea-bathing is excellent here, on account of the soft, firm, and extensive sandy ground. The climate partakes of the dry, cooling, and bracing character of Margate, but having a southern aspect, it is somewhat more sheltered and soothing. It is highly beneficial in summer to persons suffering from dyspepsia, scrofula, or chronic bronchial catarrh. The constitution will acquire more tone and resisting power against disease here than in the more relaxing and enclosed Hastings. It should never be forgotten that the principal aim of an autumn or summer sea resort is directed towards steeling the system for the winter, and *preventing* morbid dispositions from being developed into diseases. The abundance and variety of charming walks and excursions into the neighbourhood, and the plentiful accommodation, render Ramsgate one of the most delightful health-resorts of Great Britain.

NEUENAHR, in the Ahr Valley (RHENISH PRUSSIA), near the village of Beul, at the foot of the Neuenahr Mountain; 225 feet above the level of the sea, east of Altenahr, 2¼ leagues distant from Sinzig station of the Cologne-Mayence Railway. The valley extends from west to east, and joins the Rhine Valley at *Sinzig*, 2½ miles south of Remagen, 15 miles south of Bonn, and 6 miles north of Brohl. Starting from the

Sinzig station, a mile from the left Rhine shore, 10 minutes' walk to the north brings us to the *Ahr Bridge*, near the former spa of Sinzig; crossing this and pursuing the road along the left shore of the Ahr for half an hour, the village of Bodendorf appears in sight; here the mountain-slopes, covered by vineyards and forests, approach nearer. After wandering for another hour, the foot of the 'Landskrone' is reached; a few minutes further the village of Heppingen is seen; after a further quarter of an hour's walk the 'Apollinaris Brunnen' is seen to issue; a quarter of an hour's further walking along the vineyards we find the spa of *Neuenahr*, on the left shore of the Ahr. *Arhweiler* lies 2 miles, and the romantic *Altenahr* 9 miles up the valley. From the bridge the park-like enclosures on both sides of the river are viewed. The climate is very mild, the valley being only exposed to easterly winds. Tuberculosis is extremely rare amongst the inhabitants.

CONTENTS IN 16 OUNCES.

	Augustenquelle	Marienaprudel	Apollinaris Brunnen
Carbonate of soda	5·99	5·62	9·65
Carbonate of magnesia	1·77	2·68	3·39
Carbonate of lime	1·68	1·61	0·45
Chloride of sodium	0·71	0·69	3·57
Sulphate of soda	0·58	0·76	2·30
Oxide of iron	0·04	} 0·06	} 0·15
Alumina	0·13		
Silica	0·17	0·19	0·06
Total	11·11 gr.	11·66 gr.	19·59 gr.
Free carbonic acid	17·79 cub. in.	15·52 cub. in.	36·45 cub. in.
Partly combined carb. ac.	6·94 „	7·00 „	10·59 „
Temperature	90½° Fahr.	102° Fahr.	70° Fahr.

The sprudel rises for a quarter of an hour every hour to a height of 24 feet, and then sinks again into the bore-hole. The bath establishment is extremely well arranged, having a long wide glass-covered corridor, and all conveniences for douche, rain, shower, and vapour baths. The springs principally promote renal, cutaneous, and mucous secretion, and improve the biliary and digestive functions. The spa is principally employed for bronchial, laryngeal, and gastric catarrhs and incipient tuberculosis. The springs contain less carbonate of soda than Ems, exercising therefore a diminished solvent effect; on the other hand, the climate has a less relaxing influence. Nevertheless, persons affected with considerable bronchial irritation will find Ems more suitable; but where a gently tonic influence is sought to be combined with the use of alkaline thermal waters, the charming Neuenahr, with its numerous interesting excursions and excellent accommodation, deserves the preference.

Physicians—Drs. Weidgen, Praessar, Schulz, Feltgen, and Schmitz.

NORDERNEY, island in the North Sea, south-west of Helgoland, belonging to Hanover, about 4 miles distant from the east Friesian coast;

20 miles north-west of *Aurich*, west of Wangeroog and of Bremerhaven; a league and a half long, with a circumference of three leagues. Lat. N. 53° 42'; long. E. nearly 8°. The railway will bring the visitor from Cologne viâ Münster to Emden, and hence a steamer performs the voyage to Norderney in 5 hours three times a week. The climate is extremely mild and equable, notwithstanding the northern position, mean annual temperature being 48°: summer, 68°; winter, $34\frac{1}{2}$°; the range from day to day from 4° to 10°. West-north-west and west winds are prevailing. Population, below 1,000. The bathing establishments at the west end are protected by a mountain ridge. The ladies' baths lie at the west-north-west, the gentlemen's at the north-north-west; the wave-strokes of the latter are stronger in consequence of the more exposed locality. The strand has a firm, dense, sandy ground, sloping down gradually, and serving as a promenade during ebb tide. From the village to the baths a fine shady walk protects the visitor during the sunny hours, besides several park-like enclosures. The sea water is conducted by press-pipes to the downs for warm, rain, and douche baths. Season, from 1st of July to middle of September. When strong wave-strokes are considered desirable, it is better to bathe in middle of August or end of June; for, in the extreme height of summer, the sea is too quiet, and hence a comparatively weak wave motion exists. This stillness of the atmosphere, moreover, causes great depression and sometimes migraine. The place is highly recommended for persons affected with bronchial catarrh and even incipient tuberculosis, who have to drink whey (brought daily from Norden), and to use inhalations of sea-water vapours.

Physicians—Drs. Wiedasch and Riefkohl.

OFEN (or BUDA), on the right shore of the Danube, connected with the opposite Pesth by a magnificent suspension-bridge; 130 miles southeast of Vienna (14 hours' railway journey). Lat. N. 47° 29'; long. E. 19° 3'. Population, 55,000. The city is built in the form of an amphitheatre on the slope of a hill, with a citadel in the centre; altitude, 461 feet. Many thermal springs arise at the foot of the Josefsberg in the north, called the upper, and at the foot of the Gerhards or Blocksberg on the south, called the lower. They provide many bath-houses, and some few of them are used for drinking. The *Kaisersbad* has a temperature of $135\frac{1}{2}$° Fahr.; its drinking spring, $141\frac{1}{2}$°; *Königsbad*, 140°; *Wäscher Brunnen* (laundress spring), 147°; *Blocksbad*, 117° to 119°; the *Raizenbad*, 115° to 117°. Composition of the *Trinkquelle*:—Sulphate of soda, 2·95; chloride of sodium, 0·82; carbonate of soda, 2·02; carbonate of magnesia, 0·46; carbonate of lime, 3·12; silica, 0·69; alumina, 0·18: total, $10\frac{1}{2}$ grains in 16 ounces; carbonic acid, 5·72 cub. inches. The other springs contain analogous ingredients; they are weak alkaline saline springs, but highly efficacious through their temperature in chronic gout, rheumatism, eczema, and psoriasis. They are recommended internally in gastric catarrh, connected with a gouty diathesis, with hepatic hypertrophy, or with an ulcerated condition of the mucous membrane of the stomach, and in obstinate constipation, especially of old atonic individuals. Bath

arrangements are deficient, but have latterly somewhat improved. The Lucas bath contains three swimming basins.
Physicians—Drs. Heinrich and Herz.

OSTEND, a fortified seaport town of BELGIUM; province, West Flanders, on the North Sea, 60 miles north of North Foreland (Kent). Lat. N. 51° 14'; long. E. 2° 55'. Population, 17,000. The citadel is separated from the sea by a stupendous stone dam 1,100 feet long, 30 high. The temperature of the sea water in summer ranges from $63\frac{1}{2}°$ to 66°. The bathing strand is equable, firm, and sandy, gradually sloping towards the sea. The bathing-places lie on the north-east and south-west side, where both sexes bathe in common, invested with a complete swimming costume. In the so-called 'Paradies,' more to the south, opposite the Pavillon du Rhin, bathing without dress is permitted. There are arrangements for warm, rain, and douche baths. That most visitors have to reside in town, somewhat distant from the sea, is to be regretted; on the other hand, the town lying below the level of the sea, allows the marine air to sweep over every portion and to impregnate the atmosphere more thoroughly with its saline exhalations than in any other higher sea-bathing localities. In consequence of this exposure the season commences very late, about the end of July, and lasts till the end of September, as it takes a considerable time for the ground to be thoroughly imbued with summer heat; but then Ostend is certainly one of the most thoroughly bracing and stimulating watering-places, forming the rendezvous represented by almost every nation.
Physicians—Drs. Verhaeghe, Noppe, von Jumné, Soenens, de Cunynck, Jansens, and Freymann.

PARTENKIRCHEN, SOUTH BAVARIA, 2,434 feet above the level of the sea, about $47\frac{1}{2}°$ N. lat., in an extensive picturesque meadow-valley, sheltered against north and north-east winds by the Alpine mountain-chains (9,000 feet high). The railway proceeds from Munich as far as *Staremberg*; thence the Würmser lake has to be crossed; and a further half-day's journey to the south brings us to this romantic locality, with its extremely mild Alpine air, and whey establishments. The *Kanitzer-brunnen* lies not far off towards the east, and contains iodine and alkaline salts, with a magnificent Curhaus. Patients are sent here suffering from tubercular diathesis or incipient consumption, to check the further progress of the malady.

PETERSTHAL, Grand Duchy of BADEN, 25 miles south of Baden-Baden, equidistant (south-east) of Strasburg, 15 miles east of *Appenweiler* station on the Freiburg-Heidelberg Railway ($3\frac{1}{2}$ hours' diligence ride), 1,251 feet above the level of the sea, lies in a continuation of the Rench Valley, enclosed by mountains 3,000 feet high. By the direction of the valley from north-east to south-west, and by the ridge of the Kniebis, sharp north and east winds are kept off. Great vicissitudes of temperature are rare; warmth increases in summer through the narrowing rocky walls, but never reaches to such a degree as to become sultry or oppressive. July is generally the warmest month. Four springs issue here. The

Stahlquelle (or Petersquelle) contains $23\frac{3}{4}$ grains of solid constituents in 16 ounces—viz. bicarbonate of lime, 11·71 gr.; bicarbonate of magnesia, $3\frac{1}{2}$; bicarbonate of iron, 0·35; bicarbonate of lithia, 0·04; bicarbonate of soda, 0·46; chloride of sodium, 0·30; sulphate of soda, 6·06; sulphate of potash, 0·57; phosphate of alumina, 0·05; organic substances, oxide of manganese and arsenic acid, traces; free carbonic acid, 33·2 cub. inches. The *Gas* (or *Sophienquelle*) contains $21\frac{1}{3}$ gr.; iron, 0·33; less carbonate of lime and sulphate of soda than the former; and 0·01 cub. inch of free nitrogen. The *Salzquelle* possesses 24·92 gr., very analogous to the first (only somewhat more magnesia and sulphate of soda); besides 34·02 cub. inches of carbonic acid, and 0·02 cub. inch of nitrogen. The springs are employed for drinking and bathing, in cases of anæmia and defective biliary secretion. The climate is extremely mild and salubrious.
Physician—Dr. Erhardt.

GRIESBACH, a village in the neighbourhood (to the east), in the narrowest portion of the *Rench* Valley, 1,500 feet high, 2 leagues north of Rippoldsau, 7 leagues east of Appenweiler station, possesses a drinking spring, which surpasses that of Petersthal by its amount of carbonate of iron (0·60 gr.) and carbonic acid gas; the composition is otherwise analogous, and accommodation perfectly satisfactory.

PUTBUS (Frederic-William sea-bath), on the south coast of the Island of *Rügen*, above 54° N. lat.; long. E. about 14°; 5 miles south-east of Bergen, 17 miles east of Stralsund. Population, 1,340. *Rostock* is the nearest railway station to the west, and *Stettin* to the east. Steam communication exists during the season between these places and the sea-bath. Being situated on the southern declivity of the coast, Putbus possesses a mild sheltered climate, the high woody shores of the opposite island of Vilm serving as a further protection. But the town lies too far from the strand, the road offers little shade, and the bathing-ground itself is rather stony; moreover, the wave-strokes are weakened by the projecting shores of the opposite island. But all artificial arrangements are perfectly satisfactory for cold, warm, and douche baths. The charms of rural life in a highly romantic landscape are combined with the amusements and social advantages of a town. Those who prefer solitude may avail themselves of the forest of *Granitz*. *Sassnitz*, lying on the sea, and sheltered to the north by the chalk mountains of the Stubnitz, covered with beech-groves, is a charming retreat, with real fishermen's life.
Physicians—Dr. Stockmann and Dr. Hohnbaum-Hornschuh.

PAU, a town of FRANCE, capital of the Basses Pyrenées, 56 miles east-south-east of Bayonne ($4\frac{1}{2}$ hours' railway journey), on the right shore of the Gave de Pau, with a remarkably high bridge of seven arches. The wild romantic scenery and mildness of climate attract many visitors. Population, 21,000. Pau was the capital of the old province of Béarn, the birthplace of Henry IV., and of General Bernadotte, afterwards King of Sweden. Lat. N. $43\frac{1}{2}°$; long. E. $\frac{1}{2}°$. It rests on elevated gravelly soil, which allows a rapid percolation of the rain-water. The views of the Western Pyrenées are grand. Every convenience and luxury of a large airy city are available here, besides the beautiful walks along the side of the Gave, and the large shaded platform within the town. The accommodation for invalids is excellent in every respect. The climate has a purely sedative character, though subject to an annual rainfall of 43 inches (119 rainy days), with rapid alternations from clear to rainy weather. The mean temperature of September, October, November, is $56 \cdot 4°$; of December, January, and February, $42 \cdot 8°$; and of March, April, and May, $54°$. The winds are modified by the softening influence of the neighbouring Atlantic on the one side, and the mountainous protection on the other. Thus the east winds are generally tempered before they arrive at Pau. In fact, the ordinary atmospheric calmness allows change of temperature to be better borne by patients. In October, the weather becomes sometimes suddenly chilly, from snow falling on the Pyrenées; in November, it becomes clear and mild; in December and January slight snow-showers occasionally occur, but the heat of the sun soon clears them away; towards the end of February, the spring rains sometimes render the weather chilly. Mild and humid westerly winds alternate with dry easterly winds in spring. In April, vegetation progresses rapidly; in May the atmosphere becomes warmer; in June it is fine and hot; in July, August, and September, the thermometer sometimes reaches $94°$ in the shade. Pau is recommended to those affected with a dry tickling cough, and very little or no healthy secretion, and in conditions of general nervous debility and dyspepsia; but there ought to be a rather vigorous constitution, as the climate has a tendency to reduce the standard of tone. Hence diseases of a mixed nervous and inflammatory character are often subdued here. The climate is neither sufficiently dry to cause irritation, nor so overcharged with dampness as to be too relaxing. There are neither fogs nor cold piercing winds. The mildness of its spring renders it particularly useful in inflammatory irritation of the larynx or trachea, but it is not beneficial if the system is relaxed, or if the disease be accompanied with profuse expectoration and dyspnœa. Season, from 1st September to 1st June.

PLOMBIÈRES, a small French town in the department of the Vosges, on the Eaugronne, 14 miles south of Epinal station (three hours' drive). Lat. N. $48°$; long. E. $6\frac{1}{2}°$. (About ten hours' journey from Paris.) It is situated in a deep valley, opening from east towards west; 1,310' above the level of the sea. The air is bracing and pure, but subject to frequent vicissitudes of temperature, a hot day being often succeeded by a cool evening. There are six comfortable bathing establishments. The temperature of the springs ranges from $80°$ to $159°$; besides a cold spring (the Savonneuses). The water contains about 2 grains of solid ingredients in 16 ounces—viz. $0 \cdot 62$ silicate of soda, $0 \cdot 03$ of potash, $0 \cdot 24$ silicate of lime and magnesia, $0 \cdot 27$ chlorides of sodium, of potassium, and of calcium, $0 \cdot 62$ sulphate of soda, $0 \cdot 0054$ arsenate of soda, $0 \cdot 08$ silica, $0 \cdot 07$ alumina, $0 \cdot 15$ nitrogenous organic matter. There is also a gas-bath called 'hell,' with a temperature of $149°$; an ascending douche (trou des Capucins), used in sterility and other diseases of the female sexual organs. The waters are chiefly used externally; but the Savonneuses, the Bourdeille (cold chalybeate), and others are occasionally employed for drinking, when they exert a tonic, stimulating, and diuretic effect. The spa is one of the most fashionable in France, and especially celebrated for the cure of chronic rheumatism and gout, tic-doloureux, sciatica, paralysis dependent on rheumatic affection of the spinal membranes, congestion of the womb, chronic diarrhœa, and dysentery. The duration of the baths is gradually prolonged to two hours, but this should never be allowed without due caution. On the other hand, since Professor Hebra, of Vienna, kept patients in warm water for 100 days (and nights), with a perfectly successful result, in certain intractable cutaneous diseases, we ought no more to look upon the prolonged warm bathing with such distrust, especially if the patient has been gradually accustomed to it. In Dr. Hebra's ingeniously contrived bed, seen here in the last exhibition, patients were able to eat, drink, sleep, and perform all natural functions for the above number of days without leaving the water. They became rid of the disease (at least for the time), and improved in general health and bulk. Most remarkably curative this ingenious contrivance showed itself in severe cases of *burn*. The most torturing and cruel dressing of these painful wounds was completely avoided, the sufferers moving freely in the water till the cure was completed. It would, therefore, be most desirable and humane to introduce these beds into the general hospitals here.

Physicians—Drs. Turk, L'Heritier, Grillot, Sibylle, and Garnier.

RECOARO, a Lombardian village, lat. N. $45\frac{1}{2}°$; long. E. $11\frac{1}{2}°$, nineteen miles north-west of *Vicenza* station (four hours' drive), west of Venice. It is greatly resorted to in summer for its chalybeate springs, and its mild bracing climate, being situated at the foot of the Alps, in the valley of Prekele, 1,465 feet over the level of the sea. It is greatly recommended as a residence from May to October, for persons inclined to phthisis, who do not wish to resort to the higher Alpine situations.

Physician—Dr. Chiminelli.

REICHENHALL, a small town of UPPER BAVARIA, in the valley of the Saalach, near the Austrian frontier, 1,407 feet over the level of the sea, 16 miles south of Traunstein, 11 miles south of *Salzburg* station (about two hours' diligence ride), scarcely an hour's ride from *Teisendorf* station. Lat. N. about 47°; long. E. $13\frac{1}{4}°$. The charming little town, extending along the left bank of the Saalach (an affluent of the Salza), lies in a wide mountain depression, surrounded by towering verdant hills. The valley is directed here from south-west to north-east, and is perfectly sheltered against violent atmospheric currents. The bathing establishment of *Achselmannstein*, with its graduation works, is scarcely ten minutes distant. The climate is very mild and bracing, extremely grateful to persons affected with irritation of the bronchial mucous membrane, the air becoming moist and impregnated with the saline particles of the graduation works. The mean temperature of spring is 56° Fahr.; of summer, 64°; and of autumn, $54\frac{1}{2}°$. The fertile plain and wild mountain scenery offer the most charming contrast.

The views presented by the road to Traunstein, enclosed and narrowed as it is by high rocks in some portions, are extremely romantic. *Mauthhausel*, about six miles distant along this road, allows a charming view, through a narrow ravine, of the gigantic snow-covered Watzmann, upwards of 9,000 feet high in the south. In an excursion to Berchtesgaden, three leagues to the east, green meadows alternate with dense luxurious forests and steep imposing mountain groups. These heights approach nearer and nearer, till Berchtesgaden is reached, almost lying at their feet. The old castle of *Fürstenstein* affords a most admirable panorama of the whole neighbouring mountain scenery. One hours' walk further (south) reaches the 'Königsee.'

Of the nineteen saline springs, the Edelquelle is the most abundant. It contains, in 16 ounces, $1798\frac{1}{2}$ grains of solid constituents—viz., chloride of sodium, 1723·10 grains; chloride of ammonium, 0·19 grain; chloride of magnesium, 13·84 grains; bromide of magnesium, 0·23 grain; sulphate of soda, 15·36 grains; sulphate of potash, 4·70 grains; sulphate of lime, 31·98 grains; carbonate of lime, 0·07 grain; carbonate of magnesia, traces; oxide of iron and alumina, 0·06 grain; silica, 0·08 grain; some free carbonic acid.

The motherlye contains $33\frac{1}{2}$ parts of solid constituents in 100; very little chloride of sodium ($\frac{3}{4}$); but a considerable quantity of chloride of magnesium (29), and of bromide of magnesium (0·57). It has therefore some resemblance with the Kreuznach motherlye. The brine is, of course, diluted with water before being used for bathing. Inhalations of the saline particles are used in the corridors of the graduation works (2,298 feet long, and almost 60 feet high): these exert a very sedative effect in cases of dry tickling laryngeal or bronchial cough. Reichenhall is generally recommended in scrophulosis without any local exudations, in anæmia from hæmorrhage or from chronic diseases, obstinate catarrhs of the mucous membranes of the chest and intestines; and, lastly, in incipient tuberculosis.

Physicians—Drs. Von Geeböck, Von Liebig, Ris, and Schmidt.

REMAGEN, on the left shore of the Rhine, the neighbouring Sinzig and *Bodendorf*, as well as the town of Hannef, are distinguished by a very mild climate. It is a well-known fact that the western valleys and river domains which terminate into the Rhine valley *below* the Rheingau have a more congenial and salubrious climate than those of the right shores, which came from the east. The excellence of the wines and the abundant vegetation in the valleys of the *Nahe*, of the *Moselle*, and of the *Ahr*, are due to their comparatively high summer temperature.

RIGI-SCHEIDECK, on the east side of the Rigi chain, in a narrow plateau 5,073 feet over the level of the sea, above 47° lat. N., $8\frac{3}{4}$° long. E. The visitor is carried by steamer through the Vierwaldstädtersee from Lucerne to Weggis, on the north-eastern shore; from here the ascent is most delightful, and offers really sublime scenery. The Curhaus is highly recommended for anæmic debilitated persons; but, being greatly exposed to bleak winds, it has to be avoided by individuals whose respiratory organs are not perfectly sound. An earthy alkaline chalybeate issues at a distance of about half a league in such abundance that from 60 to 80 baths may be administered daily.

RIGI-KALT-BAD, 4,436 feet above the level of the sea, enjoys a more sheltered situation, the north and east winds being kept off through mountain-ridges, whilst the southerly winds have a free access. The newly built Curhaus can accommodate 120 persons. A few steps to the south-west an open place is reached, containing a chapel, and a chalybeate issuing out of a rocky fissure, used for bathing and drinking; but the principal curative agency is cow or goat whey. The months of June, July, and August are the most appropriate for a course. Accommodation in every respect satisfactory.

RIPPOLDSAU, in the Grand Duchy of BADEN, 1,886 feet above the level of the Mediterranean, $1\frac{1}{2}$ league east of Griesbach and Petersthal, not far from Appenweiler station, $48\frac{1}{2}°$ North lat., $8\frac{1}{2}°$ East long., lies in a narrow valley of the Wolfach (affluent of the Kinzig), surrounded by woody mountains. The forests, rising to a height of 3,052 feet, connecting Rippoldsau with Griesbach, offer a most romantic road, with the charming view of the western declivities of the Black Forest, and the distant perspective of Strasburg and the Rhine valley in the west. The springs are distinguished by a great quantity of free carbonic acid, of sulphate of soda, carbonate of lime, of iron, and of manganese. They belong, therefore, to the class of *tonic resolvents*. The climate is not bleak, notwithstanding the high position. The air is pure, fresh, and bracing, having a really balsamic character from the exhalations of the neighbouring fir and pine forests. Persons suffering from pulmonary catarrh ought to take frequent walks along these woods. The *Josephquelle* contains $22\frac{3}{4}$ grains of solid ingredients in 16 ounces: viz. carbonate of lime, 8·93; carbonate of magnesia, 0·33; carbonate of iron, 0·28; carbonate of manganese, 0·02; sulphate of soda, 9·31; sulphate of lime, 0·42; sulphate of magnesia, 1·86; silica, 0·43; alumina, 0·03; chloride of magnesium, 0·65; sulphate of potash, 0·46; traces of phosphoric acid, arsenic and organic matter. Carbonic acid (free and partly combined), 32 cubic inches; temperature, 50° Fahr.

Social life is very simple and rural. The place is one of the most celebrated of the so-called *Kniebisbäder*, and most frequently resorted to from the middle of May till the middle of September by chlorotic, anæmic, and weakly individuals.

Physician—Dr. Feyerlin.

RÖMERBAD, near *Tüffer*, in Lower Styria, station on the South Austrian railway, 10 miles south of *Cilli*, lat. North $46\frac{1}{4}°$, long. East 15°, north-east of Trieste, west of Töplitz, 755 feet above the level of the Adriatic, with luxurious vegetation, near the border of the Sann valley. The climate is very mild. The three springs possess a temperature of $93\frac{1}{2}°$ Fahr., and less than 3 grains of solid constituents; among these, chloride of sodium, 0·42; chloride of magnesium, 0·29; sulphate of soda,

0·20; carbonate of lime, 0·24; sulphate of lime, 0·10; carbonate of magnesia, 0·05; silica, 0·63; carbonic acid, 4·84 cubic inches. Bathing takes place here in large basins (so-called Gehbäder); but separate baths can also be had, besides ascending, descending, and side-douches, in hyperæmia and swelling of the womb, catamenial derangements, &c. The baths are also used with great advantage in nervous debility, chronic rheumatism and gout, neuralgia, &c.
Physician: Dr. Bunzel.

ROHITSCH, in STYRIA, 3 leagues south-east of *Pöltschach* station (on the Trieste-Vienna Railway), north of Cilli and of Tüffer, about 46½° lat. N., and 16° long. E., is situated in a most fertile and lovely landscape. It contains five springs of almost identical composition. The *Tempelbrunnen* (exclusively used for drinking) contains in 16 ounces 44 grains of solid ingredients: viz. 15½ sulphate of soda, 5¾ carbonate of soda, 11¾ carbonate of lime, nearly 10 carbonate of magnesia, 0·09 carbonate of iron, 0·72 chloride of sodium, 0·14 silica, and 51 cubic inches of carbonic acid in 100 of the gaseous contents. The climate almost possesses Italian mildness, and attracts visitors from May to September, principally in cases of the so-called abdominal plethora, when the blood accumulates too much in the portal system, and ushers in the numerous derangements based on deficient or morbid secretions of bile, as acidity, irregular alvine action, constipation, alternating with diarrhœa, gastric distension, &c. However, as an exciting effect is produced by the great amount of carbonic acid, persons inclined to cerebral congestion have to avoid the spa, or at least use it with great caution.
Physicians—Dr. Sock and Dr. Fröhlich.

ROSENHEIM, a station on the Munich-Salzburg Railway, below 48° lat. North, about 12¼° long. East, contains bathing establishments in which the brine of Berchtesgaden and Reichenhall are jointly used. A subterranean canal of 40 miles in length conducts the brine here from the latter places; moreover, chalybeate and sulphur springs are available for drinking and bathing. Moor-baths and pine-foliage vapour-baths are also administered in cases of chronic rheumatism, neuralgia, and articular stiffness remaining after acute attacks of rheumatic fever.
Physician—Dr. Halbreiter.

ROYAN, a maritime town of FRANCE, department of the Charente Inférieure, at the mouth of the *Gironde*, below 46° lat. North, about 1° long. West, 20 miles south-west of Saintes on the Charente, north-west of Bordeaux. Population 4,000. A fort defends the harbour. Lying on the southwest coast, in a somewhat protected position, the sea-baths offer the advantage of Atlantic currents with a mild climate.
Physician—Dr. Allard.

SAINT MORITZ, Upper Engaddin, SWITZERLAND, Canton Graubünden (Grisons), the highest village of the Engaddin, 5,710 feet above the level of the sea, enjoys a magnificent situation and most extensive and romantic views in its environs. The Curhaus, with its acidulous chalybeate springs, lies about a mile distant from the village on the other side of the lake of Saint Moritz. The environs abound in the most romantic and picturesque sights of the whole of Switzerland. The very diligence journey from the *Chur* station (Coire), the most eastern point of the iron-road in Switzerland, over the Albula through Tiefenkasten, Juliers Pass, Silva Plana, &c., is full of interest and charms. The canton of Grisons, the most eastern of Switzerland, is nearly shut off from the other cantons by lofty mountain ranges. It comprises the upper valley of the Inn (Engaddin), with the sources and early affluents of the Rhine and tributaries of the Po and Adda, being a mass of mountains and narrow valleys. The climate is rendered cold and severe in the upper valleys by the snow with which they are covered during seven months of the year. Its scenery is extremely grand and magnificent, as may be imagined from its possessing 240 glaciers. Whilst a great part of the surface is covered with snow in winter, the considerable quantity and extent of lakes of the upper Engaddin contributes a peculiarly picturesque character of landscapes resembling the Norwegian, and at the same time modifies the variations and extremes of temperature prevailing in the lakeless lower Engaddin, so that it gains somewhat of the character of a coast climate. This modifying influence is further heightened by the extensive forests which surround St. Möritz on three sides; whilst on the naked heights of the Rigi (5,541 feet), in the Northern Swiss, Tyrolese, and Bavarian Alps (5,500 to 6,000 feet), in the Riesengebirge (4,400 feet), and even on the Harz Mountains (3,300 feet), the growth of trees is entirely missing. Here luxurious forests reach even 1,800 feet above the valley (7,000 feet high). The whole organic world shows the same favourable character. In the highest localities beautiful flower and vegetable gardens may be seen near palace-like residences. Mangold, spinach, cresses, radishes, and white carrots, besides the Alpine rose, accompany man to his highest habitation, as is shown in the Alpine villages of Fex and Graevesalvas (6,100 feet), and on the Juliers Pass to the south, Albula Pass to the north, and Bernina Pass (7,140 feet) to the east of St. Moritz. Agriculture, which does not extend beyond 3,700 feet in northern Switzerland, reaches here, near Pontresina, with its uppermost barley-fields, to a height of 6,000 feet. The snow-line (the lower border of eternal snow) does not extend below 9,450 feet. On the Bavarian Alps 7,100 feet is considered the limit; in the Swiss Alps generally 8,200 feet; on the Mont Blanc, 8,900 feet; on the Pyrenees, 8,400 feet; Monte Rosa, 9,200 feet. Nearly half a year a snow cover 1 to 5 feet deep protects the fields (five months and twenty-two days on an average). In the summer months, from 1856 to 1859, the thermometer did not sink once beyond the freezing point, but exhibited an average from 64° to 77° Fahr. On an average of nine years between the 12th and 21st of June the last snow fell, and between the 7th and 10th of September the first. About the 20th of June the rose-coloured Alpine rose, *Rhododendron ferrugineum*, displays its flaming blossoms, surrounded by brilliant numbers of flowers, worthily opening the summer flora.

Average Temperature of Four Years at St. Moritz.

Time and Hour	June 21-30	July 1-10	July 11-20	July 21-31	August 1-10	August 11-20	August 21-31	September 1-10
Morning, from 5 to 6 o'clock	42°	42°	44°	45°	45°	43½°	40°	39°
Afternoon, from 1 to 2	60	60	64	62	64	62	58½	54
Evening, 9	47	47	51	51	51	50	46	43½
Mean	50¼	50½	53	53	53	51	48	45½
Daily difference	18	18	20	17	19	18½	18½	15

Sometimes, the temperature remains suitable till the latter part of September, and might induce prolongation of the season—the relation between clear and wet days, and the predominance of south-westerly winds, being even more favourable in September than in the earlier summer months. The water has a cooling, acidulous, astringent taste. The old spring contains 11 grains of solid constituents in 16 ounces : viz. carbonate of lime, 5½; carbonate of magnesia, nearly 1 ; carbonate of iron, 0·18 ; carbonate of manganese, 0·03 ; carbonate of soda, 1·46 ; sulphate of soda, 2 ; chloride of sodium, 0·29 ; sulphate of potash, 0·12 ; silica, 0·29 ; phosphoric acid, 0·03 ; traces of bromine, iodine, fluorine ; 39½ cubic inches of carbonic acid. Temperature, 42°. The new spring is mostly used for drinking, similarly composed, but contains 13·46 grains of solid constituents, somewhat more lime and magnesia, and 0·25 grains of iron, 40½ cubic inches of carbonic acid (the Stahlbrunnen of Schwalbach contains 0·64 grains of iron and 50¼ cubic inches of carbonic acid ; Weinbrunnen 0·44 grains and 45½ cubic inches of carbonic acid).

The effect of the water is tonic and stimulating. St. Moritz is indicated in general debility, anæmia, and cutaneous atony (disposition to profuse perspiration, to rheumatism), in scrofula, neuralgia, gastric spasms, chronic gastric catarrh or fluor albus, in tardy digestion, acidity, vesical catarrh, sexual debility, sterility. It is contra-indicated in febrile, congestive and inflammatory diseases, hæmoptysis, tuberculosis, diseases of the heart, epilepsy, and gravidity.

Children affected with helminthiasis or scrophulosis take the water with great benefit. Weakly persons ought to acclimatise themselves for a few days before commencing the course. Baths are used with a somewhat low temperature—between 68° and 92¾° Fahr. ; average, 81° to 86° Fahr. But the great amount of carbonic acid causes soon a feeling of warmth and comfort to spread over the surface of the body. After bathing, mostly rest in bed is enjoined for some time, without sleep. The course lasts from three to four weeks. Compared with Schwalbach, St. Moritz is certainly a weaker chalybeate, containing only a quarter of a grain of carbonate of iron in a pound of water, with a greater quantity of lime and solid ingredients, thus diminishing the proportion of iron still more. The Stahlbrunnen possesses more than half a grain of iron in a total of 4·6 grains—thus above the eighth of its contents; whilst in St. Moritz, ¼ of a grain in a total of 13 grains amounts only to the fifty-second part of the contents. If, therefore, a considerable degree of anæmia prevails, requiring a corresponding amount of the restorative metal to effect a cure, Schwalbach deserves the preference. But in many conditions of mental and bodily exhaustion, resulting from excessive wear and tear, and shown by lassitude and inaptitude for any exertion, sluggish circulation, great irritability, failing appetite, deficient nutrition, and sanguification, a course of three weeks in St. Moritz, with a contemplation of the great and varied magnificence of the wondrous landscape and environs, affords such a thorough stimulus to the nervous centres, that metamorphosis is greatly improved, and thus the whole organism sooner restored to its healthy equilibrium than at any other less favoured locality. Only a few hours' ride to the village of Maria offers, I might say, an almost intoxicating variety of charms to the astonished and bewildered eye. Beautiful green lakes alternate with Alpine rocks, sometimes covered with verdure, at other times towering naked one over the other, with their beautiful Alpine glow in the twilight. Approaching the village, the interesting road to Italy, with its serpentine course, is looked down on from a giddy height; a little further, and you walk up a mountain with soft velvety grass, down which glacier torrents rush constantly with a sound of wild velocity. Having walked up this charming slope for an hour and a half, you stand all at once before a lofty glacier. The unaccustomed eye thinks the snow so near that it might almost be swept off apparently by a high pole, and still the mountain is four miles distant. There is an absolute *embarras de richesse*. People have to deliberate daily what excursion to choose in order to explore the greatest portion of the unique mountain scenery. If we consider the very great advantage change of scene and of air exercises on the organic functions of the human economy, I must look upon a few weeks' residence among these grandees of nature's works as more recreative and restorative to soul and body than double and treble the time spent in more monotonous localities, where the mind finds frequently time and opportunity of recurring to its ordinary thoughts and association of ideas. The bracing action of the Alpine air is another advantage of high order. Dr. Brügger, the intelligent physician of St. Moritz, says as regards the diseases of the inhabitants: ' Digestive derangements, as gastric catarrh, acidity, flatulence, abnormal innervation, tardy peristaltic action based on muscular atony, and sluggish abdominal circulation, rarely incommode the inhabitants of these high Alpine regions. Chlorosis, olygæmia, and plethora serosa are likewise rare. Scrophulosis and tuberculosis are only known here as exotic products; the former mostly disappears during a prolonged sojourn in this Alpine air. Phthisical disposition is generally weakened and often arrested for a long time in its development. Advanced consumption, however, proceeds rapidly here towards a fatal issue. Gout is not frequent; intermittent fever and scurvy are perfectly absent. Diseases of the nervous system and sexual atony are much rarer here than in lower localities.'

SCHINZNACH Bath, a quarter of a league from the village of Schinznach, lies in a charming friendly valley of the Aar, 1,060 feet over the level of the Mediterranean, at the foot of the Wülpelsberg, canton Aargau, station on the railway which connects Zurich with Aarau, about three-quarters of a league distant from Brugg, three leagues from Aarau, and two from Baden. It simply consists of a large Curhaus with a small promenade; and with a charming wood in the north-west, intercepted by many footpaths, and stretching to the shore of the Aar. Flower and vegetable gardens surround the building on the south side. Further on, a fine alley of poplars extends along the Aar. Accommodation in every respect satisfactory.

The water contains, in 16 ounces, $20\frac{1}{3}$ grains of solid constituents—viz., sulphate of potash, 0·68; sulphate of soda, 9·87; sulphate of lime, 1·20; chloride of potassium, 5·48; chloride of magnesium, 1·14; magnesia, 0·64; carbonate of magnesia, 0·03; carbonate of lime, 1·09; oxide of iron, 0·008; alumina, 0·07; silica 0·09. Gaseous contents: carbonic acid, 2·38 cubic inches; sulphuretted hydrogen, 1·72 cubic inches; nitrogen, small quantity. Temperature, 94° to 96° Fahr.

The spa is particularly renowned for the cure of certain cutaneous diseases, as prurigo, sycosis, eczema, and also of milder cases of psoriasis The ioduretted saline water of the neighbouring *Wildegg*, south of Schinznach, between Aarau and Brugg, is often taken internally, while prolonged baths are used externally. Schinznach is also used with advantage in helminthiasis, in lead and arsenic poisoning, and in diseases produced by excessive employment of mercury. In scrofulous and carious diseases, in necrosis, in chronic rheumatism, especially of the hip-joint, the use of this spa is beneficial. In masked tertiary syphilis the dormant character of the original disease becomes more prominent, and, through the influence of the sulphur-water, the organism becomes more disposed to respond to the action of the specific anti-syphilitic remedies, which often produce a speedy cure afterwards, when they seemed to be inert before the course of the sulphur-water. Schinznach is contra-indicated in sanguine temperaments, and in all congestive and inflammatory conditions. Season, from middle of May to end of September.

Physicians—Dr. Hemmann and Dr. Amsler.

WILDEGG Spring, one league to the south of Schinznach, contains, in 16 ounces, 104·94 grains of solid constituents—viz., chloride of sodium, $75\frac{1}{4}$; chloride of potassium, 0·04; chloride of calcium, 2·81; chloride of magnesium, 12·38; iodide of sodium, 0·30; bromide of sodium, 0·006; sulphate of lime, 13·48; carbonate of lime, 0·63; oxide of iron, 0·003; carbonic acid, 2·3 cubic inches. Temperature, 66° Fahr. It resembles Adelheidsquelle in its composition; but though containing less bromide of sodium, and no carbonate of soda, it is distinguished by a greater amount of chloride of sodium (more than double, though Bauer found only 59 grains), and through its chlorides of calcium and magnesium, which are absent in Adelheidsquelle. It is therefore extremely useful in obstinate cases of scrophulosis. Schönlein ordered the water to chlorotic and scrofulous children, mixed with acorn coffee, or with milk and sugar. In secondary and tertiary syphilis, a drachm of iodide of potassium is sometimes dissolved in a bottle of the Wildegg water (with gradual increase to two drachms); and a month's course of a tumbler-full every morning is said to be sufficient for curing the most inveterate cases, especially if the skin is the organ principally affected.

SCHEVENINGEN, a fishing village of 6,000 inhabitants, in SOUTH HOLLAND, on the North Sea; lat. N. 52°, long. E. $4\frac{1}{2}°$; two miles and a half north-west of the Hague, with which it is connected by a beautiful triple alley with very ancient oaks, and an adjoining forest. Numerous residences are available in the charming villas, or in the bathing establishment. The neighbouring forest gives it a marked preference over the bare Ostend. The sexes have different bathing-places—the ladies on the south side of the great bathing establishment, the gentlemen on the north side. Accommodation is excellent.

Physician—Dr. Mess.

The Hague may be reached by rail in about two hours from Rotterdam, and in about six from Ostend. Considering the ease and rapidity with which Rotterdam may now be reached by the London and Harwich line, this fashionable and excellent North Sea bath deserves to be more frequently resorted to. Its exposed and yet sheltered position, its rural aspect, and fine bathing-ground, are all reasons for rendering it a very bracing and restorative watering-place. Another advantage is the proximity of the interesting capital of Holland, with its 82,000 inhabitants; its celebrated hotels, Paulez Old Doelen, de Belle Vue (considered among the best in Europe); its unrivalled collection of paintings; its palace in the wood, approached through a magnificent plantation of beeches and oaks, grouped round lakes of water; besides numerous promenades, and objects of diversion and amusement.

SODEN, near *Aschaffenburg* station (BAVARIA), north-west of Würzburg; lat. N. 50°, long. E. $10\frac{1}{4}°$; in the Spessart, lies in a valley 440 feet over the level of the sea, and is protected against violent winds by surrounding hills and mountain ranges, only open to the southwest: hence its climate is mild, moist, and equable, resembling that of its namesake in the Taunus, near Frankfort. Chloride of sodium and calcium, with bromide of magnesium, are the prominent ingredients. *Spring* No. 1 contains 111·91 grains of chloride of sodium; 3·8 chloride of potassium; 4·96 chloride of magnesium; 39·47 chloride of calcium; 0·51 bromide of magnesium; 0·0006 iodide of magnesium; 5·46 sulphate of lime; 0·89 carbonate of lime; 0·03 carbonate of magnesia; 0·03 carbonate of iron; 0·03 silica; traces of phosphoric and boracic acid, of ammonia, manganese, and organic substance; carbonic acid, 1·27. Temperature, $54\frac{1}{2}°$. *Spring* No. 2 contains only 40 grains of chloride of sodium; 1 chloride of potassium; $2\frac{1}{3}$ chloride of magnesium; $18\frac{2}{3}$ chloride of calcium; and only 0·17 bromide of magnesium; 2 sulphate of lime; and agrees even with delicate children requiring anti-scrofulous remedies. The former is more adapted for external use.

Physician.—Dr. Herrmann.

STACHELBERG, Canton *Glarus*, Switzerland; below 47° lat. N., $9\frac{1}{2}°$

long. E.; south-west of Pfäfers, a league and a half south of *Glarus* station, situated in the background of the *Linth Valley*, at the foot of the steep Braunwald Mountains, 2,044 feet over the level of the sea, with a magnificent panorama. The valley is enclosed by the gigantic snow-covered Tödi and Bifertenstock. On clear days the climate is very mild and equable; winds scarcely ever penetrate; nevertheless, winter clothes are sometimes requisite in summer, in consequence of rain occasionally following hot days, and suddenly lowering the temperature. The spring issues out of a grotto in the high mountain rocks, and contains 4·19 grains of solid ingredients in 16 ounces—viz., sulphuret of sodium, 0·36; sulphuret of hydrate of calcium, 0·32; sulphate of soda, 1; sulphate of potash, 0·03; sulphite of soda, 0·12; chloride of sodium, 0·04; carbonate of lithia, 0·02; carbonate of lime, 0·32; carbonate of magnesia, 0·17; alumina, with phosphoric acid, 0·33; silica, 0·09; organic substance, 0·64; free carbonic acid, 57·8 cubic inches in 100 of gas; half combined, 51; nitrogen, 16 cubic inches; sulphuretted hydrogen, 1·45.

The water is used internally against chronic bronchial and gastric catarrhs; externally, in chronic rheumatism and various cutaneous diseases. The cure establishment consists of two great buildings, connected by a covered gallery. Accommodation is still somewhat defective. Season, June, July, and August.

Physician—Dr. König.

STEBEN, in Upper Frankonia, BAVARIA, 1,786 feet over the level of the sea, on a plateau, and connected with the north-western portion of the Fichtel Mountains, fifteen miles north-west of *Hof* station (Bamberg-Leipzig Railway), three and a half hours' diligence ride. The climate is very bleak, but tonic, there being no shelter against east and north-east winds. The drinking spring contains 3·85 grains of solid ingredients in 16 ounces—viz., 0·49 carbonate of soda; 0·69 carbonate of magnesia; 1·67 carbonate of lime; 0·31 carbonate of iron; 0·02 chloride of sodium; 0·07 sulphate of soda; 0·47 silica; 0·11 organic matter; free carbonic acid, 29·3 cubic inches. Moor-baths are also available. There are pleasant walks near the springs. Residences in the village (Untersteten). In cases of spermatorrhœa, this spa is often chosen on account of its bracing climate.

Physician—Dr. Reichel.

STREITBERG (BAVARIA,) between Bamberg and Erlangen, two leagues east of *Forchheim* station near the entrance of the so-called ' Fränkische Schweiz.' The village lies on the southern slope of the Streitberg, 1,800 feet over the level of the sea, in a most charming valley, sheltered by semicircular hills against north-east and westerly winds, being only open towards the south-west. The climate is therefore very mild and equable, and the whey-establishment is frequently used by persons affected with incipient tuberculosis. Accommodation ample, as well in the cur-establishments as in the hotels.

Physician—Dr. Weber.

SULZA, between *Kösen* and *Weimar* stations of the Thuringian Railroad, has very strong saline springs, and recommends itself to those scrofulous patients who wish to live in a retired locality. The *Mühlbrunnen* contains—sulphate of soda, 34·51 grains; sulphate of lime, 12·96; chloride of sodium, 29·44; chloride of potassium, 1·008; chloride of magnesium, 8·99; bromide of magnesium, 0·76; iodide of magnesium, traces; carbonate of iron, 1·001; traces of carbonate of magnesia, of carbonate of lithia, of silica, of alumina, and of organic matter; carbonic acid, 19 to 20 cubic inches. Temperature, 64°.
Physician—Dr. Beyer.

SULZBRUNN, ioduretted spring, one league south of Kempten, on the Augsburg-Lindau Railway, in BAVARIA, north-east of Lindau; below 48° lat. N. It lies 2,671 feet above the level of the sea, and is sheltered by the Alpine range, which borders the valley of the Iller, and stretches from the south-west to the north-east. The Bodelsberg forms a further protection. The climate is therefore peculiarly favourable, the mean temperature of summer being 62° Fahr.; of autumn, 43½°; of spring, 43¾; of winter, 34°. Of the five springs, the first and second are enclosed in one stream under the name of *Römerquelle*, and contain, in 16 ounces—chloride of sodium, 14½ grains; chloride of potassium, 0·13; chloride of calcium, 0·26; chloride of magnesium, 1; iodide of magnesium, 0·11; bromine, traces; carbonate of lime, 2·48; silica, 0·03; oxide of iron, 0·01; chloride of ammonium, 0·02; free carbonic acid, 1·47 cubic inches. There is a drinking and bathing establishment, with excellent arrangements and accommodation — very useful in all forms of scrophulosis.
Physicians—Dr. Faist, Dr. Hertel.

SWINEMÜNDE, in the island of *Usedom*, one of the most frequented Baltic Sea baths, thirty-six miles north-north-west of Stettin, on the Swiene, the outlet of the great haff in the Baltic; population, 4,600; south-east of Heringsdorf; below 54° N. lat., 16¼° E. long. Natural sea-baths are taken at the west of the harbour; and about a mile to the north-east of the town, the 'Plantage,' a park-like promenade, stretching from the town to the strand, encloses the establishment for warm and douche baths. Bathing season, from June to September. Temperature of the sea at that time, from 61° to 66°. Climate analogous to that of Heringsdorf.
Physicians—Dr. Kind, Dr. Schultze, Dr. Moser, Dr. Lendel, Dr. Cohn.

SYLT, an island on the west coast of SCHLESWIG, or rather the village of *Westerland*, on the east coast of the Downs, contains friendly residences for sea-bathers. Three Down-passages lead to the bathing-strand. From *Husum* station of the Altona-Tönningen Railway, a steamer passes three times a week to the islands of Föhr and of Sylt. From *Nösse*, the landing-place on the south-eastern point of the island, the guests are carried in an hour to Westerland by omnibus. This North Sea bath offers the advantages of a thorough maritime climate, with strong wave-strokes, and must therefore exercise a very bracing effect on persons possessed with strong con-

stitutions, but debilitated by exhausting labour or disease. N. lat. nearly 55°; E. long. 8½°.
Physician—Dr. Jenner.

SAINT SAUVEUR is situated on the Gave de Pau, in the lovely valley of Laverdan, between Barèges and Cauterets, south of *Tarbes*, 4,620 feet over the level of the sea. Notwithstanding this high situation, the climate is far from bleak, nor is it subject to sudden or extreme vicissitudes of temperature. The water of the chief spring, which feels like a soapy liquid, possesses a temperature of 86° to 97° Fahr., and only 1½ grain of constituents in 16 ounces—viz., sulphuret of sodium, 0·19; sulphate of soda, 0·29; chloride of sodium, 0·56; silica, 0·38; lime, 0·01; magnesia, 0·001; caustic soda, 0·089; nitrogen, 0·104 cubic inch. It lies on the road which leads to the celebrated Cirque de Gavarnie. The baths are very mild and soothing, and have an especially sedative effect on the nervous system. They are particularly recommended in neuralgia, migraine, and nervous cardialgia. Though the composition of the water does not materially differ from that of Barèges, the effects are different—probably in consesequence of the lower temperature of the baths here. It is also recommended in cases of uterine infiltration, with chronic fluor albus. The neighbouring chalybeate of Viscos assists in improving the general tone of the system. Considering the most romantic scenery of the environs, the pure, bracing, and still mild Alpine air, with the soothing baths and the tonic beverage, no wonder a great benefit is derived in many derangements of the constitution requiring a thorough change of climate, as well as of dietetic and therapeutic influences.

SALZBRUNN (*Obersalzbrunn*), in the Waldenburg circle of UPPER SILESIA, 1,215 feet over the level of the sea; population, 2,000; forty-five miles south-west of Breslau, six miles south of *Freiburg* station, five miles north-west of Waldenburg, one league north of *Altwasser* station. The village extends in a charming wide valley from south to north, along the Salzach, a distance of three miles (with the names of Ober-Nieder and Neusalzbrunn), forming two rows of houses, surrounded by orchards, meadows, and fields. Park-like enclosures stretch on a rising ground towards the Annenthurm. The centre of the place is occupied by tasteful private residences and large hotels. The climate is bracing and mild, the valley being only exposed to north-west winds. Charming excursions may be made to Wilhelmsburg, which affords picturesque views of the Riesengebirge and of the Schneekoppe, to Altwasser, &c. The Oberbrunnen contains, in 16 ounces, 17·17 grains of solid ingredients—carbonate of soda, 8·14; of lime, 2·33; of magnesia, 1·88; of iron, 0·03; of lithia, 0·01; of strontia, 0·02; sulphate of soda, 2·94; chloride of sodium, 1·16; phosphate of soda, 0·005; bromide of sodium, 0·006; silica, 0·33; alumina, 0·002; carbonic acid 36½ inches.

Mühlbrunnen contains 15½ grains and 40 cubic inches of carbonic acid. Salzbrunn formerly enjoyed a great reputation for the cure of incipient tuberculosis, being often designated *cold Ems*; but severe winds, incidental to its high position, and the abundance of carbonic acid, somewhat contraindicate its use to persons suffering from any considerable amount of deep-seated pulmonary mischief—but it is extremely beneficial in chronic pulmonary catarrh, particularly if connected with abdominal plethora. The carbonate and sulphate of soda promote the function of the intestinal canal. Hæmorrhoidal fulness, with its concomitant digestive disturbance and subsequent thoracic oppression, find a great relief here; also chronic catarrh of the bladder. If, notwithstanding the above facts, Salzbrunnen is frequently resorted to by phthisical patients, this is principally due to its excellent whey-establishment, and to the frequent use of warm ass's, cow's, or goat's milk, fresh from milking, as introduced by Dr. Zemplin. He prefers the addition of milk in almost all *nervous* diseases. Indeed, milk, possessing the most analogous nutriment to the animal body, is preeminently suitable when the weakened innervation impedes the reception of ordinary food. In *abdominal* diseases, however, whey is more appropriate, its constituents being less concentrated; it possesses likewise reparative substances, the osmazome accompanying its lactates being the finest extract of animal matter extant. In deeply sunk digestive and assimilative function this mild nutriment seems to act as a congenial stimulant of the alimentary absorbents, followed by an increased mobility of the sluggish and distended veins. Hence we witness such excellent results in diseases characterised by heightened venosity with profuse tough mucous secretion. This being rendered looser and prepared for excretion, the intestinal mucous membrane becomes materially freer from oppression, digestion rapidly assumes a more normal condition, and the whole habit of the patient is invigorated. The combination of whey with an alkaline spa adds to its beneficial effect. This action explains the utility of this combination in abdominal as well as in chest diseases. When the respiratory process is obstructed by the formation of tubercles, vicarious respiration takes place by skin and abdomen. Here again the high locality and thinner air prove advantageous in checking the further deposit of new tubercles by the necessary deeper inspirations.

Physicians—Dr. Valentiner, Dr. Biefel, Dr. Hoffmann, Dr. Straehler.

SALZHAUSEN, in the Wetterau, near Nidda, Grand Duchy of HESSE, 461′ above the level of the sea, five leagues east-north-east of *Nauheim* station, equidistant north-east of *Friedberg* station, on the high road which leads from the Wetterau to the Vogelsberg. The valley is surrounded by moderate heights, and only open to the south. Charming forests abound in the neighbourhood. The Curhaus possesses a large covered gallery for exercise in unfavourable weather. There are eight saline springs; the principal, No. 2, contains 98⅔ grains of solid ingredients—viz., chloride of sodium, 73·45; chloride of calcium, 2·57; chloride of potassium, chloride of iron and loss, 1·83; chloride of magnesium, 8·79; sulphate of lime, 11·17; iodide of sodium 0·59. No. 1 contains no iodine; but bromide of sodium, 0·003; free carbonic acid, 4·3 cubic inches. Temperature, 57° to 59° Fahr. The climate is mild, on account of its sheltered position. The spa has proved efficacious in cutaneous diseases of scrofulous character, inveterate

ulcers, in eczema, &c. The neighbouring graduation works are useful for inhalations in chronic laryngeal irritation.
Physicians—Dr. Prinz, Dr. Strack.

SALZUNGEN, a town of 3,000 inhabitants, in the Duchy of SACHSEN-MEININGEN-HILDBURGHAUSEN, 778' over the level of the sea. Station on the Thuringian Railway, twelve miles south of Eisenach, five miles west of the Liebenstein chalybeate; 51° lat. N., 10½° long. E.; intersected by the Armbach on the left shore of the Werra; bordered on its other bank by the south-western declivity of the Thuringer Forest. The friendly valley is surrounded by woody heights in its direction from east to west; saline and bathing establishments adjoin the town. To the south, a large lake of forty acres exists, with numerous saline springs, which were formerly conducted to the salt works. The climate is mild and salubrious, and considerably impregnated with saline exhalations. The Stadtbrunnen contains 365 grains of solid constituents; among these, 334 of chloride of sodium, 3 chloride of potassium, $7\frac{1}{2}$ chloride of magnesium, 0·41 chloride of calcium, $2\frac{3}{4}$ sulphate of soda, 4 sulphate of lime, 0·12 sulphate of magnesia, $2\frac{1}{2}$ carbonate of lime, $\frac{1}{4}$ carbonate of magnesia, and traces of iron, iodine, &c.; carbonic acid, 4·7 cub. inches. Temperature, $54\frac{1}{4}°$. The Bernhards-brunnen contains 2002 grains of chloride of sodium, 0·09 chloride of magnesium, 0·10 carbonate of iron, $8\frac{1}{4}$ cub. inches carbonic acid. Temperature, $54\frac{1}{4}°$. Saline, vapour and douche-baths are used, besides baths of pine-foliage and of moor. In atrophy, scrophulosis, chronic catarrh, articular stiffness, Salzungen will prove useful.
Physician—Dr. Wagner.

SALCOMBE, a watering-place in the county of Devon, two miles east-north-east of *Sidmouth* station. Population, 434. It is situated within a creek, and protected by the surrounding uplands. It possesses a mild and equable winter climate, in which orange and lemon trees are able to mature their fruit in the open air. In the year 1774, an agave had been flourishing for twenty-eight years without being covered in winter; but there is a great want of sheltered walks, counterbalancing to some extent its climatic advantages.

SCARBOROUGH, a seaport town in the North Riding of Yorkshire, on the southern slope of a headland extending into the North Sea; lat. N. 54° 17'; long. W. 0° 23'; on the North Midland Railway, $42\frac{1}{4}$ miles north-east of York, $233\frac{3}{4}$ miles from King's Cross station (from seven to eight hours' journey). Population, 18,000 (12,900 in 1851). Altitude, 174 feet. Mean temperature, June, 59·1°; January, 38·1°. The ravine separating the two parts of the town is spanned over by a cast-iron bridge, leading to extensive pleasure grounds, saloon, and music-hall. The old castle stands on a promontory 270 feet high. It is justly called the Queen of British Watering-places, with its airy cliffs, its extensive sands, its bracing breezes and charming aspect, and the pleasant walks and drives. The north sands are generally in a better condition than the south; but the bather must be extremely cautious on the former against the strong outward current, which has often proved fatal even to experienced swimmers. The south sands are more broken up by springs. Though somewhat protected to the north-east by the upland, Scarborough is subject to rather sudden vicissitudes of temperature, even in summer, which ought to make visitors of delicate health doubly cautious in their dress. It possesses also two mineral springs, considered as aperient and alterative and somewhat tonic. Temperature, 49°. The *north well* yields 46 grains of solid ingredients in a pint — viz., $3\frac{1}{2}$ chloride of sodium, 18 sulphate of magnesia, 18 sulphate of lime, and $6\frac{1}{2}$ carbonate of lime. The *south well* possesses 66 grains of solid constituents — viz., 10 more of sulphate of lime and of magnesia; each contains, besides, about a quarter of a grain of iron. The new assembly-room and promenade adjacent to the wells and the lofty bridge of communication, greatly add to the convenience of Scarborough. The sands are generally so hard that the carriages swiftly run along them a great distance from the shore; they shelve so very gradually that the machines have to be driven very far into the water to procure a good plunge. Altogether, Scarborough may be selected as one of the most bracing and charming sea-baths for persons of somewhat vigorous constitution. The sands are never quite dry; the sea is colder than at the south bathing-places, but, in the same proportion, the sojourn here is more bracing and restorative, especially if the bather only rests a very short time in the water, so as to ensure a thorough reaction.

SIDMOUTH, a seaport town in Devonshire, at the mouth of the Sid, in the English Channel, thirteen miles east-south-east of Exeter, with which it is connected by railway. Population, 3,300. It is picturesquely sheltered by lofty hills from the north-west, and partially from the north, where luxuriant groves are available to the visitor; it is open to the sea towards the south; whilst easterly and westerly winds are checked by Peak and Salcombe Hills. The climate is mild and relaxing; snow is scarcely ever seen in the town, though occasionally perceived on the neighbouring hills. Severe storms occasionally happen in the early part of the year. Invalids should reside at some elevated houses in a more inland situation. It is well adapted for consumptive patients in the early stages, with great nervous irritability, but not otherwise too reduced in health; for where a bracing climate is required, Sidmouth would be unsuitable. It is greatly recommended for its sea-bathing in summer.

SWANSEA, a seaport town of SOUTH WALES, County Glamorgan, on the west side of the Tawy, at its mouth in Swansea Bay. Lat. N. 51°; long. W. 3°. Population, 33,900. The harbour, at the mouth of the river, is nearly enclosed by two piers. It communicates with London by the South Wales Railway. From the beauty of its situation it is frequently resorted to as a watering-place.

TARASP, in the Lower Engaddin, on the right shore of the Inn, Canton Grisons, 4,608 feet over the level of the sea, separated from the surrounding country by the deep valley of the Inn on the north, by the towering Piz-Pisog on the south, to the east and west by the ravines of the Scarlbach and the Plafua, twenty-eight leagues distant from *Chur* station (eighteen hours' diligence journey viâ Saint Moritz), the only Catholic German-speaking village of the Lower Engaddin. After the Inn has broken in its rapid course through the rocks of Ardetz, it bends towards the north, cuts deeply into the slate mountains, and flows round the plateau on which the village stands. A smaller upland rises above it, and is approached by very steep steps. A small lake, surrounded by meadows, separates the plateau from the Schlossberg. The panorama of the landscape, in which meadows alternate with fruit-gardens, rocks, ravines with their torrents, lakes, and woods, is extremely charming to the eye. Between the commune and the northerly Lutheran commune of *Schuls*, on the other side of the Inn, most powerful springs issue from the ground. The new Curhouse offers most excellent accommodation. The climate is mild. The prevailing winds are tempered by the towering mountains, whilst the shadow of the southern heights and of the luxuriant foliage creates refreshing coolness even in high summer. Sixteen ounces contain the following amount of ingredients:—Carbonate of lime, 12·45 ; carbonate of magnesia, 5·07 ; carbonate of iron, 0·15 ; carbonate of soda, 27·22 ; chloride of sodium, 29·40 ; iodide of sodium, 1·53 ; sulphate of soda, 16·54 ; sulphate of potash, 2·99 ; silica, 0·24 ; phosphoric acid, 0·0023 ; alumina, 0·0015 ; fluor, manganese, traces ; free and half combined carbonic acid, 34·88 ; perfectly free carbonic acid, 15·39 grains. Temperature, 43° F. *Tarasp* thus combines ingredients of saline and alkaline spas, and certainly belongs to the most useful mineral waters. They stimulate and promote the functions of the intestinal canal, of the liver, and of the lymphatic vessels, whilst the tone of the muscular and nervous system becomes increased. Robust persons with phlegmatic temperaments, whose liver has been overtaxed by luxurious living or sedentary habits, find particular benefit there. It is also useful in obstruction of the portal system, in hæmorrhoidal complaints, in chlorosis of leucophlegmatic individuals, who do not bear pure chalybeates, in goître, abnormal stoutness, in chronic gout and rheumatism without deposits, in obstinate hoarseness if not based on organic disease. It is often compared with Carlsbad, and considered analogous in its effects. However, though both possess somewhat similar constituents, Tarasp contains more carbonate and less sulphate of soda, considerably more chloride of sodium, besides a great amount of iodide of sodium ; further, a greater quantity of iron and of carbonic acid. These apparently superior solvent agents are somewhat counterbalanced by the presence of carbonate of lime. The high temperature of Carlsbad plays, no doubt, an important part in the remarkable cures observed there. Indeed, the composition of the Tarasp springs is so excellent, the Alpine air so bracing and restorative, the scenery so charming and picturesque, that they require to borrow no extraneous reputation ; their difficulty of access has hitherto been the great obstacle to their more general employment, but this defect grows less and less every year. A much nearer road from Tyrol will soon be available. In cases of intense hepatic obstruction, Carlsbad will still remain unique. Its happy combination of solvents and antacids, and of purgatives absorbed by the system with the warm fluid, cannot fail to exert a powerful reaction. But it will only be resorted to where its use is absolutely indicated; for a certain strength of constitution is required to elaborate the healing agents. On the other hand, Tarasp appears more as a promoter of the natural, dormant, or oppressed functions of the glandular and vascular system. No doubt, its course, when indicated, sends the patient to his home in a more vigorous and cheerful condition. The intestinal canal was not so much the focus of its action, but rather the general assimilative process and organic metamorphosis.

Physician—Dr. Killias.

TEGERNSEE, a village and lake of UPPER BAVARIA, thirty-one miles south of Munich, two and a half hours' diligence ride from the *Holzkirchen* station, north of Kreuth, 2487' above the level of the sea, is surrounded by a circle of mountains covered with the most charming and variegated woods, and offering an ever-changing series of beautiful walks. It is frequently resorted to in summer for its picturesque scenery and salubrious climate, as a bracing and reparative health-resort by delicate persons inclined to pulmonary diseases.

Physician—Dr. Rosener.

TEINACH, a village of 500 inhabitants, in the Black Forest circle of Würtemberg, five miles south of Calw, 25 miles west-south-west of *Stuttgardt* (its nearest station), situated in a wild romantic valley, surrounded by woody hills; 1,223 feet above the level of the sea. The climate is mild, and the air impregnated with exhalations of fir-trees, peculiarly grateful to tuberculous patients. The neighbouring Zavelstein, 1,800 feet high, possesses an excellent whey establishment. The road from Calw rises first along the shore of the Nagold, the eastern boundary of the Black Forest, and then diverges westward into the fertile meadow valley of the Teinach, where the Castle of Zavelstein appears as a charming eminence, with Teinach at its feet. All the buildings belonging to the cure-establishment, with two hotels, form an enclosed whole, connected with each other by covered passages. Gardens and promenades along the valley and along the mountains abound in the environs. At the border of the forest, at about the third of the height of the northern mountain, the lovely *Wilhelmshöhe* is erected, forming a reunion for the guests, and offering an excellent view of the valley and of the Castle of Zavelstein. There are five springs. The *Bachquelle* contains 13·9 grains of solid ingredients in 16 ounces—viz., carbonate of lime, $5\frac{1}{2}$; carbonate of magnesia, $1\frac{1}{3}$; carbonate of soda, $4\frac{1}{2}$; carbonate of iron, 0·05; carbonate of manganese, 0·008; sulphate of soda, 1·10; sulphate of potash, 0·24; chloride of sodium, 0·56; silica, 0·44; free carbonic acid, 38·72 cubic inches. The ascending gases consist, in 100 volumes, of—90·46 carbonic acid; 9·53 nitrogen; 0·01 oxygen. The *Dintenquelle* (ink-spring) is a pure chalybeate, only imbued with 0·88 grains of solids in 16 ounces—amongst these, 0·13 of carbonate of iron; carbonic acid, 1·37 cubic inches. The springs exhibit, on the whole, a tonic and stimulating effect, promoting the secretions of the mucous membranes, counteracting acidity and profuse discharges. They are therefore indicated in general debility, hypochondriasis, difficult and painful menstruation, fluor albus, gastric dyspepsia, pulmonary and vesical catarrh. The alkaline (Bachquelle), lime (Hirschquelle), and acidulous (Dächleinsquelle) springs, and the more chalybeate (Dintenquelle), all display here their various peculiar action, and approach, on the whole, the effects of alkaline chalybeates, being distinguished by the charming and salubrious climate, which greatly co-operates in the curative results.

Physicians—Drs. Epting and Zipperlen.

TIEFENAU, near Elgg, Canton Zürich, not far from the *Elgg* and *Aadorf* stations of the St. Gall-Winterthur Railway, in a romantic spot, surrounded by pine-forests, 1,800 feet over the level of the sea, on the slope of the Schaumberg, possesses a hydropathic establishment, often resorted to after a course of mercury in secondary syphilis, to promote general metamorphosis, and strengthen the reactive power of the organism; for it occasionally happens that prolonged anti-syphilitic courses of treatment incapacitate the body at last from properly absorbing and elaborating the requisite remedies. In such cases, this and other favoured localities are sought to restore the former vigour, by exercise in the open air, by contemplation of nature's beautiful works, and by internal and external application of the pure element. After such a course, old syphilitic remains are apt to yield rapidly to a gentle mercurial treatment, when previously this drug seemed to have lost all curative power.

Physician—Dr. Winkler.

TÖPLITZ, or TOPLIKA, a village of NORTHERN CROATIA, with 900 inhabitants, nine miles south-south-east of the town of *Warasdin*; above 46° N. latitude, 16½° E. longitude; in the charming Bjedna Valley, possesses warm springs, arising in the midst of a park, known to the Romans under the name of *Thermæ Jassæ*. *Friedau*, the nearest railroad station of the South Austrian Railway, is 20 miles distant to the north-west, and connected with the spa by a well-built open road. The *Bettina*, which runs from west to east into the Drau, is bordered on its left (northern) shore by the flat forerunners of the Matzel Mountain, and on the right (southern) shore by the lofty Warasdiner Mountain. The spa lies in a pleasant locality on the southern declivity of the former mountain, a few minutes' walk from the northern bank of the river; the climate is therefore mild, salubrious, and sheltered. Very interesting excursions may be made into the environs. Warasdin, on the right shore of the Drau, is a very pleasant town, possessing an old fortress, a castle, and various other attractive objects. The spring contains 7·13 grains of constituents in 16 ounces—viz., carbonate of lime, 2⅕; carbonate of magnesia, 0·59; carbonate of iron, 0·04; sulphate of potash, 0·28; sulphate of soda, 1·34; sulphate of lime, 0·23; chloride of sodium, 0·79; chloride of magnesium, 0·14; alumina, 0·01; silica, 0·37; sulphuretted hydrogen, 0·11 cubic inch; carbonic acid, free and half combined, 3·94 cubic inches. Temperature, 135½° Fahr. There are large basins for bathing in common, as well as separate bathing cabinets, besides the extremely efficacious sulphur moor-baths. As a sulphurous thermal spring, Töplitz is distinguished by having so few ingredients to counteract or modify the effect of the sulphurous compounds, and may therefore be looked upon as a *pure sulphur spa*, with a highly pronounced alterative action on the cutaneous and sero-fibrous systems. It enjoys a great reputation in chronic, arthritic, and neuralgic complaints, in uterine excitement, and in certain chronic cutaneous diseases.

Physician—Dr. Rakovec.

TRAVEMÜNDE, a fortified town in the north of GERMANY; lat. N. below 54°; nine miles north of *Lübeck*, on the left bank of the Trave, which enters here into the Baltic. Population, 4,000. The sea-baths are about ¼ of a league to the east of the town. The bathing-ground is firm and gently sloping, in a sheltered bay. There are besides excellent arrangements for warm sea, sulphur, and pine-foliage baths; ample accommodation in the bath establishment, as well as on the east and harbour sides of the town, with an open view of the sea, and an uninterrupted access of marine air. The climate is bracing, but not bleak. Travemünde deserves recommendation for the other curative agents it offers, besides those provided by nature. In cases of chronic rheumatism without articular deposits, especially in stiffness remaining after protracted fits of gout, or acute rheumatism, the baths of pine foliage might advantageously precede sea-bathing. Patients of this class would greatly benefit by having their cutaneous and muscular system first made more supple by the pine foliage and sulphur baths; then after a transition of warm sea-baths, gradually taken in lower and lower temperature, they should ultimately conclude the course by *short* baths in the sea itself.

Physicians—Drs. Lieboldt and Hanssen.

TRIEST (*Tergeste*), the principal seaport city of the AUSTRIAN empire, Illyria, on the Gulf of Triest, at the north-east extremity of the Adriatic Sea, 73 miles east-north-east of the opposite Venice. Lat. N. 45° 33; long. E. 13° 46'. Population, 65,000. Mean temperature of the year, 55°: winter, 39·4° (Fahr.); summer, 71·4°. The old town is built on the declivity of a steep hill, enclosed by walls, and the new town on a plain bordering the sea. The spacious *Corso* winds between the two, and opens into several large and well-built squares. The arrangements for warm and cold sea-baths are excellent, but only suited to vigorous, hardened individuals, as the hot depressing south wind (sirocco) has free entrance, and is often followed in too rapid alternation by northern blasts from the glaciers. This wind (cora) sometimes rages ten to fifteen days in winter and latter part of autumn. The summer is unfavourably distinguished by intense radiating heat, often giving way to sudden cold. Spring is subject to frequent rains, and considerable vicissitudes of temperature. The winter is most trying, through intense cold and violent atmospheric changes. Autumn is the best season, changes being rarer, temperature being on an average 70° to 72° Fahr. during the day, and not sinking below 59° in the evening. The moisture of the air is considerably less than in Venice and any other point of the south coast. The town possesses so many charms and social advantages that it would be tempting, as a frequent resort for sea-baths, without the above climatic relations. As, however, no malaria prevails to produce endemic or epidemic diseases, persons with sound constitutions will be all the more invigorated and braced against the future inroads of disease by a short course of sea-bathing here. Weakly individuals have to avoid a lengthy sojourn altogether.

VENICE, on the opposite side of the Adriatic, has excellent arrangements for warm sea-baths in the various hotels during the whole year. In summer, open baths are taken on the coast of the Lido, under the protection of tents; the bathers have to remain during the day in the adjoining restaurant or coffee-house, or the relaxing heat of the summer would somewhat counterbalance the favourable effects of sea-bathing.

TEIGNMOUTH, a maritime town of Devonshire, on both sides of the Teign, at its mouth in the English Channel, twelve and a half miles south-south-east of Exeter, south of Exmouth, north-east of Plymouth, on the South Devon Railway, 209 miles south-west of Paddington station (six to seven hours' journey). Population, 6,000. The position is very picturesque. Many resort there for sea-bathing in *summer*, as it is considered less relaxing than other southern bathing-places. The temperature is 5° lower there than in London; but as a *winter* residence the climate is not mild and steady enough for invalids, though the temperature is 6° higher than in London. In the year 1858, the mean barometric pressure was 29·93°; the highest temperature, 78·7°; the lowest, 23·8°; thus showing an extreme range of 55°. Mean temperature of the year, 50·6°. Rainfall, 54·6 inches. As a general rule, the south-western climate of England is mild, but rather humid, consequently more relaxing and soothing than tonic—hence beneficial in chronic affections of the throat, trachea, and bronchi, with a dry tickling cough; but in congestive condition of the mucous surfaces, with profuse expectoration and a languid and relaxed condition of the system, the disease will be aggravated by this climate. But benefit will arise in gastritic dyspepsia and dysmenorrhœa, based on nervous irritability: injurious in atonic dyspepsia (which is a common complaint of the inhabitants), in menorrhagia or leucorrhœa— in fact, wherever profuse secretions prevail. Even when useful, the sojourn ought not be prolonged too much. Whenever the patient commences to flag, he ought to resort to a more bracing air. The winter temperature of the south coast of Devonshire is 3° to 4° higher than that of London (5° in the very sheltered places); this is most marked in November, December, and January. In February the difference is reduced to 3°, and in March and April to less than 1°. The days are comparatively warmer on the south-western than on the southern coast, the nights being nearly equal in both. The *range* of daily temperature is about the same on both coasts; but, as regards continuance of the same temperature, Devonshire has the advantage of nearly three-fourths of a degree, the whole variation of successive days being only three degrees; this distinction is very important. According to a more or less sheltered position against northerly and easterly winds, these advantages will vary. Most of these situations labour under the defect of not offering sufficient exercise ground. Sometimes, at a little distance from the coast, places may be met with more protected than the sea-girt localities—for instance, the village of Lympstone, about two miles from Exmouth; and Bishopsteignton, about the same distance from Teignmouth. These partake of the mildness of the maritime climate, without being exposed to the southerly gales of the coast. But as we recede from the seashore the night chills become more intense, and the range of temperature more considerable.

TORQUAY, a market town of Devonshire, situated on the steep shore of a cove of Torbay, on its north side, eighteen and a half miles south of Exeter, 220 miles south-west of Paddington station (six and a half hours' journey). Lat. N. 50° 24'; long. W. 3° 26'. Population, 16,000. Through the elegance of its mansions, and the beauty of its scenery, it is called the 'City of Villas.' Whilst enjoying the general character of the Devonshire climate, its atmosphere is less moist and more equable, as it forms a portion of a promontory, or imperfect peninsula, projecting into the Atlantic towards the west, and thus offering nearly half of its circumference to the contact of the sea currents. Hence only four degrees of difference prevail between the warmest and coldest of ten places, the mean difference of succeeding years being only one and a half. The westerly winds have to travel over such a large extent of sea before touching *terra firma*, that they impart a dominant moisture to Cornwall and Devonshire.

According to Mr. Vivian, the mean annual temperature, even at Woodfield, is the highest in Great Britain (52°); the climate being more equable, less vicissitude prevails, and thus the summer is cooler (61°) and the winter (44°) warmer than at most other parts of the island. The rainfall is two inches below the general average—sixteen less than at Penzance, four less than at Clifton. The air is drier than at any analogous place mentioned in the Registrar General's Report, except Chichester; it surpasses Brighton by nearly 3°, London by more than 2° during the last quarter of the year, and Clifton by more than 3°. Another peculiar advantage lies in the circumstance that the east wind is a sea breeze. As regards the longevity of its inhabitants, it is only surpassed by Cumberland, and exceeds the general average by a proportion of 300 to 220. Torquay is 2·6° cooler in summer than Clifton (though 4·1° warmer in winter); it is half a degree cooler in summer than Hastings (5° warmer in winter). Queenstown, in the south of Ireland, is the only town in Great Britain approximating the temperature of Torquay in all seasons. The climate is well suited for out-door exercise, being sheltered against even the northeast winds, which generally are so injurious in spring and early summer. The beauty of the environs is attractive enough for inducing frequent excursions. For persons affected with irritable thoracic organs, or with incipient phthisis, Torquay is unrivalled in England as a winter resort. According to Dr. Radcliffe Hall, the first effect on consumptive patients is sedative, the restlessness, irritability, and night perspirations yielding after a few days. Digestion generally becomes torpid at first, appetite diminished, with general feeling of debility; but these symptoms yield to ordinary treatment in a few weeks. A convalescent from pneumonia or pleurisy finds the freedom of breathing increased, and evening feverishness lessened. Asthmatic invalids are either exactly suited there, or not at all. In heart disease, Torquay will agree when the patient suffering from over-impulse of the heart, and dispnœa on slight exertion, be of florid complexion, with a dry and hard skin; but when the patient is flabby and pallid, frequently faintish, with a soft, cool, easily perspiring skin, Torquay will be unsuitable. The climate tends to allay the irritation of the mucous membranes, to lessen inflammation in general, and to promote gently the functions of the skin.

According to Mr. Vivian's Table, the following difference exists in the respective temperatures of—

	Annual	Winter	Spring	Summer	Autumn
Torquay (Woodfield)	52·1°	44·0°	50·0°	61·2°	53·1°
Cove	51·9	44·1	50·1	61·3	52·2
Penzance	51·8	44·0	49·6	60·2	53·3
Undercliff	51·3	41·8	49·6	60·6	53·5
Clifton	51·2	39·9	49·7	63·8	51·4
Exeter	51·2	41·4	49·5	62·0	51·9
Hastings	50·4	39·0	47·4	61·7	52·2
London	50·3	39·1	48·7	62·3	51·3
Sidmouth	50·1	40·3	48·1	60·2	51·6
Chiswick	49·9	38·6	48·5	62·2	50·1
Nice	59·4	47·8	56·2	72·2	61·6
Rome	. .	46·8	. .	. .	. .
Madeira	64·9	60·6	62·3	69·5	67·3
Bute	48·25	39·6	46·6	58·0	48·5

The accommodation in Torquay for visitors increases every year; new buildings, mostly of a detached character, rise in various positions of the beautiful, undulating, and well-sheltered environs. The absence of fogs, and the comparative dryness—probably from the limestone rocks forming a great portion of the ground, and partly from the two streams passing on either side and attracting the rain—serve as great advantages for ordinary and healthy mortals. The village of *Tor*, behind Torquay, situated on a higher position, is colder and damper, and less protected from northerly winds. But the little *Vale of Upton*, beyond Tor, protected from southerly and northerly winds, would be a most eligible situation, according to Sir James Clark, for establishing a *Madeira village*. If houses were built along the base of the hills bounding this vale, and the intervening space well drained and laid out in pleasure-grounds for exercise, Upton would, in his opinion, form one of the best winter residences in Devonshire for invalids. Compared with the more southern climates, Torquay offers a less amount of winter-warmth than Nice or Rome. This is a point of great and vital importance in some cases of extreme pulmonary irritation, apt to be aggravated by any diminution of temperature. The mutability of the British climate, the 'frequent change' with narrow range, however unpleasant and inconvenient, is very useful in hardening the constitution of the healthy, and thus indirectly assists in prolongation of life. But the advanced pulmonary invalid requires a sedative, calm, and equable warmth, to keep off new causes of irritation, which might institute a fresh process of inflammation, of tubercular deposit and fever, and thus turn the evenly-poised balance against him. Numerous invalids will therefore not fail to turn their hopeful steps towards distant climes, with a view of warding off the dreaded fatal termination. But they should bear in mind that if, perhaps, their disorder is less inclined to progress in very warm localities, their general health has an equally less prospect of improving. Moreover the *grand* transitions, *with long intervals*, as occurring in many favourite far-off health-resorts, often impart such shocks to the human machine as to undermine the health and curtail life, undoing in a few moments the advantages of months, unless the invalids exercise the greatest care in all their doings. Apart from this, the journey itself is a frequent source of deterioration in weakly persons. If to this be added a less palatable and nutritious food than the invalid is accustomed to obtain in his own home, amongst the circle of his fond relatives and friends, delicate individuals with greatly impaired strength should certainly prefer a home winter residence—at least in all those cases in which the journey itself is likely to demand a great amount of exertion, sacrifice of comfort, or of bodily strength.

TUNBRIDGE WELLS, a town of Kent, five miles south-southwest of Tunbridge, forty-six miles south-east of London Bridge (from $1\frac{1}{4}$ to $1\frac{3}{4}$ hour's railway journey). Altitude, 289 feet; population, 17,000. The pump-room and baths of the chalybeate springs are in a small valley enclosed by sloping hills — Mounts Ephraim, Pleasant, and Zion. Its varied attractions of picturesque and truly wild scenery, 'the salubrious waters which perpetually flow from its iron substrata, and the bracing and finely-scented airs which pass over its thymy commons and umbrageous woods, are so many securities to the valetudinarian and lover of nature.' In quoting these rapturous expressions, Dr. James Johnson expresses his gratification at the beauty of the numerous detached buildings, with gardens and lawns, commanding extensive views of wild or cultivated country, of furze-clad common bestrewed with broom, and of primeval rocks and forests. The water of the Tunbridge wells is perfectly transparent, with a distinctly chalybeate odour and taste, neither acidulous nor saline, but fresh and agreeable to the palate, without any air-bubbles: temperature, 50°. F. A gallon contains $7\frac{1}{2}$ grains of solid ingredients, and amongst these a grain of iron (thus a pint holds only $\frac{1}{8}$ of a grain), with about $1\frac{1}{2}$ cubic inch of carbonic acid, and $\frac{1}{8}$ an inch of nitrogen. The other portions consist of some chloride of sodium, of potassium, of magnesium, and some carbonate of lime. The strength of the water varies with dry or wet seasons. The iron continued in a perfect solution at a temperature of 140° Fahr. Though the quantity of iron is small, its intimate combination and persistent solubility, and the small amount of other ingredients, render the water purely tonic and stimulant, correcting acidity and dyspepsia, and increasing the red globules of the blood. Exercise on the common is to be preferred to that on the fashionable but more sheltered parade. The water is unsuited, when the secretions are vitiated or the bowels constipated, or in states of plethora, inflammation, or congestion of an important organ. Increase of appetite and spirits, followed by general improvement of strength, are signs of its agreement, as also a glow of heat after taking exercise, and increased renal function. To prevent constipation, an aperient pill (as pil. aloes cum myrrh) is recommended to be taken overnight, rather than saline purgatives with the chalybeate in the morning. Atonic dyspepsia, chlorosis, and levelopment of scrofula after sea-bathing indicate the use of the springs. However useful in simple debility, the springs frequently injure if taken *to allay feelings* of debility which may be based on a local inflammatory or congestive condition. The hills encircling the glen in which the water rises do not ensure complete protection from north and east winds. *Crowboro' Common*, at the Beacon, seven miles from Tunbridge Wells, stands at an elevation of 800 feet above the level of the sea, and must have some influence on the air coming from that direction. Probably the proximity of the sea likewise exercises some effect on the purification of the air, though it is distant enough to prevent direct entrance of marine exhalations. A great peculiarity of this fashionable watering-place lies in the quality popularly ascribed to it—viz., that people whose overwrought nervous system causes distressing sleeplessness, enjoy here *a sound nightly sleep*. This cannot be solely ascribed to the relaxation and change, as many persons have actually found the above relief only here, and at no other health-resort. Of course this can only apply to those cases in which no organic or morbid impediment obstructs the action of the brain.

VERNET, a village of the *Pyrenées Orientales*, at the foot of the Canigou, two miles distant from Villefranche, four from Prades, and sixteen from Perpignan. It is situated on the right bank of the River *Tet*, at a considerable height, commanding a view of a rich and fertile valley, and possesses a mild and equable climate, so that baths are administered during the whole year. There are two bathing establishments; the larger, *Établissement des Commandants*, is reached by crossing the River Castel. The temperature of the springs varies from 66·20° to 136·40° F. The other, *Etablissement Mercader*, on the Castel Road, possesses springs of equal properties; the water is colourless and limpid, unctuous to the touch, and of a sulphurous smell and taste. The *Torrent* contains, in 16 ounces, 1·97 grains of solid ingredients, viz.— sulphuret of sodium, 0·31 ; carbonate of soda, 0·80 ; carbonate of potash, 0·06 ; sulphate of soda, 0·13 ; chloride of sodium, 0·11 ; sulphate of lime, carbonate of lime, and carbonate of magnesia 0·63 ; alumina with traces of oxide of iron, 0·007 ; silica, 0·37 ; glairy organic matter, 0·10. A Gothic building is erected in the former more fashionable establishment, called a *vaporarium*, enclosing a small friendly saloon, in the form of a rotunda, heated by an ascending spring : eight cabinets surround this rotunda, for general and local vapour-baths. The patient sits on a cane-bottomed chair, and can inhale fresh unimpregnated air by means of an elastic mouthpiece. The spa is recommended in chronic pulmonary catarrh, in imperfectly-healed wounds from firearms, in indolent ulcers, and in chronic rheumatism; they are contra-indicated by inflammatory or congestive conditions of important organs. The mean temperature of October was in the morning (at nine o'clock) 56°, at noon 61°, and in the evening 59°; in November, morning (at nine) 43°, noon 51°, evening 45°. This shows a great mildness of climate, enabling a considerable extension of the bathing season.

VICHY, on the right bank of the *Allier*, 733 feet above the level of the sea, at the foot of the Auvergne Mountains, lies in a charming fertile valley, enclosed by an amphitheatre of hills, which are abundantly covered with fruit-trees and vineyards, about 12 hours' railway ride from Paris, and about 8 hours' ride from Lyons (to its north-west). Lat. N. above 46°; long. E. about 5½°. A promenade with an avenue of plane-trees separates the old from the more fashionable and convenient new town. The climate is very mild. The principal ingredient is bicarbonate of soda: in 16 ounces—

	Grains	Temperature
La Source des Mesdumes contains	30¾	62·6°
„ d'Hauterive (nearly)	37	59°
Grand Puits Carré	37½	111·2°
Grande-Grille	37½	107·6°
De l'Hôpital	38·6	87·8°
Puits Chomel	39	109·4°
Célestins	39¼	59°

The waters are all largely impregnated with carbonic acid gas, and to some extent with nitrogen and oxygen, besides some organic matter containing free sulphur. The other ingredients are (in Grande-Grille) chloride of sodium, 4·11 grains; bicarbonate of potash, 2·70 grains: bicarbonate of magnesia, 2·32 grains; bicarbonate of lime, 3·33 grains; bicarbonate of strontia, 0·02 grains; bicarbonate of iron, 0·03 grains; sulphate of soda, 2·23 grains; phosphate of soda, 0·99 grains; arsenate of soda, 0·015 grains; silica, 0·53 grains; total, 53·81 grains; free carbonic acid, 6·97 grains. The 'Hôpital' contains a total of 56 grains; carbonic acid, 8·19 grains; and is the mildest and least stimulating of all the springs, scarcely ever disagreeing even with the most delicate digestive organs. It is somewhat more alkaline, and contains more phosphate of soda and less chloride of sodium than the Grande-Grille, which takes the next place as regards facility of agreement. The springs have a particularly excellent effect in cases of atonic dyspepsia, in irritation of the mucous membrane of the duodenum, and the biliary ducts. By their deobstruent effect they strengthen the function of the liver. The great distinction of *this king of alkaline spas* consists not only in the great amount of bicarbonate of soda, but in the comparatively small quantity of other modifying ingredients. In all diseases based on an increase of organic acidity Vichy stands unrivalled. It counteracts dyspepsia with præcordial oppression and abdominal distension, and increases the function of the kidneys by its solvent effect on lithic acid; it has even been found useful in *diabetes*. It has a strongly curative effect in removing the morbid products of gout, by producing critical paroxysms. Compared with Carlsbad, a greater amount of alkalies are introduced into the organism by the latter, but a portion of these is combined with acids, which are subject to different modes of decomposition in the laboratory of the organic metamorphosis. The sulphur, forming an important element of the protein compounds, must produce a more normal condition in cases of retarded or sluggish venous circulation. Hence the combination of sulphate and of carbonate of soda with the digestive chloride of sodium must have a more powerful disintegrating influence on the morbidly stagnant albuminous and fibrinous particles of the venous blood, and must combat the excessive production of animal substance more energetically than Vichy. In such cases of chronic gout in which Carlsbad possesses too little soda to neutralise the excessive acidity, and where Vichy cannot sufficiently stem the progress of venous dyscrasia and the frequent returns of gouty paroxysms, both remedies might be combined with the most excellent result. Thus in *Warmbrunn*, the action of the sulphur-spring is heightened by the addition of Vichy water with most satisfactory effects. In *lithiasis* and *vesical catarrh*, Vichy stands unique. The water does not dissolve large concretions so as to render lithotomy unnecessary, but it may often prevent the formation of stone. That the too prolonged use of alkalies is injurious requires no explanation. No more than a certain degree of urinary alkalescence ought to be allowed, and the condition of the urinary secretion ought to be frequently ascertained by testing it with litmus-paper before and after the addition of a few drops of diluted acid. In vesical catarrh due to gravel, Vichy is extremely useful; but if the irritation of the bladder is connected with stricture or prostatic enlargement, these ailments must be removed before the employment of the Vichy water. After the cure of vesical catarrh relapses may be prevented by the use of chalybeates, especially in lymphatic torpid individuals. In vesical piles, especially of persons with irritable constitution and with inflammatory states of the urinary organs, Vichy must be avoided. Only after the removal of the inflammatory conditions, Grande-Grille may be taken in small doses with whey or warm milk; if taken cold it might provoke hæmorrhoidal congestion through its carbonic acid. But if the vesical piles are more of a passive nature produced by general or local atony, la Grande-Grille may be used more boldly. It is requisite, especially for patients who suffer from urinary complaints, that the alvine functions be kept in good order. Vichy is also very useful in chronic gonorrhœa, which sometimes disappears in a four-weeks' course after all other remedies have proved unavailing.

Physicians—Drs. Durand-Fardel, Alquié, Willemin, Nicolas, and Noyer.

WARMBRUNN, a town of the Hirschberger Circle, in Silesia, 1,100 feet above the level of the sea, 4 miles south-west of Hirschberg, 15 miles south-east of Flinsberg, 30 miles west of *Freiburg* station ($7\frac{1}{4}$ hours' diligence ride), south-west of Breslau. This pleasant town is situated on both shores of the *Zacken*, in a broad charming valley, stretching from south-west to north-east on the northern slope of the *Riesengebirge*. The gardens surrounding the houses and the fields, extending to the mountains, give the place a very pleasant appearance. By the protection of the Sudetten ranges towards the south, of the Gröbelberg towards the east, and of the Ottilienberg to the west, the roughest winds are kept off or tempered; whilst the cold blasts descending from the highest mountain-peaks sometimes occasion sudden vicissitudes of temperature, against which the patients have to be on their guard. South-west winds prevail most; next in frequency are the south-east winds; north winds scarcely ever appear. Mean temperature of the year, 47° F.: of summer, 59°. Rheumatic and pulmonary affections are frequently met with among the inhabitants. The climate is milder than that of the other Silesian spas, but occasionally rough and changeable. July and August are the best months for a course. Warmbrunn was formerly reckoned among the sulphurous thermæ, but later researches have shown that the hepatic gas developed over the spring is probably due to a decomposition taking place in the ascending gases between organic particles and portions of sulphate of soda, in a similar manner as in bottles containing sulphate of soda-water, into which organic particles have been introduced—as little leaves or straw. The spring-water itself developed no gaseous sulphuretted hydrogen whilst heated with nitrogen, nor when the boiling was continued till the fluid was completely evaporated. The spa belongs more to the so-called indifferent (akratic) thermæ.

In 16 ounces the following substances are contained:—

	Kleines Bassin	New Spring
Sulphate of soda	1·72	2
Chloride of sodium	0·55	0·59
" ammonium	0·05	—
Iodide of sodium	—	0·033
Bromide of sodium	—	0·0004
Carbonate of soda	0·81	1·20
" lime	0·16	0·14
" iron, magnesia Phosphate of alumina	0·06	—
Organic substances	0·17	—
Silica	0·55	0·64
Total	4·07	4·62
Nitrogen	0·46 cub. in.	traces
Carbonic acid	0·13	"
Sulphuretted hydrogen	traces	
Temperature	97° F.	105° F.

The new spring has a more solvent and stimulating effect than the old, and greatly resembles the springs of Teplitz in composition and action : whilst the relation between azote and carbonic acid is as 2 to 1 in the old springs, it is as 2 to $1\frac{1}{2}$ in the new one, over which the new massive bathing establishment is built. The thermal water is conducted into subterranean air-tight pipes, where it is allowed to cool. With different cranes hot or cooled mineral water runs into the basins—hence every degree of temperature can easily be produced. Before bathing in the large basins, preparatory cabinet-baths are taken, which are less exciting and are administered with a lower temperature : douche is combined with the baths. In the yard of the former convent-buildings, baths are given with different additions—as of malt, iron, sea-salt, motherlye, &c. The large basin possesses a temperature of $90\frac{1}{2}°$ to $99\frac{1}{2}°$—the small from 95° to 100°. Both are connected by beautifully-laid-out gardens. There are rooms for inhalation and for electrical therapeutics. Excellent whey is also available in appropriate cases. Lying in the same latitude with Aix-la-Chapelle, it is one of the most eastern spas ($16\frac{1}{2}°$ long. East), and enjoys a great reputation for the cure of chronic rheumatism, gout, and articular stiffness. It is also beneficial in hyperæmia of the respiratory mucous membrane, with a loose puffy atonic condition of the tissue, probably in consequence of the sulphuretted hydrogen hovering over the water. It is further indicated in herpetic diseases which have not yet taken a too severe hold of the system, and when they are neither kept up by an unduly increased venosity (so well adapted to Carlsbad) nor by a torpid state of cutaneous degenerative tendency, against which mud-baths are so extremely useful.

Warmbrunn proves particularly beneficial in removing the consequences of gouty paroxysms, whilst pure alkaline spas are more indicated in chronic athritic dyscrasia. As regards hæmorrhoidal complaints, it proves serviceable in those cases in which the predominance of venous blood in the portal system is accompanied by general atony of the abdominal nerves, so that the vascular system lacks the energy of producing a critical discharge through the rectum.

WÄGGIS, on the northern shore of the Vierwaldstädter Lake, east of Lucerne ; lat. North above 47°; long. East. $8\frac{1}{2}°$; 1,350 feet above the level of the sea. It is situated on the southern declivity of the Rigi, surrounded by the most magnificent scenery, and completely protected against severe winds. The climate is very mild and moderately moist and exhilarating. Not only real chesnut, but fig and almond trees thrive here in the open air. In the year 1795 the rain from the Rigi precipitated such a quantity of mud towards the village that thirty-one houses were driven into the lake. The mean temperature of the year amounts to $51\frac{1}{2}°$ Fahr. : spring, 51° F.; summer, 68° F. ; autumn, $59\frac{1}{4}°$ F. It is resorted to as one of the most charming summer residences and whey establishments in cases of incipient tuberculosis.

WEISSENBURG, in the Canton of Berne, on the southern slope of the Stockhorn chain, 2,759 feet above the level of the sea, five leagues southwest of *Thun*, is situated in a deep narrow side-ravine of the *Simmer* valley, through which the wild Bunschibach rushes. The climate is distinguished by its humidity. The shelter against north and east winds allows the air to be readily impregnated with the watery vapours of the torrent. The temperature is very changeable; mornings and evenings are mostly cool, but in clear days the atmosphere is extremely mild and pleasant. A saline earthy thermal spring issues at the foot of a rock near the left shore of the Bunschibach, with a temperature of 77° Fahr. It contains in 16 ounces— sulphate of lime, $17\frac{1}{8}$ gr.; sulphate of magnesia, $5\frac{1}{2}$; sulphate of strontia, nearly $\frac{1}{4}$; sulphate of soda, above $\frac{1}{2}$; sulphate of potash, about $\frac{1}{8}$; phosphate of lime, $\frac{1}{4}$; carbonate of lime, $\frac{4}{5}$; carbonate of magnesia, $\frac{3}{8}$; chloride of sodium, $\frac{1}{8}$; silicate of soda, $\frac{1}{4}$; silica, $\frac{1}{3}$; oxide of iron, $\frac{1}{50}$. As regards gaseous contents, 1,000 grammes contain—carbonic acid, 2·53 cubic centimetres; nitrogen, 0·99; oxygen, 0·46. The spa is resorted to in such chronic plumonary catarrhs which follow the inflammatory irritation of the mucous membrane, and are characterised by a dry tickling cough, with very sparing expectoration. It is especially adapted to young people with very excitable nervous and vascular systems, and to plethoric but weakly persons of middle age who have a great tendency to renewed obstinate attacks of bronchitis.

Physician.—Dr. Müller.

WEISSENSTEIN, on the ridge of the foremost Jura chain, above the town of *Solothurn*, 3,949 feet above the level of the sea, with most charming and magnificent Alpine views, contains thirty comfortably-arranged rooms and three bathing-cabinets for whey-drinking and whey-baths. The establishment is particularly exposed to east and west winds, and therefore subject to frequent changes of temperature. Walks into the environs are most attractive; but the climate is unsuited for pulmonary invalids, and more adapted to cases of anæmia after exhausting diseases, when the Alpine air is most able to restore the pristine vigour of the organism.

WILDUNGEN, in the Principality of Waldeck, twenty minutes' walk from the village of Nieder Wildungen, 300 feet above the level of the sea, four leagues west of *Wabern* station (which is reached in an hour and a half from Cassel, and in four-and-a-half hours from Frankfort). The charming valley of Wildungen, intersected by the Wilde and surrounded by woody forests, offers most pleasant and variegated shady promenades to the visitors. A great and most convenient establishment has lately been built, with eighty rooms and suitable saloons. The climate is mild and salubrious: season, from June to September. From the eight springs that issue here, those most in use are the *Stadtbrunnen* (Victorquelle), the *Salzbrunnen* (Helenenquelle), arising half a league from the town at an altitude of 740 feet, and the Stahlbrunnen.

In 16 ounces are contained:—

	Victorquelle (Stadtbrunnen)	Helenenquelle (Salzbrunnen)	Stahlbrunnen
Bicarbonate of soda	0·49 gr.	6·49 gr.	..
,, iron	0·16	0·14	0·58 gr.
,, manganese	0·01	0·009	0 069
,, lime	5·47	9·75	0·98
,, magnesia	4·11	10·47	1·38
Sulphate of lime	..	..	0·07
,, soda	0·52	0·10	0·04
,, potash	;0·08	0·21	0·05
Chloride of sodium	0·59	8·01	0·05
Silica	0·15	0·23	0·08
Phosphate of soda			
Borate of soda			
Bromide of sodium			
Nitrate of soda	traces	traces	traces
Bicarbonate of lithia			
,, baryta, alumina, and organic matter			
Total	11·09 gr.	35·15 gr.	3·30 gr.
Free carbonic acid	19·26 gr.	19·55 gr.	18·06 gr.

The carbonic acid gas forms a layer of one and a half feet high over the mirror of the spring, within which the bottles are filled for exportation. The 'Salzbrunnen' (which contains more soda, magnesia, and lime) has a considerably milder effect than the Stadtbrunnen. The spa is particularly recommended in chronic diseases of the uropoietic organs—in gravel, lithiasis, excessive mucosity, spasms of the bladder, and chronic inflammation of the prostatic gland. Hufeland narrates (in 1832) how his own illness was cured by Wildungen: retention of urine, which had lasted for twelve weeks, was succeeded by vesical blennorrhage; a profuse secretion of tough gelatinous phlegm with difficult micturition persisted, and produced great debility and emaciation; uva ursi bark and other remedies brought no relief. At last he took Wildungen water with an infusion of quassia, and in a short time the discharge got gradually less, and disappeared completely within four weeks. He subsequently drank daily for a whole year a glass of the water. He attributed his cure to the combination of soda, lime, carbonic acid, and iron: he probably used the Salzbrunnen. These springs have at all times enjoyed a great reputation as lithontriptics. They are considered especially curative in those cases of lithiasis which exhibit an atonic character of the urinary organs; they are thought the best means for promoting the expulsion of calculi. In catarrh and hæmorrhoids of the bladder (after the removal of the inflammatory stage), in painful or deficient menstruation, in chronic leucorrhœa, gonorrhœa, sterility, &c., they are found extremely useful.

Physicians—Drs. Doehne, Roerig, Von Lingelsheim, Krueger, and Schauer of Berlin.

WIPFELD, a borough in Under-Franconia (BAVARIA), on an eminence on the right shore of the River Main, five miles east of *Bergtheim* station (Bamberg-Würzburg Railroad), fifteen miles north-east of Würzburg, below lat. 50° N. The *Ludwigsbad* lies opposite Wipfeld, 800 yards distant from the left shore of the Main, at an altitude of 550 feet, in a very pleasant country. The climate is described as very mild, and suitable to persons affected with pulmonary diseases: mean summer temperature, $63\frac{1}{2}°$ Fahr. The Ludwigsquelle contains carbonate of lime, 2·30 grains; carbonate of magnesia, 0·71; carbonate of iron, traces; sulphate of lime, 4·60; sulphate of magnesia, 2·12 extractive substance, 0·25 — total, 9·98 grains. Carbonic acid, 1·28 cubic inch; sulphuretted hydrogen, 0·92. Temperature, $56\frac{3}{4}°$ Fahr. The sulphur-spring contains 17 grains of solid constituents (10 of sulphate of lime; 3·2 cubic inches of carbonic acid; 0·6 sulphuretted hydrogen). The sulphur-mud greatly assists the curative means of the spa; it possesses considerable quantities of humus acid, sulphuretted hydrogen, but little sulphur—also some carburetted and phosphoretted hydrogen. According to Scherer, 16 ounces slowly dried lose 12 ounces of humidity, and furnish 2·7 cubic inches of sulphuretted hydrogen, and 17 cubic inches of carbonic acid; 100 grains of the solid mass, freed from roots, contain—carbonate of lime, 24·09 grains; sulphate of lime, 6·34; carbonate of magnesia, 4·72; alumina, 10·30; oxide of iron, 2·90; silica, 12·00; sulphur, 0·81; humus acid, 25·50; bituminous resin, 0·80; extractive substance, 4·00; remnants of carbon and silica, 8·51. Whey and herb-juices are also administered in appropriate cases. Wipfeld is recommended in cases of chronic rheumatism and neuralgia.

Physician—Dr. Froehlich.

WHITBY, a seaport town in the North Riding of Yorkshire, on the tidal river *Esk*, bordered here by five piers, and crossed by an iron swing-bridge, 21 miles north-north-west of Scarborough, on the terminus of the York Railway. Lat. N. 54° 29'; long. E. 0° 36'. Population, 12,000. A new town has been lately built on the West Cliff, with excellent accommodation for the visitors. The sea view from here is most extensive and interesting. The sands stretch to a distance of three miles, and are of a very good condition. Numerous wooded and sheltered walks are available for pedestrian exercise. Several chalybeate springs drop down the cliffs at intervals. The *Bagdale* spa, in the town itself, contains 2·92 grains of solid ingredients in 16 ounces—viz.: sulphate of lime, 0·46; carbonate of lime, 0·20; carbonate of magnesia, 0·34; chloride of potassium, 0·53; carbonate of potash, 0·04; chloride of sodium, 0·42; carbonate of iron, 0·22; carbonate of manganese, traces. Those who are vigorous enough to bear the pure and bracing air of this beautiful locality will find it a most agreeable tonic summer residence.

. WIGHT (ISLE OF), in the English Channel, off the south coast of England, separated from the mainland of Hampshire by the Solent and Spithead. Its length from east to west is 22½ miles; greatest breadth at the centre, 13½ miles. Population, 55,000. It is one of the finest parts of Great Britain, and presents almost every variety of landscape in miniature. The north coast has an undulating surface, well wooded in many parts. It rises towards the centre, where it is traversed by a range of chalk hills from east to west. The highest of these (St. Catherine's Hill) is 830 feet above the level of the sea. The south coast (termed the back of the island) is distinguished by most romantic scenery, by precipitous cliffs, and ravines or 'chines.' The Culver Cliff, Shanklin, Luccombe, and Blackgang chines are on this side. The Needle rocks are on the western extremity. The island is almost separated into two equal portions by the *Medina* river, the eastern being the more fertile. Wide downs are found on the west. The principal towns are, besides the capital, *Newport* in the north, Yarmouth, Cowes, Ryde, and Ventnor. For sea-bathing the island offers very inferior accommodation; but besides its great charms and attractions for the ordinary visitor, it has acquired a great reputation for the mildness of climate of that south-eastern portion called the *Undercliff*, and extending from Niton to Bonchurch in the west (five miles). Its average width is a quarter of a mile. It has been formed by a landslip from a range of chalkcliffs, which bound it on the land side, where they constitute a steep wall from 90 to 120 feet high. The breadth of the landslip varies from a quarter to half a mile. It consists of a series of terraces formed of limestone-rock, intersected here and there by 'chines' (deep fissures). The origin of the landslip is supposed to be due to the action of the sea on the outside, and various hidden springs on the inside, gradually wasting the foundation of blue marl, till all at once the cliff pushed downwards and forwards to assume its present romantic aspect. The protecting downs on the background rise to a height of 500 to 700 feet. They are formed of chalk and sandstone with clayey deposit on the north, and greensand overlaid by Wealden clay on the south. They shelter the invalid against north, north-east, and west winds, and to some extent against south-west winds; but south and southeast winds enter freely. The variety and beauty of the walks, and the nature of the soil, allowing a ready percolation of the rain, render the place equally attractive and salubrious. A certain dryness and astringency of the air prevents it from being too relaxing. The altitude of the Undercliff is 50 to 60 feet. Through this elevation the strong sea atmosphere is tempered and less felt than at other southern places—as at Hastings, for instance, which is almost completely cut off from land-breezes by the encircling hills at the background. Annual temperature, 51·35°: winter, 41·89°; spring, 49·66°; summer, 60·63°; autumn, 53·58°. Annual rainfall, 23·48 inches.

It affords a most desirable winter and spring residence for consumptive patients who wish to enjoy a mild and equable climate, to avoid the northeasterly winds, and to have at the same time an abundance of charming places to resort to for exercise and diversion. Children with tuberculous disposition or scrofulous swellings are greatly benefited by wintering here. *Bonchurch* (with 564 inhabitants), at the east end, exhibits a combination of cliffs and knolls, intermingled with the most luxuriant foliage. The numerous ivy-covered spots deprive the winter of its barren appearance. Whilst Bonchurch (eight and a half miles south-east of Newport) has a more rural character, with its elegant villas and beautiful residences, the neighbouring *Ventnor* (about four miles east of Niton : population, 3,208) has a more town-like appearance, with all its hotels and shops, and regular lines of houses for visitors. The village of *St. Lawrence*, on the other side of Ventnor, closes the most favourable district for a winter sojourn of delicate individuals. Several short ridges project from the main range of hills towards the sea, breaking the violence of south-westerly winds. The eastern portion, from Bonchurch to St. Lawrence (about three miles), is the most sheltered ; the western is somewhat more open to south-westerly winds, though not varying in temperature. The Undercliff may be considered as a lofty natural terrace, screened by a mountainous wall on the north, and open to the full influence of the sun on the south. *Newport*— in the interior of the island, to the north of the chain of hills (seventeen miles south-south-east of Southampton), on the Medina river, with a population of 3,800—though only a few miles distant, exhibits a great difference in climate; 33·6 inches of rainfall annually in the latter locality to 23·48 in Ventnor. Annual temperature of Newport, 49·73° (less in winter, spring, and autumn, and higher in summer), and of Ventnor 51·35°. The soil of the Undercliff consists chiefly of the detritus of sandstone and chalk from the overhanging cliff; it has therefore the property of drying soon after rain. The climate is so equable, dry, and mild that the invalid need scarcely miss a day where he is prevented from taking outdoor exercise. The perpendicular cliffs are considered as playing a double part: whilst they keep off the northern blasts from the back, their exposure to the solar rays in front causes a great absorption of heat during the day, which radiates at night, and prevents the temperature from a too great fall. According to Sir James Clark, it surpasses in mildness and equability all the places of the south and south-west coast, except Torquay. With almost an identical temperature, Torquay has a soft but humid and relaxing climate, and is therefore preferable in cases of great bronchial and laryngeal irritation with sparing and difficult expectoration. That of the Undercliff is dry sometimes, sharp and bracing, with a smaller range of temperature. It is more suitable to delicate persons with profuse expectoration, tendency to excessive action of the skin, and reduced in strength. The best season is from November to May ; the climate remains pleasant up to the middle of August. A sea breeze usually sets in about seven in the morning. The lightness and buoyancy felt here is to be ascribed to the open and undulating surface, favouring a free circulation and frequent renewal of the atmosphere. From middle of August till middle of October the air becomes relaxing and depressing. *Niton*, at the western extremity beyond the Undercliff, is a pleasant rural summer residence.

Cowes (*East*), on the right bank of the River Medina, a hamlet with 1,900 inhabitants, four miles north of Newport, near Her Majesty's marine residence ; and *Cowes* (*West*), a town at the mouth of the left bank of the River Medina, at the northern extremity of the island, 10½ miles south-south-east of Southampton, and 11 miles west-south-west of Portsmouth, with a population of 4,500, and a good bathing establishment, are suitable for a summer residence. The hamlet of *Sandown* on the south-eastern coast, 2 miles south of Brading, attracts many visitors in summer, through its beautiful bay and fine sands. *Shanklin*, to the south of Sandown, 2 miles north of Bonchurch, elevated and finely sheltered, is one of the handsomest summer retreats in England. The Shanklin chine is a romantic chasm of the cliff, covered with verdure, and opening to the sea. A small cascade at the upper end heightens the interest of the scenery.

Ryde, on the north-east coast of the lozenge-shaped ' *Garden of England*,' opposite and five miles south-west of Portsmouth, with a population of 9,200, is the most favourable spot for a summer residence. It is built on the slope of a dry gravelly hill facing the north, with many open spaces. Residences, with gardens and lawns, alternate with charming walks of a wild or rural character. It is indeed a lovely place, which combines the advantages of a marine climate with that of the most recreating and diverting country retreat. It is recommended as the most eligible summer residence, whenever simple sea-air is sought to be employed as a curative means.

WORTHING, a town in Sussex, on the English Channel, 10 miles west of Brighton, 61 miles south-west of London (two hours' railway journey), east of Littlehampton and of Bognor. Population, 5,800, with fine sands extending for some miles along the sea on either side. Being situated only a few feet above the level of the sea, and sheltered from the north and north-east winds, and partly from the east and north-west winds, by the lofty Southdown Hills, which range in a nearly circular form from east to west about a mile to the north of the town, it enjoys a mild and soft climate, but of a somewhat relaxing character. The town is open to due south and south-west winds. The soil consists of a rich loam over a stratum of sand and pebbles, resting on a foundation of chalk. It offers numerous sheltered pleasant walks, and excellent accommodation for sea-bathing. It is milder than Brighton as a winter climate, but occasionally subject to fogs. Children with scrofulous cachexia or phthisical tendency are greatly benefited here; also cases of chronic rheumatism, bronchial irritation, and spasmodic asthma, find relief here on account of the sedative and rather agreeable climate.

ZAIZON'S IODURETTED SPRINGS, five miles east of *Kronstadt*, in *Transylvania*, below 46° lat. N., 26½° long. E., at an altitude of 1,700 feet, on the south-eastern slope of the great range of Carpathian Mountains, are distinguished by their very considerable amount of *iodide of sodium*. The neighbouring mountains, rising to a height of 8,000 feet, render the place cool, though they oppose the entrance of severe winds, and thus prevent sudden vicissitudes of temperature. In 16 ounces the springs contain :—

	Ferdinand-brunnen	Ludwig-brunnen (Chalybeate)
Chloride of sodium	4·69 gr.	0·47 gr.
Iodide of sodium	1·91	—
Bicarbonate of soda	10·11	4·18
,, lime	3·51	4·40
,, magnesia	0·84	1·18
,, iron	0·11	1·19
Sulphate of soda	0·15	0·39
Silica	0·12	0·21
Sulphate of potash	—	0·59
Phosphate of alumina	—	0·49
Total	21·47	13·10
Free carbonic acid	19·69 cub. in.	30 cub. in.

This spa has acquired a great reputation for the cure of scrofulous and glandular swellings, and anæmia combined with sluggishness of the lymphatic system. If the analysis should become confirmed by the highest chemical authorities, we would have here, in the extreme corner of south-eastern Germany, the most powerful ioduretted and the most potent chalybeate springs of all those used for curative purposes. An excellent whey-establishment is likewise available for those who suffer from delicacy of thoracic organs.

Physician—Dr. Fabricius.

INDEX.

ABERYSTWITH, 280
Achselmannstein, 277
Acidulous springs, origin of, 10, 13
Adelheidsquelle, 183. Analysis of, 185
Æolus-bath, 365
Aix-la-Chapelle, 200. Analysis of Kaiserquelle (Elisenbrunnen), 203
Aix-les-Bains, 277
Akratopegæ (chemically indifferent springs), 27
Alexandersbad, 278
Alexisbad, 278
Algiers, 280
Alpine climate, 282
Altwasser, 278
Amélie-les-Bains, 279
Apenrade, 279
Arnstadt, 279
Artificial medicated baths, 276
Ascending douches, 7
Askerne spa, 280
Ausbaden (out-bathing), 52
Aussee, 280

BADEN (Austria), 168. Analysis of springs, 170
Baden-Baden, 239. Analysis of Ursprung, 240
Baden (Switzerland), 286
Badenweiler, 287
Bagnères-de-Bigorre, 287
Bagnères-de-Luchon, 288
Barèges, 289
Barking, 321
Barnes, 321
Bath, 290
Bath-eruption, 8
Baths, effects of, 23
Baths, saline, effects of on the healthy organism, 263

Battersea, 321
Bayswater, 320
Berg, 292
Berka, 293
Bertrich, 293
Berwick (North), 295
Bex, 293
Biarritz, 294
Bilin, 85
Blackheath, 319
Blackpool, 296
Blankenberghe, 295
Bocklet, 129. Analysis of the springs, 130
Bonchurch, 413
Bordeaux, 297
Botzen, 294
Boulogne-sur-Mer, 295
Bournemouth, 296
Bow, 320
Brighton, 296
Brighton Pumproom, 5
Brompton, 319
Brückenau, 133. Analysis of s'eel spring, 134
Burtscheid, 208
Buxton, 292

CAIRO, 301
Camberwell, 321
Cannes, 336
Canstadt, 40. Analysis of Sulzerainquelle, 40
Cape of Good Hope, 339
Carbonic acid, 4. Free (formation of), 13
Carlsbad, 90. Analysis of the Sprudel, 94
Castellamare, 300
Cauterets, 300
Chalybokrenæ (Steel springs), 209
Charlottenbrunnen, 298
Cheltenham, 303
Chemically indifferent spas, 5, 27

Chiswick, 321
Clapham, 321
Clapton, (Upper) 320
Clarens, 298
Clifton, 304
Coimbra, 302
Colberg, 299
Cold water, effects of, 26
Cowes (East), 414
Cowes (West), 414
Cranz, 299
Cuxhaven, 299

DALSTON, 320
Denmark Hill, 321
Deptford, 319
Dieppe, 305
Doberan, 305
Douches, ascending, 7
Dover, 307
Driburg, 216. Analysis of spring, 217
Dürkheim, 306

EARTHQUAKES, their relations to thermae, 10
East Ham, 321
East Wickham, 319
Eaux-Bonnes, 308
Eaux-Chaudes, 309
Eilsen, 198
Ems, 230. Analysis of Kesselbrunnen, 232
Etretat, 309

FACHINGEN water, 4, 86
Fécamp, 310
Florence, 349
Föhr, 310
Forest Hill, 321
Franzensbad, 112. Analysis of Franzensbrunnen, 113

E E

418   INDEX.

FRI
Friedrichshaller water, 89
Fulham, 321

GAIS, 310
Gastein, 54. Analysis of its mineral water, 60
Geilnau, 87
Genoa, 349
Giessbach, 343
Ginseng, Vale of, 339
Glairine, 6
Grape-cure, 52, 307
Great Britain, 312. Climate of, 314
Greenwich, 319
Griesbach, 380
Grindelwald, 344
Gros-Caillou, 6

HAGUE, the, 390
Hackney, 320
Hall (Austria), Analysis of the mineral water, 185
Hallein, 69
Halokrenæ (cold saline springs), 119
Halopegæ (saline springs), 119
Halothermæ, (warm saline springs), 119
Hammersmith, 321
Hampstead Hill, 320
Harrogate, 336
Hastings, 338
Hatcham, 321
Havre de Grace, 334
Heat of warm springs, causes of, 12
Heiden, 330
Heilbrunn, 183
Heinrichsbad, 332
Helgoland, 333
Hendon, 319
Heppingen, 87
Heringsdorf, 334
Highbury, 321
Highgate Hill, 320
Hofgastein, 57
Hofragaz, 44
Homburg, 136. Analysis of its springs, 138
Hyères, 335

ILMENAU, 340
Imnau, 340
Interlaken, 341

ISC
Ischia, 345
Ischl, 70. Analysis of its mineral water, 71
Italy, climate of, 346

JERSEY, 355

KENSINGTON, 319
Kiel, 356
Kingsland, 320
Kissingen, 121. Analysis of its springs, 124
Kochbrunnen (Wiesbaden), 153
Königsdorff-Jastrzemb, 356
Kösen, 356
Krankenheil, 357
Krenæ, or cold springs, 9
Kreuznach, 175. Analysis of Elisenquelle, 178
Kronthal, 358

LABASSÈRE, 359
Landeck, 359
Langenbrücken, 359
Langenschwalbach, 218
Leamington, 365
Leghorn, 365
Leuk, 360
Liebenzell, 361
Lippik, 361
Lippspringe, 362
London, climate of, 313
Lowestoft, 366
Lucca, 365
Luhatschowitz, 363
Lymington, 366

MADEIRA Islands, 366
Magnesia, Solution of, in carbonic acid, 6
Malaga, 368
Malvern, 373
Margate, 376
Marienbad, 102. Analysis of Kreuzbrunnen, 104
Matlock, 374
Meinberg, 198. Analysis of its springs, 200
Mentone, 369
Meran, 371
Mergentheim, 372
Meyringen, 344
Milan, 350
Mineral waters, characteristics of, 17
Misdroy, 372

MON
Mondorf, 372
Montpellier, 297
Montreux, 299
Mudbaths, 193

NAPLES, 350
Nauheim, 259. Analysis of its springs, 260
Nenndorf, 190. Mudbaths of, 193. Analysis of its springs, 195
Neuenahr, 376
Newport, 414
Nice, 370
Nitrogen, effects of, 36
Norderney, 377
Nunhead, 321

OEYNHAUSEN, 243
Analysis of its water, 244
Ofen, 378
Ostend, 379
Ottilienquelle, 363

PALERMO, 353
Partenkirchen, 379
Pau, 380
Peckham, 321. Peckham Rye, 361
Pegæ, or mineral springs, 9
Petersthal, 379
Pfäfers, 42. Analysis of its mineral water, 48
Pikrokrenæ (cold bitter springs), 85
Pikropegæ (bitter springs), 85
Pikrothermæ (warm bitter springs), 85.
Pisa, 352
Plaistow, 321
Plombières, 381
Pozzuoli, 351
Püllna, 88
Purulent absorption, 207
Putbus, 380
Putney, 321
Pyrmont, 210. Analysis of its springs, 213

RAGAZ, 45
Railway Travelling, influence of, on health, 324
Ramsgate, 376

INDEX. 419

REC

Recoaro, 382
Regent's Park, 320
Reichenhall, 382
Remagen, 383
Rigi-Kaltbad, 384
Rigi-Schiedeck, 383
Rippoldsau, 384
Rohitsch, 385
Rome, 352
Römerbad, 384
Rosenheim, 385
Royan, 385
Ryde, 415

SAIDSCHÜTZ, 87
St. John's Wood, 320
St. Lawrence, 414
St. Leonards, 338
St. Moritz, 385
St. Sauveur, 393
Salcombe, 395
Saline baths, effects of, on the healthy organism, 263
Salzbrunn, 393
Salzhausen, 394
Salzungen, 395
Scarborough, 395
Schevingen, 390
Schinznach, 388
Schlangenbad, 236. Analysis of Schachtbrunnen, 237
Schwalbach, 218. Analysis of its springs, 220
Schwalheim, 275
Sea-air, influence of, 254
Sea-bathing, remarks on, 253
Sea-water, solid ingredients of, 252
Seidlitz, 38
Shepherd's Bush, 321
Shooter's Hill, 319
Sidmouth, 396
Snaresbrook, 321
Soden (near Frankfort), 146. Analysis of its springs, 148
Soden (Bavaria), 390

SPA

Spa, 225. Analysis of its springs, 226
Springs, cold, 9 ; hot, 9
Stachelberg, 390
Stamford Hill, 320
Steben, 391
Steel springs, 209
Stoke Newington, 320
Stratford, 321
Streitberg, 391
Sulza, 392
Sulzbrunn, 392
Swansea, 396
Swinemünde, 392
Sylt, 392
Synkratopegæ (springs with efficient ingredients), 27

TARASP, 396
Tegernsee, 398
Teignmouth, 401
Teinach, 398
Temperature, medical effects of, 22
Tension of evaporating bodies, 21
Teplitz, 74. Analysis of its mineral water, 77
Theiokrenæ (cold sulphur springs), 160
Theiopegæ (sulphur springs), 160
Theiothermæ (warm sulphur springs), 160
Thermæ, or hot springs, 9
Thermal springs, origin of, 10, 11
Thermal springs, composition of, 12
Tiefnau, 399
Töplitz, 399
Torquay, 402
Travemünde, 400
Triest, 400
Tropical influence, 210
Trouville, 334
Tunbridge Wells, 404

UNDERCLIFF, 413

VAP

VAPOURS, effects of, 25
Venice, 354
Ventnor, 414
Vernet 405
Vernex, 299
Vevay, 298
Vichy, 406
Victoria Park, 320

WÄGGIS, 409
Walthamstow, 321
Wandsworth, 321
Wanstead, 321
Warmbrunn, 407
Warmth, effects of, in the digestive canal, 26
Warmth of air, diminution of, 9
Water, its changes, 9. Mechanical effects of, 26
Weilbach, 160. Analysis of its spring, 161
Weissbad, 332
Weissenburg, 409
Weissenstein, 410
Westbourne Grove, 320
West Ham, 321
Whey: difference of composition between ewe's, cow's, and goat's whey, 312
Whey-cure, 311
Whitby, 412
Wiesbaden, 150. Analysis of the Kochbrunnen, 153
Wight (Isle of), 413
Wildbad, 29. Analysis of its mineral water, 32
Wildbad-gastein, 59
Wildegg, 389
Wildungen, 410
Willesden, 319
Wipfeld, 412
Wormwood Scrubs, 319
Worthing, 415

ZAIZON'S ioduretted springs, 415

39 Paternoster Row, E.C.
London, *March* 1876.

GENERAL LIST OF WORKS
PUBLISHED BY
MESSRS. LONGMANS, GREEN, AND CO.

	PAGE		PAGE
Arts, Manufactures, &c.	26	Mental & Political Philosophy	8
Astronomy & Meteorology	17	Miscellaneous & Critical Works	12
Biographical Works	7	Natural History & Physical Science	19
Chemistry & Physiology	24	Poetry & the Drama	36
Dictionaries & other Books of Reference	15	Religious & Moral Works	29
Fine Arts & Illustrated Editions	25	Rural Sports, Horse & Cattle Management, &c.	37
History, Politics, Historical Memoirs, &c.	1	Travels, Voyages, &c.	32
Index	41 to 44	Works of Fiction	35
		Works of Utility & General Information	39

HISTORY, POLITICS, HISTORICAL MEMOIRS, &c.

The History of England from the Accession of James II.

By the Right Hon. Lord Macaulay.

STUDENT'S EDITION, 2 *vols. cr. 8vo.* 12*s.*
PEOPLE'S EDITION, 4 *vols. cr. 8vo.* 16*s.*
CABINET EDITION, 8 *vols. post 8vo.* 48*s.*
LIBRARY EDITION, 5 *vols. 8vo.* £4.

Critical and Historical Essays contributed to the Edinburgh Review.

By the Right Hon. Lord Macaulay.

CHEAP EDITION, *crown 8vo.* 3*s.* 6*d.*
STUDENT'S EDITION, *crown 8vo.* 6*s.*
PEOPLE'S EDITION, 2 *vols. crown 8vo.* 8*s.*
CABINET EDITION, 4 *vols.* 24*s.*
LIBRARY EDITION, 3 *vols. 8vo.* 36*s.*

A

Lord Macaulay's Works.
Complete and uniform Library Edition.
Edited by his Sister, Lady Trevelyan.
8 vols. 8vo. with Portrait, £5. 5s.

The History of England from the Fall of Wolsey to the Defeat of the Spanish Armada.
By J. A. Froude, M.A.
CABINET EDITION, 12 vols. cr.8vo. £3. 12s.
LIBRARY EDITION, 12 vols. 8vo. £8. 18s.

The English in Ireland in the Eighteenth Century.
By J. A. Froude, M.A.
3 vols. 8vo. £2. 8s.

Journal of the Reigns of King George the Fourth and King William the Fourth.
By the late Charles Cavendish Fulke Greville, Esq.
Edited by H. Reeve, Esq.
Fifth Edition. 3 vols. 8vo. price 36s.

The Life of Napoleon III.
derived from State Records, Unpublished Family Correspondence, and Personal Testimony.
By Blanchard Jerrold.
In Four Volumes 8vo. with numerous Portraits and Facsimiles. VOLS. I. and II. price 18s. each.
*** The Third Volume is now in the press.

Recollections and Suggestions, 1813–1873.
By John Earl Russell, K.G.
New Edition, revised and enlarged. 8vo. 16s.

Introductory Lectures on Modern History delivered in Lent Term 1842 ; with the Inaugural Lecture delivered in December 1841.
By the late Rev. Thomas Arnold, D.D.
8vo. price 7s. 6d.

On Parliamentary Government in England: its Origin, Development, and Practical Operation.
By Alpheus Todd.
2 vols. 8vo. £1. 17s.

The Constitutional History of England since the Accession of George III. 1760–1870.
By Sir Thomas Erskine May, K.C.B. D.C.L.
Fifth Edition. 3 vols. crown 8vo. 18s.

Democracy in Europe; a History.
By Sir Thomas Erskine May, K.C.B. D.C.L.
2 vols. 8vo. [*In the press.*

Lectures on the History of England from the Earliest Times to the Death of King Edward II.
By W. Longman, F.S.A.
Maps and Illustrations. 8vo. 15s.

The History of the Life and Times of Edward III.
By W. Longman, F.S.A.
With 9 Maps, 8 Plates, and 16 Woodcuts. 2 vols. 8vo. 28s.

History of England under the Duke of Buckingham and Charles the First, 1624–1628. By S. Rawson Gardiner, late Student of Ch. Ch.
2 vols. 8vo. with two Maps, 24s.

Popular History of France, from the Earliest Times to the Death of Louis XIV. By Elizabeth M. Sewell, Author of 'Amy Herbert' &c.
Crown 8vo. [Nearly ready.

The History of Prussia, from the Earliest Times to the Present Day; tracing the Origin and Development of her Military Organisation. By Captain W. J. Wyatt.
Vols. I. & II. A.D. 700 to A.D. 1525. 8vo. 36s.

History of Civilisation in England and France, Spain and Scotland. By Henry Thomas Buckle.
3 vols. crown 8vo. 24s.

A Student's Manual of the History of India from the Earliest Period to the Present. By Col. Meadows Taylor, M.R.A.S.
Second Thousand. Cr. 8vo. Maps, 7s. 6d.

Studies from Genoese History. By Colonel G. B. Malleson, C.S.I. Guardian to His Highness the Mahárájá of Mysore.
Crown 8vo. 10s. 6d.

The Native States of India in Subsidiary Alliance with the British Government; an Historical Sketch. By Colonel G. B. Malleson, C.S.I. Guardian to the Mahárájá of Mysore.
With 6 Coloured Maps, 8vo. price 15s.

The History of India from the Earliest Period to the close of Lord Dalhousie's Administration. By John Clark Marshman.
3 vols. crown 8vo. 22s. 6d.

Indian Polity; a View of the System of Administration in India. By Lieut.-Colonel George Chesney.
Second Edition, revised, with Map. 8vo. 21s.

Waterloo Lectures; a Study of the Campaign of 1815. By Colonel Charles C. Chesney, R.E.
Third Edition. 8vo. with Map, 10s. 6d.

Essays in Modern Military Biography.
By Colonel Charles C. Chesney, R.E.
8vo. 12s. 6d.

The British Army in 1875; *with Suggestions on its Administration and Organisation.*
By John Holms, M.P.
New and Enlarged Edition. Crown 8vo. with Diagrams, 4s. 6d.

The Oxford Reformers— John Colet, Erasmus, and Thomas More; being a History of their Fellow-Work.
By Frederic Seebohm.
Second Edition. 8vo. 14s.

The New Reformation, a Narrative of the Old Catholic Movement, from 1870 *to the Present Time; with an Historical Introduction.*
By Theodorus.
8vo. price 12s.

The Mythology of the Aryan Nations.
By Geo. W. Cox, M.A. late Scholar of Trinity College, Oxford.
2 vols. 8vo. 28s.

A History of Greece.
By the Rev. Geo. W. Cox, M.A. late Scholar of Trinity College, Oxford.
Vols. I. and II. 8vo. Maps, 36s.

The History of the Peloponnesian War, by Thucydides.
Translated by Richd. Crawley, Fellow of Worcester College, Oxford.
8vo. 10s. 6d.

The Tale of the Great Persian War, from the Histories of Herodotus.
By Rev. G. W. Cox, M.A.
Fcp. 8vo. 3s. 6d.

General History of Greece to the Death of Alexander the Great; with a Sketch of the Subsequent History to the Present Time.
By the Rev. George W. Cox, M.A. Author of 'The Aryan Mythology' &c.
Crown 8vo. with Maps, 7s. 6d.

General History of Rome from the Foundation of the City to the Fall of Augustulus, B.C. 753—A.D. 476.
By the Very Rev. C. Merivale, D.D. Dean of Ely.
With 5 Maps, crown 8vo. 7s. 6d.

History of the Romans under the Empire.
By Dean Merivale, D.D.
8 vols. post 8vo. 48s.

The Fall of the Roman Republic; a Short History of the Last Century of the Commonwealth.
By Dean Merivale, D.D.
12mo. 7s. 6d.

The Sixth Oriental Monarchy; or the Geography, History, and Antiquities of Parthia. Collected and Illustrated from Ancient and Modern sources.
By Geo. Rawlinson, M.A.
With Maps and Illustrations. 8vo. 16s.

The Seventh Great Oriental Monarchy; or, a History of the Sassanians: with Notices Geographical and Antiquarian.
By Geo. Rawlinson, M.A.
With Map and 95 Illustrations. 8vo. 28s.

Encyclopædia of Chronology, Historical and Biographical; comprising the Dates of all the Great Events of History, including Treaties, Alliances, Wars, Battles, &c. Incidents in the Lives of Eminent Men, Scientific and Geographical Discoveries, Mechanical Inventions, and Social, Domestic, and Economical Improvements.
By B. B. Woodward, B.A. and W. L. R. Cates.
8vo. 42s.

The History of Rome.
By Wilhelm Ihne.
Vols. I. and II. 8vo. 30s. Vols. III. and IV. in preparation.

History of European Morals from Augustus to Charlemagne.
By W. E. H. Lecky, M.A.
2 vols. 8vo. 28s.

History of the Rise and Influence of the Spirit of Rationalism in Europe.
By W. E. H. Lecky, M.A.
Cabinet Edition, 2 vols. crown 8vo. 16s.

Introduction to the Science of Religion: Four Lectures delivered at the Royal Institution; with two Essays on False Analogies and the Philosophy of Mythology.
By F. Max Müller, M.A.
Crown 8vo. 10s. 6d.

The Stoics, Epicureans, and Sceptics.
Translated from the German of Dr. E. Zeller, by Oswald J. Reichel, M.A.
Crown 8vo. 14s.

Socrates and the Socratic Schools.
Translated from the German of Dr. E. Zeller, by the Rev. O. J. Reichel, M.A.
Crown 8vo. 8s. 6d.

Plato and the Older Academy.
Translated, with the Author's sanction, from the German of Dr. E. Zeller by S. Frances Alleyne and Alfred Goodwin, B.A. Fellow of Balliol College, Oxford.
Post 8vo. [*Nearly ready.*

Sketch of the History of the Church of England to the Revolution of 1688. By T. V. Short, D.D. sometime Bishop of St. Asaph.
New Edition. Crown 8vo. 7s. 6d.

The Historical Geography of Europe.
By E. A. Freeman, D.C.L.
8vo. Maps. [*In the press.*

The Student's Manual of Ancient History: containing the Political History, Geographical Position, and Social State of the Principal Nations of Antiquity.
By W. Cooke Taylor, LL.D.
Crown 8vo. 7s. 6d.

The Student's Manual of Modern History: containing the Rise and Progress of the Principal European Nations, their Political History, and the Changes in their Social Condition.
By W. Cooke Taylor, LL.D.
Crown 8vo. 7s. 6d.

The History of Philosophy, from Thales to Comte.
By George Henry Lewes.
Fourth Edition, 2 vols. 8vo. 32s.

The Crusades.
By the Rev. G. W. Cox, M.A.
Fcp. 8vo. with Map, 2s. 6d.

The Era of the Protestant Revolution.
By F. Seebohm, Author of 'The Oxford Reformers.'
With 4 Maps and 12 Diagrams. Fcp. 8vo. 2s. 6d.

The Thirty Years' War, 1618-1648.
By Samuel Rawson Gardiner.
Fcp. 8vo. with Maps, 2s. 6d.

The Houses of Lancaster and York; with the Conquest and Loss of France.
By James Gairdner.
Fcp. 8vo. with Map, 2s. 6d.

Edward the Third.
By the Rev. W. Warburton, M.A.
Fcp. 8vo. with Maps, 2s. 6d.

The Age of Elizabeth.
By the Rev. M. Creighton, M.A., late Fellow and Tutor of Merton College, Oxford.
Fcp. 8vo. with Maps, 2s. 6d.

BIOGRAPHICAL WORKS.

The Life and Letters of Lord Macaulay.
By his Nephew, G. Otto Trevelyan, M.P.
2 vols. 8vo. with Portrait, price 36s.

The Life of Sir William Fairbairn, Bart. F.R.S. Corresponding Member of the National Institute of France, &c.
Partly written by himself; edited and completed by William Pole, F.R.S. Member of Council of the Institution of Civil Engineers.
[In the press.

Arthur Schopenhauer, his Life and his Philosophy.
By Helen Zimmern.
Post 8vo. with Portrait, 7s. 6d.

The Life, Works, and Opinions of Heinrich Heine.
By William Stigand.
2 vols. 8vo. with Portrait of Heine, price 28s.

Memoirs of Baron Stockmar.
By his Son, Baron E. Von Stockmar. Translated from the German by G. A. M. Edited by F. Max Müller, M.A.
2 vols. crown 8vo. 21s.

Admiral Sir Edward Codrington, a Memoir of his Life; with Selections from his Correspondence.
Abridged from the larger work, and edited by his Daughter, Lady Bourchier.
With Portrait, Maps, &c. Crown 8vo. price 7s. 6d.

Life and Letters of Gilbert Elliot, First Earl of Minto, from 1751 to 1806, when his Public Life in Europe was closed by his Appointment to the Vice-Royalty of India.
Edited by the Countess of Minto.
3 vols. post 8vo. 31s. 6d.

Autobiography.
By John Stuart Mill.
8vo. 7s. 6d.

Isaac Casaubon, 1559-1614.
By Mark Pattison, Rector of Lincoln College, Oxford.
8vo. price 18s.

Biographical and Critical Essays, reprinted from Reviews, with Additions and Corrections.
By A. Hayward, Q.C.
Second Series, 2 vols. 8vo. 28s. Third Series, 1 vol. 8vo. 14s.

The Memoirs of Sir John Reresby, of Thrybergh, Bart. M.P. for York, &c. 1634-1689. Written by Himself. Edited from the Original Manuscript by James J. Cartwright, M.A.
8vo. price 21s.

Lord George Bentinck; a Political Biography. By the Right Hon. B. Disraeli, M.P.
New Edition. Crown 8vo. 6s.

Essays in Ecclesiastical Biography. By the Right Hon. Sir J. Stephen, LL.D.
Cabinet Edition. Crown 8vo. 7s. 6d.

Leaders of Public Opinion in Ireland; Swift, Flood, Grattan, O'Connell. By W. E. H. Lecky, M.A.
Crown 8vo. 7s. 6d.

Dictionary of General Biography; containing Concise Memoirs and Notices of the most Eminent Persons of all Ages and Countries. By W. L. R. Cates.
New Edition, 8vo. 25s. Supplement, 4s. 6d.

Life of the Duke of Wellington. By the Rev. G. R. Gleig, M.A.
Crown 8vo. with Portrait, 5s.

The Rise of Great Families; other Essays and Stories. By Sir Bernard Burke, C.B. LL.D.
Crown 8vo. 12s. 6d.

Memoirs of Sir Henry Havelock, K.C.B. By John Clark Marshman.
Crown 8vo. 3s. 6d.

Vicissitudes of Families. By Sir Bernard Burke, C.B.
2 vols. crown 8vo. 21s.

MENTAL and POLITICAL PHILOSOPHY.

Comte's System of Positive Polity, or Treatise upon Sociology. Translated from the Paris Edition of 1851-1854, and furnished with Analytical Tables of Contents. In Four Volumes, each forming in some degree an independent Treatise:—
Vol. I. *General View of Positivism and Introductory Principles.* Translated by J. H. Bridges, M.B. *formerly Fellow of Oriel College, Oxford.* 8vo. price 21s.
Vol. II. *The Social Statics, or the Abstract Laws of Human Order.* Translated by Frederic Harrison, M.A. 8vo. *price* 14s.
Vol. III. *The Social Dynamics, or the General Laws of Human Progress* (the Philosophy of History). Translated by E. S. Beesly, M.A. *Professor of History in University College, London.* 8vo.
[*Nearly ready.*
Vol. IV. *The Synthesis of the Future of Mankind.* Translated by Richard Congreve, M.D., and an *Appendix*, containing the Author's *Minor Treatises*, translated by H. D. Hutton, M.A. *Barrister-at-Law.* 8vo. [*In the press.*

Order and Progress: Part I. Thoughts on Government; Part II. Studies of Political Crises. By Frederic Harrison, M.A. of Lincoln's Inn.
8vo. 14s.

'We find from this book—a large part, and by far the more valuable part, of which is new—that Mr. HARRISON has devoted careful attention to what we shall call the constructive problems of political science. Whoever has mistaken him for a commonplace Radical, either of the Chartist or the Trades Unionist type, has been wrong.... The best political thinkers for a quarter of a century or upwards have more or less vaguely felt that one grand problem they had to solve was how our governing apparatus may be made to yield good government; but we are not aware that any writer has looked it more fully in the face, or more carefully scanned it with a view to a solution, than Mr. HARRISON.'
LITERARY WORLD.

Essays, Political, Social, and Religious. By Richd. Congreve, M.A.
8vo. 18s.

Essays, Critical and Biographical, contributed to the Edinburgh Review. By Henry Rogers.
New Edition. 2 vols. crown 8vo. 12s.

Essays on some Theological Controversies of the Time, contributed chiefly to the Edinburgh Review. By Henry Rogers.
New Edition. Crown 8vo. 6s.

Democracy in America. By Alexis de Tocqueville. Translated by Henry Reeve, Esq.
New Edition. 2 vols. crown 8vo. 16s.

A 2

On Representative Government. By John Stuart Mill.
Fourth Edition, crown 8vo. 2s.

On Liberty. By John Stuart Mill.
Post 8vo. 7s. 6d. crown 8vo. 1s. 4d.

Principles of Political Economy. By John Stuart Mill.
2 vols. 8vo. 30s. or 1 vol. crown 8vo. 5s.

Essays on some Unsettled Questions of Political Economy. By John Stuart Mill.
Second Edition. 8vo. 6s. 6d.

Utilitarianism. By John Stuart Mill.
Fourth Edition. 8vo. 5s.

A System of Logic, Ratiocinative and Inductive. By John Stuart Mill.
Eighth Edition. 2 vols. 8vo. 25s.

Examination of Sir William Hamilton's Philosophy, and of the principal Philosophical Questions discussed in his Writings. By John Stuart Mill.
Fourth Edition. 8vo. 16s.

Dissertations and Discussions. By John Stuart Mill.
4 vols. 8vo. price £2. 6s. 6d.

Analysis of the Phenomena of the Human Mind. By James Mill. New Edition, with Notes, Illustrative and Critical.
2 vols. 8vo. 28s.

The Law of Nations considered as Independent Political Communities; the Rights and Duties of Nations in Time of War. By Sir Travers Twiss, D.C.L. F.R.S.
New Edition, revised; with an Introductory Juridical Review of the Results of Recent Wars, and an Appendix of Treaties and other Documents. 8vo. price 21s.

Church and State; their relations Historically Developed.
By T. Heinrich Geffcken, Professor of International Law at the University of Strasburg. Translated from the German by E. Fairfax Taylor. [*In the press.*

A Systematic View of the Science of Jurisprudence.
By Sheldon Amos, M.A.
8vo. 18s.

A Primer of the English Constitution and Government.
By Sheldon Amos, M.A.
Second Edition. Crown 8vo. 6s.

Outlines of Civil Procedure. Being a General View of the Supreme Court of Judicature and of the whole Practice in the Common Law and Chancery Divisions under all the Statutes now in force. With Introductory Essay, References, Time Table, and Index. Designed as a Systematic and Readable Manual for Students, and as a Handbook of General Practice.
By Edward Stanley Roscoe, Barrister-at-Law.
12mo. price 3s. 6d.

Principles of Economical Philosophy.
By H. D. Macleod, M.A. Barrister-at-Law.
Second Edition, in 2 vols. Vol. I. 8vo. 15s. Vol. II. Part I. price 12s.

The Institutes of Justinian; with English Introduction, Translation, and Notes.
By T. C. Sandars, M.A.
Fifth Edition. 8vo. 18s.

Lord Bacon's Works,
Collected and Edited by R. L. Ellis, M.A. J. Spedding, M.A. and D. D. Heath.
New and Cheaper Edition. 7 vols. 8vo. £3. 13s. 6d.

Letters and Life of Francis Bacon, including all his Occasional Works. Collected and edited, with a Commentary, by J. Spedding.
7 vols. 8vo. £4 4s.

The Nicomachean Ethics of Aristotle. Newly translated into English. By R. Williams, B.A.
8vo. 12s.

The Politics of Aristotle; Greek Text, with English Notes. By Richard Congreve, M.A.
New Edition, revised. 8vo. 18s.

The Ethics of Aristotle; with Essays and Notes. By Sir A. Grant, Bart. M.A. LL.D.
Third Edition. 2 vols. 8vo. price 32s.

Bacon's Essays, with Annotations. By R. Whately, D.D.
New Edition. 8vo. 10s. 6d.

Picture Logic; an Attempt to Popularise the Science of Reasoning by the combination of Humorous Pictures with Examples of Reasoning taken from Daily Life. By A. Swinbourne, B.A.
Second Edition; with Woodcut Illustrations from Drawings by the Author. Fcp. 8vo. price 5s.

Elements of Logic. By R. Whately, D.D.
New Edition. 8vo. 10s. 6d. cr. 8vo. 4s. 6d.

Elements of Rhetoric. By R. Whately, D.D.
New Edition. 8vo. 10s. 6d. cr. 8vo. 4s. 6d.

An Outline of the Necessary Laws of Thought: a Treatise on Pure and Applied Logic. By the Most Rev. W. Thomson, D.D. Archbishop of York.
Twelfth Thousand. Crown 8vo. 6s.

An Introduction to Mental Philosophy, on the Inductive Method. By J. D. Morell, LL.D.
8vo. 12s.

Philosophy without Assumptions. By the Rev. T. P. Kirkman, F.R.S. Rector of Croft, near Warrington.
8vo. price 10s. 6d.

Ueberweg's System of Logic, and History of Logical Doctrines. Translated, with Notes and Appendices, by T. M. Lindsay, M.A. F.R.S.E.
8vo. 16s.

The Senses and the Intellect.
By A. Bain, LL.D.
Third Edition, 8vo. 15s.

The Emotions and the Will.
By Alexander Bain, LL.D. Professor of Logic in the University of Aberdeen.
Third Edition, thoroughly revised, and in great part re-written. 8vo. price 15s.

Mental and Moral Science; a Compendium of Psychology and Ethics.
By A. Bain, LL.D.
Third Edition. Crown 8vo. 10s. 6d. Or separately: Part I. Mental Science, 6s. 6d. Part II. Moral Science, 4s. 6d.

On the Influence of Authority in Matters of Opinion.
By the late Sir George Cornewall Lewis, Bart.
New Edition, 8vo. 14s.

Hume's Treatise on Human Nature.
Edited, with Notes, &c. by T. H. Green, M.A. and the Rev. T. H. Grose, M.A.
2 vols. 8vo. 28s.

Hume's Essays Moral, Political, and Literary.
By the same Editors.
2 vols. 8vo. 28s.

*** *The above form a complete and uniform Edition of* HUME'S *Philosophical Works.*

MISCELLANEOUS & CRITICAL WORKS.

Miscellaneous and Posthumous Works of the late Henry Thomas Buckle.
Edited, with a Biographical Notice, by Helen Taylor.
3 vols. 8vo. £2. 12s. 6d.

Short Studies on Great Subjects.
By J. A. Froude, M.A.
CABINET EDITION, 2 vols. crown 8vo. 12s.
LIBRARY EDITION, 2 vols. demy 8vo. 24s.

Manual of English Literature, Historical and Critical.
By Thomas Arnold, M.A.
New Edition. Crown 8vo. 7s. 6d.

Lord Macaulay's Miscellaneous Writings.
LIBRARY EDITION, 2 vols. 8vo. Portrait, 21s.
PEOPLE'S EDITION, 1 vol. cr. 8vo. 4s. 6d.

Lord Macaulay's Miscellaneous Writings and Speeches.
Students' Edition. Crown 8vo. 6s.

Speeches of the Right Hon. Lord Macaulay, corrected by Himself.
People's Edition. Crown 8vo. 3s. 6d.

The Rev. Sydney Smith's Essays contributed to the Edinburgh Review.
Authorised Edition, complete in One Volume. Crown 8vo. 2s. 6d. sewed, or 3s. 6d. cloth.

The Wit and Wisdom of the Rev. Sydney Smith.
Crown 8vo. 3s. 6d.

German Home Life; a Series of Essays on the Domestic Life of Germany.
Reprinted, with Revision and Additions, from FRASER'S MAGAZINE. 1 vol. crown 8vo. [Nearly ready.

The Miscellaneous Works of Thomas Arnold, D.D. Late Head Master of Rugby School and Regius Professor of Modern History in the Univ. of Oxford.
8vo. 7s. 6d.

Realities of Irish Life.
By W. Steuart Trench.
Cr. 8vo. 2s. 6d. sewed, or 3s. 6d. cloth.

Lectures on the Science of Language.
By F. Max Müller, M.A. &c.
Eighth Edition. 2 vols. crown 8vo. 16s.

Chips from a German Workshop; being Essays on the Science of Religion, and on Mythology, Traditions, and Customs.
By F. Max Müller, M.A.
4 vols. 8vo. £2. 18s.

Southey's Doctor, complete in One Volume.
Edited by Rev. J. W. Warter, B.D.
Square crown 8vo. 12s. 6d.

Lectures delivered in America in 1874.
By Charles Kingsley, late Rector of Eversley.
Crown 8vo. 5s.

Families of Speech.
Four Lectures delivered at the Royal Institution.
By F. W. Farrar, D.D.
New Edition. Crown 8vo. 3s. 6d.

Chapters on Language.
By F. W. Farrar, D.D.
New Edition. Crown 8vo. 5s.

A Budget of Paradoxes.
By Augustus De Morgan.
Reprinted, with Author's Additions, from the Athenæum. 8vo. 15s.

Apparitions; a Narrative of Facts.
By the Rev. B. W. Savile, M.A. Author of 'The Truth of the Bible' &c.
Crown 8vo. price 4s. 6d.

The Oration of Demosthenes on the Crown.
Translated by the Right Hon. Sir R. P. Collier.
Crown 8vo. 5s.

Miscellaneous Writings of John Conington, M.A.
Edited by J. A. Symonds, M.A. With a Memoir by H. J. S. Smith, M.A.
2 vols. 8vo. 28s.

Recreations of a Country Parson.
By A. K. H. B.
Two Series, 3s. 6d. each.

Landscapes, Churches, and Moralities.
By A. K. H. B.
Crown 8vo. 3s. 6d.

Seaside Musings on Sundays and Weekdays.
By A. K. H. B.
Crown 8vo. 3s. 6d.

Changed Aspects of Unchanged Truths.
By A. K. H. B.
Crown 8vo. 3s. 6d.

Counsel and Comfort from a City Pulpit.
By A. K. H. B.
Crown 8vo. 3s. 6d.

Lessons of Middle Age.
By A. K. H. B.
Crown 8vo. 3s. 6d.

Leisure Hours in Town.
By A. K. H. B.
Crown 8vo. 3s. 6d.

The Autumn Holidays of a Country Parson.
By A. K. H. B.
Crown 8vo. 3s. 6d.

Sunday Afternoons at the Parish Church of a Scottish University City.
By A. K. H. B.
Crown 8vo. 3s. 6d.

The Commonplace Philosopher in Town and Country.
By A. K. H. B.
Crown 8vo. 3s. 6d.

Present-Day Thoughts.
By A. K. H. B.
Crown 8vo. 3s. 6d.

Critical Essays of a Country Parson.
By A. K. H. B.
Crown 8vo. 3s. 6d.

The Graver Thoughts of a Country Parson.
By A. K. H. B.
Three Series, 3s. 6d. each.

DICTIONARIES and OTHER BOOKS of REFERENCE.

A Dictionary of the English Language.
By R. G. Latham, M.A. M.D. Founded on the Dictionary of Dr. S. Johnson, as edited by the Rev. H. J. Todd, with numerous Emendations and Additions.
4 vols. 4to. £7.

Thesaurus of English Words and Phrases, classified and arranged so as to facilitate the expression of Ideas, and assist in Literary Composition.
By P. M. Roget, M.D.
Crown 8vo. 10s. 6d.

English Synonymes.
By E. J. Whately. Edited by Archbishop Whately.
Fifth Edition. Fcp. 8vo. 3s.

Handbook of the English Language. For the use of Students of the Universities and the Higher Classes in Schools.
By R. G. Latham, M.A. M.D. &c. late Fellow of King's College, Cambridge; late Professor of English in Univ. Coll. Lond.
The Ninth Edition. Crown 8vo. 6s.

A Practical Dictionary of the French and English Languages.
By Léon Contanseau, many years French Examiner for Military and Civil Appointments, &c.
Post 8vo. 7s. 6d.

Contanseau's Pocket Dictionary, French and English, abridged from the Practical Dictionary, by the Author.
Square 18mo. 3s. 6d.

A New Pocket Dictionary of the German and English Languages.
By F. W. Longman, Balliol College, Oxford. Founded on Blackley and Friedländer's Practical Dictionary of the German and English Languages.
Square 18mo. price 5s.

A Dictionary of Roman and Greek Antiquities. With 2,000 Woodcuts from Ancient Originals, illustrative of the Arts and Life of the Greeks and Romans.
By Anthony Rich, B.A.
Third Edition. Crown 8vo. 7s. 6d.

New Practical Dictionary of the German Language; German - English and English-German. By Rev. W. L. Blackley, M.A. and Dr. C. M. Friedländer.
Post 8vo. 7s. 6d.

The Mastery of Languages; or, the Art of Speaking Foreign Tongues Idiomatically. By Thomas Prendergast.
Second Edition. 8vo. 6s.

A Greek-English Lexicon. By H. G. Liddell, D.D. Dean of Christchurch, and R. Scott, D.D. Dean of Rochester.
Sixth Edition. Crown 4to. 36s.

A Lexicon, Greek and English, abridged for Schools from Liddell and Scott's Greek - English Lexicon.
Fourteenth Edition. Square 12mo. 7s. 6d.

An English-Greek Lexicon, containing all the Greek Words used by Writers of good authority. By C. D. Yonge, M.A.
New Edition. 4to. 21s.

Mr. C. D. Yonge's New Lexicon, English and Greek, abridged from his larger Lexicon.
Square 12mo. 8s. 6d.

A Latin-English Dictionary. By John T. White, D.D. Oxon. and J. E. Riddle, M.A. Oxon.
Fifth Edition, revised. 1 vol. 4to. 28s.

White's College Latin-English Dictionary; abridged from the Parent Work for the use of University Students.
Third Edition, Medium 8vo. 15s.

A Latin-English Dictionary adapted for the use of Middle-Class Schools. By John T. White, D.D. Oxon.
Square fcp. 8vo. 3s.

White's Junior Student's Complete Latin - English and English-Latin Dictionary.
Square 12mo. 12s.

Separately { ENGLISH-LATIN, 5s. 6d.
LATIN-ENGLISH, 7s. 6d.

M'Culloch's Dictionary, Practical, Theoretical, and Historical, of Commerce and Commercial Navigation.
Edited by H. G. Reid.
8vo. 63s.
Supplement, price 5s.

A General Dictionary of Geography, Descriptive, Physical, Statistical, and Historical; forming a complete Gazetteer of the World. By A. Keith Johnston.
New Edition, thoroughly revised.
[*In the press.*

The Public Schools Manual of Modern Geography. Forming a Companion to 'The Public Schools Atlas of Modern Geography' By Rev. G. Butler, M.A.
[*In the press.*

The Public Schools Atlas of Modern Geography. In 31 Maps, exhibiting clearly the more important Physical Features of the Countries delineated. Edited, with Introduction, by Rev. G. Butler, M.A.
Imperial 8vo. price 5s. cloth; or in imperial 4to. 3s. 6d. sewed & 5s. cloth.

The Public Schools Atlas of Ancient Geography. Edited, with an Introduction on the Study of Ancient Geography, by the Rev. G. Butler, M.A.
Imperial Quarto. [*In the press.*

ASTRONOMY and METEOROLOGY.

The Universe and the Coming Transits; Researches into and New Views respecting the Constitution of the Heavens. By R. A. Proctor, B.A.
With 22 Charts and 22 Diagrams. 8vo. 16s.

Saturn and its System. By R. A. Proctor, B.A.
8vo. with 14 Plates, 14s.

The Transits of Venus; A Popular Account of Past and Coming Transits, from the first observed by Horrocks A.D. 1639 to the Transit of A.D. 2012. By R. A. Proctor, B.A.
Second Edition, revised and enlarged, with 20 Plates (12 Coloured) and 27 Woodcuts. Crown 8vo. 8s. 6d.

Essays on Astronomy. A Series of Papers on Planets and Meteors, the Sun and Sun-surrounding Space, Stars and Star Cloudlets. By R. A. Proctor, B.A.
With 10 Plates and 24 Woodcuts. 8vo. 12s.

The Moon; her Motions, Aspect, Scenery, and Physical Condition. By R. A. Proctor, B.A.
With Plates, Charts, Woodcuts, and Lunar Photographs. Crown 8vo. 15s.

The Sun; Ruler, Light, Fire, and Life of the Planetary System. By R. A. Proctor, B.A.
Second Edition. Plates and Woodcuts. Cr. 8vo. 14s.

A 3

The Orbs Around Us; a Series of Familiar Essays on the Moon and Planets, Meteors and Comets, the Sun and Coloured Pairs of Suns.
By R. A. PROCTOR, B.A.
Second Edition, with Chart and 4 Diagrams. Crown 8vo. 7s. 6d.

Other Worlds than Ours; The Plurality of Worlds Studied under the Light of Recent Scientific Researches.
By R. A. PROCTOR, B.A.
Third Edition, with 14 Illustrations. Cr. 8vo. 10s. 6d.

Brinkley's Astronomy. Revised and partly re-written, with Additional Chapters, and an Appendix of Questions for Examination.
By JOHN W. STUBBS, D.D. and F. BRUNNOW, Ph.D.
With 49 Diagrams. Crown 8vo. 6s.

Outlines of Astronomy.
By Sir J. F. W. HERSCHEL, Bart. M.A.
Latest Edition, with Plates and Diagrams. Square crown 8vo. 12s.

The Moon, and the Condition and Configurations of its Surface.
By EDMUND NEISON, Fellow of the Royal Astronomical Society &c.
Illustrated by Maps and Plates.
[*Nearly ready.*

Celestial Objects for Common Telescopes.
By T. W. WEBB, M.A. F.R.A.S.
New Edition, with Map of the Moon and Woodcuts. Crown 8vo. 7s. 6d.

'By universal consent of observers in this country, Mr. WEBB's *Celestial Objects* has taken the place of a standard text-book. With a book so well known and so highly appreciated, we have little more to do than to mention the appearance of a new edition, which we know has been wanted for some time, and which those who survey the glories of the heavens will be anxious to obtain.'
THE STUDENT.

A New Star Atlas, for the Library, the School, and the Observatory, in 12 Circular Maps (with 2 Index Plates).
By R. A. PROCTOR, B.A.
Crown 8vo. 5s.

Larger Star Atlas, for the Library, in Twelve Circular Maps, photolithographed by A. Brothers, F.R.A.S. With 2 Index Plates and a Letterpress Introduction.
By R. A. PROCTOR, BA.
Second Edition. Small folio, 25s.

Dove's Law of Storms, considered in connexion with the ordinary Movements of the Atmosphere.
Translated by R. H. SCOTT, M.A.
8vo. 10s. 6d.

Air and Rain; the Beginnings of a Chemical Climatology. By R. A. Smith, F.R.S.
8vo. 24s.

Air and its Relations to Life, 1774–1874; a Course of Lectures delivered at the Royal Institution of Great Britain in 1874, with some Additions. By Walter Noel Hartley, F.C.S. Demonstrator of Chemistry at King's College, London.
Small 8vo. with Illustrations, 6s.

Nautical Surveying, an Introduction to the Practical and Theoretical Study of. By J. K. Laughton, M.A.
Small 8vo. 6s.

Schellen's Spectrum Analysis, in its Application to Terrestrial Substances and the Physical Constitution of the Heavenly Bodies. Translated by Jane and C. Lassell; edited, with Notes, by W. Huggins, LL.D. F.R.S.
With 13 Plates and 223 Woodcuts. 8vo. 28s.

NATURAL HISTORY and PHYSICAL SCIENCE.

Professor Helmholtz' Popular Lectures on Scientific Subjects. Translated by E. Atkinson, F.C.S.
With many Illustrative Wood Engravings. 8vo. 12s. 6d.

Ganot's Natural Philosophy for General Readers and Young Persons; a Course of Physics divested of Mathematical Formulæ and expressed in the language of daily life. Translated by E. Atkinson, F.C.S.
Second Edition, with 2 Plates and 429 Woodcuts. Crown 8vo. 7s. 6d.

The Correlation of Physical Forces. By the Hon. Sir W. R. Grove, F.R.S. &c.
Sixth Edition, with other Contributions to Science. 8vo. 15s.

Weinhold's Introduction to Experimental Physics, Theoretical and Practical; including Directions for Constructing Physical Apparatus and for Making Experiments. Translated by B. Loewy, F.R.A.S. With a Preface by G. C. Foster, F.R.S.
With 3 Coloured Plates and 404 Woodcuts. 8vo. price 31s. 6d.

Ganot's Elementary Treatise on Physics, Experimental and Applied, for the use of Colleges and Schools. Translated and edited by E. Atkinson, F.C.S.
Seventh Edition, with 4 Coloured Plates & 758 Woodcuts. Post 8vo. 15s.

*** *Problems and Examples in Physics*, an Appendix to the Seventh and other Editions of Ganot's Elementary Treatise. 8vo. price 1s.

Text-Books of Science, Mechanical and Physical, adapted for the use of Artisans and of Students in Public and Science Schools. Small 8vo. Woodcuts.

The following Text-Books in this Series may now be had:—

Anderson's *Strength of Materials*, 3s. 6d.
Armstrong's *Organic Chemistry*, 3s. 6d.
Barry's *Railway Appliances*, 3s. 6d.
Bloxam's *Metals*, 3s. 6d.
Goodeve's *Mechanics*, 3s. 6d.
——— *Mechanism*, 3s. 6d.
Griffin's *Algebra & Trigonometry*, 3s. 6d.
Notes on the same, with Solutions, 3s. 6d.
Jenkin's *Electricity & Magnetism*, 3s. 6d.
Maxwell's *Theory of Heat*, 3s. 6d.
Merrifield's *Technical Arithmetic*, 3s. 6d.
Key, 3s. 6d.
Miller's *Inorganic Chemistry*, 3s. 6d.
Preece and Sivewright's *Telegraphy*, 3s. 6d.
Shelley's *Workshop Appliances*, 3s. 6d.
Thorpe's *Quantitative Analysis*, 4s. 6d.
Thorpe and Muir's *Qualitative Analysis*, 3s. 6d.
Watson's *Plane & Solid Geometry*, 3s. 6d.

*** *Other Text-Books*, in extension of this Series, in active preparation.

Principles of Animal Mechanics. By the Rev. S. Haughton, F.R.S.
Second Edition. 8vo. 21s.

Fragments of Science. By John Tyndall, F.R.S.
New Edition, crown 8vo. 10s. 6d.

Heat a Mode of Motion. By John Tyndall, F.R.S.
Fifth Edition, Plate and Woodcuts. Crown 8vo. 10s. 6d.

Sound. By John Tyndall, F.R.S.
Third Edition, including Recent Researches on Fog-Signalling; Portrait and Woodcuts. Crown 8vo. 10s. 6d.

Researches on Diamagnetism and Magne-Crystallic Action; including Diamagnetic Polarity. By John Tyndall, F.R.S.
With 6 Plates and many Woodcuts. 8vo. 14s.

Contributions to Molecular Physics in the domain of Radiant Heat. By John Tyndall, F.R.S.
With 2 Plates and 31 Woodcuts. 8vo. 16s.

Six Lectures on Light, delivered in America in 1872 and 1873. By John Tyndall, F.R.S.
Second Edition, with Portrait, Plate, and 59 Diagrams. Crown 8vo. 7s. 6d.

Notes of a Course of Nine Lectures on Light, delivered at the Royal Institution. By *John Tyndall, F.R.S.*
Crown 8vo. 1s. sewed, or 1s. 6d. cloth.

Notes of a Course of Seven Lectures on Electrical Phenomena and Theories, delivered at the Royal Institution. By *John Tyndall, F.R.S.*
Crown 8vo. 1s. sewed, or 1s. 6d. cloth.

A Treatise on Magnetism, General and Terrestrial. By *H. Lloyd, D.D. D.C.L.*
8vo. price 10s. 6d.

Elementary Treatise on the Wave-Theory of Light. By *H. Lloyd, D.D. D.C.L.*
Third Edition. 8vo. 10s. 6d.

The Comparative Anatomy and Physiology of the Vertebrate Animals. By *Richard Owen, F.R.S.*
With 1,472 Woodcuts. 3 vols. 8vo. £3. 13s. 6d.

Sir H. Holland's Fragmentary Papers on Science and other subjects. Edited by the *Rev. J. Holland.*
8vo. price 14s.

Kirby and Spence's Introduction to Entomology, or Elements of the Natural History of Insects.
Crown 8vo. 5s.

Light Science for Leisure Hours; Familiar Essays on Scientific Subjects, Natural Phenomena, &c. By *R. A. Proctor, B.A.*
First and Second Series. 2 vols. crown 8vo. 7s. 6d. each.

Homes without Hands; a Description of the Habitations of Animals, classed according to their Principle of Construction. By *Rev. J. G. Wood, M.A.*
With about 140 Vignettes on Wood. 8vo. 14s.

Strange Dwellings; a Description of the Habitations of Animals, abridged from 'Homes without Hands.' By *Rev. J. G. Wood, M.A.*
With Frontispiece and 60 Woodcuts. Crown 8vo. 7s. 6d.

Insects at Home; a Popular Account of British Insects, their Structure Habits, and Transformations. By *Rev. J. G. Wood, M.A.*
With upwards of 700 Woodcuts. 8vo. 21s.

Insects Abroad; being a Popular Account of Foreign Insects, their Structure, Habits, and Transformations. By *Rev. J. G. Wood, M.A.*
With upwards of 700 Woodcuts. 8vo. 21s

Out of Doors; a Selection of Original Articles on Practical Natural History.
By Rev. J. G. Wood, M.A.
With 6 Illustrations from Original Designs engraved on Wood. Crown 8vo. 7s. 6d.

Bible Animals; a Description of every Living Creature mentioned in the Scriptures, from the Ape to the Coral.
By Rev. J. G. Wood, M.A.
With about 112 Vignettes on Wood. 8vo. 14s.

The Polar World: a Popular Description of Man and Nature in the Arctic and Antarctic Regions of the Globe.
By Dr. G. Hartwig.
With Chromoxylographs, Maps, and Woodcuts. 8vo. 10s. 6d.

The Sea and its Living Wonders.
By Dr. G. Hartwig.
Fourth Edition, enlarged. 8vo. with many Illustrations, 10s. 6d.

The Tropical World.
By Dr. G. Hartwig.
With about 200 Illustrations. 8vo. 10s. 6d.

The Subterranean World.
By Dr. G. Hartwig.
With Maps and Woodcuts. 8vo. 10s. 6d.

The Aerial World; a Popular Account of the Phenomena and Life of the Atmosphere.
By Dr. George Hartwig.
With Map, 8 Chromoxylographs, and 60 Woodcuts. 8vo. price 21s.

Game Preservers and Bird Preservers, or 'Which are our Friends?'
By George Francis Morant, late Captain 12th Royal Lancers & Major Cape Mounted Riflemen.
Crown 8vo. price 5s.

A Familiar History of Birds.
By E. Stanley, D.D. late Ld. Bishop of Norwich.
Fcp. 8vo. with Woodcuts, 3s. 6d.

Rocks Classified and Described.
By B. Von Cotta.
English Edition, by P. H. LAWRENCE (with English, German, and French Synonymes), revised by the Author. Post 8vo. 14s.

Excavations at the Kesslerloch near Thayngen, Switzerland, a Cave of the Reindeer Period.
By Conrad Merk. Translated by John Edward Lee, F.S.A. F.G.S. Author of 'Isca Silurum' &c.
With Sixteen Plates. Royal 8vo. 7s. 6d.

The Origin of Civilisation, and the Primitive Condition of Man; Mental and Social Condition of Savages.
By Sir J. Lubbock, Bart. M.P. F.R.S.
Third Edition, with 25 Woodcuts. 8vo. 18s.

The Native Races of the Pacific States of North America. By Hubert Howe Bancroft.

Vol. I. *Wild Tribes, their Manners and Customs;* with 6 Maps. 8vo. 25s.
Vol. II. *Native Races of the Pacific States.* 8vo. 25s.
Vol. III. *Myths and Languages.* 8vo. price 25s.
Vol. IV. *Antiquities and Architectural Remains,* with Map. 8vo. 25s.
Vol. V. *Aboriginal History and Migrations;* Index to the Entire Work. With 2 Maps, 8vo. 25s.
** This work may now be had complete in 5 volumes, price £6. 5s.

The Ancient Stone Implements, Weapons, and Ornaments of Great Britain. By John Evans, F.R.S.

With 2 Plates and 476 Woodcuts. 8vo. 28s.

The Elements of Botany for Families and Schools. Eleventh Edition, revised by Thomas Moore, F.L.S.

Fcp. 8vo. with 154 Woodcuts, 2s. 6d.

The Rose Amateur's Guide. By Thomas Rivers.

Tenth Edition. Fcp. 8vo. 4s.

On the Sensations of Tone, as a Physiological Basis for the Theory of Music. By H. Helmholtz, Professor of Physiology in the University of Berlin. Translated by A. J. Ellis, F.R.S.

8vo. 36s.

A Dictionary of Science, Literature, and Art. Re-edited by the late W. T. Brande (the Author) and Rev. G. W. Cox, M.A.

New Edition, revised. 3 vols. medium 8vo. 63s.

The History of Modern Music, a Course of Lectures delivered at the Royal Institution of Great Britain. By John Hullah.

New Edition. Demy 8vo. 8s. 6d.

The Transition Period of Musical History; a Second Course of Lectures on the History of Music from the Beginning of the Seventeenth to the Middle of the Eighteenth Century, delivered at the Royal Institution. By John Hullah.

New Edition, 1 vol. demy 8vo.
[*In the Spring.*

The Treasury of Botany, or Popular Dictionary of the Vegetable Kingdom; with which is incorporated a Glossary of Botanical Terms. Edited by J. Lindley, F.R.S. and T. Moore, F.L.S.

With 274 Woodcuts and 20 Steel Plates. Two Parts, fcp. 8vo. 12s.

A General System of Descriptive and Analytical Botany.

Translated from the French of Le Maout and Decaisne, by Mrs. Hooker. Edited and arranged according to the English Botanical System, by J. D. Hooker, M.D. &c. Director of the Royal Botanic Gardens, Kew.

With 5,500 Woodcuts. *Imperial 8vo. 31s.6d.*

Loudon's Encyclopædia of Plants; comprising the Specific Character, Description, Culture, History, &c. of all the Plants found in Great Britain.

With upwards of 12,000 Woodcuts. *8vo. 42s.*

Handbook of Hardy Trees, Shrubs, and Herbaceous Plants; containing Descriptions &c. of the Best Species in Cultivation; with Cultural Details, Comparative Hardiness, suitability for particular positions, &c. Based on the French Work of Decaisne and Naudin, and including the 720 Original Woodcut Illustrations. By W. B. Hemsley.

Medium 8vo. 21s.

Forest Trees and Woodland Scenery, as described in Ancient and Modern Poets.

By William Menzies, Deputy Surveyor of Windsor Forest and Parks, &c.

With Twenty Chromolithographic Plates. *Folio, price £5. 5s.*

CHEMISTRY and PHYSIOLOGY.

Miller's Elements of Chemistry, Theoretical and Practical.

Re-edited, with Additions, by H. Macleod, F.C.S.

3 vols. 8vo.

PART I. CHEMICAL PHYSICS, 15s.
PART II. INORGANIC CHEMISTRY, 21s.
PART III. ORGANIC CHEMISTRY, New Edition in the press.

Health in the House, Twenty-five Lectures on Elementary Physiology in its Application to the Daily Wants of Man and Animals.

By Mrs. C. M. Buckton.

New Edition. *Crown 8vo. Woodcuts, 2s.*

Outlines of Physiology, Human and Comparative. By J. Marshall, F.R.C.S. Surgeon to the University College Hospital.
2 vols. cr. 8vo. with 122 Woodcuts, 32s.

Select Methods in Chemical Analysis, chiefly Inorganic. By Wm. Crookes, F.R.S.
With 22 Woodcuts. Crown 8vo. 12s. 6d.

A Dictionary of Chemistry and the Allied Branches of other Sciences. By Henry Watts, F.C.S. assisted by eminent Scientific and Practical Chemists.
6 vols. medium 8vo. £8. 14s. 6d.

Supplement completing the Record of Discovery to the year 1873.
8vo. price 42s.

The FINE ARTS and ILLUSTRATED EDITIONS.

Poems. By William B. Scott.
I. Ballads and Tales. II. Studies from Nature. III. Sonnets &c.
Illustrated by Seventeen Etchings by L. Alma Tadema and William B. Scott.
Crown 8vo. 15s.

Half-hour Lectures on the History and Practice of the Fine and Ornamental Arts. By W. B. Scott.
Third Edition, with 50 Woodcuts. Crown 8vo. 8s. 6d.

A Dictionary of Artists of the English School: Painters, Sculptors, Architects, Engravers, and Ornamentists; with Notices of their Lives and Works. By Samuel Redgrave.
8vo. 16s.

A 4

In Fairyland; Pictures from the Elf-World. By Richard Doyle. With a Poem by W. Allingham.
With 16 coloured Plates, containing 36 Designs. Second Edition, folio, 15s.

The New Testament, illustrated with Wood Engravings after the Early Masters, chiefly of the Italian School.
Crown 4to. 63s.

Lord Macaulay's Lays of Ancient Rome. With 90 Illustrations on Wood from Drawings by G. Scharf.
Fcp. 4to. 21s.

Miniature Edition, with Scharf's 90 Illustrations reduced in Lithography.
Imp. 16mo. 10s. 6d.

Moore's Irish Melodies,
Maclise's Edition, with 161
Steel Plates.
Super royal 8vo. 31s. 6d.

Sacred and Legendary Art.
By Mrs. Jameson.

6 *vols. square crown 8vo. price* £5. 15s. 6d.
as follows:—

Legends of the Saints and Martyrs.
New Edition, with 19 Etchings and 187 Woodcuts. 2 vols. 31s. 6d.

Legends of the Monastic Orders.
New Edition, with 11 Etchings and 88 Woodcuts. 1 vol. 21s.

Legends of the Madonna.
New Edition, with 27 Etchings and 165 Woodcuts. 1 vol. 21s.

The History of Our Lord, with that of his Types and Precursors. Completed by Lady Eastlake.
Revised Edition, with 13 Etchings and 281 Woodcuts. 2 vols. 42s.

The USEFUL ARTS, MANUFACTURES, &c.

Industrial Chemistry; a Manual for Manufacturers and for Colleges or Technical Schools. Being a Translation of Professors Stohmann and Engler's German Edition of Payen's 'Précis de Chimie Industrielle,' by Dr. J. D. Barry. Edited, and supplemented with Chapters on the Chemistry of the Metals, by B. H. Paul, Ph.D.
8vo. with Plates and Woodcuts.
[*In the press.*

Gwilt's Encyclopædia of Architecture, with above 1,600 *Woodcuts.*
New Edition (1876), *with Alterations and Additions, by Wyatt Papworth.*
8vo. 52s. 6d.

The Three Cathedrals dedicated to St. Paul in London; their History from the Foundation of the First Building in the Sixth Century to the Proposals for the Adornment of the Present Cathedral. By W. Longman, F.S.A.
With numerous Illustrations. Square crown 8vo. 21s.

Lathes and Turning, Simple, Mechanical, and Ornamental.
By W. Henry Northcott.
With 240 Illustrations. 8vo. 18s.

Hints on Household Taste in Furniture, Upholstery, and other Details.
By Charles L. Eastlake, Architect.
New Edition, with about 90 Illustrations. Square crown 8vo. 14s.

Handbook of Practical Telegraphy.
By R. S. Culley, Memb. Inst. C.E. Engineer-in-Chief of Telegraphs to the Post-Office.
Sixth Edition, Plates & Woodcuts. 8vo. 16s.

A Treatise on the Steam Engine, in its various applications to Mines, Mills, Steam Navigation, Railways and Agriculture.
By J. Bourne, C.E.
With Portrait, 37 Plates, and 546 Woodcuts. 4to. 42s.

Catechism of the Steam Engine, in its various Applications.
By John Bourne, C.E.
New Edition, with 89 Woodcuts. Fcp. 8vo. 6s.

Handbook of the Steam Engine.
By J. Bourne, C.E. forming a KEY to the Author's Catechism of the Steam Engine.
With 67 Woodcuts. Fcp. 8vo. 9s.

Recent Improvements in the Steam Engine.
By J. Bourne, C.E.
With 124 Woodcuts. Fcp. 8vo. 6s.

Encyclopædia of Civil Engineering, Historical, Theoretical, and Practical.
By E. Cresy, C.E.
With above 3,000 Woodcuts. 8vo. 42s.

Ure's Dictionary of Arts, Manufactures, and Mines.
Seventh Edition, re-written and greatly enlarged by R. Hunt, F.R.S. assisted by numerous Contributors.
With 2,100 Woodcuts. 3 vols. medium 8vo. price £5. 5s.

Practical Treatise on Metallurgy,
Adapted from the last German Edition of Professor Kerl's Metallurgy by W. Crookes, F.R.S. &c. and E. Röhrig, Ph.D.
3 vols. 8vo. with 625 Woodcuts. £4 19s.

Treatise on Mills and Millwork.
By Sir W. Fairbairn, Bt.
With 18 Plates and 322 Woodcuts. 2 vols. 8vo. 32s.

Useful Information for Engineers.
By Sir W. Fairbairn, Bt.
With many Plates and Woodcuts. 3 vols. crown 8vo. 31s. 6d.

The Application of Cast and Wrought Iron to Building Purposes.
By Sir W. Fairbairn, Bt.
With 6 Plates and 118 Woodcuts. 8vo. 16s.

The Theory of Strains in Girders and similar Structures, with Observations on the application of Theory to Practice, and Tables of the Strength and other Properties of Materials. By Bindon B. Stoney, M.A. M. Inst. C.E.
New Edition, royal 8vo. with 5 Plates and 123 Woodcuts, 36s.

Practical Handbook of Dyeing and Calico-Printing. By W. Crookes, F.R.S. &c.
With numerous Illustrations and Specimens of Dyed Textile Fabrics. 8vo. 42s.

Occasional Papers on Subjects connected with Civil Engineering, Gunnery, and Naval Architecture. By Michael Scott, Memb. Inst. C.E. & of Inst. N.A.
2 vols. 8vo. with Plates, 42s.

Mitchell's Manual of Practical Assaying. Fourth Edition, revised, with the Recent Discoveries incorporated, by W. Crookes, F.R.S.
crown 8vo. Woodcuts, 31s. 6d.

Naval Powers and their Policy: with Tabular Statements of British and Foreign Ironclad Navies; giving Dimensions, Armour, Details of Armament, Engines, Speed, and other Particulars. By John C. Paget.
8vo. price 10s. 6d. cloth.

Loudon's Encyclopædia of Gardening; comprising the Theory and Practice of Horticulture, Floriculture, Arboriculture, and Landscape Gardening.
With 1,000 Woodcuts. 8vo. 21s.

Loudon's Encyclopædia of Agriculture; comprising the Laying-out, Improvement, and Management of Landed Property, and the Cultivation and Economy of the Productions of Agriculture.
With 1,100 Woodcuts. 8vo. 21s.

Reminiscences of Fen and Mere. By J. M. Heathcote.
With 27 Illustrations and 3 Maps. Square 8vo. price 28s.

RELIGIOUS and MORAL WORKS.

An Exposition of the 39 *Articles, Historical and Doctrinal.*
By E. H. Browne, D.D. Bishop of Winchester.
New Edition. 8vo. 16s.

Historical Lectures on the Life of Our Lord Jesus Christ.
By C. J. Ellicott, D.D.
Fifth Edition. 8vo. 12s.

An Introduction to the Theology of the Church of England, in an Exposition of the 39 *Articles.* By Rev. T. P. Boultbee, LL.D.
Fcp. 8vo. 6s.

Three Essays on Religion: Nature; the Utility of Religion; Theism.
By John Stuart Mill.
Second Edition. 8vo. price 10s. 6d.

Sermons Chiefly on the Interpretation of Scripture.
By the late Rev. Thomas Arnold, D.D.
8vo. price 7s. 6d.

Sermons preached in the Chapel of Rugby School; with an Address before Confirmation.
By the late Rev. Thomas Arnold, D.D.
Fcp. 8vo. price 3s. 6d.

Christian Life, its Course, its Hindrances, and its Helps; Sermons preached mostly in the Chapel of Rugby School.
By the late Rev. Thomas Arnold, D.D.
8vo. 7s. 6d.

Christian Life, its Hopes, its Fears, and its Close; Sermons preached mostly in the Chapel of Rugby School.
By the late Rev. Thomas Arnold, D.D.
8vo. 7s. 6d.

Religion and Science, their Relations to Each Other at the Present Day; Three Essays on the Grounds of Religious Beliefs.
By Stanley T. Gibson, B.D. Rector of Sandon, in Essex; and late Fellow of Queen's College, Cambridge.
8vo. price 10s. 6d.

Notes on the Earlier Hebrew Scriptures.
By Sir G. B. Airy, K.C.B.
8vo. price 6s.

Synonyms of the Old Testament, their Bearing on Christian Faith and Practice.
By Rev. R. B. Girdlestone.
8vo. 15s.

The Primitive and Catholic Faith in Relation to the Church of England. By the Rev. B. W. Savile, M.A. Rector of Shillingford, Exeter.
8vo. price 7s.

The Eclipse of Faith; or *a Visit to a Religious Sceptic.*
By Henry Rogers.
Latest Edition. Fcp. 8vo. 5s.

Defence of the Eclipse of Faith.
By Henry Rogers.
Latest Edition. Fcp. 8vo. 3s. 6d.

A Critical and Grammatical Commentary on St. Paul's Epistles.
By C. J. Ellicott, D.D.
8vo. Galatians, 8s. 6d. Ephesians, 8s. 6d. Pastoral Epistles, 10s. 6d. Philippians, Colossians, & Philemon, 10s. 6d. Thessalonians, 7s. 6d.

The Life and Epistles of St. Paul.
By Rev. W. J. Conybeare, M.A. and Very Rev. J. S. Howson, D.D.
LIBRARY EDITION, *with all the Original Illustrations, Maps, Landscapes on Steel, Woodcuts, &c.* 2 vols. 4to. 42s.
INTERMEDIATE EDITION, *with a Selection of Maps, Plates, and Woodcuts.* 2 vols. square crown 8vo. 21s.
STUDENT'S EDITION, *revised and condensed, with 46 Illustrations and Maps.* 1 vol. crown 8vo. 9s.

An Examination into the Doctrine and Practice of Confession.
By the Rev. W. E. Jelf, B.D.
8vo. price 3s. 6d.

Evidence of the Truth of the Christian Religion derived from the Literal Fulfilment of Prophecy.
By Alexander Keith, D.D.
40th Edition, *with numerous Plates.* Square 8vo. 12s. 6d. or in post 8vo. with 5 Plates, 6s.

Historical and Critical Commentary on the Old Testament; with a New Translation.
By M. M. Kalisch, Ph.D.
Vol. I. Genesis, 8vo. 18s. or *adapted for the General Reader*, 12s. Vol. II. Exodus, 15s. or *adapted for the General Reader*, 12s. Vol. III. Leviticus, Part I. 15s. or *adapted for the General Reader*, 8s. Vol. IV. Leviticus, Part II. 15s. or *adapted for the General Reader*, 8s.

The History and Literature of the Israelites, according to the Old Testament and the Apocrypha.
By C. De Rothschild and A. De Rothschild.
Second Edition. 2 vols. crown 8vo. 12s. 6d.
Abridged Edition, in 1 vol. fcp. 8vo. 3s. 6d.

Ewald's History of Israel.
Translated from the German by J. E. Carpenter, M.A. with Preface by R. Martineau, M.A.
5 vols. 8vo. 63s.

Ewald's Antiquities of Israel.
Translated from the German by Henry Shaen Solly, M.A.
8vo. 12s. 6d.

The Types of Genesis, briefly considered as revealing the Development of Human Nature.
By Andrew Jukes.
Third Edition. Crown 8vo. 7s. 6d.

The Second Death and the Restitution of all Things; with some Preliminary Remarks on the Nature and Inspiration of Holy Scripture.
By Andrew Jukes.
Fourth Edition. Crown 8vo. 3s. 6d.

History of the Reformation in Europe in the time of Calvin.
By the Rev. J. H. Merle D'Aubigné, D.D. Translated by W. L. R. Cates, Editor of the Dictionary of General Biography.
6 vols. 8vo. price £4. 10s.
*** VOLS. VII. & VIII. completing the Work, are preparing for publication.

Commentaries, by the Rev. W. A. O'Conor, B.A. Rector of St. Simon and St. Jude, Manchester.
Crown 8vo.
Epistle to the Romans, price 3s. 6d.
Epistle to the Hebrews, 4s. 6d.
St. John's Gospel, 10s. 6d.

Some Questions of the Day.
By Elizabeth M. Sewell, Author of 'Amy Herbert,' 'Passing Thoughts on Religion,' &c.
Crown 8vo. 2s. 6d.

An Introduction to the Study of the New Testament, Critical, Exegetical, and Theological.
By the Rev. S. Davidson, D.D. LL.D.
2 vols. 8vo. price 30s.

Thoughts for the Age.
By Elizabeth M. Sewell.
New Edition. Fcp. 8vo. 3s. 6d.

Preparation for the Holy Communion; the Devotions chiefly from the works of Jeremy Taylor.
By Elizabeth M. Sewell.
32mo. 3s.

Bishop Jeremy Taylor's Entire Works; with Life by Bishop Heber.
Revised and corrected by the Rev. C. P. Eden.
10 vols. £5. 5s.

Hymns of Praise and Prayer.
Collected and edited by Rev. J. Martineau, LL.D.
Crown 8vo. 4s. 6d. 32mo. 1s. 6d.

Spiritual Songs for the Sundays and Holidays throughout the Year. By J. S. B. Monsell, LL.D.
9th Thousand. Fcp. 8vo. 5s   18mo. 2s.

Lyra Germanica; Hymns translated from the German by Miss C. Winkworth.
Fcp. 8vo. 5s.

Lectures on the Pentateuch & the Moabite Stone; with Appendices. By J. W. Colenso, D.D. Bishop of Natal.
8vo. 12s.

Endeavours after the Christian Life; Discourses. By Rev. J. Martineau, LL.D.
Fifth Edition. Crown 8vo. 7s. 6d.

Supernatural Religion; an Inquiry into the Reality of Divine Revelation.
Sixth Edition carefully revised, with 80 pages of New Preface. 2 vols. 8vo. 24s.

The Pentateuch and Book of Joshua Critically Examined. By J. W. Colenso, D.D. Bishop of Natal.
Crown 8vo. 6s.

TRAVELS, VOYAGES, &c.

The Indian Alps, and How we Crossed them: being a Narrative of Two Years' Residence in the Eastern Himalayas, and Two Months' Tour into the Interior, towards Kinchinjunga and Mount Everest. By a Lady Pioneer.
With Illustrations from Original Drawings made on the spot by the Authoress. Imperial 8vo. 42s.

Tyrol and the Tyrolese; being an Account of the People and the Land, in their Social, Sporting, and Mountaineering Aspects. By W. A. Baillie Grohman.
With numerous Illustrations from Sketches by the Author. Crown 8vo. 14s.

'The Frosty Caucasus;' an Account of a Walk through Part of the Range, and of an Ascent of Elbruz in the Summer of 1874. By F. C. Grove.
With Eight Illustrations engraved on Wood by E. Whymper, from Photographs taken during the Journey, and a Map. Crown 8vo. price 15s.

A Journey of 1,000 *Miles through Egypt and Nubia to the Second Cataract of the Nile. Being a Personal Narrative of Four and a Half Months' Life in a Dahabeeyah on the Nile.* By Amelia B. Edwards.
With numerous Illustrations from Drawings by the Authoress, Map, Plans, Facsimiles, &c. Imperial 8vo.
[In the Autumn.

Over the Sea and Far Away; being a Narrative of a Ramble round the World. By Thos. Woodbine Hinchliff, M.A. F.R.G.S. President of the Alpine Club, Author of 'Summer Months among the Alps,' &c.

1 vol. medium 8vo. with numerous Illustrations. [*Nearly ready.*

Discoveries at Ephesus. Including the Site and Remains of the Great Temple of Diana. By J. T. Wood, F.S.A.

1 vol. imperial 8vo. copiously illustrated. [*In the press.*

Through Bosnia and the Herzegovina on Foot during the Insurrection, August and September 1875; with a Glimpse at the Slavonic Borderlands of Turkey. By Arthur J. Evans, B.A. F.S.A.

Post 8vo. with Map and numerous Illustrations. [*In the press.*

Italian Alps; Sketches in the Mountains of Ticino, Lombardy, the Trentino, and Venetia. By Douglas W. Freshfield, Editor of 'The Alpine Journal.'

Square crown 8vo. Illustrations. 15s.

A 5

Memorials of the Discovery and Early Settlement of the Bermudas or Somers Islands, from 1615 *to* 1685. Compiled from the Colonial Records and other original sources. By Major-General J. H. Lefroy, R.A. C.B. F.R.S. Hon. Member New York Historical Society, &c. Governor of the Bermudas.

8vo. with Map. [*In the press.*

Here and There in the Alps. By the Hon. Frederica Plunket.

With Vignette-title. Post 8vo. 6s. 6d.

The Valleys of Tirol; their Traditions and Customs, and How to Visit them. By Miss R. H. Busk.

With Frontispiece and 3 Maps. Crown 8vo. 12s. 6d.

Two Years in Fiji, a Descriptive Narrative of a Residence in the Fijian Group of Islands; with some Account of the Fortunes of Foreign Settlers and Colonists up to the time of British Annexation. By Litton Forbes, M.D.

Crown 8vo. 8s. 6d.

Eight Years in Ceylon.
By Sir Samuel W. Baker, M.A. F.R.G.S.
New Edition, with Illustrations engraved on Wood by G. Pearson. Crown 8vo. Price 7s. 6d.

The Rifle and the Hound in Ceylon.
By Sir Samuel W. Baker, M.A. F.R.G.S.
New Edition, with Illustrations engraved on Wood by G. Pearson. Crown 8vo. Price 7s. 6d.

Meeting the Sun; a Journey all round the World through Egypt, China, Japan, and California.
By William Simpson, F.R.G.S.
With Heliotypes and Woodcuts. 8vo. 24s.

The Dolomite Mountains. Excursions through Tyrol, Carinthia, Carniola, and Friuli.
By J. Gilbert and G. C. Churchill, F.R.G.S.
With Illustrations. Sq. cr. 8vo. 21s.

The Alpine Club Map of the Chain of Mont Blanc, from an actual Survey in 1863-1864.
By A. Adams-Reilly, F.R.G.S. M.A.C.
In Chromolithography, on extra stout drawing paper 10s. or mounted on canvas in a folding case, 12s. 6d.

The Alpine Club Map of the Valpelline, the Val Tournanche, and the Southern Valleys of the Chain of Monte Rosa, from actual Survey.
By A. Adams-Reilly, F.R.G.S. M.A.C.
Price 6s. on extra Stout Drawing Paper, or 7s. 6d. mounted in a Folding Case.

Untrodden Peaks and Unfrequented Valleys; a Midsummer Ramble among the Dolomites.
By Amelia B. Edwards.
With numerous Illustrations. 8vo. 21s.

The Alpine Club Map of Switzerland, with parts of the Neighbouring Countries, on the scale of Four Miles to an Inch.
Edited by R. C. Nichols, F.S.A. F.R.G.S.
In Four Sheets, in Portfolio, price 42s. coloured, or 34s. uncoloured.

The Alpine Guide.
By John Ball, M.R.I.A. late President of the Alpine Club.
Post 8vo. with Maps and other Illustrations.

Eastern Alps.
Price 10s. 6d.

Central Alps, including all the Oberland District.
Price 7s. 6d.

Western Alps, including Mont Blanc, Monte Rosa, Zermatt, &c.
Price 6s. 6d.

Introduction on Alpine Travelling in general, and on the Geology of the Alps.
Price 1s. Either of the Three Volumes or Parts of the 'Alpine Guide' may be had with this Introduction prefixed, 1s. extra. The 'Alpine Guide' may also be had in Ten separate Parts, or districts, price 2s. 6d. each.

Guide to the Pyrenees, for the use of Mountaineers. By Charles Packe.
Second Edition, with Maps &c. and Appendix. Crown 8vo. 7s. 6d.

How to See Norway; embodying the Experience of Six Summer Tours in that Country. By J. R. Campbell.
With Map and 5 Woodcuts, fcp. 8vo. 5s.

WORKS of FICTION.

Higgledy-Piggledy; or, Stories for Everybody and Everybody's Children. By the Right Hon. E. H. Knatchbull-Hugessen, M.P. Author of 'Whispers from Fairyland' &c.
With 9 Illustrations from Original Designs by R. Doyle, engraved on Wood by G. Pearson. Crown 8vo. price 6s.

Whispers from Fairyland. By the Rt. Hon. E. H. Knatchbull-Hugessen, M.P. Author of 'Higgledy-Piggledy' &c.
With 9 Illustrations from Original Designs engraved on Wood by G. Pearson. Crown 8vo. price 6s.

'A series of stories which are certain of a ready welcome by all boys and girls who take delight in dreamland, and love to linger over the pranks and frolics of fairies. The book is dedicated to the mothers of England, and more wholesome food for the growing mind it would be unreasonable to desire, and impossible to procure. .... This welcome volume abounds in vivacity and fun, and bears pleasant testimony to a kindly-hearted Author with fancy, feeling, and humour.' MORNING POST.

The Folk-Lore of Rome, collected by Word of Mouth from the People. By Miss R. H. Busk.
Crown 8vo. 12s. 6d.

Becker's Gallus; or Roman Scenes of the Time of Augustus.
Post 8vo. 7s. 6d.

Becker's Charicles: Illustrative of Private Life of the Ancient Greeks.
Post 8vo. 7s. 6d.

Novels and Tales. By the Right Hon. Benjamin Disraeli, M.P.
Cabinet Editions, complete in Ten Volumes, crown 8vo. 6s. each, as follows :—

Lothair, 6s.	Venetia, 6s.
Coningsby, 6s.	Alroy, Ixion, &c. 6s.
Sybil, 6s.	Young Duke, &c. 6s.
Tancred, 6s.	Vivian Grey, 6s.
Henrietta Temple, 6s.	
Contarini Fleming, &c. 6s.	

The Modern Novelist's Library.

Atherstone Priory, 2s. boards; 2s. 6d. cloth.
Mlle. Mori, 2s. boards; 2s. 6d. cloth.
The Burgomaster's Family, 2s. and 2s. 6d.
MELVILLE'S Digby Grand, 2s. and 2s. 6d.
———— Gladiators, 2s. and 2s.6d.
———— Good for Nothing, 2s. & 2s. 6d.
———— Holmby House, 2s. and 2s. 6d.
———— Interpreter, 2s. and 2s. 6d.
———— Kate Coventry, 2s. and 2s. 6d.
———— Queens Maries, 2s. and 2s. 6d.
———— General Bounce, 2s. and 2s. 6d.
TROLLOPE'S Warden, 1s. 6d. and 2s.
———— Barchester Towers, 2s. & 2s. 6d.
BRAMLEY-MOORE'S Six Sisters of the Valleys, 2s. boards; 2s. 6d. cloth.
Elsa: a Tale of the Tyrolean Alps. Translated from the German of Mme. Von Hillern by Lady Wallace. Price 2s. boards; 2s. 6d. cloth.

Tales of Ancient Greece. By the Rev. G. W. Cox, M.A.

Crown 8vo. 6s. 6d.

Stories and Tales. By Elizabeth M. Sewell. Cabinet Edition, in Ten Volumes:—

Amy Herbert, 2s. 6d.
Gertrude, 2s. 6d.
Earl's Daughter, 2s. 6d.
Experience of Life, 2s. 6d.
Cleve Hall, 2s. 6d.
Ivors, 2s. 6d.
Katharine Ashton, 2s. 6d.
Margaret Percival, 3s. 6d.
Laneton Parsonage, 3s. 6d.
Ursula, 3s. 6d.

POETRY and THE DRAMA.

Ballads and Lyrics of Old France; with other Poems. By A. Lang, M.A.

Square fcp. 8vo. 5s.

The London Series of French Classics. Edited by Ch. Cassal, LL.D. T. Karcher, LL.B. and Léonce Stiévenard.

The following Plays, in the Division of the Drama in this Series, are now ready:—
CORNEILLE'S Le Cid, 1s. 6d.
VOLTAIRE'S Zaire, 1s. 6d.
LAMARTINE'S Toussaint Louverture, double volume, 2s. 6d.

Milton's Lycidas and Epitaphium Damonis. Edited, with Notes and Introduction, by C. S. Jerram, M.A.

Crown 8vo. 2s. 6d.

Lays of Ancient Rome; with Ivry and the Armada. By the Right Hon. Lord Macaulay.

16mo. 3s. 6d.

Lord Macaulay's Lays of Ancient Rome. With 90 Illustrations on Wood from Drawings by G. Scharf.

Fcp. 4to. 21s.

Miniature Edition of Lord Macaulay's Lays of Ancient Rome, with Scharf's 90 Illustrations reduced in Lithography.

Imp. 16mo. 10s. 6d.

Horatii Opera, Library Edition, with English Notes, Marginal References and various Readings. Edited by Rev. J. E. Yonge, M.A.
8vo. 21s.

Southey's Poetical Works with the Author's last Corrections and Additions.
Medium 8vo. with Portrait, 14s.

Bowdler's Family Shakspeare, cheaper Genuine Edition.
Complete in 1 vol. medium 8vo. large type, with 36 Woodcut Illustrations, 14s. or in 6 vols. fcp. 8vo. price 21s.

Poems by Jean Ingelow.
2 vols. Fcp. 8vo. 10s.
FIRST SERIES, containing 'Divided,' 'The Star's Monument,' &c. 16th Thousand. Fcp. 8vo. 5s.
SECOND SERIES, 'A Story of Doom,' 'Gladys and her Island,' &c. 5th Thousand. Fcp. 8vo. 5s.

Poems by Jean Ingelow. First Series, with nearly 100 *Woodcut Illustrations.*
Fcp. 4to. 21s.

The Æneid of Virgil Translated into English Verse. By J. Conington, M.A.
Crown 8vo. 9s.

RURAL SPORTS, HORSE and CATTLE MANAGEMENT, &c.

Annals of the Road, being a History of Coaching from the Earliest Times to the Present. By Captain Malet. With Practical Hints on Driving and all Coaching matters, by Nimrod.
Reprinted from the SPORTING MAGAZINE by permission of the Proprietors. 1 vol. medium 8vo. with Coloured Plates, uniform with Mr. Birch Reynardson's 'Down the Road.' [On May 1.

Down the Road; or, Reminiscences of a Gentleman Coachman. By C. T. S. Birch Reynardson.
Second Edition, with 12 Coloured Illustrations from Paintings by H. Alken. Medium 8vo. price 21s.

Blaine's Encyclopædia of Rural Sports; Complete Accounts, Historical, Practical, and Descriptive, of Hunting, Shooting, Fishing, Racing, &c.
With above 600 Woodcuts (20 from Designs by JOHN LEECH). 8vo. 21s.

A Book on Angling: a Treatise on the Art of Angling in every branch, including full Illustrated Lists of Salmon Flies. By Francis Francis.
Post 8vo. Portrait and Plates, 15s.

Wilcocks's Sea-Fisherman: comprising the Chief Methods of Hook and Line Fishing, a glance at Nets, and remarks on Boats and Boating.
New Edition, with 80 Woodcuts. Post 8vo. 12s. 6d.

The Ox, his Diseases and their Treatment; with an Essay on Parturition in the Cow.
By J. R. Dobson, Memb. R.C.V.S.
Crown 8vo. with Illustrations 7s. 6d.

Youatt on the Horse.
Revised and enlarged by W. Watson, M.R.C.V.S.
8vo. Woodcuts, 12s. 6d.

Youatt's Work on the Dog, revised and enlarged.
8vo. Woodcuts, 6s.

Horses and Stables.
By Colonel F. Fitzwygram, XV. the King's Hussars.
With 24 Plates of Illustrations. 8vo. 10s. 6d.

The Dog in Health and Disease.
By Stonehenge.
With 73 Wood Engravings. Square crown 8vo. 7s. 6d.

The Greyhound.
By Stonehenge.
Revised Edition, with 25 Portraits of Greyhounds, &c. Square crown 8vo. 15s.

Stables and Stable Fittings.
By W. Miles, Esq.
Imp. 8vo. with 13 Plates, 15s.

The Horse's Foot, and how to keep it Sound.
By W. Miles, Esq.
Ninth Edition. Imp. 8vo. Woodcuts, 12s. 6d.

A Plain Treatise on Horse-shoeing.
By W. Miles, Esq.
Sixth Edition. Post 8vo. Woodcuts, 2s. 6d.

Remarks on Horses' Teeth, addressed to Purchasers.
By W. Miles, Esq.
Post 8vo. 1s. 6d.

The Fly-Fisher's Entomology.
By Alfred Ronalds.
With 20 coloured Plates. 8vo. 14s.

WORKS of UTILITY and GENERAL INFORMATION.

Maunder's Treasury of Knowledge and Library of Reference; comprising an English Dictionary and Grammar, Universal Gazetteer, Classical Dictionary, Chronology, Law Dictionary, Synopsis of the Peerage, Useful Tables,&c.
Fcp. 8vo. 6s.

Maunder's Biographical Treasury.
Latest Edition, reconstructed and partly rewritten, with about 1,000 additional Memoirs, by W. L. R. Cates.
Fcp. 8vo. 6s.

Maunder's Scientific and Literary Treasury; a Popular Encyclopædia of Science, Literature, and Art.
New Edition, in part rewritten, with above 1,000 new articles, by J. Y. Johnson.
Fcp. 8vo. 6s.

Maunder's Treasury of Geography, Physical, Historical, Descriptive, and Political.
Edited by W. Hughes, F.R.G.S.
With 7 Maps and 16 Plates. Fcp. 8vo. 6s.

Maunder's Historical Treasury; General Introductory Outlines of Universal History, and a Series of Separate Histories.
Revised by the Rev. G. W. Cox, M.A.
Fcp. 8vo. 6s.

Maunder's Treasury of Natural History; or Popular Dictionary of Zoology.
Revised and corrected Edition. Fcp. 8vo. with 900 Woodcuts, 6s.

The Treasury of Bible Knowledge; being a Dictionary of the Books, Persons, Places, Events, and other Matters of which mention is made in Holy Scripture.
By Rev. J. Ayre, M.A.
With Maps, 15 Plates, and numerous Woodcuts. Fcp. 8vo. 6s.

The Theory and Practice of Banking.
By H. D. Macleod, M.A.
Third Edition, revised throughout. 8vo price 12s.

The Elements of Banking.
By Henry Dunning Macleod, Esq. M.A.
Crown 8vo. 7s. 6d.

Modern Cookery for Private Families, reduced to a System of Easy Practice in a Series of carefully-tested Receipts.
By Eliza Acton.
With 8 Plates & 150 Woodcuts. Fcp. 8vo. 6s.

A Practical Treatise on Brewing; with Formulæ for Public Brewers, and Instructions for Private Families.
By W. Black.
Fifth Edition. 8vo. 10s. 6d.

English Chess Problems.
Edited by J. Pierce, M.A. and W. T. Pierce.
With 608 Diagrams. Crown 8vo. 12s. 6d.

The Theory of the Modern Scientific Game of Whist.
By W. Pole, F.R.S.
Seventh Edition. Fcp. 8vo. 2s. 6d.

The Correct Card; or, How to Play at Whist: a Whist Catechism.
By Captain A. Campbell-Walker.
Fcp. 8vo. [Nearly ready.

The Cabinet Lawyer; a Popular Digest of the Laws of England, Civil, Criminal, and Constitutional.
Twenty-fourth Edition, corrected and extended. Fcp. 8vo. 9s.

Pewtner's Comprehensive Specifier; a Guide to the Practical Specification of every kind of Building-Artificer's Work.
Edited by W. Young.
Crown 8vo. 6s.

Chess Openings.
By F. W. Longman, Balliol College, Oxford.
Second Edition, revised. Fcp. 8vo. 2s. 6d.

Hints to Mothers on the Management of their Health during the Period of Pregnancy and in the Lying-in Room.
By Thomas Bull, M.D.
Fcp. 8vo. 5s.

The Maternal Management of Children in Health and Disease.
By Thomas Bull, M.D.
Fcp. 8vo. 5s.

INDEX.

Acton's Modern Cookery.......................... 40
Aird's Blackstone Economised 39
Airy's Hebrew Scriptures 29
Alpine Club Map of Switzerland 34
Alpine Guide (The) 34
Amos's Jurisprudence 10
——— Primer of the Constitution............ 10
Anderson's Strength of Materials 20
Armstrong's Organic Chemistry 20
Arnold's (Dr.) Christian Life 29
——————— Lectures on Modern History 2
——————————— Miscellaneous Works 13
——————————— School Sermons 29
——————————— Sermons 29
——— (T.) Manual of English Literature 12
Atherstone Priory.................................... 36
Autumn Holidays of a Country Parson ... 14
Ayre's Treasury of Bible Knowledge 39

Bacon's Essays, by *Whately* 11
——— Life and Letters, by *Spedding* ... 11
——— Works 10
Bain's Mental and Moral Science............ 12
——— on the Senses and Intellect 12
——— Emotions and Will...................... 12
Baker's Two Works on Ceylon 34
Ball's Guide to the Central Alps 34
———Guide to the Western Alps............ 35
———Guide to the Eastern Alps 34
Bancroft's Native Races of the Pacific..... 23
Barry on Railway Appliances 20
Becker's Charicles and Gallus.................. 35
Black's Treatise on Brewing 40
Blackley's German-English Dictionary...... 16
Blaine's Rural Sports 37
Bloxam's Metals 20
Boultbee on 39 Articles........................... 29
Bourne's Catechism of the Steam Engine . 27
——— Handbook of Steam Engine...... 27
——— Treatise on the Steam Engine ... 27
——— Improvements in the same......... 27
Bowdler's Family Shakspeare................... 37
Bramley-Moore's Six Sisters of the Valley . 36
Brande's Dictionary of Science, Literature, and Art 23
Brinkley's Astronomy 12
Browne's Exposition of the 39 Articles...... 29
Buckle's History of Civilisation 3
——— Posthumous Remains 12
Buckton's Health in the House 24
Bull's Hints to Mothers......................... 40
———Maternal Management of Children . 40
Burgomaster's Family (The) 34
Burke's Rise of Great Families 8

Burke's Vicissitudes of Families............... 8
Busk's Folk-lore of Rome 35
——— Valleys of Tirol 33

Cabinet Lawyer....................................... 40
Campbell's Norway 35
Cates's Biographical Dictionary............... 8
——— and *Woodward's* Encyclopædia ... 5
Changed Aspects of Unchanged Truths ... 14
Chesney's Indian Polity 3
——— Modern Military Biography....... 4
——— Waterloo Campaign 3
Codrington's Life and Letters 7
Colenso on Moabite Stone &c. 32
———'s Pentateuch and Book of Joshua. 32
Collier's Demosthenes on the Crown 13
Commonplace Philosopher in Town and Country, by A. K. H. B. 14
Comte's Positive Polity 8
Congreve's Essays................................... 9
——— Politics of Aristotle 11
Conington's Translation of Virgil's Æneid 37
——— Miscellaneous Writings......... 13
Contanseau's Two French Dictionaries ... 15
Conybeare and *Howson's* Life and Epistles of St. Paul... 30
Corneille's Le Cid 36
Counsel and Comfort from a City Pulpit... 14
Cox's (G. W.) Aryan Mythology 4
——— Crusades 6
——— History of Greece 4
——— General History of Greece 4
——— School ditto 4
——— Tale of the Great Persian War.. 4
——— Tales of Ancient Greece ... 36
Crawley's Thucydides............................. 4
Creighton's Age of Elizabeth 6
Cresy's Encyclopædia of Civil Engineering 27
Critical Essays of a Country Parson........ 14
Crookes's Chemical Analysis 25
——— Dyeing and Calico-printing......... 28
Culley's Handbook of Telegraphy............ 27

Davidson's Introduction to the New Testament... 31
D'Aubigné's Reformation 31
De Caisne and *Le Maout's* Botany 24
De Morgan's Paradoxes 13
De Tocqueville's Democracy in America... 9
Disraeli's Lord George Bentinck 8

A 6

42 NEW WORKS PUBLISHED BY LONGMANS & CO.

Disraeli's Novels and Tales	35
Dobson on the Ox	38
Dove's Law of Storms	18
Doyle's (R.) Fairyland	25
Eastlake's Hints on Household Taste	26
Edwards's Rambles among the Dolomites	34
———— Nile	32
Elements of Botany	23
Ellicott's Commentary on Ephesians	30
———————————— Galatians	30
————— ———————— Pastoral Epist.	30
———————————— Philippians, &c.	30
———————————— Thessalonians	30
———— Lectures on Life of Christ	29
Elsa : a Tale of the Tyrolean Alps	36
Evans' (J.) Ancient Stone Implements	23
———— (A. J.) Bosnia	33
Ewald's History of Israel	30
———— Antiquities of Israel	31
Fairbairn's Application of Cast and Wrought Iron to Building	27
———————— Information for Engineers	27
———————— Life	7
———————— Treatise on Mills and Millwork	27
Farrar's Chapters on Language	13
———— Families of Speech	13
Fitzwygram on Horses and Stables	38
Forbes's Two Years in Fiji	33
Francis's Fishing Book	37
Freeman's Historical Geography of Europe	6
Freshfield's Italian Alps	33
Froude's English in Ireland	2
———— History of England	2
———— Short Studies	12
Gairdner's Houses of Lancaster and York	6
Ganot's Elementary Physics	20
———— Natural Philosophy	19
Gardiner's Buckingham and Charles	3
———————— Thirty Years' War	6
Geffcken's Church and State	10
German Home Life	13
Gibson's Religion and Science	29
Gilbert & Churchill's Dolomites	34
Girdlestone's Bible Synonyms	29
Goodeve's Mechanics	20
———— Mechanism	20
Grant's Ethics of Aristotle	11
Graver Thoughts of a Country Parson	14
Greville's Journal	2
Griffin's Algebra and Trigonometry	20
Grohman's Tyrol and the Tyrolese	32
Grove (Sir W. R.) on Correlation of Physical Forces	19
———— (F. C.) The Frosty Caucasus	32
Gwilt's Encyclopædia of Architecture	26
Harrison's Order and Progress	9
Hartley on the Air	19
Hartwig's Aerial World	22
———— Polar World	22

Hartwig's Sea and its Living Wonders	22
———— Subterranean World	22
———— Tropical World	22
Haughton's Animal Mechanics	20
Hayward's Biographical and Critical Essays	7
Heathcote's Fen and Mere	28
Heine's Life and Works, by Stigand	7
Helmholtz on Tone	23
Helmholtz's Scientific Lectures	19
Helmsley's Trees, Shrubs, and Herbaceous Plants	24
Herschel's Outlines of Astronomy	18
Hinchliff's Over the Sea and Far Away	33
Holland's Fragmentary Papers	21
Holms on the Army	4
Hullah's History of Modern Music	23
———— Transition Period	23
Hume's Essays	12
———— Treatise on Human Nature	12
Ihne's History of Rome	5
Indian Alps	32
Ingelow's Poems	37
Jameson's Legends of Saints and Martyrs	26
———— Legends of the Madonna	26
———— Legends of the Monastic Orders	26
———— Legends of the Saviour	26
Jelf on Confession	30
Jenkin's Electricity and Magnetism	20
Jerram's Lycidas of Milton	35
Jerrold's Life of Napoleon	2
Johnston's Geographical Dictionary	17
Jukes's Types of Genesis	31
———— on Second Death	31
Kalisch's Commentary on the Bible	30
Keith's Evidence of Prophecy	30
Kerl's Metallurgy, by *Crookes* and *Röhrig*	27
Kingsley's American Lectures	13
Kirby and *Spence's* Entomology	21
Kirkman's Philosophy	11
Knatchbull-Hugessen's Whispers from Fairy-Land	35
———— Higgledy-Piggledy	35
Lamartine's Toussaint Louverture	36
Landscapes, Churches, &c. by A. K. H. B.	14
Lang's Ballads and Lyrics	36
Latham's English Dictionary	15
———— Handbook of the English Language	15
Laughton's Nautical Surveying	19
Lawrence on Rocks	22
Lecky's History of European Morals	5
———— Rationalism	5
———— Leaders of Public Opinion	8
Lee's Kesslerloch	22
Lefroy's Bermudas	33
Leisure Hours in Town, by A. K. H. B.	14
Lessons of Middle Age, by A. K. H. B.	14
Lewes's Biographical History of Philosophy	6

NEW WORKS PUBLISHED BY LONGMANS & CO.

Lewis on Authority	12
Liddell and *Scott's* Greek-English Lexicons	16
Lindley and *Moore's* Treasury of Botany	23
Lloyd's Magnetism	21
——— Wave-Theory of Light	21
Longman's (F. W.) Chess Openings	40
——— German Dictionary	15
——— (W.) Edward the Third	2
——— Lectures on History of England	2
——— Old and New St. Paul's	26
Loudon's Encyclopædia of Agriculture	28
——— Gardening	28
——— Plants	24
Lubbock's Origin of Civilisation	22
Lyra Germanica	32
Macaulay's (Lord) Essays	1
——— History of England	1
——— Lays of Ancient Rome 25,	36
——— Life and Letters	7
——— Miscellaneous Writings	12
——— Speeches	12
——— Works	2
McCulloch's Dictionary of Commerce	16
Macleod's Principles of Economical Philosophy	10
——— Theory and Practice of Banking	39
——— Elements of Banking	39
Mademoiselle Mori	36
Malet's Annals of the Road	37
Malleson's Genoese Studies	3
——— Native States of India	3
Marshall's Physiology	25
Marshman's History of India	3
——— Life of Havelock	8
Martineau's Christian Life	32
——— Hymns	31
Maunder's Biographical Treasury	39
——— Geographical Treasury	39
——— Historical Treasury	39
——— Scientific and Literary Treasury	39
——— Treasury of Knowledge	39
——— Treasury of Natural History	39
Maxwell's Theory of Heat	20
May's History of Democracy	2
——— History of England	2
Melville's Digby Grand	36
——— General Bounce	36
——— Gladiators	36
——— Good for Nothing	36
——— Holmby House	36
——— Interpreter	36
——— Kate Coventry	36
——— Queens Maries	36
Menzies' Forest Trees and Woodland Scenery	24
Merivale's Fall of the Roman Republic	5
——— General History of Rome	4
——— Romans under the Empire	4
Merrifield's Arithmetic and Mensuration	20
Miles on Horse's Foot and Horse Shoeing	38
——— on Horse's Teeth and Stables	38
Mill (J.) on the Mind	10
——— (J. S.) on Liberty	9
——— on Representative Government	9
——— Utilitarianism	9
——— Autobiography	7
Mill's Dissertations and Discussions	9
——— Essays on Religion &c.	29
——— Hamilton's Philosophy	9
——— System of Logic	9
——— Political Economy	9
——— Unsettled Questions	9
Miller's Elements of Chemistry	24
——— Inorganic Chemistry	20
Minto's (Lord) Life and Letters	7
Mitchell's Manual of Assaying	28
Modern Novelist's Library	36
Monsell's ' Spiritual Songs '	32
Moore's Irish Melodies, illustrated	26
Morant's Game Preservers	22
Morell's Elements of Psychology	11
——— Mental Philosophy	11
Müller's Chips from a German Workshop.	13
——— Science of Language	13
——— Science of Religion	5
Nelson on the Moon	18
New Reformation, by *Theodorus*	4
New Testament, Illustrated Edition	25
Northcott's Lathes and Turning	26
O'Conor's Commentary on Hebrews	31
——— Romans	31
——— St. John	31
Owen's Comparative Anatomy and Physiology of Vertebrate Animals	21
Packe's Guide to the Pyrenees	35
Paget's Naval Powers	28
Pattison's Casaubon	7
Payen's Industrial Chemistry	26
Pewtner's Comprehensive Specifier	40
Pierce's Chess Problems	40
Plunket's Travels in the Alps	33
Pole's Game of Whist	40
Preece & *Sivewright's* Telegraphy	20
Prendergast's Mastery of Languages	16
Present-Day Thoughts, by A. K. H. B.	14
Proctor's Astronomical Essays	17
——— Moon	17
——— Orbs around Us	18
——— Other Worlds than Ours	18
——— Saturn	17
——— Scientific Essays (New Series)	21
——— Sun	17
——— Transits of Venus	17
——— Two Star Atlases	18
——— Universe	17
Public Schools Atlas of Ancient Geography	17
——— Atlas of Modern Geography	17
——— Manual of Modern Geography	17
Rawlinson's Parthia	5
——— Sassanians	5
Recreations of a Country Parson	14
Redgrave's Dictionary of Artists	25
Reilly's Map of Mont Blanc	34
——— Monte Rosa	34
Reresby's Memoirs	8

Reynardson's Down the Road 37
Rich's Dictionary of Antiquities 15
River's Rose Amateur's Guide 23
Rogers's Eclipse of Faith..................... 30
————— Defence of Eclipse of Faith 30
————— Essays................................... 9
Roget's Thesaurus of English Words and Phrases 15
Ronald's Fly-Fisher's Entomology 38
Roscoe's Outlines of Civil Procedure......... 10
Rothschild's Israelites 30
Russell's Recollections and Suggestions ... 2

Sandars's Justinian's Institutes 10
Savile on Apparitions........................... 13
————— on Primitive Faith 30
Schellen's Spectrum Analysis 19
Scott's Lectures on the Fine Arts 25
————— Poems 25
————— Papers on Civil Engineering 28
Seaside Musing, by A. K. H. B. 14
Seebohm's Oxford Reformers of 1498......... 4
————— Protestant Revolution 6
Sewell's Questions of the Day 31
————— Preparation for Communion 31
————— Stories and Tales 36
————— Thoughts for the Age 31
————— History of France 3
Shelley's Workshop Appliances 20
Short's Church History 6
Simpson's Meeting the Sun..................... 34
Smith's (Sydney) Essays 12
————— Wit and Wisdom 13
————— (Dr. R. A.) Air and Rain 19
Southey's Doctor 13
————— Poetical Works........................ 37
Stanley's History of British Birds 22
Stephen's Ecclesiastical Biography........... 8
Stockmar's Memoirs 7
Stonehenge on the Dog........................ 38
————— on the Greyhound 38
Stoney on Strains 28
Sunday Afternoons at the Parish Church of a University City, by A. K. H. B. 14
Supernatural Religion 32
Swinbourne's Picture Logic 11

Taylor's History of India 3
————— Manual of Ancient History 6
————— Manual of Modern History 6
————— *(Jeremy)* Works, edited by *Eden*. 31
Text-Books of Science........................... 20
Thomson's Laws of Thought 11
Thorpe's Quantitative Analysis 20

Thorpe and *Muir's* Qualitative Analysis ... 20
Todd (A.) on Parliamentary Government... 2
Trench's Realities of Irish Life 13
Trollope's Barchester Towers.................. 36
————— Warden 36
Twiss's Law of Nations 10
Tyndall's American Lectures on Light ... 20
————— Diamagnetism........................ 20
————— Fragments of Science............... 20
————— Lectures on Electricity 21
————— Lectures on Light 21
————— Lectures on Sound.................. 20
————— Heat a Mode of Motion 20
————— Molecular Physics................... 20

Ueberweg's System of Logic 11
Ure's Dictionary of Arts, Manufactures, and Mines 27

Voltaire's Zaire................................... .-

Walker on Whist ....
Warburton's Edward the Third ....
Watson's Geometry 20
Watts's Dictionary of Chemistry 25
Webb's Objects for Common Telescopes ... 18
Weinhold's Experimental Physics............ 19
Wellington's Life, by *Gleig* 8
Whately's English Synonymes 15
————— Logic 11
————— Rhetoric 11
White and *Riddle's* Latin Dictionaries ... 16
Wilcocks's Sea-Fisherman 38
Williams's Aristotle's Ethics.................. 11
Wood's (T. G.) Bible Animals 22
————— Homes without Hands ... 21
————— Insects at Home 21
————— Insects Abroad............... 21
————— Out of Doors 22
————— Strange Dwellings 21
————— (J. T.) Ephesus 33
Wyatt's History of Prussia 3

Yonge's English-Greek Lexicons 16
————— Horace................................. 37
Youatt on the Dog 38
————— on the Horse 38

Zeller's Plato..................................... 6
————— Socrates 5
————— Stoics, Epicureans, and Sceptics... 5
Zimmern's Life of Schopenhauer 7

www.ingramcontent.com/pod-product-compliance
Lightning Source LLC
Chambersburg PA
CBHW020835020526
44114CB00040B/783